Cleft Palate and Craniofacial Anomalies

The Effects on Speech and Resonance

Cleft Palate and Craniofacial Anomalies

The Effects on Speech and Resonance

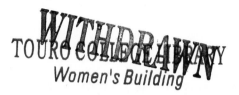

Ann W. Kummer, Ph.D.

Field Service Professor
Department of Pediatrics
University of Cincinnati Medical Center
Director, Speech Pathology Department
Cincinnati Children's Hospital Medical Center
The Craniofacial Center
Cincinnati, Ohio

With Contributions

SINGULAR
™
THOMSON LEARNING

Australia Canada Mexico Singapore Spain United Kingdom United States

WB

SINGULAR

THOMSON LEARNING

Cleft Palate and Craniofacial Anomalies: The Effects on Speech and Resonance
by Ann W. Kummer, Ph.D.

Business Unit Director:
William Brotmiller

Executive Marketing Manager:
Dawn Gerrain

Executive Production Manager:
Karen Leet

Acquisitions Editor:
Marie Linville

Channel Manager:
Tara Carter

Production Editor:
Sandy Doyle

Editorial Assistant:
Kristin Banach

COPYRIGHT © 2001 by Singular, an imprint of Delmar, a division of Thomson Learning, Inc. Thomson Learning™ is a trademark used herein under license

Printed in the USA
8 9 10 11 XXX 09 08 07 06

For more information contact Singular,
401 West "A" Street, Suite 325
San Diego, CA 92101-7904

Or find us on the World Wide Web at http://www.singpub.com

Library of Congress Cataloging-in-Publication Data
Kummer, Ann W.
Cleft palate and craniofacial anomalies : the effects on speech and resonance / by Ann W. Kummer, with contributions.
p. ; cm.
Includes bibliographical references and index.
ISBN 0-7693-0077-4 (hardcover ; alk. paper)
1.Cleft palate—Complications. 2. Face—Abnormalities—Complications. 3. Skull—Abnormalities—Complications. 4. Speech disorders. I. Title. [DNLM: 1. Cleft Palate—complications. 2. Cleft Palate—therapy. 3. Craniofacial Abnormalities—complications. 4. Craniofacial Abnormalities—therapy. 5. Speech Disorders—etiology. WV 440 K96c 2000]
RD763.K86 2000
617.5'225—dc21   00-032189

NOTICE TO THE READER

Publisher does not warrant or guarantee any of the products described herein or perform any independent analysis in connection with any of the product information contained herein. Publisher does not assume, and expressly disclaims, any obligation to obtain and include information other than that provided to it by the manufacturer.

The reader is expressly warned to consider and adopt all safety precautions that might be indicated by the activities herein and to avoid all potential hazards. By following the instructions contained herein, the reader willingly assumes all risks in connection with such instructions.

The Publisher makes no representation or warranties of any kind, including but not limited to, the warranties of fitness for particular purpose or merchantability, nor are any such representations implied with respect to the material set forth herein, and the publisher takes no responsibility with respect to such material. The publisher shall not be liable for any special, consequential, or exemplary damages resulting, in whole or part, from the readers' use of, or reliance upon, this material.

2/01/07

CONTENTS

PREFACE

To begin a discussion regarding craniofacial anomalies, I am reminded of the Far Side cartoon by Gary Larson that can be found below. In the cartoon, two female insects are sitting across from each other in a waiting room. One is holding a larva and she says to the other, "Well, Frank's hoping for a male, and I'd like a little female, but we'll both be content if it just has six eyes and eight legs." It seems that this cartoon represents a familiar human sentiment. We all want the same thing for our children; maybe not six eyes and eight legs, but certainly 10 fingers, 10 toes and intact faces.

THE FAR SIDE   **By GARY LARSON**

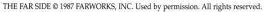
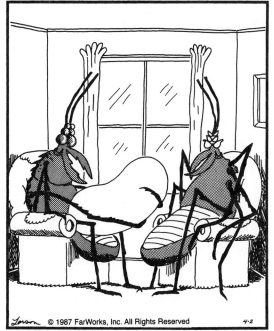

"Well, Frank's hoping for a male and I'd like a little female. . . . But, really, we'll both be content if it just has six eyes and eight legs."

Unfortunately, we don't always get our wish. Cleft lip or palate is the fourth most common birth defect and the most common facial birth defect. In fact, about 1 in every 750 children born in the United States each year is born with a cleft of the lip or palate. About half of these children have other associated malformations that often occur with clefting. In fact, more than 200 recognized syndromes include palatal clefting as a manifestation. In addition to clefts and their associated malformations, many children are born each year with other craniofacial anomalies.

Although current medical technology is not advanced enough to prevent the occurrence of these birth defects, most of the speech and physical impairments associated with craniofacial anomalies can be improved or even corrected with the help of a team of various professionals. To provide the type of care that these patients require this group of professionals must be specialists within their fields. They must have a thorough understanding of the current methods of evaluation and treatment of this population for quality care.

Purpose

The purpose of this book is to inform, to educate, and to excite students in speech pathology and in the medical and dental professions regarding the important role that they can play in the habilitation of individuals with a history of cleft or craniofacial anomalies. It is hoped that this book will spark an interest in students to become involved in evaluating and treating individuals with a history of cleft or craniofacial anomalies. With the work of educated and dedicated professionals, even children with significant anomalies can usually grow up to be normal, productive, and happy individuals. What a great feeling it is to be able to make a difference in the lives of others!

Although this book is primarily written as a textbook, it is also intended to be a source of information for working professionals, including those who have little experience in this area. The glossary provides a source of quick information that will allow the reader to understand and speak the jargon of this specialty area. Although this book is intended to be a source of didactic and theoretical information, it is also written as a practical guide on "how to do it." Therefore, many of the chapters provide practical information on procedures. Hopefully, this book will serve as a ready reference and resource to guide professionals in the delivery of quality care for this population of individuals.

Terminology

Service providers must be sensitive to the emotional and psychological needs of the patient. Sensitivity to the feelings of the patient is often overlooked by well-meaning service providers. It is easy to forget that we deal with real people, not just interesting cases. This lack of sensitivity is sometimes reflected in the terminology used in the literature and in daily use. I recall listening to a speech given by an adult who was born with a cleft palate. As he described his childhood, he pointed out that being called a "cleft palate child" evoked very negative feelings. Fortunately, this type of phrase is becoming "politically incorrect," just as the term "harelip" has in the past. Using an anomaly as an adjective to describe an individual is certainly insensitive to the feelings of a person born with this anomaly. As service providers, it is important to be careful about the way that individuals with craniofacial anomalies are described.

Since we are discussing terminology, the phrase "child (individual, patient or subject) with a cleft" is also used frequently to describe individuals who were born with a cleft of the lip or palate. Unless the cleft has not been repaired, this phrase is not technically correct. The phrase "children born with cleft palates" is also used periodically in the literature. This seems awkward because it would be very unusual indeed for a child to have more than one cleft palate. We certainly would never use the phrase "children born with spina bifidas" or "children born with cerebral palsies." Therefore, when speaking of more than one child, the correct phrase is "children with a repaired cleft palate" or " children with a history of cleft palate." The reader will note that the word "child" is frequently used throughout the text for an individual with this anomaly. This is used because the speech and resonance disorders secondary to cleft lip/palate and craniofacial anomalies are usually addressed during childhood. However, it should be understood that this information also applies to adults with the same anomalies. Finally, the terms "speech pathology" and "speech pathologist" are used throughout the book. Although language is a big part of this profession, it is not a major focus of this book. Therefore, it is hoped that the reader will understand and forgive the use of the shorter, abbreviated terms in this book.

How to Use This Book

This book was written in a purposeful sequence so that the information from each chapter builds on the information from previous chapters. The first section of the text provides basic information on the normal anatomy of the orofacial structures and the normal physiology of the velopharyngeal valve. After the normal structures and function are described, information on clefts and craniofacial anomalies is discussed in subsequent chapters. The various causes of these anomalies, including the genetic bases, are reviewed. Once the student has completed the first section, there should be a firm understanding of normal and abnormal facial and velopharyngeal features and the potential causes of abnormalities.

The second section of the text includes chapters on the various problems associated with clefts and craniofacial anomalies. In particular, this section covers the effects of these anomalies on feeding, dentition, language, cognition, phonology, articulation, resonance, hearing, dentition, and psychosocial development.

After completing the second section, the reader will have an understanding of the number, types, and complexity of the problems that occur secondary to clefts and craniofacial anomalies. It will then be apparent to the reader that there is a need for multidisciplinary management of these patients in an interdisciplinary setting. This leads naturally to the third section of this book in which the importance of a team approach is covered. This section is short, but important, because it emphasizes the fact that services from several disciplines are needed for these patients. The reader will complete this section with an understanding that quality patient care necessitates interdisciplinary interaction and collaboration in the assessment and treatment of patients with clefts and craniofacial anomalies.

The fourth part covers the various diagnostic methods used for assessing speech, resonance and velopharyngeal function. This section includes the perceptual examination of speech and resonance, the physical examination of the oral cavity, and instrumental measures for evaluating resonance and velopharyngeal function.

The fifth and final section of this book discusses the treatment of speech and resonance disorders secondary to clefts, craniofacial anomalies and velopharyngeal dysfunction. This section includes surgical management, prosthetic management, and speech therapy.

At the end of the book, the reader will find appendixes that contain resource information. In addition, a glossary of terms is found at the back of the text. The first time that a technical or medical term is used in this book, it is printed in italics and a definition is given in the text. All of these words are also listed in the glossary. The student may find studying the glossary of terms helpful in learning much of the information in the book.

The author and contributors are grateful for the opportunity to present this information to you and we are hopeful that you will be educated, enlightened, and inspired. Let the adventure begin.

ACKNOWLEDGMENTS

I would like to acknowledge my colleague and good friend, Linda Lee, Ph.D. Dr. Lee volunteered to review this entire manuscript as a favor. She provided outstanding feedback and offered many suggestions that have helped to improve the quality of this book. For that I am very grateful.

I would like to acknowledge Janet H. Middendorf, M.A., another colleague and good friend. She helped me complete this book in many ways, including picking up my patients and clinics when life became too hectic.

I would like to thank Tracy Stehlin, my outstanding administrative coordinator and friend, and Vickie Shell, our temporary assistant, for their help in organizing and scanning illustrations. Thanks also to Joey Wolfenbarger for his technical knowledge and his help in preparing illustrations and to Dr. Robin Cotton for allowing me to use many of his drawings.

Finally, I would like to acknowledge and thank the staff of the Speech Pathology Department at Cincinnati Children's Hospital Medical Center. They are truly the best in the country! Their patience with me during this busy time, and their interest, encouragement, and support kept me going to the finish line.

CONTRIBUTORS

David A. Billmire, M.D.*
Associate Professor of Clinical Surgery
University of Cincinnati College of Medicine
Director, Craniofacial and Pediatric Plastic
Surgery Division
Children's Hospital Medical Center
Cincinnati, Ohio

Richard Campbell, D.M.D., M.S.*
Assistant Professor of Clinical Pediatrics
University of Cincinnati College of Medicine
Director, Orthodontics
Division of Pediatric Dentistry
Children's Hospital Medical Center
Cincinnati, Ohio

Julia Corcoran, M.D.*
Assistant Professor of Clinical Surgery
University of Cincinnati College of Medicine
Attending Physician
Children's Hospital Medical Center
Cincinnati, Ohio

Murray Dock, D.D.S., M.S.D.
Associate Professor of Clinical Pediatric
University of Cincinnati College of Medicine
Director, Residency Training Program
Division of Pediatric Dentistry
Children's Hospital Medical Center
Cincinnati, Ohio

Robert J. Hopkin, M.D.*
Assistant Professor of Pediatrics
University of Cincinnati College of Medicine
Division of Human Genetics
Children's Hospital Medical Center
Cincinnati, Ohio

Claire K. Miller, M.S.
Speech Pathologist III
Speech Pathology Department
Children's Hospital Medical Center
Cincinnati, Ohio

Howard Saal, M.D.*
Associate Professor of Pediatrics
University of Cincinnati College of Medicine
Head, Clinical Genetics Services
Division of Human Genetics
Children's Hospital Medical Center
Cincinnati, Ohio

Janet R. Schultz, Ph.D., ABBP*
Professor
Psychology Department
Xavier University
Team Psychologist
Craniofacial Center of Children's Hospital
    Medical Center
Cincinnati, Ohio

J. Paul Willging, M.D.*
Asssociate Professor
Department of Pediatric Otolaryngology—
    Head and Neck Surgery
University of Cincinnati College of Medicine
Children's Hospital Medical Center
Cincinnati, Ohio

David Zajac, Ph.D.
Assistant Professor
Department of Dental Ecology and the
    Craniofacial Center
University of North Carolina at Chapel Hill
Chapel Hill, North Carolina

*Denotes member of the team of The Craniofacial Center, Children's Hospital Medical Center, Cincinnati, Ohio

DEDICATION

This book is dedicated to the three people who have influenced me most in my life and have helped me to be the best that I can be. Without their love and support, I would never have had a career and certainly would not have had the opportunity to write this book.

The first dedication is to my father, who was a wonderful, caring and talented otolaryngologist whom I always admired. Dad, I always wanted to be just like you when I grew up.

The next dedication is to my mother, who is the kindest, most thoughtful and most caring person that I have ever known. Mom, now that I am grown up, I strive to be more like you.

The final dedication is to my husband, who has supported me, encouraged me, and helped me to focus and succeed in my career. John, you have allowed me to spread my wings and fly. For that I will be eternally grateful.

With all my love, Ann

PART I

Normal and Abnormal Craniofacial Features

CHAPTER

1

Anatomy and Physiology: The Orofacial Structures and Velopharyngeal Valve

CONTENTS

To understand patterns of clefting and various craniofacial anomalies, it is important to be aware of how these structures should normally be formed. In addition, knowledge about the function of the oral structures and the velopharyngeal valve is essential before the speech pathologist will be able to evaluate abnormal speech and velopharyngeal dysfunction.

This chapter reviews the basic anatomy of the structures of the orofacial and velopharyngeal complex as they relate to speech production. The physiology of the velopharyngeal mechanism is also described in detail. The interested reader is referred to other sources for more detailed information on anatomy and physiology of the speech articulators (Cassell & Elkadi, 1995; Cassell, Moon, & Elkadi, 1990; Dickson, 1972, 1975; Dickson & Dickson, 1972; Dickson, Grant, Sicher, Dubrul, & Paltan, 1974, 1975; Huang, Lee, & Rajendran, 1998; Kuehn, 1979; Maue-Dickson, 1977, 1979; Maue-Dickson & Dickson, 1980; Moon & Kuehn, 1996, 1997).

Anatomy

The structures that are important for normal speech and resonance include facial structures, oral structures, and pharyngeal structures. Unfortunately, these are the structures that are commonly affected by anomalies related to a craniofacial syndrome or cleft lip and/or cleft palate. Before the examiner can fully appreciate abnormalities of structure that occur with these malformations or deformations, a thorough understanding of normal structure is important. In addition, the examiner needs to know the terminology of various aspects of the orofacial and velopharyngeal structures. This section describes these structures, beginning with the outside facial features, then moving to the oral cavity, and concluding with the posterior velopharyngeal structures.

Nose and Nasal Cavity

Although the facial structures are familiar to all, some aspects of the face are important to point out for a thorough understanding of congenital anomalies and clefting. The facial landmarks can be seen on Figure 1–1A. Starting with the nose, the *nasal root* is where the nose begins at the level of the eyes. The *nasal bridge*, also known as the *nasion*, is the bony structure that is located between the eyes and corresponds with the nasofrontal suture. The nostrils are separated by the *columella* (little column), which is the tissue that is under the nasal tip and between the nostrils. The columella is at the lower end of the nasal septum and consists of cartilage and mucosa. Ideally, the columella is straight and backed by a straight nasal septum. It must also be long enough so that the nasal tip is not depressed or flattened.

The nostrils are frequently referred to as *nares*, although the individual nostril is a *naris*. The *ala nasi* (Latin for "wing") is the outside curved side of the nostril, which consists of cartilage. The *alae* are the two curved sides of the nostril. The *alar rims* surround the opening to the nostril on either side and the *alar base* is the area where the ala meets the upper lip. The *nasal sill* is the base of the nostril opening. The *piriform aperture*, which literally means pear-shaped opening, is the opening to the nostril or nasal cavity.

The nasal cavity is divided into two sections by the nasal septum. As can be seen in Figure 1–2, the *nasal septum* consists of the vomer bone, the perpendicular plate of the ethmoid, and the quadrangular cartilage. It is covered with *mucous membrane*, which is the lining tissue of the nasal cavity, oral cavity, and the pharynx. It consists of stratified squamous epithelium and lamina propria and is also known as *mucosa*. (This should not be confused with *mucus*, which is the clear, viscid secretion of the mucous membranes.) The *vomer* is positioned

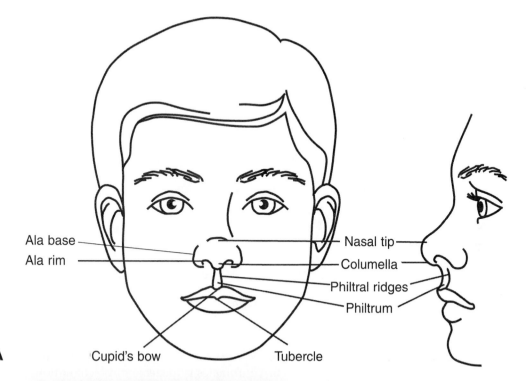

Ala base

Ala rim

Nasal tip

Columella

Philtral ridges

Philtrum

Cupid's bow

Tubercle

A

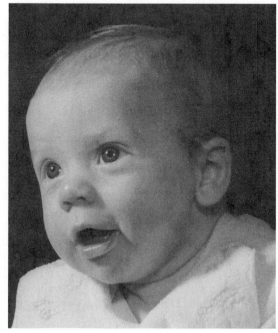

B

Figure 1-1. Normal facial landmarks. **A.** Note the structures on the diagram. **B.** Normal face. Try to locate the normal structures on this infant's face.

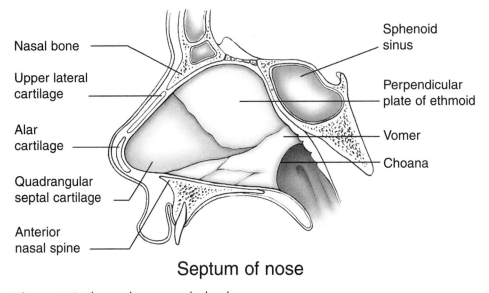

Nasal bone

Upper lateral cartilage

Alar cartilage

Quadrangular septal cartilage

Anterior nasal spine

Sphenoid sinus

Perpendicular plate of ethmoid

Vomer

Choana

Septum of nose

Figure 1–2. The nasal septum and related structures.

posteriorly and is perpendicular to the palate. As such, the lower portion of the vomer fits in a groove formed by the median palatine suture line on the nasal aspect of the maxilla. The *perpendicular plate of the ethmoid* is between the vomer and the quadrangular cartilage. It projects down to join the vomer. The *quadrangular cartilage* forms the anterior nasal septum and projects anteriorly to the columella. It is not uncommon for the nasal septum to be less than perfectly straight, particularly in adults. The *anterior nasal spine* is the anterior point of the maxilla that corresponds to the base of the columella.

Attached to the lateral walls of the nose are the superior, middle, and inferior *turbinates* (also called *concha*) (Figure 1–3). The turbinates are bony structures that are covered with mucosa. The superior and middle turbinates are parts of the ethmoid bone. The inferior turbinate, which is the largest, consists of part of the sphenoid bone. The superior, middle, and inferior *nasal meatuses* are the openings or passageways that lie directly under their re-

spective turbinates. The purpose of the turbinates is to create turbulent airflow within the nose to increase humidification and to deflect air superiorly in the nose for the sense of smell. The *choana* is a funnel-shaped opening at the back of the nasal cavity that leads to the nasopharynx. There is a choana on each side of the posterior part of the vomer.

Upper Lip

The features of the upper lip can be seen on Figure 1–1A. An examination of the upper lip reveals the *philtrum*, which is a long dimple or indentation that courses from the columella down to the upper lip. The philtrum is bordered by the *philtral columns* on each side. These columns are actually embryological fusion lines that are formed as the segments of the upper lip fuse. The philtrum and philtral columns course downward from the nose, and terminate at the edge of the upper lip.

The top of the upper lip is called the *cupid's bow* due to its characteristic shape, which in-

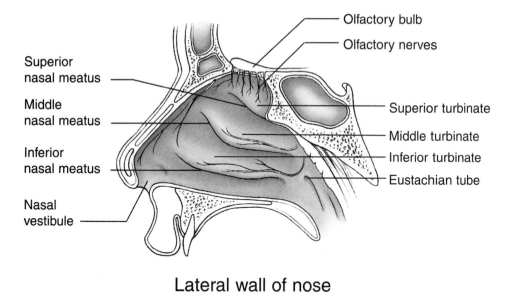

Lateral wall of nose

Figure 1–3. The lateral wall of the nose showing the turbinates.

cludes a rounded configuration with an indentation in the middle. The upper and lower lips are both highlighted by the *white roll*. This white border tissue surrounds the red portion of the lip, which is called the *vermilion*. On the upper lip, the inferior border of the midsection of the vermilion comes to a point and is somewhat prominent. Therefore, it is referred to as the *tubercle*. In its naturally closed position, the upper lip rests over and slightly in front of the lower lip, although the inferior border of the upper lip is inverted. Figure 1–1A shows a diagram of the normal facial landmarks. The student is encouraged to identify the same structures on the photo of the normal infant face shown in Figure 1–1B.

Oral Cavity

Beginning with the gross anatomy first, the palate can be separated into two main parts: the hard palate and the soft palate (Figure 1–4). The *hard palate* is a bony structure that separates the oral cavity from the nasal cavity. The *velum*, frequently referred to as the *soft palate*, is the part of the palate that is muscular and is located in the back of the mouth, just posterior to the hard palate. At the posterior edge of the velum is the pendulous *uvula*.

The tongue resides within the arch of the mandible and fills the oral cavity when the mouth is closed. With the mouth closed, the slight negative pressure within the oral cavity ensures that the tongue adheres to the palate and the tip rests against the alveolar ridge. The *dorsum* is the top of the tongue and the *ventral surface* is the lower surface of the tongue.

At the back of the oral cavity are bilateral paired curtainlike structures called *faucial pillars*. As the velum curves downward toward the tongue on both sides, it forms the anterior faucial pillar. Just behind the anterior pillar is the posterior faucial pillar. These structures contain muscles that assist with velopharyngeal and lingual movement. The *palatine tonsils* (or simply the *tonsils*) are found between the

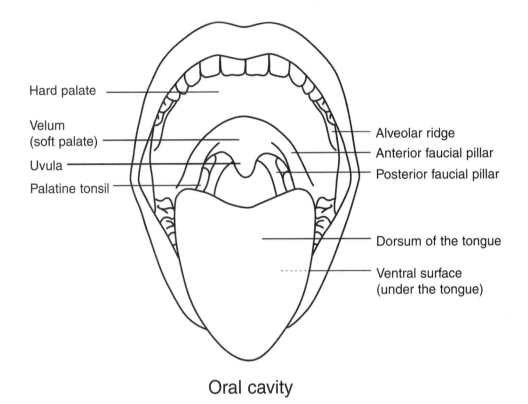

Oral cavity

Figure 1–4. The structures of the oral cavity.

anterior and posterior faucial pillars on both sides. Although the tonsils are bilateral, differences in size are common, so that it is not unusual for one tonsil to be larger than the other. The *lingual tonsils* are masses of lymphoid tissue that are located at the base of the tongue and extend to the epiglottis (Figure 1–5). The *oropharyngeal isthmus* is the opening from the oral cavity to the pharynx and is bordered superiorly by the velum, laterally by the faucial pillars, and inferiorly by the base of the tongue.

Hard Palate

The hard palate forms a rounded dome on the upper part of the oral cavity called the *palatal vault*. In addition to serving as the roof of the mouth, it also serves as the floor of the nasal cavity. The outer portion of the hard palate is called the *alveolar ridge, alveolus,* or simply the gum ridge (see Figure 1–4). This ridge forms the base and the bony support for the teeth. The bony frame of the hard palate is covered by a mucoperiosteum. *Mucoperiosteum* consists of a mucous membrane and periosteum. As noted before, mucous membrane is a lining that consists of stratified squamous epithelium and lamina propria. *Periosteum* is a thick, fibrous tissue that covers the surface of bone. The mucosal covering of the hard palate has multiple ridges running transversely, which are called the *rugae*. There is a slight elevation of the mucosa in the middle of the anterior part

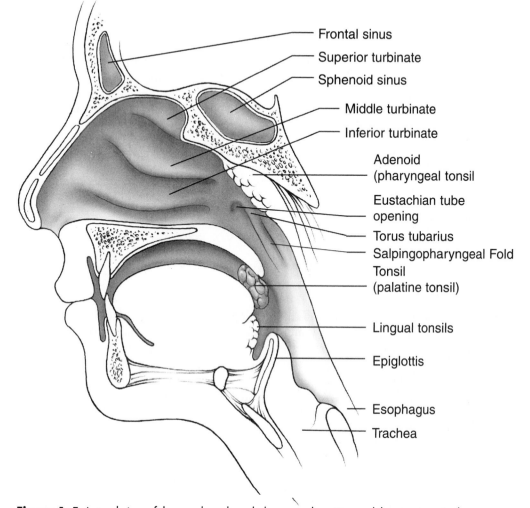

Figure 1–5. Lateral view of the nasal, oral, and pharyngeal cavities and the structures in these areas.

of the hard palate, just in the area of the incisive foramen. This is called the *incisive papilla*. A narrow ridge, called the palatine *raphe* (pronounce rayfay), forms the midline of the hard palate and runs from the incisive papilla posteriorly over the entire length of the mucosa of the hard palate. At the junction of the hard and soft palate, bilateral midline depressions can

often be seen. These are called the *foveae palati* and are the openings to minor salivary glands.

The hard palate is made up of fused bony segments that are separated by the incisive foramen and embryological fusion lines (Figure 1–6). By definition, a *foramen* is a hole or opening in a bony structure that allows blood vessels and nerves to pass through to the area on

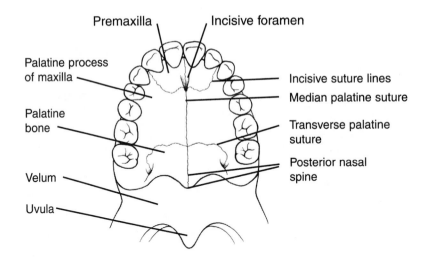

Figure 1-6. Bony structures of the hard palate.

the other side. The *incisive foramen* is located in the alveolar ridge area of the maxillary arch, just behind the central incisors. This foramen is located at the tip of a triangular-shaped bone called the *premaxilla*. The premaxilla is bordered on either side by the *incisive suture lines*. The dental arch of this bony segment contains the central and lateral maxillary incisors.

Behind the incisive suture lines are the paired *palatine processes* of the maxilla, which form the anterior three quarters of the maxilla. These paired bones terminate at the *transverse palatine suture line* (also known as the *palatomaxillary suture line*). Behind the transverse palatine suture line are the paired *horizontal plates* of the palatine bones. These bones form the posterior portion of the hard palate and end with the protrusive *posterior nasal spine*. The palatine processes of the maxilla and the horizontal plates of the palatine bones are both paired because they are separated in the midline by the *median palatine suture* (also known as the *intermaxillary suture line*). This suture line begins at the incisive foramen and ends at the posterior nasal spine. It should be noted that a prominent longitudinal

ridge on the oral surface of the hard palate in the area of this suture line is sometimes found in some Caucasians, particularly those who are of northern European descent. It is also reportedly common in the North American Indian and Eskimo populations. This is called a *torus palatinus* (or *palatine torus*). This finding is a normal variation rather than an abnormality.

The sphenoid and temporal bones provide bony attachment for the velopharyngeal musculature. The *pterygoid process* of the sphenoid bone contains the medial pterygoid plate, the lateral pterygoid plate, and the pterygoid hamulus, all of which provide attachments for muscles in the velopharyngeal complex.

Velum

The velum is attached to the posterior border of the hard palate and is held in place by its internal muscles. During normal nasal breathing, the velum drapes down from the hard palate and rests against the base of the tongue, thus opening the pharynx to the nasal cavity. It elevates during speech and other activities to close against the pharyngeal wall, thus closing off the nasal cavity.

The velum has an oral surface and a nasal surface. The oral surface of the velum is covered by a mucous membrane and it has fine vessels under the mucosa. A thin white line, called the *median palatine raphe,* can be seen coursing down the midline of the velum on the oral surface. The nasal surface of the velum consists of pseudostratified, ciliated columnar epithelium anteriorly, and stratified, squamous epithelium posteriorly in the area where the velum contacts the posterior pharyngeal wall during closure activities (Ettema & Kuehn, 1994; Kuehn & Kahane, 1990; Moon & Kuehn, 1996, 1997).

In looking at the internal structure of the velum, the anterior portion has very few muscle fibers. Instead, it consists of the tensor tendon, glandular tissue, *adipose* (fat) tissue, and the velar aponeurosis. The *palatine aponeurosis,* also known as the *velar aponeurosis* (Figure 1–7), is located in the anterior part of the velum, just below the nasal surface. It consists of a sheet of fibrous connective tissue and fibers from the tensor veli palatini tendon. The velar aponeurosis has its attachment on the posterior border of the hard palate and courses about 1 cm posteriorly through the velum. The velar aponeurosis provides an anchoring point for the velopharyngeal muscles. In addition, it adds stiffness to that portion of the velum (Cassell & Elkadi, 1995; Ettema & Kuehn, 1994; Moon & Kuehn, 1986). The medial portion of the velum contains most of the muscle fibers. The posteri-

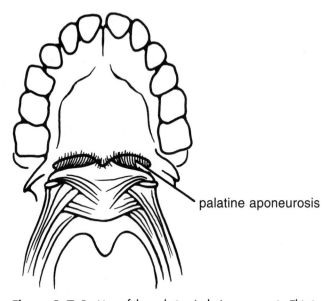

palatine aponeurosis

Figure 1–7. Position of the palatine (velar) aponeurosis. This is a sheet of fibrous tissue that is located just below the nasal surface of the velum and consists of periosteum, fibrous connective tissue and fibers from the tensor veli palatini tendon. It provides an anchoring point for the velopharyngeal muscles and adds stiffness to the velum.

or portion consists of the same glandular and adipose tissue as can be found in the anterior portion. The muscle fibers taper off as they reach the posterior portion of the velum, so that few fibers are found in this section.

Uvula

The *uvula* is a teardrop-shaped structure that is typically long and slender. It hangs freely from the posterior border of the velum. The uvula consists of mucosa on the surface and connective, glandular, and adipose tissue underneath. In addition, the uvula is very vascular, with more vascular tissue than the connecting velum. It has been theorized that this vascularity provides a warming function for this pendulous structure. The uvula is not a contributor to velopharyngeal function and has no known function.

Pharynx

The throat area between the esophagus and the nasal cavity is called the *pharynx*. The pharynx is divided into several sections, as can be seen in Figure 1–8. These sections include the *oropharynx*, which is at the level of the oral cavity or just posterior to the mouth; the *nasopharynx*, which is above the oral cavity and velum and is just posterior to the nasal cavity; and the *hypopharynx*, which is below the oral cavity and extends from the epiglottis inferiorly to the esophagus. The back wall of the throat is called the *posterior pharyngeal wall* and the side walls of the throat are called the *lateral pharyngeal walls*. The *adenoids* (also called the *pharyngeal tonsil*) consist of lymphoid tissue and are found on the posterior pharyngeal wall of the nasopharynx, just behind the velum. Adenoids are usually present in children, but they atrophy with age; therefore, adults have little if any adenoid tissue.

The eustachian tube connects the middle ear with the pharynx. On each side of the pharynx, the pharyngeal opening of the eustachian tube is lateral and slightly above the level of the velum during phonation. The *torus tubarius* is a ridge that is located posterior to the eustachian tube opening and is caused by a projection of the cartilaginous portion of the tube. In the adult, the opening of the eustachian tube is about the size of the diameter of a pencil. The tube is closed at rest, but it opens whenever the individual swallows or yawns.

The *salpingopharyngeal folds* are found on both sides of the pharynx (see Figure 1–5). These folds originate from the torus tubarius at the opening to the eustachian tube and then course downward to the lateral pharyngeal wall. The folds consist primarily of glandular and connective tissue (Dickson, 1975).

Muscles of the Velopharyngeal Mechanism

The velopharyngeal sphincter requires the coordinated action of several different muscles, all of which are paired with one on each side of the midline (Moon & Kuehn, 1996) (Figure 1–9). Many of the muscles in the velopharyngeal complex have their attachments at the medial and lateral pterygoid plates and the pterygoid hamulus of the pterygoid process of the sphenoid bone. Each muscle has been studied extensively and its function defined. However, control of the velopharyngeal valve is very complex, requiring the interaction not only of these muscles, but also the articulators, particularly the tongue. Therefore, much more remains to be learned about the dynamics of the muscles and their interactions during speech.

The *levator veli palatini* muscles provide the main muscle mass of the velum and are primarily responsible for velar elevation (Bell-Berti, 1973). The levator veli palatini muscles from

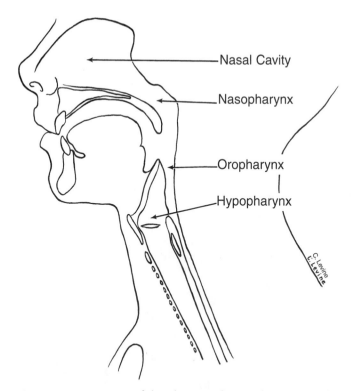

Figure 1–8. Sections of the pharynx. The *oropharynx* is at the level of the oral cavity or just posterior to the mouth. The *nasopharynx* is above the oral cavity and velum and is just posterior to the nasal cavity. The *hypopharynx* is below the oral cavity and extends from the epiglottis inferiorly to the esophagus.

each side of the head course medially to inter-digitate in the middle of the velum and blend together to create the *levator sling*. Contraction of the levator muscles forces the free edge of the soft palate to move in a superior and posterior direction in order to close against the posterior pharyngeal wall. On each side of the nasopharynx, the levator veli palatini muscle originates from the apex of the petrous portion of the temporal bone at the base of the skull. The muscle then courses through an area that is anterior and medial to the carotid canal and inferior to the eustachian tube (Moon & Kuehn,

1996, 1997) so that it enters the velum at a 45° angle. The paired muscles then insert into the upper surface of the palatal aponeurosis and into the medial raphe of the velum. The levator veli palatini muscles take up the middle 40% of the entire velum (Boorman & Sommerlad, 1985).

The upper fibers of the *superior pharyngeal constrictor* muscles are thought to be responsible for the medial displacement of the lateral pharyngeal walls to effectively narrow the velopharyngeal port (Iglesias, Kuehn, & Morris, 1980; Shprintzen, McCall, Skolnick, & Lencione,

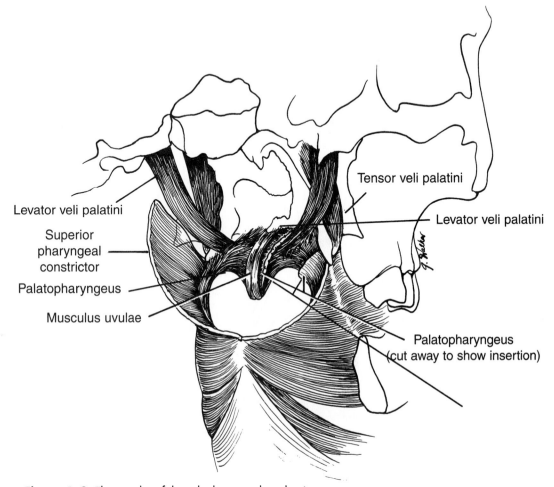

Figure 1–9. The muscles of the velopharyngeal mechanism.

1975; Skolnick, McCall, & Barnes, 1973). The paired superior pharyngeal constrictor muscles are located in the upper pharynx and arise from the pterygoid hamulus, pterygomandibular raphe, posterior tongue, posterior mandible, and palatine aponeurosis. They insert posteriorly in the pharyngeal raphe in the midline of the posterior pharyngeal wall.

The *musculus uvulae* muscles contract during phonation and create a bulge on the posterior part of the nasal surface of the velum. It has been postulated that the bulge serves two purposes (Kuehn, Folkins, & Linville, 1988; Moon & Kuehn, 1996, 1997). The first purpose is to provide additional stiffness to the nasal side of the velum during contraction, which prevents velar distortion. The second purpose is to fill in the area of contact between the velum and posterior pharyngeal wall in midline, which helps to assure a firm velopharyngeal seal (Huang, Lee, & Rajendran, 1997; Kuehn et al., 1988). It has also been suggested that the musculus uvulae may have an extensor effect on the nasal aspect of the velum, displacing it toward the posterior pharyngeal wall (Huang et al., 1997). The paired musculus uvulae muscles are located in the midline of the posterior velum and originate from the area of the palatal aponeurosis. They are the only intrinsic muscles of the velum and, as such, they are contained solely within the velum and do not extend beyond its borders (Moon & Kuehn, 1996). They are positioned side by side and extend to the free edge of the soft palate, superficial to the levator veli palatini. It should be noted that the name of this muscle is somewhat misleading in that it does not exist within the uvula. In fact, the uvula contains very few muscle fibers and does not contribute to velopharyngeal closure (Ettema & Kuehn, 1994; Kuehn & Kahane, 1990; Moon & Kuehn, 1996, 1997).

The *palatoglossus* muscles act antagonistically to the levator veli palatini to depress the velum or elevate the tongue. As such, these muscles are felt to be responsible for the rapid downward movement of the velum during connected speech when a nasal consonant is produced. On each side, the palatoglossus muscle arises from the palatal aponeurosis of the anterior half of the soft palate and inserts into the posterior lateral aspect of the tongue. It is contained within the anterior faucial pillar, and may be subject to possible damage during tonsillectomy.

The function of the *palatopharyngeus* muscle is not well understood. The horizontal fibers of these muscles are thought to be associated with the sphincteric action of pulling the lateral pharyngeal walls medially to narrow the pharynx and assist with closure (Cassell & Elkadi, 1995). The vertical fibers may assist in the lowering of the velum, and could also assist with the elevation of the larynx and the lower portion of the pharynx (Moon & Kuehn, 1996, 1997). Some authors have suggested that this muscle functions as a muscular "hydrostat," which squeezes the posterior aspect of the velum so that it conforms to the shape of the posterior pharyngeal

wall, thus resulting in a better velopharyngeal seal (Ettema & Kuehn, 1994; Moon & Kuehn, 1997; Smith & Kier, 1989). The palatopharyngeus muscle originates from the palatal aponeurosis and posterior border of the hard palate and then courses down through the posterior faucial pillars to the pharynx. A few of the vertical fibers of this muscle reach the thyroid cartilage of the larynx.

The paired *salpingopharyngeus* muscle cannot have a significant role in achieving velopharyngeal closure given its size and location. This muscle arises from the inferior border of the torus tubarius, which is at the upper level of the pharynx. It courses vertically along the lateral pharyngeal wall and under the salpingopharyngeal fold.

In the entire length of the velum, muscle fibers are found in only about 40% of this structure, and primarily in the midsection (Ettema & Kuehn, 1994). There are muscle fibers from the levator veli palatini, the musculus uvulae, and the palatopharyngeus muscles in this section. This is also the area of the velum where the musculus uvulae is most cohesive and overlies the levator sling. It is important to stress that the muscles of the velopharyngeal mechanism do not work in isolation. In fact, each motor movement is probably the result of the synergistic activities of several muscles. For example, the position and force of closure of the velopharyngeal valve varies with different activities, as will be discussed later. These variations are probably due to variations in the relative contribution of the levator veli palatini, palatoglossus, and palatopharyngeus muscles (Moon, Smith, Folkins, Lemke, & Gartlan, 1994). The complexity of the interaction of the muscles of the velopharyngeal mechanism has been studied, but further research is needed before this interaction is fully understood.

The *tensor veli palatini* muscles are thought to be responsible for opening the eustachian tubes in order to enhance middle ear aeration and drainage (Maue-Dickson, Dickson, &

Rood, 1976). Although these muscles are the main contributors to the palatal aponeurosis, the tensor is not positioned in a way to either raise or lower the velum. Therefore, these muscles probably contribute little, if at all, to velopharyngeal closure. The tensor veli palatini muscle on each side originates from the membranous portion of the eustachian tube cartilage and the scaphoid fossa spine of the sphenoid bone (Barsoumian, Kuehn, Moon, & Canady, 1998). Additional slips arise from the lateral aspect of the medial pterygoid plate and the spine of the sphenoid. It then courses vertically down from the skull base to pass around the pterygoid hamulus. This redirects the muscle tendon 90° medially where it contributes to the palatine aponeurosis in the superior and anterior region of the velum.

Velopharyngeal Motor and Sensory Innervation

The motor and sensory innervation of the velopharyngeal mechanism arises from the cranial nerves in the medulla. The following section describes the specific innervation for motor movement and sensation.

Motor innervation for the muscles that contribute to velopharyngeal closure comes from the pharyngeal plexus. The *pharyngeal plexus* is a network of nerves that lies along the posterior wall of the pharynx and consists of the pharyngeal branches of the glossopharyngeal nerve (CN IX) and the vagus nerve (CN X). Innervation of the velar muscles with these nerves occurs through the brainstem nuclei ambiguus and retrofacialis (Cassell & Elkadi, 1995; Kennedy & Kuehn, 1989; Moon & Kuehn, 1996). The palatoglossus muscle has also been found to receive innervation from the hypoglossal nerve (CN XII) (Cassell & Elkadi, 1995). The tensor veli palatini, which does not contribute to velopharyngeal closure, receives motor innervation from the mandibular division of the trigeminal nerve (CN V).

Sensory innervation of both the hard and soft palate is believed to derive from the greater and lesser palatine nerves, which arise from the maxillary division of the trigeminal nerve (CN V). The faucial and pharyngeal regions of the oral cavity are innervated by the glossopharyngeal nerve (CN IX). The facial nerve (CN VII) and vagus nerve (CN X) might also contribute to sensory innervation. Although the peripheral distribution of sensory fibers may travel along different cranial nerve routes, they all appear to terminate in the spinal nucleus of the trigeminal nerve (Cassell & Elkadi, 1995). It has been reported that the cutaneous sensory nerve endings are more prolific in the anterior portion of the oral cavity, but diminish in quantity as they course toward the posterior regions of the mouth (Cassell & Elkadi, 1995).

Physiological Subsystems for Speech

Speech is the result of the coordination of several physiological subsystems. These include respiration, phonation, resonance, and articulation. The velopharyngeal valve must function in coordination with the other subsystems of speech for speech to be produced normally and with good intelligibility.

To understand the importance of these subsystems and the need for coordination, it may be helpful to review how sound is produced. Every instrument that is capable of producing sound needs at least three components: (1) a vibrating mechanism that can be set in motion to produce sound, (2) a stimulating mechanism that can set the vibration in motion, and (3) a resonating mechanism to reinforce or amplify the sound. In human speech, the vocal folds are the vibrating bodies, the force of breath pressure is the stimulating force, and the cavities of the vocal tract provide the mechanism for resonating the sound energy (Baken, 1987). The acoustic product is then altered by the velopharyngeal valve and by changing the size and shape of the oral cavity through the movement and placement of the articulators.

Respiration

Respiration is essential for life support, but is it also important for speech. The air pressure from the lungs is what provides the initiating force for phonation and the air pressure for speech. During quiet breathing, the inspiratory and expiratory phases are relatively long in duration. During speech, however, there is a quick period of inspiration prior to the initiation of an utterance. Air pressure through expiration is then maintained under the vocal folds during the entire phrase or sentence. The expiratory phase is relatively long and varies, depending on the length of the produced utterance. On the other hand, inspiration occurs very quickly during times of purposeful pauses. Both the inspiratory and expiratory phases must be controlled by the speaker during speech production.

Phonation

Phonation is the sound that is generated by the vocal folds as they begin to vibrate. This sound, called voice, is used for the production of all vowel sounds. It is used for only about half of the consonant sounds, however. Therefore, the vocal folds must vibrate for voiced sounds (e.g., /b/), stop vibrating abruptly for voiceless sounds (e.g., /p/) and then vibrate again for the next vowel or voiced consonant. This requires a great deal of neuromotor coordination and control.

Phonation is initiated when subglottal air pressure from the lungs passes through the glottis, forcing the gently approximated vocal folds apart. This sets the vocal folds into vibration, resulting in a type of buzzing sound. During phonation, there is continuous adduction (or closing) of the vocal folds as they vibrate for voiced phonemes and periodic ab-duction (or opening) of the vocal folds with pauses and the production of voiceless sounds. Air pressure must be maintained throughout the utterance so that it can continue to provide the force for phonation.

Resonance

Once phonation has begun, the air pressure from the lungs and sound energy from the vocal folds travel in a superior direction in the vocal tract. The sound energy vibrates throughout the cavities of the supraglottic tract, beginning with the pharyngeal cavity and then including the oral cavity or nasal cavity. The resultant vibration of sound energy adds the resonance quality to the speech.

Several factors can affect the vibration and the overall acoustic product of the voice. These factors include the size, the shape, and the wall thickness of the cavities of the vocal tract. There are significant variations among individuals in these factors, some which are determined by age and gender. For example, women and children usually have a shorter vocal tract than men, and therefore, they have higher formant frequencies in their vocal product. Variations in these factors cause some frequencies to be amplified, while other frequencies are attenuated. The changes in vibration that result from all of these factors enhance the resonance and give the perception of the timbre or vocal quality (Sataloff, 1992).

Once the sound energy and air pressure reach the pharyngeal cavity, the velopharyngeal valve regulates and directs the focus of resonance. During the production of oral speech sounds (all sounds with the exception of m, n, and ng), the velopharyngeal valve closes, thus blocking off the nasal cavity from the oral cavity. This allows the sound energy and air pressure to be directed anteriorly into the oral cavity. The velopharyngeal valve opens with the production of nasal sounds so that the sound energy can resonate primarily in the nasal cavity. The velopharyngeal valve is therefore very important for normal speech because it is responsible for regulating and directing the transmission of sound energy and air pressure in the cavities of the vocal tract.

Articulation

The sound that results from phonation and resonance is further altered for individual speech sounds by the articulators. The *articulators* are structures that include the lips, the jaws (including the teeth), the tongue, and even the velum. The articulators alter the acoustic product for different speech sounds in two ways. First, they can vary the size and shape of the oral cavity through movement and articulatory placement. In addition, the articulators can modify the manner in which the sound, and particularly the airstream, is released.

Both vowels and oral consonants require oral resonance for production, and many consonants also require oral air pressure. For the production of vowels, the tongue and jaws modify the size and shape of the oral cavity, but there is no constriction of the sound energy or air pressure. The differentiation of vowel sounds is determined by tongue height (high, mid, or low), tongue position (front, central, back), and lip rounding (present or absent). On the other hand, consonants are produced by partial or complete obstruction of the oral cavity, which results in a build-up of air pressure in the oral cavity. Intraoral air pressure provides the force for the production of all pressure-sensitive consonants (plosives, fricatives, and affricates). *Plosive sounds* (p, b, t, d, k, g) are produced with a build-up of intraoral pressure and then a sudden release. *Fricative sounds* (f, v, s, z, sh, th) require a gradual release of air pressure through a small or restricted opening. *Affricate sounds* (ch, j) are a combination of a plosive and fricative, and as such, they require a build-up of intraoral air pressure and then a gradual release through a narrow opening. Consonants are differentiated not only by the manner of production (plosives, fricatives, affricates, liquids, and glides), but also by the place of production (bilabial, labio-dental, lingual-alveolar, palatal, velar, and glottal) and the voicing (voiced or voiceless).

Stress and Intonation

In connected speech, articulation is influenced by the stress of individual phonemes and the intonation of the utterance. *Stress* is related to increased muscular effort and subglottic pressure during the production of a syllable. Stressed syllables are produced with greater articulatory precision and are longer in duration than unstressed syllables. In addition, they tend to be higher in pitch and intensity. *Intonation* refers to the frequent changes in pitch throughout an utterance, as controlled by subtle changes in vocal fold length and mass. These changes influence the rate of vibration of the vocal folds and the tension of the muscles of the larynx. Although there are changes in pitch throughout connected speech, the pitch of the voice tends to drop to a lower frequency at the end of each statement and rise to a higher frequency at the end of a question. Both stress and intonation are used for emphasis and also to help to convey meaning. For example, the words "desert" and "dessert" have different meanings that are conveyed through differences in the place of stress. When the sentence "Well that's just fine" is uttered as if it has an exclamation point, it has a different meaning than when it is spoken as if it has a period at the end. The differences in meaning are conveyed by differences in the intonation and stress.

Coordination of Processes

Speech is a very complicated process that requires the coordination of the subsystems of respiration, phonation, resonance, and articulation. During speech, all movements must be done quickly and with good accuracy. In addition, the action of every muscle is influenced by the actions of other muscles in the system, the movements of each structure are influenced by movements of other structures, and every phoneme is influenced by other phonemes around it (Lubker, 1975). At the same time, speech production must also be produced in conjunction with cognition and language function for communication. Any errors or breakdown in this coordinated process can be symptomatic of a communication disorder. Therefore, the complexity of speech production cannot be overstated.

Physiology of the Velopharyngeal Valve

Normal velopharyngeal closure is accomplished by the coordinated action of the velum (soft palate), the lateral pharyngeal walls, and the posterior pharyngeal wall (Moon & Kuehn, 1996). These structures function as a valve that serves to close off the nasal cavity from the oral cavity during speech, as well as singing, whistling, blowing, sucking, swallowing, gagging, and vomiting. Although the relative contributions of these structures to closure can vary among individuals, all are important for normal velopharyngeal function.

Velar Movement

When inactive, the velum is low in the pharynx and rests against the base of the tongue (Figure 1–10A). This position contributes to a patent pharynx, which is important for the unobstructed movement of air between the nasal cavity and lungs during normal nasal breathing. During the production of oral speech, the velum raises in a superior and posterior direction to contact the posterior pharyngeal wall or, in some cases, the lateral pharyngeal walls (Figure 1–10B). As it elevates, it has a type of "knee action" where it bends to provide maximum contact with the posterior pharyngeal

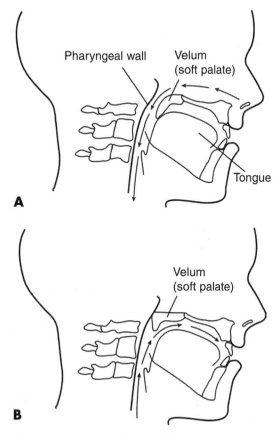

A

B

Figure 1–10. Lateral view of the velum and posterior pharyngeal wall. **A.** The velum rests against the base of the tongue during normal nasal breathing, resulting in a patent airway. **B.** The velum elevates during speech and closes against the posterior pharyngeal wall. This allows the air pressure from the lungs and the sound from the larynx to be redirected from a superior direction to an anterior direction to enter the oral cavity for speech.

wall over a large surface. The point where the velum bends is called the *velar dimple*. This is usually located at about 80% back the length of the velum (Mason & Simon, 1977) and can be seen through an intraoral examination. An examination of the nasal surface of the velum through endoscopy would reveal a muscular bulge on that side of the velar dimple, called the *velar eminence*. This bulge results from the contraction of the musculus uvulae muscles. In fact, it could be said that the musculus uvulae muscles form the "patella" of the levator "knee." The contraction of the musculus uvulae muscles is felt to provide internal stiffness to the velum. In addition, the bulk that this bulge provides in this area helps to achieve velopharyngeal closure in the midline.

As the velum elevates, it also elongates through a process called *velar stretch* (Bzoch, 1968; Mourino & Weinberg, 1975; Pruzansky & Mason, 1962; Simpson & Austin, 1972; Simpson & Chin, 1981; Simpson & Colton, 1980). Due to this stretch factor, the velum is actually longer during function than it is at rest. Therefore, the effective length of the velum is the distance between the posterior border of the hard palate and the point on the posterior pharyngeal wall where it contacts during speech. This is measured in a line on the same plane as the hard palate (Mason & Simon, 1977). The amount of velar stretch and effective length of the velum varies among individuals and is dependent on the size and configuration of the pharynx. Simpson and Colton (1980) reported that the amount of velar stretch is highly correlated with the "need ratio," which they defined as the pharyngeal depth divided by the velar length at rest. However, velar stretch even varies with different speech sounds, since the point of contact may be different.

When nasal phonemes are produced, the velum is pulled down so that the sound energy can enter the nasal cavity. The lowering of the velum is probably accomplished as a result of muscle contraction, gravity, and tissue elasticity (Moon & Kuehn, 1996). Given the speed with which the velum must be lowered for nasal phonemes and then raised for oral phonemes, muscle involvement, specifically of the palatoglossus muscle, appears to be the most likely source of this movement.

Lateral Pharyngeal Wall Movement

The lateral pharyngeal walls contribute to velopharyngeal closure by moving medially to close against the velum or, in some cases, to meet in midline behind the velum (Figure 1–11). Both lateral pharyngeal walls move during closure, but there is great variation among normal speakers in the extent of movement (Shprintzen, Rakof, Skolnick, & Lavorato, 1977). In addition, there is often asymmetry in movement so that one side may move significantly more than the other side. Although some lateral wall movement can be noted from an intraoral perspective, the point of greatest medial displacement occurs near the level of the hard palate (Iglesias et al., 1980) and velar eminence (Shprintzen et al., 1975). This area is well above the area that can be seen from an intraoral inspection. In fact, at the oral cavity level, the lateral walls may actually appear to bow outward during speech.

Posterior Pharyngeal Wall Movement

During velar movement, the posterior pharyngeal wall may move forward to assist in achieving contact, although this forward movement may be slight (Iglesias et al., 1980). Some posterior pharyngeal wall movement is noted in most normal speakers, but its contribution to closure seems to be much less than that of the velum and lateral pharyngeal walls. Some normal as well as abnormal speakers have a defined area on the posterior pharyngeal wall that bulges forward during speech. This is called Passavant's ridge, and is discussed in the next section.

Passavant's Ridge

A *Passavant's ridge*, first reported by Gustav Passavant in the 1800s, is a shelflike ridge that projects from the posterior pharyngeal wall into the pharynx (Figure 1–12). Passavant's ridge

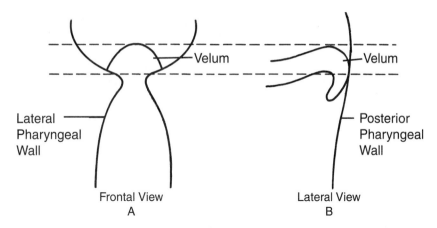

Figure 1–11. A. Frontal view of the lateral pharyngeal walls. The lateral pharyngeal walls (LPWs) move medially to close against the velum on both sides. **B.** Lateral view of the velum as it contacts the posterior pharyngeal wall (PPW). (Reprinted with permission from "Lateral Defects in Velopharyngeal Insufficiency," by R. T. Cotton and F. Quattromani, 1977, p. 469. *Archives of Otolaryngology, 103,* 469–470.)

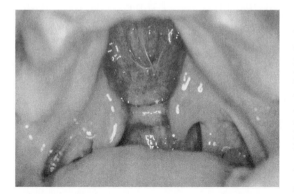

Figure 1–12. Passavant's ridge as noted during phonation. This patient has an open palate from surgical removal of the maxilla due to cancer. During phonation, the Passavant's ridge presents as a bulge of muscle on the posterior pharyngeal wall.

occurs in coordination with velopharyngeal closure. Its presence is associated with active lateral pharyngeal wall motion and is also synchronous with velar movement (Glaser, Skolnick, McWilliams, & Shprintzen, 1979).

Passavant's ridge is discussed in the physiology section rather than anatomy section because it is not a permanent structure. Instead, it is a dynamic structure that occurs inconsistently in some individuals during velopharyngeal activities, such as speech, whistling, blowing, and swallowing (Glaser et al., 1979), but disappears during nasal breathing or when velopharyngeal activity ceases (Skolnick & Cohn, 1989). Because Passavant's ridge is a localized projection, it should not be confused with the generalized anterior movement of the posterior pharyngeal wall during speech.

Passavant's ridge is thought to be formed by the contraction of specific fibers of the superior pharyngeal constrictor muscles, and possibly fibers of the palatopharyngeus muscles in the posterior pharynx (Dickson & Dickson, 1972; Finkelstein et al., 1993). This forms the muscular ridge, which projects from the posterior pharyngeal wall. Passavant's ridge extends from one lateral pharyngeal wall to the other lateral pharyngeal wall on the opposite side. The vertical location of the ridge is variable among individuals. Although it is across from the free margin of the velum, it is often well below the site of velopharyngeal contact. A study by Glaser et al. (1979) of 43 individuals found that the ridge was located opposite the velar eminence in 5%, opposite the vertical portion of the velum in 58%, opposite the uvula in 25%, and below the uvula in 12%. The orientation of the ridge is also variable among individuals. The ridge can be found to point in a superior, anterior, or inferior direction. Although the location and orientation of the ridge is variable among various speakers, it appears to be in a consistent location for each individual speaker. However, the size of the ridge appears to vary according to the speech sound being produced and the overall degree of velar activity (Skolnick & Cohn, 1989). The size has also been found to be affected by fatigue (Calnan, 1957).

Passavant's ridge is not a prerequisite for normal velopharyngeal function or normal speech, and it is probably not a compensatory mechanism either. When it is found in individuals with velopharyngeal dysfunction, it does not seem to be correlated with gap size or type of cleft palate (Massengill, Walker, & Pickrell, 1969). In addition, the formation of Passavant's ridge does not appear to be associated with the degree of velopharyngeal closure necessary for the specific speech sound. Instead, it has been found to be closely related to the tongue position for vowel production (Honjo, Kojima, & Kumazawa, 1975). When an individual demonstrates a Passavant's ridge, it is inconsistent in appearance and its appearance is often delayed, occurring after velopharyngeal closure has been achieved. It is often located well below the level of velar and lateral pharyngeal wall movement. Therefore, the significance of Passavant's ridge as a compensatory mechanism remains quite doubtful.

Reports of the prevalence of Passavant's ridge in normal speakers range from as little as 9.5% to as high as 80% (Calnan, 1957; Casey & Emrich, 1988; Finkelstein et al., 1991; Mass-

engill et al., 1969; Skolnick & Cohn, 1989; Skolnick, Shprintzen, McCall, & Rakoff, 1975). This variation in the reported prevalence may be due to the fact that Passavant's ridge is more prominent, and therefore is more easily identified, when the head is hyperextended (Glaser et al., 1979). In a look at the collective results of several studies, Casey and Emrich (1988) found that Passavant's ridge probably occurs in about 23% of individuals with history of cleft and 15% of normal speakers.

Variations in Velopharyngeal Closure Patterns Among Normal Speakers

In looking at the entire velopharyngeal mechanism, it is important to recognize that this is a three-dimensional tube that includes the anterior-posterior dimension, the vertical dimension, and the horizontal dimension. During closure, there must be coordinated movement of all structures in all dimensions so that the velopharyngeal valve can achieve closure like a sphincter. This can be seen in Figure 1–13, which shows an inferior view of the entire sphincter. It should be noted that the relative contribution of these structures varies in both normal and abnormal speakers.

In a population of normal and abnormal speakers, specific patterns of velopharyngeal closure can be identified, based on the extent of movement of the soft palate and pharyngeal walls (Croft, Shprintzen, & Rakoff, 1981a; Finkelstein, Talmi, Nachmani, Hauben, & Zohar, 1992; Igawa, Nishizawa, Sugihara, & Inuyama, 1998; Shprintzen et al., 1977; Siegel-Sadewitz & Shprintzen, 1982; Skolnick & Cohn, 1989; Skolnick et al., 1973; Witzel & Posnick, 1989). The prevalence of the different patterns of closure is similar in frequency in both normal and abnormal speakers (Croft, Shprintzen, & Rakoff, 1981). Minor differences in muscular orientation are felt to be responsible for the different contribution of the lateral and posterior pharyngeal walls to velopharyngeal closure

Inferior View

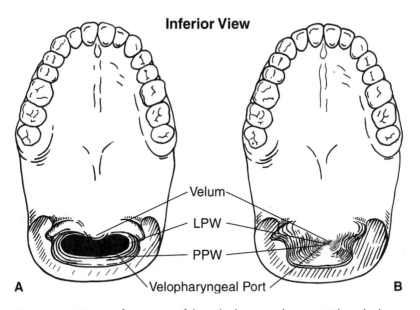

Figure 1–13. An inferior view of the velopharyngeal port. **A.** The velopharyngeal port is open for nasal breathing. **B.** The velopharyngeal port is closed for speech.

(Finkelstein et al., 1992). The basic patterns of normal velopharyngeal closure can be seen in Figure 1–14.

The *coronal pattern* of closure is the most common and is accomplished by the posterior movement of the soft palate to close against a broad area of the posterior pharyngeal wall. There may also be anterior movement of the posterior pharyngeal wall. With this closure pattern, there is minimal contribution of the lateral pharyngeal walls to closure. Witzel and Posnick (1989) studied 246 individuals who underwent nasopharyngoscopy for evaluation of velopharyngeal function. (*Nasopharyngoscopy* is an endoscopic procedure in which a scope is inserted through the nose until it reaches the nasopharynx, allowing visual observation and analysis of the velopharyngeal mechanism.) In this study, they found that 68% of their patients demonstrated a coronal pattern of closure

The next most common pattern of closure is the *circular pattern*. This pattern occurs when the soft palate moves posteriorly, the posterior pharyngeal wall moves anteriorly, and the lateral pharyngeal walls move medially. In this case, all the velopharyngeal structures contribute to closure, and the closure pattern resembles a true sphincter. Witzel and Posnick (1989) found this pattern in 23% of the individuals in their study. Another 5% had a circular pattern with Passavant's ridge. Although Passavant's ridge seems to be most common in individuals with a circular pattern of closure, it is also found with the other patterns of velopharyngeal closure (Skolnick & Cohn, 1989).

The least common pattern of closure is the *sagittal pattern*. This was found in only 4% of the patients in the Witzel and Posnick study (1989). With this pattern, the lateral pharyngeal walls move medially to meet in midline behind

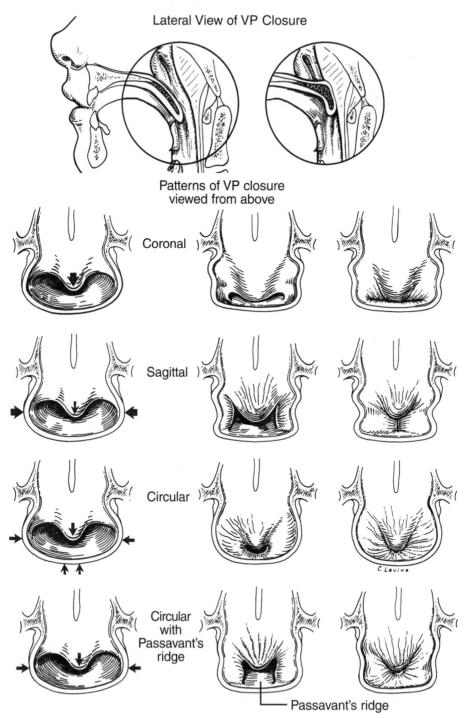

Lateral View of VP Closure

Patterns of VP closure
viewed from above

Coronal

Sagittal

Circular

Circular
with
Passavant's
ridge

Passavant's ridge

C. Levine

Figure 1-14. Patterns of velopharyngeal closure as viewed from above. The nasal surface of the velum is at the top of each diagram.

the velum. There is minimal posterior displacement of the soft palate to effect closure.

To try to explain the differences in movement patterns, Finkelstein and colleagues studied 42 consecutive individuals who were undergoing *uvulopalatopharyngoplasty* (UPPP), which is the partial excision of the velum and uvula to resolve sleep apnea. The velopharyngeal valve was studied through an oral examination and also through an endoscopic examination. They found that individuals with a deep oropharynx tended to show a sagittal or circular pattern of closure, while individuals with a flat oropharynx showed a coronal pattern of closure. These researchers concluded that there must be differences in muscular orientation among individuals to account for the different pharyngeal configurations at rest and during speech.

The variations in the basic patterns of closure among individuals are important to recognize and understand. This is particularly true in the evaluation process, because the basic pattern of closure may have an impact on the diagnosis of velopharyngeal dysfunction and on the type of intervention that is ultimately recommended (Siegel-Sadewitz & Shprintzen, 1982; Skolnick et al., 1973). For example, on a lateral *videofluoroscopy* (which is a radiographic procedure), it may appear as if there is inadequate velopharyngeal closure with the sagittal pattern of closure, even when closure is complete, since the velum does not close against the posterior pharyngeal wall. Therefore, evaluating all of the velopharyngeal structures and their contribution to closure is important so that the basic closure pattern can be identified and considered when making treatment recommendations.

Variations in Velopharyngeal Closure With Type of Activity

Velopharyngeal closure occurs during several activities, in addition to speech. These activities include blowing, whistling, singing, swallowing, gagging, and vomiting. If these activities are categorized into pneumatic and nonpneumatic functions, a characteristic and distinct closure pattern can be identified for each category (Flowers & Morris, 1973; Matsuya, Yamaoka & Miyasaki, 1979; McWilliams & Bradley, 1965; Shprintzen, Lencione, McCall, & Skolnick, 1974). In fact, there seems to be a separate neurological mechanism for closure during nonspeech activities versus closure for speech.

Nonpneumatic activities include swallowing, gagging, and vomiting. With these activities, the velum raises very high in the pharynx and the lateral pharyngeal walls close tightly along their entire length. Closure appears to be almost exaggerated and is very firm, as viewed through videofluoroscopy. This type of closure is necessary because the purpose of closure in these cases is to allow substances to pass through the oral cavity, while preventing nasal regurgitation. In swallowing, velopharyngeal closure is further assisted by the back of the tongue, which raises against the velum, thus pushing the velum up and back (Flowers & Morris, 1973). It is important to note that velopharyngeal closure may be complete for nonpneumatic activities, but insufficient for speech or other pneumatic activities (Shprintzen et al., 1975).

Pneumatic activities are activities that utilize an airstream following velopharyngeal closure. These would include blowing, whistling, singing, and speech. Sucking may also be included with this generalized pattern of closure. With these activities, closure occurs lower in the nasopharynx and appears to be less exaggerated than with nonpneumatic activities. The maximum medial excursion of the lateral pharyngeal walls is usually at the level of the velum and just below the plane of the levator eminence. At the oral level, the lateral walls may actually bow outward during velopharyngeal closure.

It would be tempting to assume that closure for all pneumatic activities is about the same. If that were true, then the use of blowing and sucking exercises would be beneficial in improving velopharyngeal function for speech. Unfortunately, the closure patterns for all of these pneumatic activities are also physiologically different from each other (McWilliams & Bradley, 1965). Blowing, for example, requires generalized movements of the velopharyngeal structures. On the other hand, speech requires precise, rapid movements of these structures and the point of contact even varies during speech, as will be discussed in the next section. When comparing velopharyngeal closure during singing and speech, the velopharyngeal port is closed longer and tighter in singing than in speech, particularly on the higher pitches (Austin, 1997).

Timing of Velopharyngeal Closure

Voice onset and velopharyngeal closure must be closely coordinated during speech. In fact, the velopharyngeal valve must be completely closed before phonation is initiated for an oral sound or there will be a negative effect on resonance. Therefore, velar movement must begin prior to the onset of phonation so that it is completely closed when phonation begins.

The timing of closure for an oral sound has been found to be somewhat dependent on the type of phoneme. Kent and Moll (1969) found some evidence to suggest that the velar elevating gesture for a stop begins earlier and is executed more rapidly when the stop is voiceless rather than voiced. Therefore, the timing of closure requires constant fine adjustments throughout an utterance, depending on the phonemic needs. In addition, missed timing may have implications for the perception of resonance or nasality.

The production of nasal consonants during an utterance has an additional effect on velopharyngeal function and timing. The velum remains elevated and closure is maintained throughout the utterance as long as oral consonants or vowels are being produced. As a nasal consonant (m, n, ng) is produced, the velum lowers quickly and the pharyngeal walls move away from midline, thus opening the velopharyngeal valve to allow for nasal resonance. Closure is quickly obtained again for the following vowel or oral consonant.

Although gravity may explain the lowering of the velum at the end of an utterance, it does not explain the quick downward movement of the velum for the production of nasal sounds. It has been postulated that the lowering of the velum is actually accomplished by a combination of gravity, tissue elasticity, and muscle contraction, most probably contraction of the palatoglossus muscles (Fritzell, 1979; Kuehn & Azzam, 1978). Contraction of the palatoglossus may occur only in instances that require quick lowering of the velum, as in the production of nasal phonemes in connected speech (Moon & Kuehn, 1997).

Variations in Velopharyngeal Closure With Phonemes

Even as velopharyngeal closure is maintained throughout oral speech, there are systematic variations in the height of velar contact and the degree of closure. This variation is due primarily to the type of phoneme being produced and its phonetic environment (Flowers & Morris, 1973; McWilliams & Bradley, 1965; Moll, 1962; Moon & Kuehn, 1997; Shprintzen et al., 1975; Simpson & Chin, 1981).

The height of velar closure is affected by the movement and height of the tongue during articulation of the sound, and also by the phoneme's requirements for intraoral air pressure. In general, velar heights are greater for consonants than for vowels. High-pressure consonants (plosives, fricatives, and affricates), especially those that are voiceless, have the greatest heights when compared to other consonants. High vowels have a higher velar height than low vowels (Moll, 1962; Moon & Kuehn, 1997), possibly due to the elevation of the tongue during the production of these sounds.

The same factors that increase the height of velar contact during speech also increase the firmness of closure. Therefore, velopharyngeal closure is much tighter on consonants than on vowels and it is most firm on high-pressure consonants. High vowels are associated with a greater degree of closure force than low vowels (Moll, 1962; Moon, Kuehn, & Huisman, 1994). Moll (1962) has shown that vowels adjacent to a nasal consonant, particularly when preceding the consonant, have less closure force than those adjacent to oral consonants.

Considering all of these factors, changes in velar position are the result of the interaction of a number of variables, including vowel height and the type of consonant (Lubker, 1975; Seaver & Kuehn, 1980). Therefore, velar position must be changed and coordinated with each syllable production (Karnell, Linville, & Edwards, 1988).

Effect of Rate and Fatigue on Velopharyngeal Closure

Rapid speech can affect the efficiency of velar movement, thus compromising velopharyngeal closure. It has been shown that when speech rate increases, the height of closure decreases and is less firm (Moll & Shriner, 1967), presumably due to the difficulty in achieving appropriate height and contact with the rapid rate. Therefore, as speech rate increases, it becomes more hypernasal.

Muscular fatigue can also affect the height and firmness of closure. Even normal speakers become more "nasal" when they are tired. Young children are often described as "whiny" at the end of the day, especially when they are tired. The term "whiny" actually describes an increase in hypernasality due to velar fatigue.

Changes in Velopharyngeal Function With Growth

The maturational changes in the craniofacial skeleton result in changes in the dimensions and relationships of the bony and pharyngeal structures. This necessarily affects the movement of the oral and velopharyngeal structures and has an impact on the acoustic product of speech. There are three basic stages of speech production: one based on the vocal tract anatomy of the infant, another based on the anatomy of the child, and the third based on the anatomy of the adult.

Although the cranium approaches adult size relatively early in childhood, the facial bones continue to grow into adolescence or early adulthood. The growth of the mandible and maxillary bones is somewhat affected by the development of dentition. As these structures grow and mature, they move down and forward relative to the cranium. Both the maxilla and mandible are similar in size in males and females until around 14 years of age. After that age, these facial bones continue to grow in males, while there is very little additional growth in females (Ursi, Trotman, McNamara, & Behrents, 1993). Although there are changes in the size of these structures, this occurs with relatively minor changes in shape, despite occlusal stages (Kent & Vorperian, 1995).

The size of the pharynx changes greatly during maturation. The newborn pharynx is estimated to be approximately 4 cm long. In fact, the velum and epiglottis are in close proximity, which enables breathing to continue during feeding. In contrast, the adult pharynx is approximately 20 cm long. The pharynx is typically longer in adult males than in females. This results in the differences in formant frequencies, which affects the perception of the voice (Kent, 1976). In addition to the increase in length, there is increase of approximately 80% in the volume of the nasopharynx from infancy to adulthood (Bergland, 1963). Since there is more vertical than horizontal growth, there is very little change in the anterior-posterior dimension of the nasopharynx (Bergland, 1963; Kent & Vorperian, 1995; Tourne, 1991). However, there is significant change in the angle of the posterior pharyngeal wall. In a newborn, the nasopharynx curves gradually to meet the oropharynx. At around age 5, the posterior pharyngeal wall of the nasopharynx and oropharynx meet at an oblique angle. By puberty and through adulthood, these sections of the posterior pharyngeal wall meet at almost a right angle (Kent & Vorperian, 1995).

Because the velum is attached to the hard palate, it also moves down and slightly forward with the growth of the maxilla. This could potentially result in an increase in the anterior-posterior (AP) dimension as well as the vertical dimension of the nasopharynx. However, the angle of the pharyngeal wall changes at the same time. In addition, the velum increases in both length and thickness and tends to stretch more to make up any difference in the structural relationships. As a result, there is little actual change in the AP dimension and the velopharyngeal mechanism is able to make fine adjustments so that the competency of closure is maintained. In addition, the maturation of the oral-motor system helps the child to improve the efficiency of the velopharyngeal mechanism and continue to achieve normal velopharyngeal closure, despite growth and changes in the structures.

Another factor that changes the relative dimensions of the pharyngeal space and can introduce some instability in velopharyngeal function is the presence and size of the adenoid tissue. The adenoid pad is positioned on the posterior pharyngeal wall in the area of velopharyngeal closure. In many young children, the adenoid tissue assists with closure to a degree so that closure is actually velar-adenoidal (Croft, Shprintzen, & Ruben, 1981; Kent & Vorperian, 1995; Skolnick et al., 1975; Subtelney & Koepp-Baker, 1956). The adenoid pad can be prominent in size until the onset of puberty. At that time, a process of involution and atrophy begins. Atrophy may occur quickly and rather suddenly with puberty in some cases.

Whether there is gradual involution of the adenoid pad or sudden atrophy, the velopharyngeal mechanism is usually able to adapt to the anatomic changes by making compensatory changes. These changes may include additional stretching and lengthening of the velum during closure to accommodate the difference in the pharyngeal dimension. In addition, there may be an increase in velar mobility and an increase in the anterior movement of the posterior pharyngeal wall during speech. Overall, a more mature pattern of velopharyngeal closure is usually adopted (Kent & Vorperian, 1995). However, if there was a history of cleft palate or tenuous velopharyngeal closure from the start, these compensations may not be possible. In these individuals, the changes that occur in the adenoid pad as the individual moves through puberty may result in the onset of velopharyngeal insufficiency (Mason & Warren, 1980; Siegel-Sadewitz & Shprintzen, 1986; Van Demark & Morris, 1983). If this occurs, surgical intervention may ultimately be required.

Summary

The anatomy of the face, oral cavity, and velopharyngeal valve is well documented, and is easy to describe and to understand. On the other hand, the physiology of the velopharyngeal mechanism, particularly as it relates to speech, is very complex and not well understood. There is still much to be learned regarding the roles of the various muscles, the interaction of velopharyngeal function with articulation, and the neuromotor controls required for coordination of velopharyngeal function with the other subsystems of speech. This information would help in our understanding not only of normal speech production, but also of the causes and possible treatment of disordered speech.

References

Austin, S. F. (1997). Movement of the velum during speech and singing in classically trained singers. *Journal of Voice, 11*(2), 212–221.

Baken, R. J. (1987). *Clinical measurement of speech and voice*. Boston: College-Hill Press.

Barsoumian, R., Kuehn, D. P., Moon, J. B., & Canady, J. W. (1998). An anatomic study of the tensor veli palatini and dilatator tubae muscles in relation to the eustachian tube and velar function. *Cleft Palate Craniofacial Journal, 35*(2), 101–110.

Bell-Berti, F. (1973). *The velopharyngeal mechanism: An electromyographic study*. Unpublished, Ph.D. thesis. City University of New York, New York.

Bergland, O. (1963). The bony nasopharynx. *Acta Odontologica Scandinavia, 21*(Suppl. 35), 1–137.

Boorman, J. G., & Sommerlad, B. C. (1985). Levator palati and palatal dimples: Their anatomy, relationship and clinical significance. *British Journal of Plastic Surgery, 38*(3), 326–332.

Bzoch, K. F. (1968). Variations in velopharyngeal valving: The factor of vowel changes. *Cleft Palate Journal, 5*, 211–218.

Calnan, I. (1957). Modern views on Passavant's ridge. *British Journal of Plastic Surgery, 10*, 89.

Casey, D. M., & Emrich, L. J. (1988). Passavant's ridge in patients with soft palatectomy. *Cleft Palate Journal, 25*(1), 72–77.

Cassell, M. D., & Elkadi, H. (1995). Anatomy and physiology of the palate and velopharyngeal structures. In R. J. Shprintzen & J. Bardach (Eds.), *Cleft palate speech management: A multidisciplinary approach* (pp. 45–62). St. Louis, MO: Mosby.

Cassell, M. D., Moon, J. B., & Elkadi, H. (1990). Anatomy and physiology of the velopharynx. In J. Bardach & H. L. Morris (Eds.), *Multidisciplinary management of cleft lip and palate*. Philadelphia: Saunders.

Croft, C. B., Shprintzen, R. J., & Ruben, R. J. (1981). Hypernasal speech following adenotonsillectomy. *Otolaryngology—Head and Neck Surgery, 89*(2), 179–188.

Croft, C. B., Shprintzen, R. J., & Rakoff, S. J. (1981). Patterns of velopharyngeal valving in normal and cleft palate subjects: A multi-view videofluoroscopic and nasendoscopic study. *Laryngoscope, 91*(2), 265–271.

Dickson, D. R. (1972). Normal and cleft palate anatomy. *Cleft Palate Journal, 9*, 280–293.

Dickson, D. R. (1975). Anatomy of the normal velopharyngeal mechanism. *Clinics in Plastic Surgery, 2*(2), 235–248.

Dickson, D. R., & Dickson, W. M. (1972). Velopharyngeal anatomy. *Journal of Speech and Hearing Research, 15*(2), 372–381.

Dickson, D. R., Grant, J. C., Sicher, H., Dubrul, E. L., & Paltan, J. (1974). Status of research in cleft palate anatomy and physiology July, 1973- Part 1. *Cleft Palate Journal, 11*, 471–492.

Dickson, D. R., Grant, J. C., Sicher, H., Dubrul, E. L., & Paltan, J. (1975). Status of research in cleft lip and palate: Anatomy and physiology, Part 2. *Cleft Palate Journal, 12*(1), 131–156.

Ettema, S. L., & Kuehn, D. P. (1994). A quantitative histologic study of the normal human adult soft palate. *Journal of Speech and Hearing Research, 37*, 303–313.

Finkelstein, Y., Lerner, M. A., Ophir, D., Nachmani, A., Hauben, D. J., & Zohar, Y. (1993). Nasopharyngeal profile and velopharyngeal valve mechanism. *Plastic and Reconstructive Surgery, 92*(4), 603–614.

Finkelstein, Y., Talmi, Y. P., Kravitz, K., Bar-Ziv, J., Nachmani, A., Hauben, D. J., & Zohar, Y. (1991). Study of the normal and insufficient velopharyngeal valve by the "Forced Sucking Test." *Laryngoscope, 101*(11), 1203–1212.

Finkelstein, Y., Talmi, Y. P., Nachmani, A., Hauben, D. J., & Zohar, Y. (1992). On the variability of velopharyngeal valve anatomy and function: A combined peroral and nasendoscopic study. *Plastic and Reconstructive Surgery, 89*(4), 631–639.

Flowers, C. R., & Morris, H. L. (1973). Oral-pharyngeal movements during swallowing and speech. *Cleft Palate Journal, 10*, 181–191.

Fritzell, B. (1979). Electromyography in the study of the velopharyngeal function—A review. *Folia Phoniatrica, 31*(2), 93–102.

Glaser, E. R., Skolnick, M. L., McWilliams, B. J., & Shprintzen, R. J. (1979). The dynamics of Passavant's ridge in subjects with and without velopharyngeal insufficiency—A multi-view videofluoroscopic study. *Cleft Palate Journal, 16*(1), 24–33.

Honjo, I., Kojima, M., & Kumazawa, T. (1975). Role of Passavant's ridge in cleft palate speech. *Archives of Otorhinolaryngology, 211*(3), 203–208.

Huang, M. H., Lee, S. T., & Rajendran, K. (1997). Structure of the musculus uvulae: Functional and surgical implications of an anatomic study. *Cleft Palate Craniofacial Journal, 34*(6), 466–474.

Huang, M. H., Lee, S. T., & Rajendran, K. (1998). Anatomic basis of cleft palate and velopharyngeal surgery: Implications from a fresh cadaveric study. *Plastic and Reconstructive Surgery, 101*(3), 613–627; Discussion 628–629.

Igawa, H. H., Nishizawa, N., Sugihara, T., & Inuyama, Y. (1998). A fiberscopic analysis of velopharyngeal movement before and after primary palatoplasty in cleft palate infants. *Plastic and Reconstructive Surgery, 102*(3), 668–674.

Iglesias, A., Kuehn, D. P., & Morris, H. L. (1980). Simultaneous assessment of pharyngeal wall and velar displacement of selected speech sounds. *Journal of Speech and Hearing Research, 23*, 429–446.

Karnell, M. P., Linville, R. N., & Edwards, B. A. (1988). Variations in velar position over time: A nasal videoendoscopic study. *Journal of Speech and Hearing Research, 31*(3), 417–424.

Kennedy, J. G., & Kuehn, D. P. (1989). Neuroanatomy of speech. In D. P. Kuehn, M. L. Lemme, & J. M. Baumgartner (Eds.), *Neural bases of speech, hearing, and language* (pp. 111–145). Boston: College-Hill Press.

Kent, R. D. (1976). Anatomical and neuromuscular maturation of the speech mechanism: Evidence from acoustic studies. *Journal of Speech and Hearing Research, 19*(3), 421–447.

Kent, R. D., & Moll, K. L. (1969). Vocal-tract characteristics of the stop cognates. *Journal of the Acoustical Society of America, 46*(6), 1549–1555.

Kent, R. D., & Vorperian, H. K. (1995). Development of the craniofacial-oral-laryngeal anatomy: A review. *Journal of Medical Speech-Language Pathology, 3*(3), 145–190.

Kuehn, D. P. (1979). Velopharyngeal anatomy and physiology. *Ear, Nose, and Throat Journal, 58*(7), 316–321.

Kuehn, D. P., & Azzam, N. A. (1978). Anatomical characteristics of palatoglossus and the anterior faucial pillar. *Cleft Palate Journal, 15*, 349–359.

Kuehn, D. P., Folkins, J. W., & Linville, R. N. (1988). An electromyographic study of the musculus uvulae. *Cleft Palate Journal, 25*(4), 348–355.

Kuehn, D. P., & Kahane, J. C. (1990). Histologic study of the normal human adult soft palate. *Cleft Palate Journal, 27*, 26–34.

Lubker, J. F. (1975). Normal velopharyngeal function in speech. *Clinics in Plastic Surgery, 2*(2), 249–259.

Mason, R. L., & Simon, C. (1977). Orofacial examination checklist. *Language, Speech, and Hearing Services in the Schools, 8*, 161–163.

Mason, R. M., & Warren, D. W. (1980). Adenoid involution and developing hypernasality in cleft palate. *Journal of Speech and Hearing Disorders, 45*(4), 469–480.

Massengill, R., Jr., Walker, T., & Pickrell, K. L. (1969). Characteristics of patients with a Passavant's pad. *Plastic and Reconstructive Surgery, 44*(3), 268–270.

Matsuya, T., Yamaoka, M., & Miyasaki, T. (1979). A fiberoscopic study of velopharyngeal closure in patients with operated cleft palates. *Plastic and Reconstructive Surgery, 63*(4), 497–500.

Maue-Dickson, W. (1977). Cleft lip and palate research: An updated state of the art. Section II. Anatomy and physiology. *Cleft Palate Journal, 14*(4), 270–287.

Maue-Dickson, W. (1979). The craniofacial complex in cleft lip and palate: An update review of anatomy and function. *Cleft Palate Journal, 16*(3), 291–317.

Maue-Dickson, W., & Dickson, D. R. (1980). Anatomy and physiology related to cleft palate: Current research and clinical implications. *Plastic and Reconstructive Surgery, 65*(1), 83–90.

Maue-Dickson, W., Dickson, D. R., & Rood, S. R. (1976). Anatomy of the eustachian tube and related structures in age-matched human fetuses with and without cleft palate. *Transactions of the*

American Academy of Ophthalmology and Otolaryngology, 82(2), 159–164.

McWilliams, B. J., & Bradley, D. P. (1965). Ratings of velopharyngeal closure during blowing and speech. *Cleft Palate Journal, 2*(1), 46–55.

Moll, K. (1962). Velopharyngeal closure on vowels. *Journal of Speech and Hearing Research, 5,* 30–37.

Moll, K. L., & Shriner, T. H. (1967). Preliminary investigation of a new concept of velar activity during speech. *Cleft Palate Journal, 4,* 58.

Moon, J. B., & Kuehn, D. P. (1996). Anatomy and physiology of normal and disordered velopharyngeal function for speech. *National Center for Voice and Speech, 9*(April), 143–158.

Moon, J. B., & Kuehn, D. P. (1997). Anatomy and physiology of normal and disordered velopharyngeal function for speech. In K. R. Bzoch (Ed.), *Communicative disorders related to cleft lip and palate* (Vol. 4, pp. 45–47). Austin, TX: Pro-Ed.

Moon, J., Kuehn, D., & Huisman, J. (1994). Measurement of velopharyngeal closure force during vowel production. *Cleft Palate Craniofacial Journal, 31,* 356–363.

Moon, J., Smith, A., Folkins, J., Lemke, J., & Gartlan, M. (1994). Coordination of velopharyngeal muscle activity during positioning of the soft palate. *Cleft Palate Craniofacial Journal, 31,* 45–55.

Mourino, A. P., & Weinberg, B. (1975). A cephalometric study of velar stretch in 8 and 10-year old children. *Cleft Palate Journal, 12,* 417–435.

Pruzansky, S., & Mason, R. (1962). The "stretch factor" in soft palate function. *Journal of Dental Research, 48,* 972.

Sataloff, R. T. (1992, December). The human voice. *Scientific American,* pp.108–115.

Seaver, E. J., & Kuehn, D. P. (1980). A cineradiographic and electromyographic investigation of velar positioning in non-nasal speech. *Cleft Palate Journal, 17*(3), 216–226.

Shprintzen, R. J., Lencione, R. M., McCall, G. N., & Skolnick, M. L. (1974). A three dimensional cinefluoroscopic analysis of velopharyngeal closure during speech and nonspeech activities in normals. *Cleft Palate Journal, 11,* 412–428.

Shprintzen, R. J., McCall, G. N., Skolnick, M. L., & Lencione, R. M. (1975). Selective movement of the lateral aspects of the pharyngeal walls during velopharyngeal closure for speech, blowing, and whistling in normals. *Cleft Palate Journal, 12*(1), 51–58.

Shprintzen, R. J., Rakof, S. J., Skolnick, M. L., & Lavorato, A. S. (1977). Incongruous movements of the velum and lateral pharyngeal walls. *Cleft Palate Journal, 14*(2), 148–157.

Siegel-Sadewitz, V. L., & Shprintzen, R. J. (1982). Nasopharyngoscopy of the normal velopharyngeal sphincter: An experiment of biofeedback. *Cleft Palate Journal, 19*(3), 194–200.

Siegel-Sadewitz, V. L., & Shprintzen, R. J. (1986). Changes in velopharyngeal valving with age. *International Journal of Pediatric Otorhinolaryngology, 11*(2), 171–182.

Simpson, R. K., & Austin, A. A. (1972). A cephalometric investigation of velar stretch. *Cleft Palate Journal, 9,* 341–351.

Simpson, R. K., & Chin, L. (1981). Velar stretch as a function of task. *Cleft Palate Journal, 18*(1), 1–9.

Simpson, R. K., & Colton, J. (1980). A cephalometric study of velar stretch in adolescent subjects. *Cleft Palate Journal, 17*(1), 40–47.

Skolnick, M. L., & Cohn, E. R. (1989). *Videofluoroscopic studies of speech in patients with cleft palate.* New York: Springer-Verlag.

Skolnick, M. L., McCall, G., & Barnes, M. (1973). The sphincteric mechanism of velopharyngeal closure. *Cleft Palate Journal, 10,* 286–305.

Skolnick, M. L., Shprintzen, R. J., McCall, G. N., & Rakoff, S. (1975). Patterns of velopharyngeal closure in subjects with repaired cleft palate and normal speech: A multi-view videofluoroscopic analysis. *Cleft Palate Journal, 12,* 369–376.

Smith, K. K., & Kier, W. M. (1989). Trunks, tongues, and tentacles: Moving with the skeletons of muscle. *American Scientist, 77,* 29–35.

Subtelney, J. D., & Koepp-Baker, H. (1956). The significance of adenoid tissue in velopharyngeal function. *Plastic and Reconstructive Surgery, 17,* 235–250.

Tourne, L. P. (1991). Growth of the pharynx and its physiologic implications. *American Journal of Orthodontics and Dentofacial Orthopediatrics, 99*(2), 129–139.

Ursi, W. J., Trotman, C. A., McNamara, J. A., Jr., & Behrents, R. G. (1993). Sexual dimorphism in normal craniofacial growth. *Angle Orthodontist, 63*(1), 47–56.

Van Demark, D. R., & Morris, H. L. (1983). Stability of velopharyngeal competency. *Cleft Palate Journal, 20*(1), 18–22.

Witzel, M. A., & Posnick, J. C. (1989). Patterns and location of velopharyngeal valving problems: Atypical findings on video nasopharyngoscopy. *Cleft Palate Journal, 26*(1), 63–67.

CHAPTER

2

Genetics and Patterns of Inheritance

Robert J. Hopkin, M.D.

CONTENTS

Craniofacial anomalies like many other conditions tend to recur in families. The risk for recurrence however is variable, depending on interactions of multiple environmental and genetic factors. The purpose of this chapter is to briefly review the modes of inheritance that may influence the occurrence of craniofacial anomalies. The first part of the chapter reviews DNA, genes, chromosomes, and the cell cycle. The second part of the chapter discusses the principles of Mendelian inheritance, including autosomal recessive, autosomal dominant, and X-linked patterns. The last portion of the chapter focuses on complex or non-Mendelian inheritance. Particular attention is placed on multifactorial inheritance, the pattern associated with most cases of cleft palate or cleft lip with or without cleft palate.

Deoxyribonucleic Acid (DNA) and Genes

Deoxyribonucleic Acid (DNA)

For centuries, scientists wondered how the information needed to organize and direct the development of an organism was transmitted from a single cell to a mature individual with complex organs and tissues. Then in 1869, Friedrich Miescher discovered a substance in cell nuclei that he called "nuclein." The name was eventually changed to deoxyribonucleic acid or DNA. In 1944, Avery, Macleod, and McCarthy demonstrated that DNA is the substance that carries hereditary information in bacteria. It is now known that the genetic information of all cells is carried on DNA (McKusick, 1997).

Deoxyribonucleic acid or *DNA* is a nucleic acid made up of building blocks called nucleotides. *Nucleotides* consist of a 5-carbon sugar (deoxyribose) chemically bonded to a phosphate group and a nitrogenous base. The nitrogenous bases can be divided into two groups: *purines*

(adenine and guanine) and *pyrimidines* (thymine, and cytosine). The nucleotides are linked together through the phosphate groups at the 5th and 3rd carbons of the sugar to form long unbranching polymers. These are arranged in an antiparallel (going in opposite directions) *double helix* (coiled ladder) such that the nitrogenous bases are paired according to specific rules. A purine is always paired with a pyrimidine. In fact adenine (A) is always paired with thymine (T) and guanine (G) is always paired with cytosine (C). For example, if one strand contains the sequence 5'GGATTCG 3', the complementary sequence would be 3'CCTAAGC5'. The numbers 5' and 3' indicate the direction of the strand. The strands are held together by hydrogen bonds between A-T pairs and C-G pairs (Strachan & Read, 1996).

Replication

The complementary nature of the double helix allows DNA to serve as a template for its own replication. *Replication*, which is the process of making two identical DNA molecules from one, is a process resulting in two double strands, each containing one original and one complimentary newly synthesized strand of DNA. This process is complex and carefully controlled, but it must take place quickly to allow for rapid cell division and growth. In humans, over 3.5×10^9 nucleotides must be precisely matched for each cell division. The process starts at several sites along a DNA molecule simultaneously. When DNA is replicated, a replication bubble forms as the double helix is unwound and the complementary strands are separated. Nucleotides are then added sequentially forming new complementary strands. The final result is two identical double helix molecules of DNA (Strachan & Read, 1996).

The process of replicating DNA is very carefully controlled to prevent errors. In addition, there are proofreading and repair mechanisms to preserve the exact sequence of nucleotides (Strachan & Read, 1996). Fortunately errors are rare; however, they do occur. When a change in the sequence of a molecule of DNA occurs, it is referred to as a *mutation*. The mutation can be as small as a substitution of a single base pair or as large as the deletion of an entire chromosome. Mutations may have important consequences for the cell and for the individual.

Genes

Long strands of DNA are organized into shorter functional units known as genes. A *gene* is a submicroscopic functional unit of heredity. It consists of a discrete segment of a DNA molecule that resides within the chromosome. A *chromosome* is a single, linear double strand of DNA with associated proteins that function to organize and compact the DNA and/or function in regulating gene activity. Thousands of genes are found in each chromosome. The order of the nucleotides in the DNA of an individual gene determines the information coded by that gene. Each gene consists of a promoter region that functions as the starting point for the gene's activity and serves as an on/off switch, a coding region that contains the information needed to make a functional protein, and regulatory elements that determine how much of that protein will be made. In addition there are segments called introns, whose functions are not understood.

Ribonucleic Acid (RNA)

The processes controlled by the genes take place outside the nucleus in the cytoplasm of the cell. However, the DNA is found primarily in the nucleus of the cells. The genetic information is transported from the nucleus to the cytoplasm as strands of *ribonucleic acid* (RNA). The DNA in a gene serves as a template for *transcription*, which is the process of creating a strand of RNA that is complementary to a given strand of DNA. RNA is similar to DNA in that it is a linear polymer composed of a 5-carbon sugar (although ribose is the sugar in RNA) bound to a phosphate group and a nitrogenous base. The nitrogenous bases differ slightly from those in DNA because RNA contains the pyrimidine uracil in place of thymine. The other nitrogenous bases are the same as in DNA. However, RNA is a single-stranded molecule in living cells. The RNA sequence of a gene is read in the cytoplasm and determines which amino acids will be incorporated into the protein. Each amino acid is specified by a group of three nucleotides called a codon. Most amino acids can be coded by more than one codon. Thus some changes in the nucleotide sequence may not result in changes in the amino acid sequence of the protein. These changes are called conservative mutations (Cummings, 1997).

The portions of a gene that determine the amino acid sequence for a polypeptide are referred to as the *coding region*. The coding region is divided into segments called *exons*. *Introns* are the segments between exons. They are removed or "spliced out" from the RNA following transcription. The exons are then spliced together to form a continuous RNA coding sequence. It is critical that the process of removing introns and splicing the remaining RNA segments together starts and stops at the correct point. An error of one nucleotide can result in an RNA transcript that codes for a nonfunctional protein.

RNA that has had the introns removed is called *messenger RNA* or *mRNA*. mRNA is transported from the nucleus to the cytoplasm to function as a template for protein synthesis. In the cytoplasm of the cell, *ribosomes* (organelles within the cell that function in protein synthesis) attach to the mRNA and translate the nucleotides into the specified amino acid sequence, forming a polypeptide. The polypeptides are then processed to form the functional proteins (Mange & Mange, 1999).

The flow of genetic information, therefore, proceeds from DNA through transcription to RNA. RNA is then translated to amino acid sequence forming a protein. Even small changes in the coding region of a gene may lead to changes in function through several mechanisms. Disease-causing mutations may disrupt gene function, leading to early termination of translation and often to an unstable or nonfunctional product. A change in the DNA can lead to disease if the change results in a change of function for the protein. Deletions and insertions of one or more nucleotides can disrupt gene function by changing, adding, or deleting important amino acids.

Nevertheless, with the exception of identical twins, no two individuals share all of the same DNA. In fact, much of the DNA in humans is variable. This variability is called *polymorphism.* Polymorphisms are very common (seen in virtually all genes) and contribute to the uniqueness of each individual. Mutations lead to new variations in the DNA. New variants that do not contribute to disease or that improve function may become more common over time, while changes that lead to disease will tend to remain rare or be eliminated (Cummings, 1997).

Chromosomes

As noted previously, chromosomes are single, linear double strands of DNA with associated proteins that function to organize and compact the DNA in a cell for cell division. The genetic material, DNA, in human cells is organized into 46 chromosomes in most cells. This can be seen in a *karotype*, which is a chromosome analysis that is done by drawing blood, growing the cells in a culture, analyzing the white blood cells, photographing the chromosomes, and then arranging the chromosomes in pairs for display and assessment. A karotype of normal human chromosomes can be seen in Figure 2–1. Together the chromosomes contain the complete set of instructions for cell replication and differentiation. This complete set of instructions is called the *genome* (Cummings, 1997).

Each chromosome has a narrowed region called a *centromere*. The centromere is critical for normal cell division; however, the location of the centromere is quite variable. In some cases it is in the middle of the chromosome, dividing it into approximately equal halves. Chromosomes with a centrally located centromere are referred to as *metacentric*. The centromere may also be off center, leading to a short (p) arm. The "p" refers to *petit*, the French word for small. The long arm is referred to as the q arm. The "q" is simply the letter after "p." Chromosomes with this structure are referred to as *submetacentric*. Finally, the centromere may be very close to one end of the chromosome. These chromosomes are *acrocentric*. The location of the centromere and the length of the chromosome give each chromosome a characteristic shape, which allows them to be distinguished from one another. Traditionally chromosomes are labeled according to length with the longest being number 1.

Each of 22 chromosomes has two copies, one from each parent. These chromosomes are called *autosomes* (and include all chromosomes with the exception of the two sex chromosomes). The 23rd pair of chromosomes are referred to as the *sex chromosomes* (X and Y) because of their role in gender determination. If a person inherits two X chromosomes (one from each parent), that person will be female. If an X (from the mother) and a Y (from the father) are inherited, the person will be male. The normal chromosomal make-up is written as 46,XX for a female or 46, XY for a male (Keagle & Brown, 1999).

Chromosomes can be specially stained to reveal a pattern of light and dark colored bands. This allows specific segments of the chromosome to be identified. The bands are labeled by

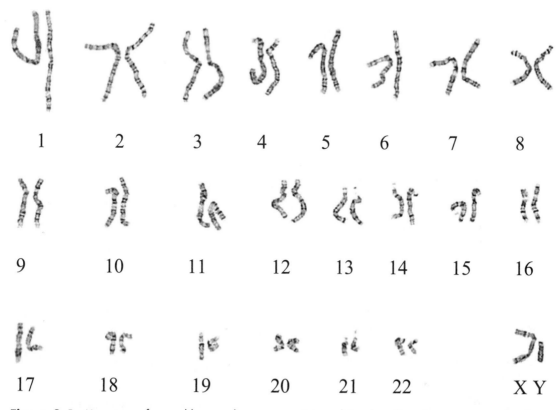

Figure 2–1. Karyotype of normal human chromosomes. It is traditional to align chromosomes so that the p arm is on top. (Karyotype provided by R. Blough, Ph.D., Division of Human Genetics, Children's Hospital Medical Center, Cincinnati, Ohio.)

the chromosome number followed by "p" or "q" to indicate which arm the band is on. Each band is also given a number that indicates its location relative to the centromere and the other bands on that arm of the chromosome. This system is used to describe the rough location of genes in gene mapping studies. For example a gene may be mapped to 1p36. This means that the gene is found on the short arm of chromosome 1 in the band labeled 36. Figure 2–2 shows an *ideogram* (a schematic drawing of the banding pattern of a chromosome) for chromosome 1. The bands can be further subdivided in some cases allowing for more specific localization to be described. Even with the best current

staining techniques, it is not possible to identify individual genes on a chromosome. The smallest bands that can be distinguished still contain multiple genes (Mange & Mange, 1999).

Cell Cycle

Cells in the body alternate between states of active division and states of nondivision. When a cell is dividing, it goes through a sequence of events called the *cell cycle*, which is the process of preparing for and undergoing cell division. The frequency of the cell cycle depends on the type of cell and the rate of growth of the organism at the time. The steps in each cycle are very similar for all types of somatic cells.

Cell division can be divided into two major processes: *mitosis*, which is the process of separating duplicated chromosomes and reconstitution of two cell nuclei, and *cytokinesis*, which is the separation of the cell cytoplasm to form two distinct cells with separate cell membranes. During mitosis, a complete identical set of chromosomes is distributed to each daughter cell. It is critical for the process to be accurate and precise for the cells to function normally. The chromosomes contain the genes and therefore the instructions that govern cell function. If errors (mutations) occur in either the process of DNA replication or the separation of the chromosomes, they often have serious consequences for the cell. The process of division takes about 1 hour. The time between cell divisions is called *interphase*. Cells spend much more time in interphase than in active division.

Mitosis takes place in the somatic cells and results in daughter cells with the same number of chromosomes (46) as the parent cell. In contrast, *meiosis* results in 23 chromosomes rather than 46. Meiosis occurs only in the production of *gametes*, which are sperm from the testes and eggs from the ovaries. If sperm and eggs each contained 46 chromosomes at conception, the new cell would contain double that number or 92 chromosomes. This would double with each generation. During meiosis cells undergo one round of DNA replication but two rounds of cell division. This produces four cells, each with a single copy of each chromosome (Griffiths, Miller, Suzuki, Lewontin, & Gelbart, 1996).

In men, meiosis occurs continuously following puberty and produces four sperm cells per original cell. This results in the availability of large numbers of mature sperm on a continual basis. In women, meiosis starts in fetal life but then arrests until puberty. Following puberty, one oocyte per menstrual cycle completes

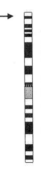

Figure 2–2. Ideogram (schematic drawing of the banding pattern) of chromosome 1: Note the light and dark bands. Each chromosome has a unique but consistent banding pattern that allows it to be distinguished from other chromosomes. The arrow indicates band 1p36.

meiosis. Errors in meiosis may have serious consequences because they result in abnormalities in every cell in a developing organism (Keagle & Brown, 1999).

Chromosomal Abnormalities

Chromosomal mutations may include changes in the number of copies of an individual chromosome. Loss of one copy of a chromosome results in *monosomy*, which is the presence of a single copy of a chromosome. The gain of one extra copy of a chromosome (for a total of 3 chromosomes) results in *trisomy*. Figure 2–3 shows a karotype of trisomy 13. Most monosomies and trisomies end in early miscarriage.

The only monosomy that commonly results in the birth of living infants is monosomy X. This results in Turner syndrome. Turner syndrome is characterized by short stature, webbed neck, and lack of sexual maturation. The presence of the Y chromosome with no X results in early miscarriage.

Survival is possible for several trisomies, including trisomy for X, 13, 18, or 21. Individuals born with trisomy X or with 47,XXY may be

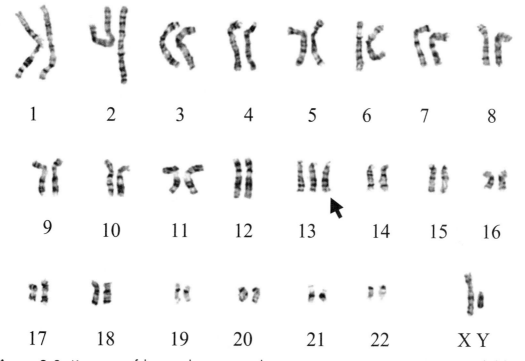

Figure 2–3. Karyotype of human chromosomes demonstrating trisomy 13. (Karyotype provided by R. Blough, Ph.D., Division of Human Genetics, Children's Hospital Medical Center, Cincinnati, Ohio.)

relatively healthy and undistinguishable from the general population. The presence of extra copies of the Y chromosome is also compatible with healthy survival. Those with trisomy 21 have Down syndrome, which is associated with mental retardation, congenital heart disease, low muscle tone, and distinct facial features. Trisomy 13 and 18 may result in live born infants; however, these infants are born with multiple severe birth defects and rarely survive more than a few weeks. Trisomy 13 is frequently associated with cleft lip and palate and other craniofacial malformations. Trisomy 18 can lead to Pierre Robin sequence and cleft palate in addition to many other malformations. Trisomies for other chromosomes result in early miscarriage.

Trisomies and monosomies result from a failure in meiosis. The abnormal number of chromosomes results from *nondisjunction*, which is the failure of one or more chromosomes to separate in cell division. Nondisjunction can be seen in both sperm and egg development. The cause of nondisjunction is not known, but the risk for nondisjunction and related chromosomal abnormalities increases with advancing maternal age. For example, the risk for trisomy 21 (which causes Down syndrome) in a pregnancy to a 20-year-old woman is approximately 1:2000. The risk for a pregnancy to a 45-year-old woman is approximately 1:20. The risk for nondisjunction rises slowly with age at first but increases more rapidly after age 35. For this reason, pregnant women over age 35 are offered chromosomal analysis through amniocentesis. The risk for nondisjunction in men remains relatively stable with advancing age (Randolph, 1999).

Mosaicism is the presence of cells with two or more different genetic contents in a single individual. This may be caused by nondisjunction in mitosis. Because errors in mitosis affect only the daughter cells descended from the cell in which the error occurred, in many cases the abnormal cells may simply be eliminated or the functions of the cell may not be seriously impaired. However, if nondisjunction occurs in mitosis early in embryonic development, it may result in serious malformations. The effect of the abnormal cells will depend on the ratio of normal versus abnormal cells and the distribution of the each cell type (Mange & Mange, 1999).

Chromosomal abnormalities, other than the gain or loss of an entire chromosome, can also occur. These include deletions, duplications, inversions, and translocations.

When part of a chromosome becomes separated and lost, this is called a *deletion*. Deletions have been reported for all chromosomes. The location of the deletion is designated by the chromosome number, a "p" (for the short arm) or "q" (for the long arm), and the number of the band where the break occurred. For example, a deletion of the short arm of chromosome 4 with a break point in band 16 in a female could be written 46, XXdel(4)(p16). Figure 2–4 shows ideograms of a normal and a deleted chromosome 4. This deletion would result in Wolf-Hirschhorn syndrome (see Chapter 4). Deletions are often accompanied by multiple malformations, including facial clefts or other craniofacial malformations. However, unlike the example above, many deletions do not result in recognizable genetic syndromes.

Pure *duplications* of part of a chromosome are rare. Like deletions, chromosomal duplications are usually associated with multiple malformations and developmental handicaps. The pattern of malformations and severity of developmental disability depend on the size and location of the duplication. Even when the size and location are known, it can be difficult to predict what malformations will result or the long-term outcome for an individual patient. Combinations of deletion and duplication frequently result from unbalanced translocations (Kaiser-Rogers & Rao, 1999) and will be discussed later in this chapter.

Inversions occur when a portion of a chromosome is turned 180° from its usual orientation. *Translocations* are the result of a transfer of genetic material between two or more chromosomes. Inversions and translocations may not be associated with any abnormalities in the individual because the total amount of genetic material may be unchanged. In that case, a problem will result only if the break points are located in areas that disrupt a gene or genes. Inversions and translocations that do not result in the gain or loss of DNA have approximately a 10% risk for associated malformations or developmental disabilities. This is not surprising, as only approximately 10% of our DNA is in genes. Translocations and inversions may, however, increase the risk for infertility or birth defects in the children of an asymptomatic individual who carries the chromosomal rearrangement.

All of the types of chromosomal abnormalities discussed above can be associated with

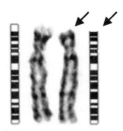

Figure 2–4. Normal and deleted human chromosome 4 with ideograms. The arrows indicate the deleted segment at 4p16. This deletion is associated with Wolf-Hirschhorn syndrome. (Photographs of chromosomes provided by R. Blough, Ph.D., Division of Human Genetics, Children's Hospital Medical Center, Cincinnati, Ohio.)

cleft palate, cleft lip, or other craniofacial malformations. Chromosomal abnormalities involve large changes in the genome and involve multiple genes. Because they involve large amounts of DNA, the changes are relatively easy to detect. It is important to identify people with chromosomal abnormalities because their needs and associated risks may be different from those of patients with isolated craniofacial malformations or single gene disorders. However, chromosomal abnormalities account for only a small portion of birth defects and genetic diseases. Smaller mutations involving only single genes are collectively common even though the individual disorders are often rare.

Chromosome Analysis

In order to discover abnormalities in the chromosomes, they must be visualized. The chromosomes are condensed enough to be easily viewed under a microscope only during certain stages of the cell cycle. Fortunately, by stimulating white blood cells to divide simultaneously, large numbers of cells can be expected to reach the same stage of the cell cycle at about the same time. This greatly improves the efficiency of chromosomal analysis. There are also chemicals that lead to arrest of cell division at certain stages of the cell cycle. Thus, the cell cycle can be controlled, to maximize the number of cells appropriate for analysis (Keagle & Gersen, 1999).

Some chromosomal rearrangements involve only very short segments that are too small to be seen using routine chromosomal analysis. With special techniques, such as *fluorescence in situ hybridization* or *FISH*, some submicroscopic segments of DNA can be identified by a cytogenetic laboratory. (*Cytogenetics* is the branch of genetics that is concerned with the structure and function of the cell, particularly the chromosomes within the cell.) This procedure involves the use of a nucleic acid probe labeled with a fluorescent dye to localize a specified DNA segment. For example, the deletion of chromosome 22q11.2, associated with Velocardiofacial syndrome (see Chapter 4), is usually not visible on chromosomal analysis, but is seen using FISH in the majority of cases. Syndromes caused by deletions large enough to contain several genes, but too small to be seen on routine cytogenetic analysis, are referred to as *contiguous gene syndromes*. In most, if not all cases, the problems associated with the syndrome are caused by the loss of function of several important genes (Kaiser-Rogers & Rao, 1999). See Table 2–1 for a list of some microdeletion contiguous gene syndromes.

Mendelian Inheritance

The common patterns of inheritance and the rules that govern them were first outlined by Mendel in 1866 in his studies on peas (McKusick, 1997). The patterns he described are known as Mendelian inheritance and include autosomal recessive, autosomal dominant, and

TABLE 2–1. Examples of microdeletion contiguous gene syndromes.

Velocardiofacial syndrome	del 22q11.2
Wolf-Hirschhorn syndrome	del 4p16.3
Cri du chat syndrome	del 5p15
Prader-Willi syndrome	del 15q11q13
Miller-Dieker syndrome	del 17p13.3
Langer-Giedion syndrome	del 8q24
Smith-Magenis syndrome	del 17p11.2
Kallmann syndrome	del Xp22.3
X-linked ichthyosis	del Xp22.3
Jacobsen syndrome	del 11q24.1
Williams syndrome	del 7q11.23

X-linked patterns. Mendel described four rules of inheritance. He discovered that:

1. Genes come in pairs, one from each parent.
2. Genes can have different *alleles*, which are variations of a gene. Some of these are dominant, and will exert their effects over the effects of the other allele. Others will be manifest only when the genes are *homozygous* (having two similar alleles). They are called recessive.
3. At meiosis, alleles segregate from each other with each gamete carrying only one allele.
4. The segregation of alleles for one trait is independent of the segregation of alleles from other genes for other traits.

These principles have remained valid with only a few modifications since they were first described.

Pedigrees

In determining a pattern of inheritance for a condition in a family, it is helpful to have a systematic way of collecting and recording the family history. A system has been developed, called a *pedigree*, which is a pictorial representation of family members and their line of descent. This system is used to record the inheritance of traits or anomalies affecting several members of a family. It allows the important findings to be recorded in a short period of time, usually on a single sheet of paper. Three sample pedigrees are illustrated on Figure 2–5. Using this system, most families can be easily described for three to four generations on a single page. In addition pedigrees can be simply and quickly hand drawn during the course of a brief interview with minimal training and a little practice (Mange & Mange, 1999).

Autosomal Recessive Inheritance

All people carry genes with mutations that are capable of causing disease. Fortunately, we in-herit two copies of each gene, one from each parent, and in many cases, one copy that functions normally is sufficient. There are approximately 100,000 different genes in each cell, but each person carries on average six to seven potentially disease-causing mutations. Therefore, the chance that both members of a couple will carry mutations in the same gene is small. Individuals who have one abnormal copy of a gene and are without detectable abnormalities are referred to as carriers. They are *heterozygous* (having two different copies of a gene). Traits that are manifest only when mutations are present in both copies of a gene are recessive traits. If a gene causing a recessive trait is on one of the autosomes, the trait is *autosomal recessive*.

Autosomal recessive traits tend to occur more frequently in isolated populations or in cases of *consanguinity*, which is mating between related individuals. The parents of affected individuals are usually unaffected. Recurrences between siblings are common, but recurrences in multiple generations of a family are rare in the absence of consanguinity. Autosomal recessive conditions are seen in both males and females in equal numbers.

The probability of two people carrying abnormalities in the same genes is increased if they are related. This is because relatives share genetic material. The closer the relationship, the more shared genetic material two individuals will have in common. Thus, consanguinity leads to increased risk for both members of a couple to carry disease-causing mutations in the same genes. This is one explanation for the high incidence of genetic disorders in isolated or inbred populations. In some populations, a relatively small number of original ancestors has led to a high frequency of carriers for certain disorders. This is known as a founder effect. In some cases, it is possible to trace family lines to a single common ancestor who brought a trait into a population. More frequently, a founder effect is implied by a high frequency of a few mutations in a large population. For ex-

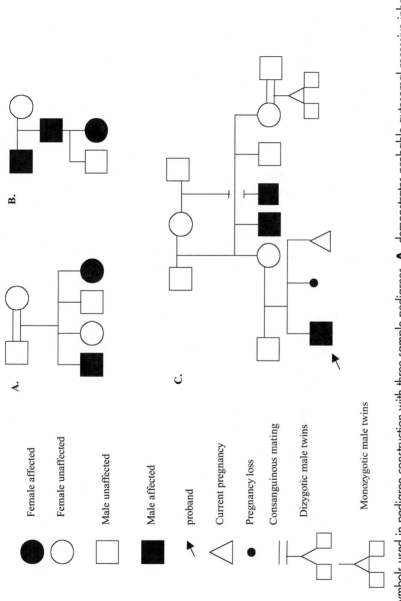

Figure 2-5. Symbols used in pedigree construction with three sample pedigrees. **A.** demonstrates probable autosomal recessive inheritance. Note recurrence in siblings with unaffected parents and consanguinity. Multifactorial inheritance cannot be ruled out based on the information given. **B.** demonstrates autosomal dominant inheritance. Note father-to-son transmission and recurrence in several generations. **C.** demonstrates X-linked recessive inheritance. Note occurrence of multiple males born to unaffected female relatives over multiple generations. In drawing a pedigree, horizontal lines connecting two individuals indicate mating between them. Children are indicated by vertical lines with squares or circles to indicate the sex of the child. If more than one child is born to a couple a horizontal line intersects the vertical line to allow each child to be appropriately recorded. If a parent has children with more than one partner additional lines can be drawn as seen in the first generation of family C. Divorce or separation can be indicated by as hash mark and space in the line connecting two individuals (not shown). If more than one trait is being recorded in a family, the affected individuals can be indicated by shading only one quadrant, for example the upper left for trait 1, the lower left for trait 2, etc. If still more traits are recorded, different colors or patterns of shading can be added.

ample, three mutations account for 98% of Tay-Sachs disease in the Ashkenazi Jewish population (Rutledge & Percy, 1997).

The chance of having an affected child is 25% for each pregnancy resulting from mating between two heterozygous carriers of an autosomal recessive condition. The other possibilities are 50% that a child will be a carrier of a single copy of the mutation and 25% that the child will be a noncarrier. This is because each parent has an approximately equal probability of passing on either the normal or abnormal allele. If two individuals with the same autosomal recessive condition have children together, all of their children will be affected because the parents only have abnormal alleles to pass on (Mueller & Cook, 1997).

Recurrence in more than one generation is uncommon because carrier frequency is low for most autosomal recessive conditions. For example, cystic fibrosis is one of the most common autosomal recessive disorders, affecting 1:2000 live births among populations of Northern European descent. The carrier frequency in that population is 1:25. That means a carrier would have a 24/25 probability of reproducing with a noncarrier in a population with random choice of partners. Testing is available for carrier status of some of the more common autosomal recessive diseases, such as cystic fibrosis, sickle cell anemia, and Tay-Sachs disease. This can help couples in making reproductive decisions if they are from a high-risk population or if there is a family history of the disorder that indicates a high probability that one or both partners may be carriers for that condition. Prenatal testing that can distinguish affected individuals from carriers is also available for some autosomal recessive conditions.

Occasionally two people with the same autosomal recessive trait will have children but the children will be unaffected. An example of this would be autosomal recessive hearing loss. This can be explained by *heterogeneity*, which occurs when mutations in different genes lead to the same abnormality or *phenotype* (Mueller & Cook, 1997). See Table 2–2 for a list of some autosomal recessive conditions that can be associated with cleft lip or cleft palate.

Autosomal Dominant Inheritance

In autosomal dominant disorders, heterozygous individuals have a recognizable phenotype, which is the group of characteristics associated with the genetic condition. Homozygous individuals also show the phenotype, but may be more severely affected. Pedigrees from families with autosomal dominant conditions demonstrate different findings than those seen in autosomal recessive inheritance.

Autosomal dominant pedigrees will frequently show that a parent is affected. If neither parent is affected, the affected individual is presumed to carry a new mutation that is causing the condition. For some autosomal dominant conditions, the new mutation rate is high and may account for a large percentage of affected individuals, as in Pfieffer syndrome (Winter & Baraitser, 1996). The chance that the offspring of an individual with a dominant condition and an unaffected partner will have an affected child is 50% for each pregnancy. The number of affected males and females is approximately equal. Two affected individuals

TABLE 2–2. Examples of autosomal recessive craniofacial syndromes.

Smith-Lemli-Opitz syndrome

Meckel-Gruber syndrome

Baller-Gerold syndrome

Oral-facial-digital syndrome type II

Insley-Astley syndrome

Dubowitz syndrome

Roberts syndrome

Toriello-Carey syndrome

Varadi-Papp syndrome

may have affected and unaffected children since each parent would have one normal and one abnormal gene. *Homozygotes* (persons with two identical copies of a gene) for autosomal dominant disorders often have a more severe phenotype than heterozygotes. For example, achondroplasia is the most common form of short-limbed dwarfism. Homozygous offspring of parents with achondroplasia have a severe phenotype, with a small chest and pulmonary hypoplasia that is incompatible with survival beyond the first few days of life (Winter & Baraitser, 1996).

Many autosomal dominant conditions have *variable expressivity* (variation in the phenotype associated with a single condition). This may cause affected individuals to be missed if the phenotype is not appropriately defined. For example, in Van der Woude syndrome, affected members of the same family may have cleft lip, cleft palate, lip pits, or a combination of these. Obviously, an individual with isolated lip pits could be missed if only individuals with cleft lip are identified when a family history is obtained. Most, if not all, autosomal dominant conditions demonstrate some degree of variable expressivity (Mueller & Cook, 1997).

Incomplete penetrance is the lack of a recognizable phenotype in an individual who carries a gene for an autosomal dominant trait. This is also common in autosomal dominant conditions. At times it may be difficult to distinguish between minimal expression due to variable expressivity and true incomplete penetrance. Some families have members who have no abnormal findings (nonpenetrance), but have transmitted the trait to their children, and other individuals who have only one feature of the condition (variable expressivity), but transmit the complete condition to their children. The factors that determine the penetrance and expressivity for a given trait are not well understood, but include different mutations in the same gene, modifying genes that interact with the gene that causes the disorder, environmental influences, and random variation (Mueller & Cook, 1997).

Many genes have more than one function and may therefore be associated with multiple seemingly unrelated abnormalities. For example, neurofibromatosis type 1 is associated with growth of large nerve sheath tumors, called neurofibromas, pigmentary abnormalities of the skin, bony dysplasias, and learning disabilities. This *pleiotropy* (the phenomenon where a single mutant gene can affect multiple, unrelated systems) can contribute to the variability in genetic syndromes because each function of a gene can have either variable expression or nonpenetrance (Mueller & Cook, 1997).

For examples of autosomal dominant disorders that are associated with craniofacial malformations see Table 2–3.

X-Linked Inheritance

X-linked inheritance refers to conditions caused by genes on the X chromosome. There are many X-linked recessive conditions and a few X-linked dominant conditions. X-linked inheritance is unique because males inherit only one

TABLE 2–3. Examples of autosomal dominant craniofacial syndromes.

Apert syndrome

Branchio-oto-renal syndrome

Crouzon syndrome

Distichiasis-lymphedema syndrome

Ectrodactyly-ectodermal dysplasia-clefting syndrome

Opitz Frias syndrome

Stickler syndrome

Treacher-Collins syndrome

Van der Woude syndrome

Waardenburg syndrome

copy of the X chromosome while females inherit two copies. Therefore, if a mutation occurs in an X-linked recessive gene, a female is likely to have mild or no effects. A male who inherits that gene is likely to be more severely affected because he has only one copy of a gene. X-linked recessive disorders affect males almost exclusively. Transmission occurs from carrier females to 50% of their sons and 50% of their daughters will be carriers. Affected males pass the gene to 100% of their daughters. There is no father-to-son transmission because fathers do not give an X chromosome to their sons (Mueller & Cook, 1997). See Table 2–4 for examples of X-linked recessive disorders.

X-linked dominant inheritance is rare with only a few disorders demonstrated. X-linked dominant disorders are characterized by having all of the daughters of affected males inherit the disorder. Sons of affected males never inherit the disorder, again because they receive the Y chromosome from the father. Affected females can transmit the disorder to offspring of both sexes. There is an excess of affected females in pedigrees for X-linked dominant disorders. Many X-linked dominant disorders are lethal to affected males. See Table 2–5 for a list of X-linked dominant disorders.

Non-Mendelian Inheritance

Many disorders that tend to recur in families do not follow the basic rules of Mendelian inheritance. The remainder of this chapter reviews some of the mechanisms involved in the inheritance of these disorders.

Multifactorial Inheritance

Some human disorders result from an interaction of multiple genes with environmental influences. This is called *multifactorial inheritance*. Environmental factors known to increase risks for birth defects are called *teratogens*. Common

TABLE 2–4. Examples of X-linked recessive craniofacial syndromes.

Chitayat syndrome

X-linked cleft palate

Oro-facial-digital syndrome type VIII

VATER with hydrocephaly

Lenz microphthalmia

Lowe syndrome

Oto-palato-digital syndrome type II

Simpson-Golabi-Behmel syndrome

SCARF syndrome

Say-Meyer syndrome

TABLE 2–5. Examples of X-linked dominant syndromes

Aarskog syndrome

Goltz syndrome

Conradi chondrodysplasia punctata

Oral-facial-digital syndrome type I

Melnick-Needles ostoedysplasty

Aicardi syndrome

Alport syndrome

Incontinentia pigmenti

X-linked hypophosphataemic rickets

Rett syndrome

examples of teratogens include ethanol, cigarette smoke, anti-epileptic medications, and congenital infections.

Multifactorial disorders can be divided into two categories; traits that demonstrate continuous variation and threshold disorders.

Some traits that exhibit continuous variation include height, weight, intelligence, and blood pressure. Disorders involving continuous traits are not easily distinguished from normal variation since, by definition, there will be large numbers of people on the border between normal and abnormal. The boundary therefore becomes subjective and a matter of definition. In many cases, "abnormal" is defined as greater than two standard deviations from the mean. Although this can be used to define abnormality, it may or may not be significant to the affected individual.

The second group of multifactorial disorders is threshold traits, such as cleft lip, pyloric stenosis, and neural tube defects. For these disorders, the trait is either present or absent; therefore, the abnormality is usually not difficult to distinguish. For example, one either has a cleft lip or does not have a cleft lip. With a threshold disorder, as the number of risk factors for the trait increases, the additive risk may cross a boundary or threshold, resulting in expression of the trait.

In the case of cleft lip only a few of the possible risk factors that contribute to the total risk have been identified. Recent evidence has lead to the estimate that variations in 4–12 genes contribute most of the genetic risk for cleft lip with or without cleft palate. Candidate genes include TGFA, RARA, BCL3, and END1 (Murray, 1995). Some environmental influences that affect risk for cleft lip have also been identified. Maternal smoking, for example raises the risk for cleft lip (Shaw et al., 1996); whereas maternal supplementation of folic acid appears to decrease recurrence risk in at least some studies (Tolarova & Harris, 1995). The interaction between genes and environmental factors may be additive in multifactorial disorders. For example, the risk attributed to a rare polymorphism of the TGFA gene is small (one to two fold). The risk associated with maternal smoking is also small (1.5 to 2 fold). In a recent study, when both heavy maternal smoking and the high risk allele of TGFA were present, the risk jumped to 3 to 11 fold compared to the control group risk (Shaw et al., 1996).

The risk for recurrence of a multifactorial trait in family members can be estimated by doing population studies and gathering empiric data looking at variables that may correlate with risk for the condition in question. In the case of cleft lip only, a few of the possible risk factors that contribute to the total risk have been identified. For example, cleft lip is more common in boys than girls. It is therefore predicted by the multifactorial model that, if a woman has cleft lip, the recurrence risk in the family will be higher than the risk if a man has cleft lip, and that the brothers of an affected individual will be at higher risk than sisters. Both of these predictions have been studied, but the results have been inconsistent. If both parents have cleft lip, the recurrence risk should be still higher because risk factors could be inherited from each parent. In fact, the more affected relatives, the higher the predicted risk. This prediction has been verified in cleft lip and cleft palate families. The estimated recurrence risk for future children in a family with one individual with cleft palate is 3 to 5%. If there are two affected first-degree relatives, the risk goes up to approximately 9 to 15%, depending on which family members have cleft lip (Curtis, Fraser, & Warburton, 1961; Wyszynski, Zeiger, Tilli, Bailey-Wilson, & Beaty, 1998).

The severity of the defect is also predicted to impact the recurrence risk. For example, one would predict that the recurrence risk in a family with a child who has a bilateral cleft lip would be higher than if the child had a unilateral cleft because the bilateral cleft is a more severe defect. Most studies have supported this prediction. The presence of cleft palate with cleft lip, on the other hand, has not been found to correlate well with recurrence risk in spite of being clinically more difficult to manage (Crawford & Sofaer, 1987).

The risk for multifactorial disorders is increased in close relatives because they tend to share similar genetic backgrounds and similar environmental risk factors. However, recurrences do not occur in a predictable pattern and are usually lower than the 25% or 50% that is predicted for Mendelian disorders. The risk is often in the range of 3–5% for first-degree relatives in families with one family member who has cleft lip, and much lower for more distant relatives. In consanguinous matings and inbred populations, recurrence risk is increased for multifactorial disorders because the amount of shared genetic material, and therefore the genetic risk, will be higher. Isolated populations will also share many environmental exposures as well.

There are several variations of the multifactorial model. These include the *oligogenic model*. According to this model, a trait may be determined by the interaction of multiple genes with little environmental influence. Usually a small number of genes contribute most of the risk. For example, one model of risk for cleft palate estimates that six major genes contribute most of the risk for nonsyndromic cleft palate (Fitzpatrick & Farrall, 1993). The major gene model assumes that abnormalities in one of several genes known to influence risk for a trait contribute most of the risk, but that the remaining risk is defined by environmental factors. This model has been suggested for isolated cleft lip recurrence risk estimation (Farrall & Holder, 1992).

Multifactorial inheritance is very difficult to study because it is complicated by heterogeniety, small effects of each risk factor, incomplete penetrance, and complex interactions. On the other hand, some of the most common human diseases demonstrate multifactorial inheritance. See Table 2–6 for examples of human diseases demonstrating multifactorial inheritance.

Anticipation

Some inherited disorders show a tendency to have more severe manifestations or earlier age of onset with succeeding generations. This phenomenon is known as *anticipation*. For many years, anticipation was assumed to be

TABLE 2–6. Examples of multifactorial traits.

Cleft lip with or without cleft palate

Cleft palate

Velo-pharyngeal insufficiency (VPI)

Diabetes mellitus

Alzheimer disease

Alcoholism

Athrosclerotic heart disease

Mental retardation

Colon cancer

Bipolar disease

due to sampling errors or ascertainment bias. Recent discoveries have proven that there is a genetic basis for anticipation in some diseases. All disorders with proven anticipation have a common mechanism. They are all caused by large expansions of triplet nucleotide repeats. The triplet repeat most commonly involved is CAG, which codes for glutamine. As the number of repeats expands, it becomes unstable so that in the next generation there is a tendency for the number of repeats to be greater. This, in turn, leads to an earlier age of onset and a more severe phenotype. Disorders caused by CAG repeats include Huntington disease, spinocerbellar ataxias, and other adult-onset neurodegenerative disorders. A second group of diseases is caused by unstable expansion of untranslated triplet repeats. Fragile X syndrome, the most common inherited form of mental retardation, is caused by a large expansion of an untranslated CGG repeat (Lindblad & Schalling, 1996).

Imprinting

Until recently it was assumed that having two working copies of each gene was always normal and that the two copies had equivalent function. Recent discoveries have demonstrated that some genes function differently, depending on whether they were inherited maternally or paternally. This phenomenon is called *imprinting*. It has only been demonstrated in a small number of disorders. These include Beckwith-Weidemann syndrome, Prader-Willi syndrome, Angelman syndrome, and Russell-Silver syndrome. If a gene is maternally imprinted, the allele inherited from the mother is not expressed. The opposite is true for genes that are paternally imprinted. It appears that imprinting is important in growth control and brain development. It may also play an important role in carcinogenesis (Tilghman, 1999).

Summary

The principles of inheritance and genetics covered in this chapter are fundamental to the understanding of most human malformations. Accurate counseling for parents and other family members regarding long-term prognosis and recurrence risks depends on correct diagnosis and identification of the appropriate patterns of inheritance. In addition, understanding of the basis of malformation syndromes often changes management. For example, the needs of a child with cleft lip caused by an unbalanced chromosomal translocation are likely to differ from those of a child with cleft lip due to multifactorial inheritance. As new insights are discovered into the causes of genetic disease, it will become increasingly important to understand these principles to optimize the treatment of each patient according to their individual risks and needs.

References

Crawford, M., & Sofaer, J. (1987). Cleft lip with or without cleft palate: Identification of sporadic cases with a high level of genetic predisposition. *Journal of Medical Genetics, 24,* 163–169.

Cummings, M. (1997). *Human heredity.* (4th ed.). Eagan, MD: West/Wadsworth.

Curtis, E., Fraser, F., & Warburton, D. (1961). Congenital cleft lip and palate. *American Journal of Diseases in Childhood, 102,* 853–857.

Farrall, M., & Holder, S. (1992). Familial recurrence-pattern analysis of cleft lip with or without cleft palate. *American Journal of Human Genetics, 50,* 270–277.

Fitzpatrick, D., & Farrall, M. (1993). An estimation of the number of susceptibility loci for isolated cleft palate. *Journal of Craniofacial Genetics and Developmental Biology, 13,* 230–235.

Griffiths, A., Miller, J., Suzuki, D., Lewontin, R., & Gelbart, W. (1996). *An introduction to genetic Analysis* (6th ed.). New York: W. H. Freeman and Company.

Kaiser-Rogers, K., & Rao, K. (1999). Structural chromosomal rearrangements. In S. Gersen & M. Keagle (Eds.), *The principles of clinical cytogenetics* (pp. 191–228). Totowa, NJ: Humana Press.

Keagle, M., & Brown, J. (1999). DNA, chromosomes, and cell division. In S. Gersen & M. Keagle (Eds.), *The principles of clinical cytogenetics* (pp. 11–30). Totowa, NJ: Humana Press.

Keagle, M., & Gersen, S. (1999). Basic laboratory proceedures. In M. Keagle & S. Gersen (Eds.), *The principles of clinical cytogenetics* (pp. 71–90). Totowa, NJ: Humana Press.

Lindblad, K., & Schalling, M. (1996). Clinical implications of unstable DNA repeat sequences. *Acta Pediatrica, 85,* 265–271.

Mange, E., & Mange, A. (1999). *Basic human genetics* (2nd ed.). Sunderland MA: Sinauer Associates, Inc.

McKusick, V. (1997). History of medical genetics. In D. Rimoin, J. Connor, & R. Pyeritz (Eds.), *Emery and Rimoin's principles and practice of medical genetics* (3rd ed., Vol. 1, pp. 1–30). New York: Churchill Livingstone, Inc.

Mueller, R., & Cook, J. (1997). Mendelian inheritance. In D. Rimoin, J. Connor, & R. Pyeritz (Eds.), *Emery and Rimoin's principles and practice of medical genetics* (3rd ed., Vol. 1, pp. 87–102). New York: Churchill Livingstone.

Murray, J. (1995). Face facts: Genes, environment, and clefts. *American Journal of Human Genetics, 57,* 227–232.

Randolph, L. (1999). Prenatal cytogenetics. In S. Gersen & M. Keagle (Eds.), *The principles of clinical cytogenetics* (pp. 259–316). Totowa, NJ: Humana Press.

Rutledge, S., & Percy, A. (1997). Gangliosidoses and related lipid storage diseases. In D. Rimoin, J. Connor, & R. Pyeritz (Eds.), *Emery and Rimoin's principles and practice of medical genetics* (3rd ed., Vol. 2, pp. 2105–2130). New York: Churchill Livingstone.

Shaw, G., Wasserman, C., Lammer, E., O'Malley, C., Murray, J., Basart, A., & Tolarova, M. M. (1996). Orofacial clefts, parental cigarette smoking, and transforming growth factor-alpha gene variants. *American Journal of Human Genetics, 58*, 551–561.

Strachan, T., & Read, A. (1996). *Human molecular genetics*. New York: Wiley-Liss.

Tilghman, S. (1999). The sins of the fathers and mothers: Genomic imprinting in mammalian development. *Cell, 96*, 185–193.

Tolarova, M., & Harris, J. (1995). Reduced recurrence of orofacial clefts after periconceptional supplementation with high-dose folic acid and multivitamins. *Teratology, 51*, 71–78.

Winter, R., & Baraitser, M. (1996). *London dysmorphology database* (1) [Compact Disc]. London: Oxford Medical Databases.

Wyszynski, D. F., Zeiger, J., Tilli, M. T., Bailey-Wilson, J. E., & Beaty, T. H. (1998). Survey of genetic counselors and clinical geneticists regarding recurrence risks for families with nonsyndromic cleft lip with or without cleft palate. *American Journal of Medical Genetics, 79*(3), 184–190.

CHAPTER

Clefts of the Lip and Palate

CONTENTS

Cleft lip and palate is the fourth most common birth defect and the most common congenital defect of the face. The prevalence of clefts is usually quoted as one in every 750 live births (Cleft Palate Foundation, 1999), although this varies with racial background. This estimate does not include the prevalence of bifid uvula, submucous cleft palate, or congenital palatal incompetence. In addition, there are about 300 recognized syndromes that include cleft palate as one of the features of the syndrome. When the cleft palate occurs as part of a syndrome, there are usually other associated craniofacial malformations (Jones, 1988; Rollnick & Pruzansky, 1981; Shprintzen, Schwartz, Daniller, & Hoch, 1985). In addition to infants with cleft lip and palate, there are infants who are born with other types of congenital craniofacial anomalies, which can also affect communication abilities.

This chapter begins by describing embryological development of the lip and palate, and the various types of clefts of the lip and palate that can occur when there is a disruption in this development. The effect of the cleft on the anatomy of the lip, palate, and adjacent structures is also described. Particular emphasis is placed on submucous cleft palate because this anomaly can cause significant problems with speech and resonance, but is not always easy to identify.

What Is a Cleft?

A *cleft* is an abnormal opening or a fissure in an anatomical structure that is normally closed. A cleft lip is the result of failure of parts of the lip to come together early in the life of a fetus. Cleft palate occurs when the parts of the roof of the mouth do not fuse normally during fetal development, leaving a large opening between the oral cavity and the nasal cavity. Clefts can vary in length and in width, depending on the degree of fusion of the individual parts. It is important to note

that, with cleft lip and palate, the structures are all there, but the structures have not fused together normally. In addition, the structures may be *hypoplastic,* or underdeveloped, in their formation.

A cleft of the lip and/or palate is a congenital malformation that occurs in utero during the first trimester of pregnancy. Most clefts are caused by a combination of genetic and environmental factors. Since a cleft is due to a disruption in embryological development, clefts typically follow the normal embryological fusion lines. Similar deformities can be found, however, following injury or *ablative surgery,* where some or all of the palate is removed due to a malignancy. Since cleft lip and palate represent an interference in the embryological development of the midface and oral cavity, they are often associated with malformations of the nose, eyes, and other facial structures. When other congenital anomalies occur along with the cleft lip and palate, they usually have a genetic etiology and are part of a multiple malformation syndrome (Jones, 1988).

A cleft lip presents with more serious cosmetic concerns than cleft palate, but a cleft palate presents with more serious speech problems. Individuals born with both cleft lip and cleft palate are at risk for problems with aesthetics, feeding, speech, resonance, and hearing. Although there are many commonalties in the appearance of the basic clefting conditions, clefts also give rise to unique anatomical and functional deviations. These deviations are due to variations in etiology, but are also due to the various forms of treatment to which the patient has been subjected. Therefore, the severity in aesthetics and function ranges from barely noticeable to severely affected and malformed.

Causes of Clefts and Basic Classification

To understand the common types of clefts and their etiology, it is important to have a basic knowledge of embryological development and the sequence of lip and palate formation. With this understanding, it is easy to see why clefts occur as they do. In addition, the embryological sequence provides a foundation for clinicians to describe and classify various types of clefts.

Embryological Development of the Lip and Palate

Embryological development of the face and palate is dependent on the formation of neural crest cells in the embryo. These cells migrate at different rates to form the structures of the skull and face. If migration of the neural crest cells fails to take place or if the migration is delayed, this can affect the formation of facial structures and can cause clefts or other craniofacial anomalies.

Embryological development of the lip and alveolus begins around 6 to 7 weeks of gesta-

tion and starts at the incisive foramen. Figure 3–1 shows the direction of embryological closure of the sutures lines. The development of the lip and alveolus proceeds in an anterior direction to first form the alveolus through the fusion of the bilateral incisive suture lines. Closure then proceeds to form the base of the anterior nose and finally the upper lip. The median and two lateral lip segments are then fused, forming the philtral lines and completing the formation of the upper lip.

Embryological development of the palate starts around 8 to 9 weeks of gestation. Prior to palate formation, the tongue is high and in the area of the nasal cavity. The palatal shelves are vertical and positioned on each side of the tongue. Around the seventh or eighth week, the tongue begins to gradually drop down. When this occurs, the palatal shelves move slowly from a vertical to a horizontal position and fuse, first with the premaxilla at the incisive foramen and then with each other. As can

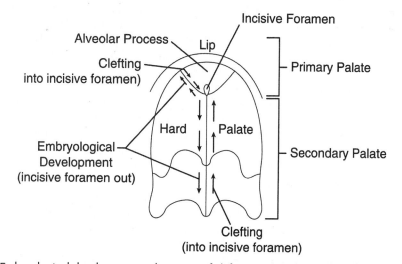

Figure 3–1. Embryological development and patterns of clefting. Embryological development proceeds from the incisive foramen out to the periphery. Clefting patterns begin at the periphery and follow the lines of normal embryological fusion toward the incisive foramen to the point of that disruption. The classification of clefts as affecting either the primary palate or secondary palate is based on embryological development, with the incisive foramen as the dividing point between the two.

be noted in Figure 3–1, the process of fusion proceeds between the palatal shelves, moving in a posterior direction from the incisive foramen along the median palatine suture line. This completes the formation of the hard palate. The vomer, forming a portion of the nasal septum, moves downward and fuses with the superior surface of the hard palate, thus completing the separation of the nasal cavity. Once the hard palate is formed, the velum and finally the uvula are formed. This process is usually complete by 12 weeks of gestation.

Causes of Clefts

Since embryological development goes from the incisive foramen out, anything that disrupts that process of fusion will cause a cleft from that point all the way to the periphery (lip or uvula). Therefore, as can be seen in Figure 3–1, clefting patterns begin at the periphery and follow the lines of normal embryological fusion toward the incisive foramen to the point of that disruption. When the cleft is complete, it follows the embryological fusion line all the way through to the incisive foramen. Clefts can occur due to disruptions or delays in cell migration or palatal shelf movement.

There are four basic causes of clefts and related craniofacial anomalies. These include chromosomal disorders and genetic disorders, which are both *endogenous* (internal) factors. In addition, clefts can be caused by environmental teratogens or by mechanical factors in utero. These are both considered *exogenous* (external) factors.

Environmental *teratogens* are substances that can cause congenital malformations. Teratogens that have been associated with cleft lip/palate include cigarette smoke, phenytoin (Dilantin), thalidomide and Valium. Certain viruses, including rubella, can also cause clefts and other malformations. Even maternal nutritional deficiencies have been

implicated in causing malformations. In particular, folic acid has been found to be important for normal embryonic and fetal development. Maternal folic acid deficiency has been associated with decreases in embryonic cell proliferation, and thus congenital malformations such as clefting.

There is evidence to show that there are differences between males and females in the timing of embryological fusion and also in the types of clefts typically presented. Cleft lip, with or without cleft palate, occurs about twice as often in males than in females and is usually more severe in males. On the other hand, cleft palate occurs about twice as frequently in females than in males (Jensen, Kreiborg, Dahl, & Fogh-Andersen, 1988; Oka, 1979; Warkany, 1971). Although the reason for these differences between males and females is not clearly understood, it has been speculated that it could be related to differences in the timing of the development of the lip and palate in the embryo. Burdi and Silvey (1969) found that, in the male human embryo, the horizontal positioning and subsequent closure of the secondary palate is more advanced and occurs earlier than in the female embryo. Because the palatal shelves are open longer in the female, there is a greater period of time during which there is susceptibility to environmental teratogens.

Mechanical interference can also affect embryonic development and cause clefts. In the case of Pierre Robin sequence, crowding in utero can cause the head to be down and the mandible to be retracted, thus restricting oral cavity space. This prevents the tongue from dropping down into the oral cavity. Because of the interference of the tongue when the palate is formed, the result is a wide, bell-shaped cleft palate.

Although various causes of clefts have been identified, the etiology of clefting in a single individual is complex and may involve a combination of factors. Several genes can contribute to clefting. These genes may lead to a genetic predisposition for the cleft, but may not cause expression of the cleft unless combined with certain environmental factors. In fact, in most cases the cause of the cleft is not due to just one factor but instead, is due to the interaction of several factors, which is called *multifactorial inheritance.*

Cleft Lip/Palate Classification

Because there are different types of clefts with different combinations, naming and classification of clefts can be a challenge. Although several classification systems have been proposed over the years, the system that has gained the most universal acceptance is the one proposed by Kernahan and Stark (1958). Kernahan and Stark recommended that clefts be classified based on embryological development, with two basic categories: clefts of the primary palate and clefts of the secondary palate with the incisive foramen as the dividing point between the two. This division can be viewed schematically on the right side of Figure 3–1.

The *primary palate* includes the structures that are anterior to the incisive foramen. These are the structures that fuse around 7 weeks of gestation and include the alveolus and also the lip (even though the terminology is primary "palate"). A cleft of the primary palate can be unilateral or bilateral, following the philtral and incisive suture lines. It can also be complete (through the entire lip and alveolus) or incomplete (as a notch in the upper lip). The *secondary palate* includes the structures that are posterior to the incisive foramen. These are the structures that fuse around 9 weeks of gestation and include the hard palate (excluding the premaxilla) and the velum. A cleft of the secondary palate can be either incomplete (such as a bifid uvula or cleft of the velum only) or complete (including the entire velum and hard palate to the incisive foramen). Technically, a cleft that extends through the hard palate can be considered unilateral if one palatal shelf is

attached to the vomer, or bilateral if neither palatal shelves are attached to the vomer so that the vomer is seen in the midline. This distinction is not usually made for clefts of the palate, however. Clefts of both the primary and secondary palate are common. When there is a combination, each section (primary palate and secondary palate) can be unilateral, bilateral, complete, or incomplete.

Although this basic classification system is used most commonly by professionals, a modification of the Kernahan and Stark classification system was later proposed by Kernahan (1971). This system is more detailed and uses a "striped –Y" figure as a means of identifying the extent of the cleft (Figure 3–2). The upper arms of the Y represent the primary palate and the base of the Y represents the secondary palate. The Y form is divided into sections that are numbered. The upper stems of the Y are divided into 3 segments with the right side numbered as 1, 2, and 3 and the left side numbered as 4, 5, and 6. The most anterior segment represents the lip, the middle segment represents the alveolus, and the posterior segment represents the area between the alveolus and the incisive foramen. The secondary palate (hard and soft palate) is also divided into three sections and these are numbered as 7, 8, and 9. When the segments affected by the cleft are darkened on the diagram, a visual representation can be made of the type and extent of the cleft. If there is a submucous cleft, the affected segments are marked with crosshatch marks. Using this figure, the extent of a cleft can be described or illustrated using the diagram.

Cleft Lip
(Clefts of the Primary Palate)

Types of Cleft Lip

There are various types of cleft lip and various degrees of severity, as can be seen in Figure

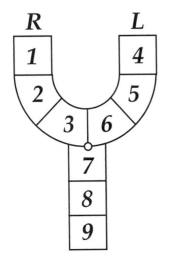

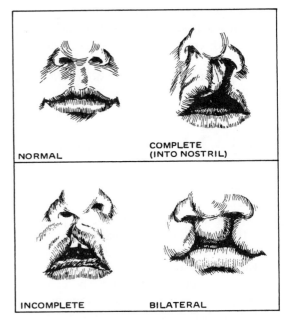

Figure 3–2. The Kernahan striped Y for cleft classification. The upper arms of the Y represent the primary palate and the base represents the secondary palate. The most anterior segment represents the lip, the middle segment represents the alveolus, and the posterior segment represents the area between the alveolus and the incisive foramen. The secondary palate (hard and soft palate) is also divided into sections to represent the areas of the velum and hard palate. The segments affected by the cleft are darkened on the diagram so that a visual representation can be made of the type and extent of the cleft. If there is a submucous cleft, the affected segments are marked with cross-hatch marks. (From "The Striped Y—A Symbolic Classification for Cleft Lip and Palate," by Desmond A. Kernahan, 1971, p. 469. *Plastic and Reconstructive Surgery, 47*(5). Reprinted with permission.)

Figure 3–3. A normal lip and basic types of cleft lip. On the drawings of clefts, note the short columella and the distortion of the ala. (From *Your Cleft Lip and Palate Child: A Basic Guide for Parents*, by G. Snyder, S. Berkowitz, K. Bzoch, and S. Stool, 1980, Fig. 1. Evansville, IN: Meade Johnson & Co. Copyright Meade Johnson & Co. 1980. Reprinted with permission.)

3–3. An incomplete cleft lip can be as minor as a small, subcutaneous notch in the vermilion with no involvement of the alveolar ridge or palate. In rare cases, a *form fruste* may occur, which is a partial or arrested form of a cleft lip. In this case, the overlying skin is intact but the underlying muscle, nasal cartilage, and oral sphincter function usually are significantly affected. In a more severe case, the cleft lip can extend through the vermilion and course up through the philtral lines to the nostril sill,

causing distortion of the nose. When the term "complete cleft lip" is used, it may refer to a complete cleft of the primary palate. In this case, it implies involvement of not only the entire lip through the nostril sil, but also the alveolus (or dental arch) all the way to the area of the incisive foramen.

In addition to incomplete or complete, a cleft lip can be unilateral (on the right or the left side) or bilateral (on both sides). If the cleft is unilateral, it most often occurs on the left side (Jensen et al., 1988; McWilliams, Morris, & Shelton, 1990). Figures 3–4, 3–5, and 3–6 illustrate a unilateral complete cleft of the lip and alveolus. Figures 3–7 and 3–8 show a bilateral incomplete cleft of the lip. A bilateral

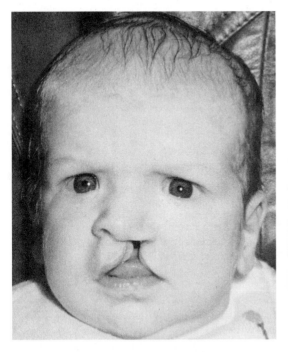

Figure 3–4. Patient with a left unilateral complete cleft of the primary palate (lip and alveolus).

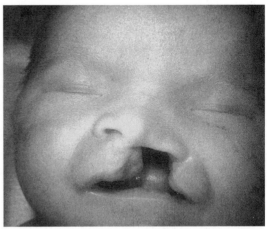

Figure 3–5. Patient with a wide left unilateral complete cleft of the primary palate (lip and alveolus).

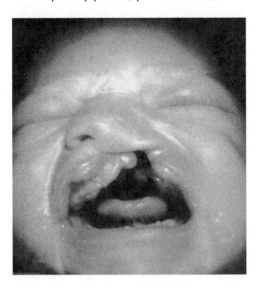

Figure 3–6. Patient with a very wide left unilateral complete cleft of the primary palate (lip and alveolus). Note the displacement of the upper lip and the distortion of the nose.

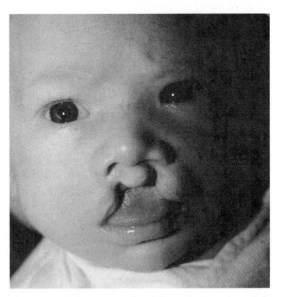

Figure 3–7. Patient with a bilateral incomplete cleft lip.

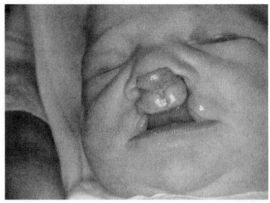

Figure 3–9. Patient with a bilateral complete cleft lip. Note the wide spread ala and the position of the prolabium and premaxilla.

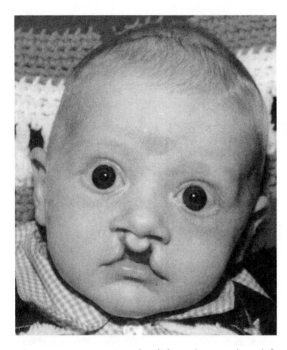

Figure 3–8. Patient with a bilateral incomplete cleft lip.

complete cleft of the lip and alveolus can be seen in Figure 3–9.

A bilateral cleft of the lip results in the complete separation of the tissue that would normally form the philtrum. The philtral tissue segment that is isolated due to the bilateral cleft is called the *prolabium*. When a bilateral cleft courses through the lip and through both incisive suture lines in the alveolus to the incisive foramen, it separates the triangular-shaped premaxilla bone. Therefore, when there is a complete bilateral cleft of the lip and alveolus, both the prolabium and the premaxilla are separated. In many cases, these structures are positioned in an extremely anterior position at birth so that they appear to extend from the tip of the nose. On Figure 3–9, the prolabium appears as tissue that is attached to the tip of the nose and the premaxilla is isolated and in an anterior position.

In rare cases, a Simonart's band may be noted with the cleft lip. A *Simonart's band* is a strand of soft tissue in the area of the cleft that is due to partial, yet incomplete embryonic fusion of the upper lip. This has no particular clinical significance and the treatment is the same as in a complete cleft lip.

By examining an unrepaired cleft lip deformity, one can see that all the structures are present, including the philtral dimple and both of the philtral ridges. The cleft passes just to the lateral side of the philtral ridge. On the cleft side, the lip is short and the cupid's bow is twisted up into the cleft. Although cleft lip can occur in isolation, it is more often found to be associated with a cleft palate.

Effects of Cleft Lip on Structure and Function

Because a complete cleft of the lip and alveolus courses through the nostril sill, the nose can be adversely affected. The nose may appear to be very wide and flattened due to the separation of the *orbicularis oris muscle*, which is the muscle that encircles the mouth and functions by closing the lips. This muscle is not only divided, but it is misaligned and curves upward along the edges of the vermilion. The wide space within the cleft can further distort the nose by spreading the nasal ala. In fact, the wider the cleft, the more distorted the nasal features will be.

The formation of the columella may also be adversely affected by a cleft lip. The columella is usually abnormally short. If the cleft is unilateral, the columella will be shortest on the cleft side and it will be positioned obliquely, with its base deviated toward the noncleft side. When the cleft is bilateral and complete, the columella may be so short that it is virtually nonexistent, giving the appearance that the prolabium and premaxilla are attached to the tip of the nose. In less common cases, as in the case of a forme fruste, the lip is intact but there is evidence of the nasal deformity and the muscle discontinuity that are typically found with cleft lip.

Upper airway obstruction is common in individuals with a history of cleft lip and palate. As a result, mouth breathing is noted more frequently in the cleft population than in the noncleft population (Drake, Davis, & Warren, 1993; Hairfield, Warren, & Seaton, 1988; Liu, Warren, Drake, & Davis, 1992; Warren & Drake, 1993). The causes of upper airway obstruction are thought to be a combination of developmental defects of the nasal cavity and the surgical correction of the cleft (Hairfield & Warren, 1989). Clefts of the lip and palate often result in nasal cavity deformities that tend to reduce the size of the nasal airway. The airway is smallest in individuals with unilateral cleft lip and palate and is largest in those with bilateral clefts. Although the nose continues to grow with age, it remains about 30% smaller than the noncleft nose (Drake et al., 1993). The lip repair can also cause nasal obstruction if it results in stenosis of the nasal vestibule. In fact, surgical correction of labial, nasal, palatal, and pharyngeal structures have the potential to compromise breathing further.

A complete cleft of the lip may result in occlusal abnormalities as the dentition is developed. This can cause specific articulation errors, particularly on anterior speech sounds. The production of anterior sounds is often affected by dental interference of tongue tip movement or crowding in the anterior portion of the oral cavity.

Cleft Palate (Clefts of the Secondary Palate)

Types of Cleft Palate

As with cleft lip, a cleft palate can be either incomplete or complete and can occur with various degrees of severity. This is shown on Figure 3–10. An incomplete cleft palate can be as slight as a bifid uvula or the cleft can extend farther into the velum. A complete cleft palate goes through the uvula and the velum, and then follows the median palatine suture line through the hard palate, all the way to the incisive foramen. The vomer bone, which is the bottom part of the nasal septum, is usually attached to the larger of the two palatal segments in a unilateral cleft, and is not attached to either segment in a bilateral cleft. A cleft palate can occur with or without a cleft lip. Isolated cleft palate (with no involvement of the lip) is more frequently associated with a syndrome, and thus with other anomalies. Figure 3–11 shows an unrepaired complete cleft of the palate with no involvement of the primary palate. Figures 3–12 and 3–13 both show a bilateral complete cleft lip and palate. The prolabium and premaxilla are isolated and in an anterior position. The vomer portion of the nasal septum can be viewed through the palate.

Some patients will demonstrate a *palatal fistula* or hole in the palate, even after the palate

Types of Cleft Palate

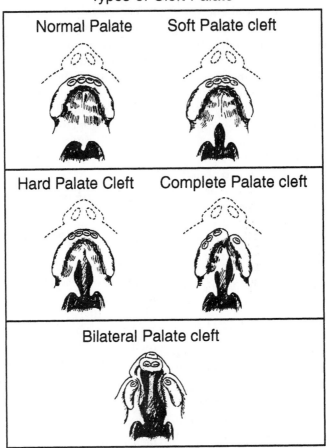

Figure 3–10. A normal palate and various types of cleft palate. (From *Your Cleft Lip and Palate Child: A Basic Guide for Parents*, by G. Snyder, S. Berkowitz, K. Bzoch, and S. Stool, 1980, p. 2. Evansville, IN: Meade Johnson & Co. Copyright Meade Johnson & Co. 1980. Reprinted with permission.)

is repaired. Although this may look like a partial cleft, it is actually due to a partial *dehiscence* (or breakdown) of the cleft repair. The fistula can be located anywhere in the hard palate or velum, but will always be located along the embryological or surgical suture lines (Figure 3–14). For more information on palatal fistulas (also called "fistulae"), see Chapter 8.

Effects of Cleft Palate on Structure and Function

With cleft palate, there are additional abnormalities of the anatomy other than the obvious. If the cleft goes entirely through the velum, the velar aponeurosis is conspicuously absent (Dickson, 1972; Koch, Grzonka, &

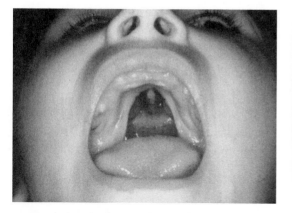

Figure 3–11. Wide unrepaired complete cleft of the secondary palate (hard palate and velum).

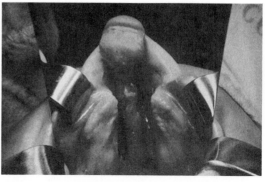

Figure 3–13. Patient with a bilateral complete cleft of the lip and palate (primary and secondary palate). Note the collapsed lateral arches and the anterior position of the premaxilla.

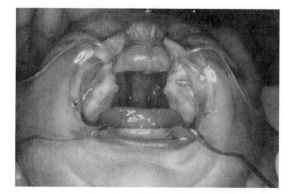

Figure 3–12. Patient with a bilateral complete cleft of the lip and palate (primary and secondary palate). Note the prolabium, premaxilla, and the nasal septum.

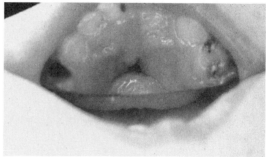

Figure 3–14. Palatal fistula. A palatal fistula is a hole in the palate that occurs after the palate is repaired. Although this may look like a partial cleft, it is actually due to a partial dehiscence (or breakdown) of the cleft repair. The fistula can be located anywhere in the hard palate or velum, but will always be located along the embryological or surgical suture lines.

Koch, 1998) and the orientation of the muscles is necessarily altered. Although the muscle origins are normal, the muscle insertions are abnormal due to the open cleft. As a result, the levator veli palatini muscle does not interdigitate in the midline. Instead, this paired muscle and the palatopharyngeus muscles are inserted onto the posterior border of the cleft

hard palate, rendering them essentially nonfunctional (Dickson, 1972; Dickson, Grant, Sicher, Dubrul, & Paltan, 1974, 1975; Kriens, 1975; Maue-Dickson, 1979; Maue-Dickson & Dickson, 1980). As a result, rather than being amuscular, the anterior one third of the velum contains the muscle fibers of the levator veli palatini and the palatopharyngeus muscles

(Dickson, 1972). This configuration of muscles has been referred to as the *cleft muscle of Veau*. Figure 3–15A shows the orientation of the velar muscles in a normal palate and velum. Figure 3–15B shows the abnormal orientation of the muscles when there is a cleft.

One goal of cleft palate surgery is to correct the orientation of the muscles in order to achieve normal function. Despite surgical attempts to normalize the muscle orientation, individuals with a repaired cleft have great variability in the insertion point of the muscles and in the muscle mass (Moon & Kuehn, 1997). Therefore, the function of the muscles following surgery can be difficult to predict. In addition, the velum may be abnormally short due to the absent aponeurosis and hypoplasia of the levator veli palatini muscles (Dickson, 1972). Due to the risk of poor velar movement or a short velum, about 20% to 30% of individuals with a history of cleft palate are likely to have velopharyngeal dysfunction (Bardach, 1995). Velopharyngeal dysfunction is the primary cause of defective speech and resonance in children with a history of cleft.

Individuals with a history of cleft palate are at high risk for otitis media and associated conductive hearing loss. This is due to malfunction of the *eustachian tube* (Bluestone, Beery, Cantekin, & Paradise, 1975; Doyle, Cantekin, & Bluestone, 1980; Paradise, Bluestone, &

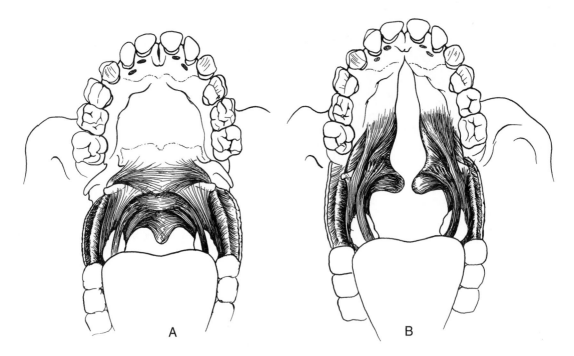

Figure 3–15. A. Illustration of normal velar musculature. Note the orientation of the muscles in midline. **B.** Abnormal muscle orientation due to a cleft palate. As a result of the cleft, the anterior one third of the velum contains the muscle fibers of the levator veli palatini and the palatopharyngeus muscles. Instead of inserting in the midline of the velum, these muscles are inserted into the posterior border of the hard palate. This abnormal orientation is called the "cleft muscle of Veau."

Felder, 1969), which connects the middle ear to the posterior pharynx. The eustachian tube is normally closed in its resting position. In response to changes in external air pressure, the individual usually swallows (or yawns) to relieve the pressure in the ears. The act of swallowing or yawning causes the tensor veli palatini muscle to contract to open the pharyngeal end of the tube. As the eustachian tube opens, it allows fluids to drain from the middle ear into the pharynx. It also results in the equalization of air pressure between the middle ear and the environment. If the tensor veli palatini muscle does not function normally, as is common when there is a history of cleft palate, this results in poor ventilation of the middle ear. This can lead to bacterial infection, inflammation, and the accumulation of fluids. The build-up of fluids impairs the conduction of sound through the ossicles, resulting in a conductive hearing loss. If this fluid build-up and inflammation become chronic, permanent damage of the middle ear, surrounding structures, and hearing can result.

As noted previously, the nasal cavity space can be compromised by developmental defects secondary to cleft lip and palate. Cleft palate alone can include abnormalities of both the cartilaginous and bony septum, causing a nasal septal deviation that can alter nasal cavity size (Wetmore, 1992). The nasopharyngeal anatomy also appears to be altered in individuals with a history of cleft palate. Smahel and colleagues (Smahel, Kasalova, & Skvarilova, 1991; Smahel & Mullerova, 1992) conducted a morphometric assessment of the pharynx of individuals with repaired cleft lip and/or palate using X-ray films. Their findings revealed significant nasopharyngeal differences in individuals with history of cleft palate. These differences included a reduction of the nasopharyngeal airway due to a decrease in depth of the nasopharyngeal bony framework and the posterior displacement of the maxilla.

The findings of reduced nasal cavity size and reduced nasopharyngeal depth can explain the high incidence of upper airway obstruction and mouth breathing in the cleft palate population.

Submucous Cleft Palate

A *submucous cleft palate* is a congenital defect that affects the underlying structures of the palate, while the structures on the oral surface are intact. This defect can involve the muscles of the velum and can also involve the bony structure of the hard palate. Like an overt cleft palate, a submucous cleft often occurs as part of a generalized syndrome of multiple malformations (Lewin, Croft, & Shprintzen, 1980). The diagnosis of submucous cleft palate is usually made by identification of one or more of the classic stigmata through an intraoral examination. Submucous cleft palate has a triad of characteristics, which include bifid uvula, zona pellucida, and a notch in the posterior border of the hard palate.

Classic Stigmata

One characteristic of a submucous cleft palate that can be seen through an intraoral examination is a bifid uvula. Instead of a single pedicle, a *bifid uvula* has two tags due to a cleft down the middle. The uvula may have two distinct pendulous structures (Figure 3–16), or it may appear as one structure with a line down the middle (Figure 3–17). In other cases, the uvula may merely have an indentation in the inferior border. At times, a bifurcation is not easily appreciated, but the uvula will appear to be *hypoplastic* (small and underdeveloped) (Figure 3–18).

A bifid uvula can be an isolated anomaly, but it is frequently associated with a submucous cleft that extends into the velum. As a re-

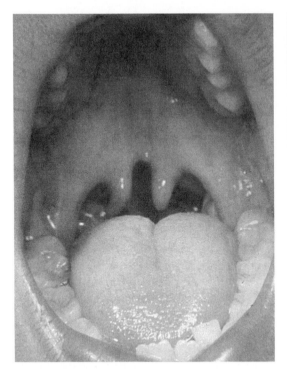

Figure 3–16. Submucous cleft palate with bifid uvula and zona pellucida.

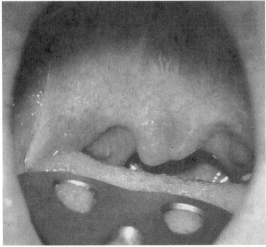

Figure 3–17. Submucous cleft palate. This type of submucous cleft is more subtle, but still very noticeable. Note the hypoplastic uvula with a faint line in the middle and the zona pellucida.

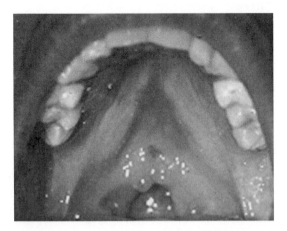

Figure 3–18. Submucous cleft with obvious diastasis of the velar musculature. Note how the muscles insert into the hard palate, resulting in an inverted "V" shape.

sult, individuals with bifid uvula may have velopharyngeal insufficiency with hypernasal speech (Shprintzen et al., 1985). Figure 3–19 shows various degrees of severity of a submucous cleft and the effect of the defect on the musculature. Some individuals demonstrate a combination of an overt cleft and a submucous cleft. This may appear as a bifid uvula with an overt cleft that extends into the velum, and then a submucous cleft that extends anterior to the overt cleft.

In addition to a bifid uvula, an inspection of the velum may reveal a *zona pellucida* (see Figures 3–16 and 3–17). This is a bluish area in the middle of the velum and is the result of thin mucosa with a lack of the normal underlying muscle mass. The velum may also appear to be in the shape of an inverted "V" at rest, but especially with phonation (see Figure 3–18). This shape is due to the *diastasis* (separation) of the paired levator veli palatini muscle with abnormal insertion of these muscles in the posterior border of the hard palate,

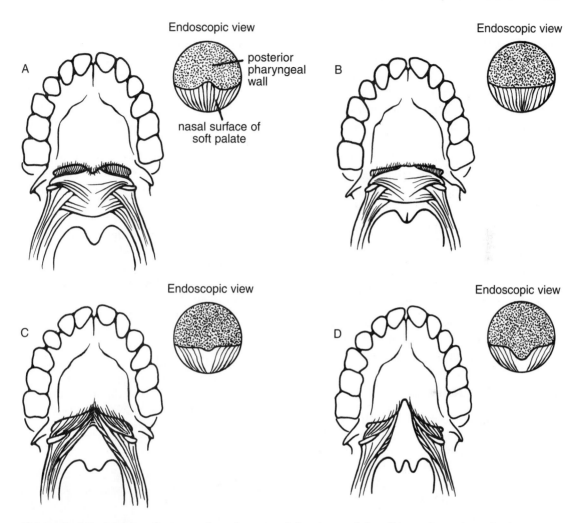

Figure 3–19. Degrees of severity of a submucous cleft palate and the effect on the uvula and velar musculature. The endoscopic view of the nasal surface of the velum can be seen in the circles. **A.** A normal velum and uvula with normal velar musculature. **B.** A bifid uvula but normal velum with no involvement of the velar musculature. This type of submucous cleft is unlikely to affect velopharyngeal function. **C.** A bifid uvula and submucous cleft that extends through the velum to the hard palate. This type of submucous cleft affects the muscle orientation of the velum and could affect velopharyngeal function and thus speech. **D.** A bifid uvula and submucous cleft that extends through the velum and partially through the hard palate. This type of submucous cleft affects the velar musculature and has the potential to affect speech.

rather than in the midline of the velum. With phonation, this abnormal muscle insertion makes the velum appear to "tent up" toward the hard palate. The submucous cleft can extend into the hard palate, all the way to the incisive foramen. When this is the case, the "V" shaped abnormality can be viewed underneath the surface of the mucoperiosteum.

At times, it is difficult to see evidence of a submucous cleft on the oral surface of the velum. In fact, a submucous cleft palate may be present, even when an intraoral examination shows an intact uvula and velum (Shprintzen et al., 1985). Palpation of the palate, however, may reveal an abnormality that cannot be appreciated though visual inspection alone. Using a gloved finger, the examiner can feel the posterior border of the hard palate at the midline. In a normal palate, the slight projection of the posterior nasal spine can often be felt. If this cannot be felt, it does not necessarily indicate an abnormality. However, if there is an appreciable notch in the posterior border of the hard palate, this is indicative of a submucous cleft palate. This notch can be small and very narrow, so it is often helpful to use the little fifth finger to be able feel it.

Occult Submucous Cleft

An *occult submucous cleft* is a defect in the velum that is not apparent on the oral surface (Kapan, 1975; Minami, Kaplan, Wu, & Jobe, 1975). In fact, it can only be appreciated by viewing the nasal surface of the velum through nasopharyngoscopy. As the word "occult" means "hidden" or "not revealed," this malformation is aptly named. The occult submucous cleft is not embryologically or genetically different from other variations of submucous clefts. Instead, the occult submucous cleft represents a point on the continuum of submucous cleft defects and cleft palate.

The diagnosis of occult submucous cleft is only pursued if the patient has velopharyngeal dysfunction of unknown etiology, as there is no obvious physical abnormality of the velum. McWilliams et al. (1990) used the term *congenital palatal insufficiency* (CPI) to describe characteristics of velopharyngeal dysfunction with no history of cleft palate, no ap-

parent evidence of submucous cleft, or other known etiology. This can be due to a discrepancy in the length of the velum and depth of the pharynx. It is possible, however, that many of these cases actually have an occult submucous cleft. With the help of nasopharyngoscopy, which is an endoscopic procedure, it is now possible to identify the velar abnormalities that commonly occur on the nasal surface only. Figure 3–20 is an endoscopic view of the velum showing the nasal surface. It can be seen that the edge of the velum has a depression rather than a rounded bulky muscle mass, thus indicating an occult submucous cleft. Figure 3–19 also shows an endoscopic view of the nasal surface of the velum and illustrates the extent of defect with each level of severity. Abnormalities of nasal surface of the velum are also frequently found by surgeons as the velum is dissected for a pharyngeal flap. In a study of 52 patients without overt cleft palate who were undergoing pharyngeal flap surgery, Trier (1983) found that 48 patients (92%) demonstrated abnormal anatomy of the velum to explain the velopharyngeal incompetence.

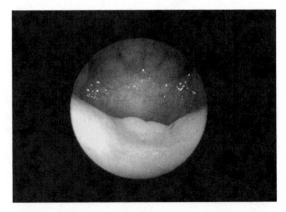

Figure 3–20. An endoscopic view of the velum showing the nasal surface. It can be seen that the edge of the velum has a depression rather than a rounded bulky muscle mass, thus indicating an occult submucous cleft.

Most individuals with an occult submucous cleft have the same abnormalities as those with an overt submucous cleft. The musculus uvulae muscles are either absent or deficient (Croft, Shprintzen, Daniller, & Lewin, 1978) and there is abnormal insertion of the muscles into the hard palate. This can be seen through nasopharyngoscopy as a V-shaped midline defect, with a flattening or depression in the area of the velar eminence.

Effect of Submucous Cleft on Function

The effect of a submucous cleft on function depends greatly on the type and extent of the defect. Abnormalities in the morphology of the velum can particularly affect velopharyngeal function and, therefore, speech. These abnormalities can also cause nasal regurgitation with swallowing, especially during the first year. With submucous cleft palate, there is an increased risk for middle-ear disease with conductive hearing loss due to abnormalities of the tensor veli palatini muscle, which can cause eustachian tube malfunction (Garcia Velasco, Ysunza, Hernandez, & Marquez, 1988; Saad, 1980; Schwartz, Hayden, Rodriquez, Shprintzen, & Cassidy, 1985).

Although individuals with a submucous cleft are at risk for dysfunction of the velopharyngeal valve, many people with this abnormality have normal speech, normal middle-ear function, and no history of nasal regurgitation with swallowing. McWilliams (1991) studied a group of 130 patients with submucous cleft, and found that 44% remained asymptomatic into adulthood. Therefore, the observation of a submucous cleft in the presence of normal speech should not be of concern. It is important, however, that the patient and the family be counseled regarding this abnormality for several reasons. The family should be informed that a full adenoidectomy with a submucous cleft is usually contraindicated due to the risk that this will cause velopharyngeal dysfunction (Shprintzen et al., 1985). In addition, the family should be counseled regarding the genetic risk for additional offspring with cleft palate or associated syndromes.

Prevalence of Submucous Cleft

In epidemiology, the term *incidence* refers to the number of new cases of a disease or disorder in a given population, such as the number of persons becoming ill with a certain disease. On the other hand, the term *prevalence* refers to a measure of existing cases of a disorder in a given population. Therefore, the term prevalence is used to refer to the number of cases of submucous cleft in the general population.

Gorlin, Cervenka, and Pruzansky (1971) reported that 1 in 80 Caucasians, or about 1.2%, have a bifid uvula. Wharton and Mowrer (1992) evaluated 709 children and found some form of uvular cleft in 2.26% of the children, while a complete bifid uvula was found in only 0.3% of the children. Bagatin (1985) found the prevalence of bifid uvula to be 0.2% in Yugoslavian children. Saad (1980) found bifid uvula in 1% of a population of 1500 children. Meskin, Gorlin, and Isaacson (1964) reported bifid uvula in about 1 of 76 people in the general population, or 1.3%. Shapiro, Meskin, Cervenka, and Pruzansky (1971) compared the occurrence of bifid uvula in four races. They reported the prevalence of bifid uvula as 10.25% (sample size of 605) in Chippewa Indians; 9.96% (sample size of 4726) of Japanese; 1.44% (sample size of 9701) of whites; and 0.27% (sample size of 2968) of blacks. It is interesting that this relative frequency by race is similar to the relative frequency of cleft lip and palate. Although these studies reported the prevalence of bifid uvula, it is important to note that children with bifid uvula often have the additional characteristics of submucous cleft palate, including velopharyngeal insufficiency and hypernasal speech (Shprintzen et al., 1985).

Several studies have attempted to determine the prevalence of submucous cleft in the general population. In a large sample of over 10,000 Denver schoolchildren, the prevalence of a complete submucous cleft (including a bony defect of the hard palate) was found to be 0.08% (Stewart, Otet, & Lagace, 1972; Weatherly-White, Sakura, Brenner, Stewart, & Ott, 1972). In a study of almost 10,000 Yugoslavian children, the prevalence of submucous cleft was found to be 0.05% (Bagatin, 1985). Gosain, Conley, Marks, and Larson (1996) summarized the results of several surveys in the literature and stated that prevalence of the classic stigmata of submucous cleft palate among the general population is between 0.02% and 0.08%.

Although a submucous cleft may be noticed at birth or soon after, especially if there are early feeding problems, an occult submucous cleft is usually not discovered until the child begins to speak and has evidence of hypernasality. In some cases, the defect is not noted for years or is never discovered, especially if it is asymptomatic and not causing any problems with speech. Therefore, the prevalence of occult submucous cleft is not known.

The prevalence of submucous cleft palate in the individuals with clefts of the primary palate has been found to be significantly greater than the prevalence of submucous cleft palate found in the general population. Kono, Young, and Holtmann (1981) found submucous cleft palate in 13% of 71 patients with clefts of the primary palate. Because of this increased prevalence, it is important for individuals with cleft lip to be thoroughly examined for submucous cleft. Early detection of submucous cleft associated with cleft lip is important for the prevention of middle-ear problems and for the proper management of velopharyngeal dysfunction if it develops.

Individuals with submucous cleft palate are at high risk for velopharyngeal dysfunction resulting in hypernasality. The occurrence of velopharyngeal dysfunction in individuals with submucous cleft has been studied with various results. Garcia and associates (1988) reported a 53% occurrence; Stewart, et al. (1972) reported a 28% occurrence; Kono and colleagues (1981) reported a 44% occurrence and Bagatin (1985) found a 25% occurrence. Overall, it is safe to say that one fourth to one half of individuals with submucous cleft will have associated velopharyngeal dysfunction. On the other hand, it is important to recognize that most individuals with a submucous cleft will have normal speech (Shprintzen et al., 1985; Stewart et al., 1972).

Treatment of Submucous Cleft

The literature and most professionals do not support the prophylactic surgical correction of the physical stigmata of submucous cleft palate, because many individuals with a submucous cleft have normal speech, swallowing, and middle-ear function. Instead, surgical correction is indicated only if there is evidence of velopharyngeal dysfunction that is affecting speech (Chen, Wu, & Noordhoff, 1994; Garcia Velasco et al., 1988; Gosain et al., 1996). It is therefore important to wait until speech has fully developed before considering surgical correction so that speech and velopharyngeal function can be adequately evaluated. For optimal speech results, however, it is best to surgically correct the defect as soon as a velopharyngeal dysfunction has been diagnosed (Abyholm, 1976).

When surgical correction is necessary and the child is still very young, a palatoplasty is often done to improve the orientation of the muscles for better function. If this is not effective, if the individual is older, or if there is significant velopharyngeal dysfunction, a common procedure for correction is the pharyngeal flap, either alone or in combination with a palatoplasty, for the best speech results (Porterfield, Mohler, & Sandel, 1976).

Facial Clefts

Although clefts usually follow embryological fusion lines, other types of facial clefts can occur. Midline (median) clefts are often associated with a spectrum of other midline problems, including *holoprosencephaly*, which is failure of the forebrain to divide into two hemispheres. Lateral clefts can occur and often begin at the mouth and then course laterally, horizontally, upward and even downward, affecting various facial structures. Figure 3–21 shows an oblique facial cleft that extends into the nose. Figure 3–22 shows a bilateral facial cleft where the defect extends into the eyes. Facial clefts are due to the failure of neural crest cell migration, which results in the lack of fusion of several facial processes, including the branchial arches.

Facial clefts are usually very severe and are accompanied by many other anomalies. For example, a midline cleft is usually accompanied by other midline defects, such as an absent corpus callosum, frontonasal *dysplasia* (abnormal tissue development), cranial base anomalies, or an *encephalocele*, which is a con-

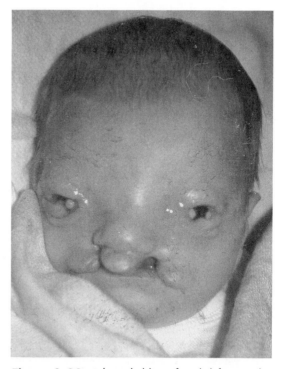

Figure 3–22. Bilateral oblique facial cleft. Note the very wide nasal bridge, hypertelorism, and the malformation of the eyes.

genital gap in the skull with herniation of brain tissue into the nose or palate. *Hypertelorism*, which is wide spacing between the eyes, is also commonly associated with midline clefts. Although facial clefts cause many aesthetic and functional problems, these types of clefts are relatively rare.

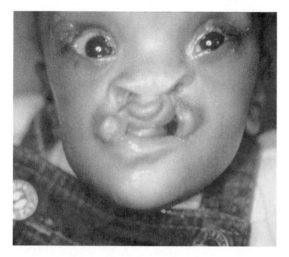

Figure 3–21. Left oblique facial cleft. Note the cleft through the nose.

Summary

Cleft lip and palate are common birth defects that manifest in a variety of ways. There are different types of clefts, such as clefts of the primary and secondary palate, and different degrees of severity. When a cleft occurs, it is the result of a disruption in embryological development. Many craniofacial syndromes include cleft palate as part of the phenotype.

Cleft lip and cleft palate potentially can affect the development of communication skills in a variety of ways. Therefore, health care providers, particularly members of a cleft palate or craniofacial team, need to be aware of the potential effects of various craniofacial anomalies on communication development so that early and appropriate intervention can be initiated.

References

Abyholm, F. E. (1976). Submucous cleft palate. *Scandinavian Journal of Plastic and Reconstructive Surgery, 10*(3), 209–212.

Bagatin, M. (1985). Submucous cleft palate. *Journal of Maxillofacial Surgery, 13*(1), 37–38.

Bardach, J. (1995). Secondary surgery for velopharyngeal insufficiency. In R. J. Shprintzen & J. Bardach (Eds.), *Cleft palate speech management: A multidisciplinary approach* (pp. 277–294). St. Louis, MO: Mosby.

Bluestone, C. D., Beery, Q. C., Cantekin, E. I., & Paradise, J. L. (1975). Eustachian tube ventilatory function in relation to cleft palate. *Annals of Otology, Rhinology, and Laryngology, 84*(3, Pt. 1), 333–338.

Burdi, A. R., & Silvey, R. G. (1969). Sexual differences in closure of the human palatal shelves. *Cleft Palate Journal, 6*, 1.

Chen, K. T., Wu, J., & Noordhoff, S. M. (1994). Submucous cleft palate. *Chang Keng I Hsueh: Chang Gung Medical Journal, 17*(2), 131–137.

Cleft Palate Foundation. (1999). Available on Website: http://www.cleft.com.

Croft, C. B., Shprintzen, R. J., Daniller, A. I., & Lewin, M. L. (1978). The occult submucous cleft palate and the musculus uvulae. *Cleft Palate Journal, 15*, 150–154.

Dickson, D. R. (1972). Normal and cleft palate anatomy. *Cleft Palate Journal, 9*, 280–293.

Dickson, D. R., Grant, J. C., Sicher, H., Dubrul, E. L., & Paltan, J. (1974). Status of research in cleft palate anatomy and physiology, Part 1. *Cleft Palate Journal, 11*, 471–492.

Dickson, D. R., Grant, J. C., Sicher, H., Dubrul, E. L., & Paltan, J. (1975). Status of research in cleft lip and palate: Anatomy and physiology, Part 2. *Cleft Palate Journal, 12*, 131–156.

Doyle, W. J., Cantekin, E. I., & Bluestone, C. D. (1980). Eustachian tube function in cleft palate children. *Annals of Otology, Rhinology, and Laryngology Supplement, 89*(3, Pt. 2), 34–40.

Drake, A. F., Davis, J. U., & Warren, D. W. (1993). Nasal airway size in cleft and noncleft children. *Laryngoscope, 103*(8), 915–917.

Garcia Velasco, M., Ysunza, A., Hernandez, X., & Marquez, C. (1988). Diagnosis and treatment of submucous cleft palate: A review of 108 cases. *Cleft Palate Journal, 25*(2), 171–173.

Gorlin, R. J., Cervenka, J., & Pruzansky, S. (1971). Facial clefting and its syndromes. *Birth Defects Original Article Series, 7*(7), 3–49.

Gosain, A. K., Conley, S. F., Marks, S., & Larson, D. L. (1996). Submucous cleft palate: Diagnostic methods and outcomes of surgical treatment. *Plastic and Reconstructive Surgery, 97*(7), 1497–1509.

Hairfield, W. M., & Warren, D. W. (1989). Dimensions of the cleft nasal airway in adults: A comparison with subjects without cleft. *Cleft Palate Journal, 26*(1), 9–13.

Hairfield, W. M., Warren, D. W., & Seaton, D. L. (1988). Prevalence of mouthbreathing in cleft lip and palate. *Cleft Palate Journal, 25*(2), 135–138.

Jensen, B. L., Kreiborg, S., Dahl, E., & Fogh-Andersen, P. (1988). Cleft lip and palate in Denmark, 1976-1981: Epidemiology, variability, and early somatic development. *Cleft Palate Journal, 25*(3), 258–269.

Jones, M. C. (1988). Etiology of facial clefts: Prospective evaluation of 428 patients. *Cleft Palate Journal, 25*(1), 16–20.

Kaplan, E. N. (1975). The occult submucous cleft palate. *Cleft Palate Journal, 12*, 356–368.

Kernahan, D. A. (1971). The striped Y—A symbolic classification for cleft lip and palate. *Plastic and Reconstructive Surgery, 47*(5), 469–470.

Kernahan, D. A., & Stark, R. B. (1958). A new classification for cleft lip and cleft palate. *Plastic and Reconstructive Surgery, 22*, 435.

Koch, K. H., Grzonka, M. A., & Koch, J. (1998). Pathology of the palatal aponeurosis in cleft palate. *Cleft Palate Craniofacial Journal, 35*(6), 530–534.

Kono, D., Young, L., & Holtmann, B. (1981). The association of submucous cleft palate and clefting of the primary palate. *Cleft Palate Journal, 18*(3), 207–209.

Kriens, O. (1975). Anatomy of the velopharyngeal area in cleft palate. *Clinical Plastic Surgery, 2*(2), 261–288.

Lewin, M. L., Croft, C. B., & Shprintzen, R. J. (1980). Velopharyngeal insufficiency due to hypoplasia of the musculus uvulae and occult submucous cleft palate. *Plastic and Reconstructive Surgery, 65*(5), 585–591.

Liu, H., Warren, D. W., Drake, A. F., & Davis, J. U. (1992). Is nasal airway size a marker for susceptibility toward clefting? *Cleft Palate Craniofacial Journal, 29*(4), 336–339.

Maue-Dickson, W. (1979). The craniofacial complex in cleft lip and palate: An update review of anatomy and function. *Cleft Palate Journal, 16*(3), 291–317.

Maue-Dickson, W., & Dickson, D. R. (1980). Anatomy and physiology related to cleft palate: Current research and clinical implications. *Plastic and Reconstructive Surgery, 65*(1), 83–90.

McWilliams, B. J. (1991). Submucous clefts of the palate: How likely are they to be symptomatic? *Cleft Palate Craniofacial Journal, 28*(3), 247–249; Discussion 250–251.

McWilliams, B. J., Morris, H. L., & Shelton, R. L. (1990). *Cleft palate speech.* Philadelphia: B.C. Decker.

Meskin, L., Gorlin, R., & Isaacson, R. (1964). Abnormal morphology of the soft palate: The prevalence of a cleft uvula. *Cleft Palate Journal, 3,* 342–346.

Minami, T., Kaplan, E. N., Wu, G., & Jobe, R. P. (1975). Velopharyngeal incompetence without overt cleft palate. A collective review and experience with 98 patients. *Plastic and Reconstructive Surgery, 55*(5), 573–587.

Moon, J. B., & Kuehn, D. P. (1997). Anatomy and physiology of normal and disordered velopharyngeal function for speech. In K. R. Bzoch (Ed.), *Communicative disorders related to cleft lip and palate.* Austin, TX: Pro-Ed.

Oka, S. W. (1979). Epidemiology and genetics of clefting: With implications for etiology. In H. K. Cooper, R. L. Harding, W. M. Krogman, M. Mazaheri, & Millard, R. T. (Eds.), *Cleft palate and cleft lip: A team approach to clinical management and rehabilitation of the patient.* Philadelphia: W.B. Saunders.

Paradise, J. L., Bluestone, C. D., & Felder, H. (1969). The universality of otitis media in 50 infants with cleft palate. *Pediatrics, 44*(1), 35–42.

Porterfield, H. W., Mohler, L. R., & Sandel, A. (1976). Submucous cleft palate. *Plastic and Reconstructive Surgery, 58*(1), 60–65.

Rollnick, B. R., & Pruzansky, S. (1981). Genetic services at a center for craniofacial anomalies. *Cleft Palate Journal, 18*(4), 304–313.

Saad, E. F. (1980). The underdeveloped palate in ear, nose and throat practice. *Laryngoscope, 90*(8, Pt. 1), 1371–1377.

Schwartz, R. H., Hayden, G. F., Rodriquez, W. J., Shprintzen, R. J., & Cassidy, J. W. (1985). The bifid uvula: Is it a marker for an otitis prone child? *Laryngoscope, 95*(9, Pt. 1), 1100–1102.

Shapiro, B. L., Meskin, L. H., Cervenka, J., & Pruzansky, S. (1971). Cleft uvula: A microform of facial clefts and its genetic basis. *Birth Defects Original Article Series, 7*(7), 80–82.

Shprintzen, R. J., Schwartz, R. H., Daniller, A., & Hoch, L. (1985). Morphologic significance of bifid uvula. *Pediatrics, 75*(3), 553–561.

Smahel, Z., Kasalova, P., & Skvarilova, B. (1991). Morphometric nasopharyngeal characteristics in facial clefts. *Journal of Craniofacial Genetics and Developmental Biology, 11*(1), 24–32.

Smahel, Z., & Mullerova, I. (1992). Nasopharyngeal characteristics in children with cleft lip and palate. *Cleft Palate Craniofacial Journal, 29*(3), 282–286.

Snyder, G., Berkowitz, S., Bzoch, K., & Stool, S. (1980). *Your cleft lip and palate child: A basic guide for parents.* Evansville, IN: Meade Johnson & Co.

Stewart, J. M., Otet, J. E., & Lagace, R. (1972). Submucous cleft palate: Prevalence in a school population. *Cleft Palate Journal, 9,* 246–250.

Trier, W. C. (1983). Velopharyngeal incompetency in the absence of overt cleft palate: Anatomic and surgical considerations. *Cleft Palate Journal, 20*(3), 209–217.

Warkany, J. (1971). *Congenital malformations; Notes and comments.* Chicago: Year Book.

Warren, D. W., & Drake, A. F. (1993). Cleft nose. Form and function. *Clinics in Plastic Surgery, 20*(4), 769–779.

Weatherly-White, R. C. A., Sakura, C. Y., Brenner, L. D., Stewart, J. M., & Ott, J. E. (1972). Submucous cleft palate incidence, natural history, and implications for treatment. *Plastic and Reconstructive Surgery, 49,* 297–304.

Wetmore, R. F. (1992). Importance of maintaining normal nasal function in the cleft palate patient. *Cleft Palate Craniofacial Journal, 29*(6), 498–506.

Wharton, P., & Mowrer, D. E. (1992). Prevalence of cleft uvula among school children in kindergarten through grade five. *Cleft Palate Craniofacial Journal, 29*(1), 10–12; Discussion 13–14.

CHAPTER

4

The Genetics Evaluation and Common Craniofacial Syndromes

Howard M. Saal, M.D.

CONTENTS

Congenital anomalies occur in 3 to 5% of all live births. They are among the most common causes of hospitalization in childhood. There are numerous causes of congenital anomalies, with contributions from both genetic and environmental factors. Craniofacial disorders make up a significant number of congenital anomalies, with 1 in 700 to 800 children born with cleft lip with or without cleft palate and 1 in 2000 children born with cleft palate (Gorlin, Cohen, & Levin, 1990; Wyszynski, Beaty, & Maestri, 1996). Other craniofacial anomalies frequently encountered are craniosynostosis, hemifacial microsomia, submucous cleft palate, and velopharyngeal insufficiency. Because there is usually a significant genetic component to the pathogenesis of most craniofacial disorders, it is important for each child born with these conditions to have a complete genetic evaluation and follow-up evaluations as the child grows and develops.

The purpose of this chapter is to first describe the components of the genetics evaluation and the information that is important to obtain to arrive at a genetics diagnosis. The reader then learns about the types and causes of dysmorphology. This chapter includes a description of the genetics of clefting and the incidence of clefts. Finally, common craniofacial syndromes are described.

The Genetics Evaluation

The purpose of the genetics evaluation is to (1) make a diagnosis; (2) determine the natural history of a condition, which will assist with anticipatory management for medical and developmental issues; (3) determine recurrence risks for the parents and other close family members, which may include information regarding availability of prenatal diagnosis for future pregnancies; and (4) provide genetic psychosocial counseling and family support, which is often the most important function of the genetic evaluation. The genetics evaluation

is an important component of the early management of the child born with a craniofacial disorder and the findings can significantly influence long-term medical and educational management.

The genetics evaluation is somewhat different from the standard medical evaluation. Greater emphasis is placed on pregnancy history and family history. Additionally, most cases of craniofacial disorders are treated as chronic conditions with a need for long-term integrated management, although occasional acute interventions are required (see Table 4–1).

Prenatal History

The prenatal history is an essential component of the genetics evaluation. In particular, it is important to determine if the fetus had any exposure to teratogens. A *teratogen* is a chemical or physical agent that can interfere with the normal embryological processes. Teratogens can include viruses, drugs, radiation, or any other outside agent that can result in abnormal fetal development. Therefore, information regarding maternal illnesses during pregnancy, such as infections, diabetes, or medications taken, can be helpful in determining a diagnosis.

If taken during pregnancy, several common medications can act as teratogens and cause orofacial and other disorders (Spranger, et al., 1982). Some of these medications are still prescribed to pregnant women, even though they are known teratogens with potential risks for the fetus. For example, anticonvulsants, such as hydantoin and valproic acid, are still prescribed during pregnancy because it is assumed that their benefit in controlling seizures outweighs the risks for fetal anomalies. Alcohol is another significant teratogen. In addition to causing developmental disabilities and growth delays, its use has been associated with cleft lip, cleft palate, and Pierre Robin sequence. For certain at-risk individuals, smoking cigarettes can increase the risk for having a child with a cleft lip.

TABLE 4–1. Elements of the clinical genetics evaluation.

Major Elements	Contributing Elements
Medical history	Pregnancy history, complications, exposures Birth weight and length Perinatal history and complications Feeding history Identification of other anomalies Major illnesses Hospitalizations Surgeries Growth Feeding difficulties Other medical problems and illnesses Medications
Developmental history	Major milestones Developmental interventions School performance Therapeutic interventions
Family history	Four-generation pedigree Consanguinity Birth defects Infertility Pregnancy loss Mental retardation Major illness
Physical examination	Growth parameters: height, weight, head circumference Dysmorphology examination Complete physical examination
Laboratory testing and referrals, as indicated	Chromosomes Other genetic studies as indicated Brain imaging studies Ophthalmology examination EEG Developmental evaluation Other medical consultations
Genetic counseling	Diagnosis Prognosis Medical interventions Developmental interventions Recurrence risks Prenatal diagnosis

(continued)

TABLE 4–1. *(continued)*

Major Elements	Contributing Elements
Psychosocial genetic counseling	Family support and education Identification of related local support groups Identification of national support groups
Follow-up genetics evaluations	Diagnosis Medical management Genetic counseling Family support

Medical and Feeding History

The medical history of the newborn with a craniofacial disorder is usually straightforward and uncomplicated. Any and all perinatal complications should be noted, especially if there are any respiratory problems, seizures, heart defects, or congenital anomalies. Knowledge of birth weight, length, and head circumference can give valuable clues to diagnosis, as many syndromes are associated with low birth weight or small head size. Other disorders, such as Beckwith-Wiedemann syndrome, are associated with large body size for gestational age. An infant who is small or large for gestational age often has other underlying medical issues that require greater attention. Although any congenital anomaly can provide a clue to diagnosis, specific birth defects that are often associated with genetic conditions include structural heart anomalies, seizures, eye anomalies, and genital anomalies.

Early feeding problems are common in infants with cleft palate, but they are usually resolved quickly with simple feeding modifications. They become significant if they persist beyond the first week of life. Children with cleft palate who have normal neurological status rarely have prolonged feeding problems, however.

Developmental History

The developmental history should include comprehensive information about early developmental milestones, especially for gross motor and language development. A history of early developmental interventions, especially those related to speech and physical therapy, should be determined. School performance information should be obtained, and should include the history of special therapies, the need for special education, and the results of any developmental or intelligence testing. It should also be noted which grades were repeated, if any, and for what reasons.

Family History

What really distinguishes the genetics evaluation from a standard medical evaluation is the comprehensiveness of the family history. A *pedigree* is developed, which is a pictorial representation of family members and their line of descent. This can be used by the geneticist to analyze inheritance, particularly for certain traits or anomalies. It is important to extend the pedigree to four generations, if information is available. Any and all medical problems in relatives are noted, with special attention to birth defects, including cleft lip, cleft palate, and congenital heart defects. Developmental disabilities and mental retardation are recorded, as are miscarriages and early deaths. It can be valuable to identify if the parents are related in any way, called *consanguinity*, because this can give insight into rare autosomal recessive disorders.

Physical Examination

The physical examination of the child with a craniofacial disorder is straightforward. As with any examination, attention is given to the growth parameters (weight, height or length, and head circumference). *Microcephaly*, which is a small head size, can indicate poor brain growth or development. Children with microcephaly often have underlying genetic conditions and are at greater risk for developmental disabilities. Poor weight gain may indicate poor feeding or possibly a genetic condition associated with small stature, such as a chromosome disorder.

In addition to the standard physical examination, the clinical geneticist is trained to perform a dysmorphology examination. Here, the physician examines the child for features that may not be familial, but rather specific to that child and often indicative of specific disorders or syndromes. This may include measurements of the eyes, ears, mouth, nose, and numerous other structures. It may be helpful to identify specific *dermatoglyphics,* which are creases on the hands or changes in the fingerprints, which also can give clues to early developmental problems. The neurologic examination is especially helpful, as it provides insight regarding the child's muscle tone, level of function, and degree of social interaction. Photographs are taken of the patient at each visit. It is often helpful to look at earlier photographs that the parents bring to the visit, as well at photographs of other family members. It is helpful to examine the parents and often siblings for features similar to those of the patient.

Laboratory Studies

After the history is reviewed and the examination is completed, it becomes necessary to determine if any laboratory studies are needed to help make a diagnosis or to confirm clinical suspicions about a suspected diagnosis. Chromosome studies can be helpful in identifying known common and rare syndromes. Usually, children with chromosome anomalies have multiple anomalies; however, there are some conditions in which there may be few specific clinical features. For example, velocardiofacial syndrome, which is discussed later in greater detail, is associated with cleft palate and/or velopharyngeal insufficiency and may present with very few features. This condition is diagnosed by finding a deletion of the long arm of chromosome 22. Many children with chromosome disorders have rare deletions or duplications, adding to the challenge of genetic counseling.

In addition to the laboratory studies, it may be helpful to obtain X rays to determine bone maturation or to identify specific skeletal syndromes. An MRI scan of the brain can be helpful in identifying structural anomalies in children with serious developmental disorders, microcephaly, or neurologic problems.

Referral to other physicians may be necessary as part of a complete genetics assessment. An ophthalmology examination should be done for all children with cleft palate, because the discovery of nearsightedness is a clue to the diagnosis of Stickler syndrome. All children with suspected heart defects, such as those with velocardiofacial syndrome, should be evaluated by a cardiologist.

Genetic Counseling

After the genetics evaluation is completed, it is time to sit with the family for genetic counseling. This is usually the longest part of the genetics evaluation, because it is necessary to educate the family regarding issues of heredity and development. Part of the process involves discussion of natural history of the suspected condition and planning for medical interventions. Because many genetic disorders have associated developmental disabilities, it is important to start planning for developmental testing, including a speech and language evaluation. It is also important to plan for developmental or school interventions, with referrals to community agencies or the school system for special services as deemed necessary.

As part of the genetic counseling process, families often have questions regarding the cause of the condition and the recurrence risks for themselves, their child, and for other family members. For many genetic disorders, recurrence risks are known and can be shared with the family.

In addition to discussing recurrence risks, it is also important to identify the prenatal testing for the condition and reproductive options. Amniocentesis can be performed for prenatal identification of chromosome anomalies and specific known genetic disorders with molecular analysis. For some birth defects, such as cleft lip, with or without cleft palate, fetal ultrasound studies are the only test available for prenatal diagnosis. Unfortunately, prenatal therapy for most birth defects is not available.

Psychosocial Counseling

Finally, the genetics evaluation should include recognition of the difficulty of having a child with a birth defect and offers of psychosocial support for the family. It is essential to identify community and national resources for the family, such as local, state, and national support groups and meetings. With the advent of the worldwide web, it is also important to identify specific web sites that will be helpful to families for identifying educational and support resources.

Dysmorphology

Dysmorphology is the study of abnormal shape or form. Any clinical abnormalities that are of significant medical or cosmetic consequence, especially those requiring medical intervention, are considered major anomalies. On the other hand, abnormal features that have clinical diagnostic implications but are of minimal medical or cosmetic significance and require no intervention are considered minor anomalies. Minor anomalies occur in less than 5% of the population. The diagnosis of many genetic and craniofacial disorders depends on the identification of specific dysmorphic features, both major and minor anomalies. It is important to understand the underlying pathogenesis of congenital anomalies.

Morphogenesis is the process of embryonic tissue formation. *Dysmorphogenesis* describes errors in this process. These errors result in *dysmorphic* (abnormally formed) features (Spranger et al., 1982). Factors that can cause these abnormalities can be related to external nongenetic forces, usually attributable to abnormal fetal environment, disruption of normal development, or intrinsic genetic or developmental abnormalities.

Malformations and Deformations

Most craniofacial anomalies are malformations. A *malformation* is a morphologic anomaly that results from an intrinsically abnormal developmental process (Spranger et al., 1982) and is due to a genetic etiology. Cleft lip and many cases of cleft palate are examples of malformations. Mental retardation may also be a malformation if it results from a genetic etiology or from a brain malformation. Genetic factors can cause a *dysplasia*, which refers to an abnormal organization of cells into tissues and the outcome of the process (Spranger et al., 1982). The *craniosynostoses* are the commonly encountered dysplasias. These usually represent the abnormal development of the cranial skeleton, with other skeletal structures or tissues often being affected as well. Communication disorders are commonly found in patients with craniofacial malformation syndromes (Cary, Stevens, & Haskins, 1992).

Some birth defects arise as a result of abnormal mechanical forces on an otherwise normal structure. An anomaly that is caused by physical forces in the fetal environment is called a *deformation* or *deformity*. Deformations usually result in the abnormal shape or form of a completely formed organ or structure (Spranger et al., 1982). Classic examples of fetal deformations include clubfoot and *plagiocephaly* (abnormal skull shape).

Deformations occur when external forces disrupt the development of an intrinsically normal structure. A *disruption* causes a morphologic defect due to an extrinsic breakdown or interference with a normal developmental process (Spranger et al., 1982). Since teratogens interfere with the normal embryological processes, they are often implicated in disruptions. Examples of teratogens that cause birth defects include alcohol, anticonvulsants (such as hydantoin, valproic acid, and carbamazipine), and vitamin A analogs (such as retinoic acid), which can cause ear anomalies, hearing loss, brain anomalies, and congenital heart defects. Physical disruption of normal development can also occur; for example, *amniotic bands*, where the amnion, the membrane surrounding the embryo and fetus, ruptures and leaves strands of tissue floating in the amniotic cavity. These strands can attach to limbs, the head, or other body parts and act as tourniquets, cutting off blood supply to developing structures. This results in amputations of limbs and digits, cleft lip, and encephalocele if the cranium is involved. Even some maternal illnesses, such as maternal diabetes, can result in disruptions that cause vertebral, heart, and even brain anomalies.

Syndromes, Sequences, and Associations

A *syndrome* is a pattern of multiple anomalies that are pathogenically related, and therefore have a common known or suspected cause (Spranger et al., 1982). Because craniofacial syndromes affect the facial features, they can cause affected individuals to look alike, even when there is no family relationship. An example of this is Down syndrome. Many children with craniofacial conditions have underlying syndromes as the cause of the specific craniofacial anomaly. Recognizing a specific syndrome is important for medical management and is a focus of genetic counseling.

In contrast to a syndrome, a *sequence* is an anomaly or a pattern of multiple anomalies that arises from a single known or presumed prior anomaly or mechanical factor (Spranger et al., 1982). As a result, one anomaly occurs due to the presence of a pre-existing anomaly. The best known and perhaps one of the best-understood example is the Pierre Robin sequence. This sequence usually includes a wide, bell-shaped cleft palate; *micrognathia*, which is a small jaw or mandible; and *glossoptosis*, which is the posterior displacement of the tongue. The initiating event for this sequence is interference with normal development of the mandible at 9 weeks gestation. The small mandible then forces the tongue to remain high in the oral cavity, thereby interfering with closure of the velum. After birth, the upper airway may be obstructed due to the glossoptosis, causing life-threatening respiratory distress. A cleft palate is not always seen in Pierre Robin sequence but is present in the majority of cases.

An *association* is a nonrandom occurrence of a pattern of multiple anomalies in two or more individuals that is not a syndrome or sequence (Spranger et al., 1982). In an association, the pathogenesis is not known, and therefore a genetic etiology cannot be discerned. An association is a diagnosis of exclusion; in other words, a genetic, developmental, or teratogenic etiology must first be excluded before making the diagnosis of an association. When no genetic etiology can be discerned, the recurrence risks for associations are no greater than the risks for the general population. An example of an association is CHARGE association.

Genetics of Cleft Lip (With or Without Cleft Palate)

As has been noted, cleft lip, with or without cleft palate (CL/P), is a very common birth defect with an incidence of 1 in 800 (Gorlin et al., 1990; Wyszynski, Beaty, & Maestri, 1996). Boys are affected more frequently than girls by a ratio of 3:2 (Wyszynski et al., 1996). A left-sided cleft lip is more common than a right-sided cleft, and both occur more frequently than bilateral CL/P.

Although most cases of CL/P are isolated, that is, there are no associated syndromes or other birth defects, there still is a substantial underlying genetic pathogenesis. This is supported by the fact that the recurrence risk for CL/P is elevated for individuals with CL/P, parents of a child with CL/P, and even for siblings of an individual born with CL/P. For parents of a child with CL/P and for the individual who is born with CL/P, the recurrence risk with each future pregnancy is in the range of 3 to 5%, or a 20- to 35-fold increase over baseline risk. After a second child is born with CL/P, the recurrence risk rises to 10 to 15%, consistent with an increased genetic contribution. With the birth of a third first-degree relative who is affected, the recurrence risk increases to 25 to 50%, consistent with dominant or recessive inheritance. The recurrence risk is also influenced by the severity of the CL/P. For a child born with bilateral cleft lip and cleft palate, the recurrence risk is 5.6% for a bilateral cleft lip and palate, 4.1% for a unilateral cleft lip and cleft palate, and 2.6% for a unilateral cleft lip without cleft palate (Fraser, 1970).

In some families, multiple individuals are affected with CL/P. This can represent a more significant underlying genetic influence or predisposition. In these families, the inheritance appears to be autosomal dominant. One syndrome, Van der Woude syndrome, has been identified with autosomal dominant inheritance of clefts. In addition to having cleft lip and or cleft palate, most individuals with this disorder also have bilateral pits in the lower lip. Because this is an autosomal dominant syndrome, the recurrence risk with Van der Woude syndrome is 50%, rather than the typical 3 to 5% when there is a nonsyndromic cleft.

There are significant racial differences in the incidence of CL/P. For Caucasian populations the incidence is 1 in 800, for African Americans it is 1 in 2000, and for Asians it is 1 in 500. The incidence of CL/P appears to be highest in American Indians, with 1 in 300 being affected. Even with these data, recurrence risks are similar among all racial and ethnic groups when only one individual in a family is affected with a CL/P (Gorlin et al., 1990; Wyszynski et al., 1996).

Although most cases of CL/P are isolated birth defects, a substantial number are caused by underlying genetic syndromes or are part of a multiple congenital anomaly disorder. Over 180 different syndromes have CL/P as a component (Winter & Baraitser, 1996). At the Craniofacial Center at Cincinnati Children's Hospital Medical Center, approximately 73% of cases are isolated and 27% are syndromic or associated with other birth defects. A great variety of disorders are associated with CL/P (Table 4–2).

The most common birth defects encountered in the Cincinnati Craniofacial Center are congenital heart defects, sensorineural hearing loss, microcephaly, and *coloboma* (a congenital defect of the eye, which most often affects the

TABLE 4–2. Syndromes associated with cleft lip with or without cleft palate.

Syndrome	Inheritance
Opitz syndrome	Autosomal dominant; X-linked recessive
Trisomy 13	Chromosomal (usually sporadic)
Wolf-Hirschhorn syndrome	Chromosomal (usually sporadic)
Hemifacial microsomia	Sporadic
Amniotic bands	Sporadic
Diabetic embryopathy	Teratogenic (maternal illness)
Fetal alcohol syndrome	Teratogenic
CHARGE association	Sporadic
Van der Woude syndrome	Autosomal dominant
Popliteal pterygium syndrome	Autosomal dominant
Oral-facial-digital syndrome type 1	X-linked dominant

iris and/or retina, but may also cause a notch of the upper or lower eyelid). Brain anomalies, including brain cysts and seizures, are also common (Table 4–2). Some patients have CL/P with multiple anomalies in what appears to be an underlying syndrome, although a diagnosis cannot be made because the pattern of anomalies is not one that has been previously described. Approximately 40–50% of patients seen by a geneticist have rare or unique syndromes, making it difficult to predict natural history and recurrence risk. These patients are diagnosed as having *provisionally unique syndromes* until other patients with the same syndromic pattern are identified and reported.

A great deal of research is under way searching for the genes that cause or predispose individuals to isolated CL/P (Murray, 1995; Stein et al., 1995). Specific genes that are active during early craniofacial development have been implicated in the etiology of CL/P, including transforming growth factor-alpha retinoic acid receptor, transforming growth factor beta, and MSX1 (Lidral et al., 1998).

Syndromes Associated With Cleft Lip (With or Without Cleft Palate)

Trisomy 13

Trisomy 13 (Figure 4–1) is a lethal chromosome disorder. The incidence of this disorder is about 1 in 5000 live births (Jones, 1997). Babies born with this disorder have 47 chromosomes instead of the normal number of 46, with an extra copy of chromosome 13. This disorder is associated with multiple serious life-endangering birth defects, including severe brain anomalies, congenital heart defects, *polydactyly* (extra fingers and/or toes), spina bifida, and severe eye defects. CL/P is seen in 60 to 80% of cases (Jones, 1997) (Figure 4–1). Many infants with trisomy 13 have a midline cleft lip and midline facial anomalies (Figure 4–2). This often denotes the presence of *holoprosencephaly*, the failure of the brain to divide into the two hemispheres. Other infants have unilateral or bilateral CL/P. Trisomy 13 is a lethal disorder, with over 90% of individuals dying before their first birthday,

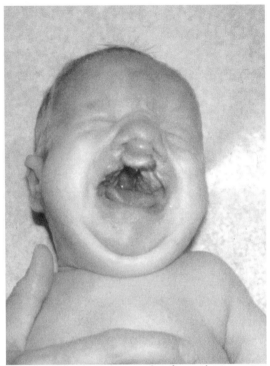

Figure 4–1. A newborn male infant with trisomy 13 and bilateral cleft lip and cleft palate. Other typical findings include a broad nose and microphthalmia.

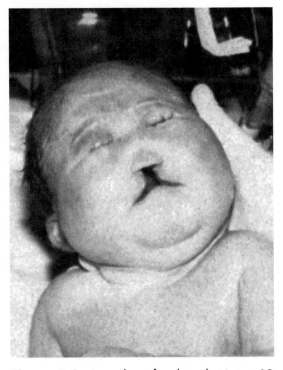

Figure 4–2. A newborn female with trisomy 13 and holoprosencephaly. Note the midline cleft lip and cleft palate.

usually from a central nervous system or cardiac event. For this reason, most patients with trisomy 13 are rarely seen in a craniofacial center. On rare occasions, a child may survive for several years. These long-term survivors are usually severely to profoundly mentally retarded and require a great deal of intervention and supervision. Feeding difficulties are usually seen in these patients, most of whom require *nasogastric tube feeding* through a tube that is placed through the nose to the stomach.

Wolf-Hirschhorn Syndrome

Wolf-Hirschhorn syndrome is a rare chromosome disorder that is caused by a deletion or missing portion of the short arm of chromo-

some 4. These patients have a very distinctive facial appearance, likened to a Greek helmet because of the presence of hypertelorism and a prominent nasal bridge. CL/P is a common feature. Most patients are very small, grow poorly, and have microcephaly. Heart defects and seizures are very common. Developmental disabilities are universal in this disorder, with most patients having severe to profound mental retardation (Jones, 1997). Most patients are expected to have significant communication disorders.

Opitz Syndrome

Opitz syndrome is a condition that has many names, including hypertelorism-hypospadias syndrome, Opitz BBB syndrome, and Opitz G syndrome. The typical manifestations are *hypertelorism* (widely spaced eyes) and *hypospadias* in affected males (where the opening of the urethra of the penis is proximal to its normal location). Other features that may be seen include imperforate anus, *cryptorchidism* (undescended testes), and inguinal hernias. One characteristic that may be very serious is that of the presence of a laryngeal cleft. This abnormality in the development of the larynx can lead to swallowing and voice disorders, aspiration pneumonia, and often requires long-term tracheostomy management. CL/P is frequently seen, and the Opitz syndrome is the second most common identifiable cause of syndromic CL/P in the Craniofacial Center at Cincinnati Children's Hospital Medical Center. Opitz syndrome is genetically *heterogeneous*, meaning that more than one gene can cause the same clinical features. A gene for Opitz syndrome has been found on chromosome 22, which is associated with autosomal dominant inheritance (Robin, Opitz, & Muenke, 1996). A second gene for Opitz syndrome is on the X chromosome and is associated with X-linked recessive inheritance. Patients with Opitz syndrome are at risk for mental retardation as well as for learning disabilities.

Patients with Opitz syndrome and normal development are not at increased risk for speech and language problems, other than those related to the cleft palate. Those with laryngeal clefts may need additional services related to any problems with voice or feeding. Individuals with developmental disabilities are not at risk for any specific speech or language disorders, but remain at risk for similar speech and language difficulties encountered in others with developmental problems.

Van der Woude Syndrome

Van der Woude syndrome is among the most common syndromic causes of CL/P. Some reports suggest that this disorder may be responsible for up to 3% of all cases of cleft lip

(Murray et al., 1990). This is an autosomal dominant disorder for which the gene has been mapped to the long arm of chromosome 1. The major manifestations are the presence of pits of the lower lip and cleft lip, cleft palate, or both (Figure 4–3). Approximately 80% of gene carriers will have lip pits (Jones, 1997). Other features described in Van der Woude syndrome include neonatal teeth and missing teeth. Development is usually normal and speech problems are usually related to the cleft palate.

Oral-Facial-Digital Syndrome Type I (OFD I)

Oral-facial-digital syndrome type I (OFD I) is one of many genetic disorders where a single mutant gene can affect multiple unrelated systems. This phenomenon is called *pleiotropy*. The

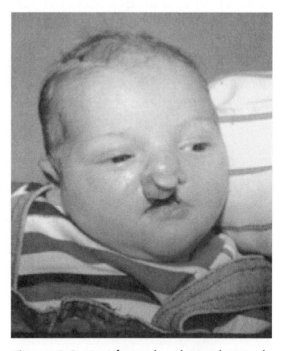

Figure 4–3. An infant male with Van der Woude syndrome and bilateral cleft lip and cleft palate. The lip pits of the lower lip are a diagnostic feature of this disorder.

gene for this condition is on the X-chromosome, and the inheritance for this condition is X-linked dominant. Therefore, affected females can have affected daughters. This is presumed to be lethal in males, and this presumption is supported by the paucity of males reported with this condition, the severe phenotype of affected males, and the diminished number of sons born to affected women (Goodship, Platt, Smith, & Burn, 1991). Infants born with this condition often have a midline cleft lip with multiple oral frenulae (oral tissue webs), cleft palate, and tongue abnormalities that include lobulations and notching of the tongue (Figure 4–4). There is hypertelorism with a broad nose and coarse and often sparse hair. The teeth may be abnormal with decreased enamel and often there are missing teeth. Digital anomalies include asymmetric short fingers, variable degrees of *syndactyly* (fusion or webbing of the digits) or *clinodactyly* (curved or bent digits). Renal anomalies may be seen, including the presence of renal cysts. Brain anomalies have been reported, including hydrocephalus and absence of the corpus callosum (Jones, 1997).

Developmental disabilities are commonly seen in this population, especially in the presence of brain anomalies (Jones, 1997). Speech and language difficulties are generally related to the cleft palate and developmental disabilities.

Genetics of Cleft Palate

Cleft palate (CP) occurs in approximately 1 in 2000 live births (Gorlin et al., 1990; Wyszynski et al., 1996). In contrast to CL/P, CP is much more likely to be associated with an underlying syndrome or other congenital anomalies. A prospective analysis of all cases of CP seen in the Craniofacial Center at Cincinnati Children's Hospital showed that approximately 55% of cases were syndromic or associated with additional anomalies. Because it can be difficult to distinguish between the malformation of cleft palate and cleft palate as a disruption of normal development, all cases of cleft palate, including those caused by Pierre Robin sequence, will be discussed as a single group of disorders.

CP is a component of numerous syndromes (Table 4–3). The London Dysmorphology Database, a computerized database of over 2500 different nonchromosomal disorders, lists 376 syndromes, excluding chromosome disorders, in which CP may be seen, many of which are quite rare. Cleft palate may occur as a malformation, but it may also be seen as part of a sequence, particularly Pierre Robin sequence (Winter & Baraitser, 1996).

A Sequence and Syndromes Associated With Cleft Palate

Pierre Robin Sequence

Pierre Robin sequence is a common cause of cleft palate. This sequence can occur in isolation, but is associated with an underlying syndrome in over 50% of cases (Tomaski, Zalzal, & Saal, 1995). This condition is not a diagnosis unto itself, but rather encompasses the pathogenesis of the cleft palate and, when recog-

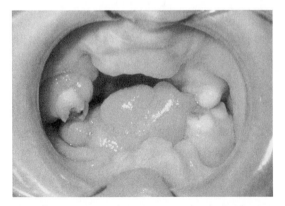

Figure 4–4. Lobulations and fissures of the tongue. This is a common characteristic of patients with oral-facial-digital syndrome type I.

TABLE 4–3. Syndromes associated with cleft palate.

Syndrome	Inheritance
Stickler syndrome	Autosomal dominant
Velocardiofacial syndrome	Autosomal dominant
Fetal alcohol syndrome	Teratogenic
Fetal hydantoin syndrome	Teratogenic
Kabuki syndrome	Possible autosomal dominant
Van der Woude syndrome	Autosomal dominant
Hemifacial microsomia	Sporadic
CHARGE association	Sporadic
Treacher Collins syndrome	Autosomal dominant
Diabetic embryopathy	Teratogenic

nized, gives some critical clues to how a newly diagnosed infant should be managed. As noted earlier in this chapter, infants born with Pierre Robin sequence are born with their tongues positioned posteriorly, often causing blockage of the pharynx and airway, a process called glossoptosis. This affects both breathing and feeding. There are many approaches to airway management in infants with Pierre Robin sequence, and often the treatment must be individualized for each child. The first approach is to place the infant in a prone position. Gravity then allows the tongue to fall forward, and for some infants this relieves the glossoptosis. Sometimes it becomes necessary to place a tube in the nose of the infant in such a way that one end of the tube is placed below the region of tongue obstruction and the other end sticks out of the nose. This tube is called a *nasopharyngeal airway*, and some infants with Pierre Robin sequence require such management until age 3 or 4 months (Tomaski et al., 1995). Some infants do not respond adequately to such conservative treatments, and require a *tracheostomy*, or placement of a tube directly in the trachea to bypass the area of upper airway obstruction (Tomaski et al., 1995). Usually the tracheostomy remains

in place until after the palate is repaired, typically at about 14 months. Unfortunately, the presence of the tracheostomy prevents most vocalizations, which often leads to further speech issues in addition to those related to the cleft palate.

Most infants with Pierre Robin sequence also have early feeding difficulty, due to difficulty coordinating breathing, sucking, and swallowing. Some infants respond to short periods of feeding with a *nasogastric tube*, a tube placed through the nose into the stomach. Other infants need a tracheostomy to feed adequately by mouth. In the most severe cases, an infant may require a feeding tube to be placed directly into the stomach for *gastrostomy (G) tube feeding*.

Stickler Syndrome

Stickler syndrome is by far the most common identifiable cause of cleft palate. This is an autosomal dominant disorder with *variable expressivity*; in other words, there is a great deal of variability in the clinical presentation of patients with this disorder. Individuals with this condition may have some or all of the clinical features associated with this disorder.

The classic presentation of Stickler syndrome (Figure 4–5) is Pierre Robin sequence, including cleft palate; early onset osteoarthritis, often in early adulthood but sometimes in later childhood, and *myopia* (nearsightedness) (Snead & Yates, 1999; Spranger, 1998). The eye problems associated with Stickler syndrome can be very severe, with most patients having moderate to high myopia. The myopia is usually progressive and patients with Stickler syndrome and myopia are at high risk for retinal detachments, and therefore must be followed closely for any vision changes (Naiglin et al., 1999). In addition, sensorineural hearing loss is very common in Stickler syndrome. Most individuals have hearing loss in the high frequencies, but the loss occasionally falls within the voice range (Nowak, 1998). Sensorineural hearing loss is also complicated by the conductive hearing loss often seen as a complication of middle-

ear effusion with a cleft palate. For these reasons, individuals with Stickler syndrome should be followed with serial audiograms.

Many individuals with Stickler syndrome also have characteristic facial features including micrognathia in infancy, a flat facial profile, *epicanthal folds* (folds of skin over the medial portion of the openings of the eyes or palpebral fissures), and midface hypoplasia. The nasal bridge is often flat, even in adulthood.

Development is usually normal in Stickler syndrome. Affected individuals do not appear to be at increased risk for any particular learning disabilities. Speech and language problems are usually related to the cleft palate, hearing loss, and in some instances, problems related to tracheostomy.

Stickler syndrome is a genetically heterogeneous disorder, meaning that mutations of different genes can cause the same clinical fea-

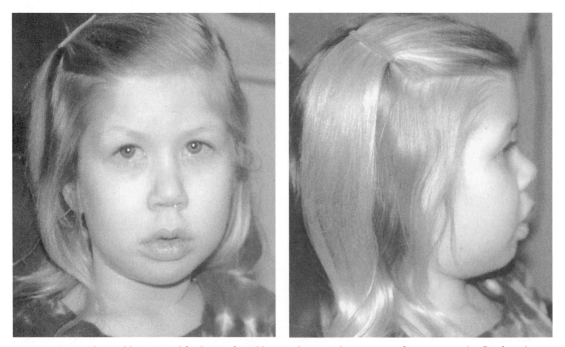

Figure 4–5. This girl has typical findings of Stickler syndrome. Characteristic features are the flat facial profile, small nose and flat nasal bridge. She was born with Pierre Robin sequence.

tures. At least four different genes may cause a form of Stickler syndrome. The most common mutation is that of a gene responsible for a particular collagen, collagen 11A1, a ubiquitous protein present in the craniofacial skeleton, the eye, and cartilage (Snead & Yates, 1999; Spranger, 1998). Clinical testing is available for gene collagen 11A1 mutations, but if negative, these tests do not exclude the other genetic causes of Stickler syndrome. Therefore, diagnosis is generally made by clinical evaluation.

Velocardiofacial Syndrome (VCF)

Velocardiofacial syndrome is a relatively common condition with an incidence of approximately 1 in 4000 live births (Demczuk & Aurias, 1995; Motzkin, Marion, Goldberg, Shprintzen, & Saenger, 1993). This is a highly variable condition; more than 160 different associated features have been reported. The most common anomalies are palate anomalies (cleft palate and/or velopharyngeal insufficiency), congenital heart defects, and dysmorphic facial features (Shprintzen et al., 1978).

The most common characteristic of velocardiofacial syndrome is velopharyngeal insufficiency. In the Velopharyngeal Insufficiency Clinic at Cincinnati Children's Hospital, velocardiofacial syndrome is diagnosed in about 20% of individuals with velopharyngeal insufficiency in the absence of overt cleft palate. Velocardiofacial syndrome is also the second most common cause of cleft palate only. The cleft palate is associated with Pierre Robin sequence; therefore, these infants must be monitored for respiratory and feeding complications.

Approximately 50% of all children with velocardiofacial syndrome followed in the Division of Human Genetics at Children's Hospital Medical Center of Cincinnati are born with congenital heart defects. These specific defects affect the formation of the aorta, the ventricular septum (the tissue that separates the two lower chambers of the heart), the pulmonary artery,

and the pulmonary valve. This group of heart defects seen in velocardiofacial syndrome is called a *conotruncal defect*, because of their location and development. In the population of children born with conotruncal heart defects, 10 to 15% have a deletion of chromosome 22 and probable velocardiofacial syndrome (Motzkin et al., 1993).

In addition to the cardiac anomalies, vascular anomalies have also been reported with velocardiotacial syndrome. In particular, tortuosity and medial displacement of the carotid arteries is commonly seen in this population (D'Antonio & Marsh, 1987; Finkelstein et al., 1993; Mac-Kenzie-Stepner et al., 1987; Ross, Witzel, Armstrong, & Thomson, 1996). The pulsation of the carotid arteries can often be viewed on the pharyngeal wall through nasopharyngoscopy. Knowledge of this syndrome and the potential for displacement of the carotid arteries in the posterior pharyngeal wall is important for the surgeon prior to placement of a pharyngeal flap, a surgical procedure that is discussed in Chapter 18.

The facial characteristics associated with velocardiofacial syndrome include microcephaly, narrow *palpebral fissures* (eye slits), a wide nasal root, a bulbous nasal tip, vertical maxillary excess, a thin upper lip, a long face, *micrognathia* (small mandible) and minor auricular anomalies (Figures 4–6 and 4–7). Additional physical features include short stature, usually below the 10th percentile, and thin, tapered fingers.

Individuals with velocardiofacial syndrome can have a myriad of medical problems, which can include kidney or urinary tract anomalies, obesity, and failure to thrive in infancy. A subgroup of patients will have what is termed the DiGeorge sequence (Stevens et al., 1990). This condition is characterized by not only the conotruncal heart defects, but also hypoplasia or absence of the thymus (the organ in the chest which is the source of T-lymphocytes) and absence or hypoplasia of the parathyroid glands (glands responsible for making parathyroid

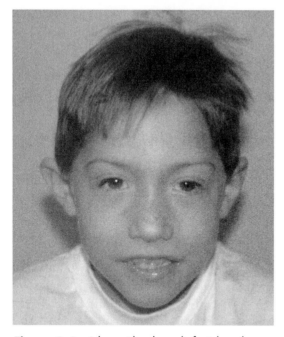

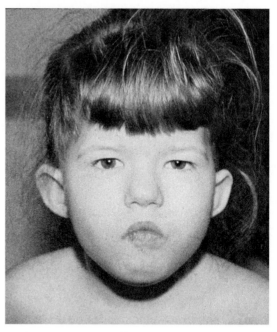

Figure 4–6. A boy with velocardiofacial syndrome. Note the narrow face and broad nasal tip.

Figure 4–7. A girl with velocardiofacial syndrome. She has a long oval face, broad nasal tip, prominent brow, and small mouth.

hormone, which helps regulate calcium levels in the blood). These individuals can have seizures from hypocalcemia and serious infections from abnormal T-lymphocyte function and abnormal immune response (Motzkin, Marion, Goldberg, Shprintzen, & Saenger, 1993; Ryan et al., 1997).

Infants with velocardiofacial syndrome often demonstrate hypotonia, and oral apraxia is often evident, even in early infancy. Most children will have problems with sucking because of poor oral-motor skills and abnormal palate function. Later feeding problems include difficulty with chewing and swallowing. Drooling is often noted due to difficulty in handling oral secretions. When speech develops, articulation disorders are common and are caused by a combination of velopharyngeal insufficiency or incompetence, and oral-motor dysfunction.

If a pharyngoplasty is needed for velopharyngeal dysfunction, the prognosis for total correction is somewhat guarded due to the pharyngeal hypotonia and oral-motor problems.

Developmental disabilities are characteristic for velocardiofacial syndrome. Most individuals with this disorder will have some degree of learning problems or mental retardation (Kok & Solman, 1995; Swillen et al., 1997). Intelligence tends to be in the low normal range (Golding-Kushner, Weller, & Shprintzen, 1985), although mild to moderate mental retardation is relatively common (Ryan et al., 1997). Language and learning disabilities are also common, with most patients having difficulty with reading comprehension and extemporaneous speech (Golding-Kushner et al., 1985). Educational goals must therefore focus on the development of language and communication skills.

Specific abnormalities of behavior and socialization are common with velocardiofacial syndrome (Swillen et al., 1999). In addition, psychiatric problems are seen in many individuals with this syndrome. There is an increased incidence of schizophrenia and schizo-affective disorders, often beginning in the second decade (Heineman-de Boer, Van Haelst, Cordia-de Haan, & Beemer, 1999; Karayiorgou et al., 1995). In addition, there is an increased incidence of depression, usually related to bipolar illness. Exactly how these conditions are related to velocardiofacial syndrome has yet to be determined.

Velocardiofacial syndrome has been shown to be associated with a 22q11 deletion, which is a deletion of part of band 11 on the long arm of chromosome 22. This is determined through *fluorescence in situ hybridization (FISH) techniques*. Although most individuals with velocardiofacial syndrome demonstrate this deletion, approximately 10% of patients with velocardiofacial syndrome do not have a demonstrable deletion on chromosome 22. It is assumed that these individuals have a mutation or genetic rearrangement of the critical gene or genes in the velocardiofacial syndrome region on chromosome 22 that cannot be detected by routine established diagnostic tests. Most identified cases represent new deletions with no prior family history, but in 10–20% of cases, one of the parents will have a deletion of chromosome 22 and will have phenotypic features of velocardiofacial syndrome.

The diagnosis of velocardiofacial syndrome is usually straightforward. However, any child with a cleft palate or velopharyngeal insufficiency and a congenital heart defect should be evaluated for this disorder. Not all patients have the classic presentation, and some patients may present with just velopharyngeal insufficiency and learning disabilities. Also, any child with a conotruncal heart defect should be tested for a deletion on chromosome 22 as well (Ryan et al., 1997).

Fetal Alcohol Syndrome (FAS)

The efforts of Jones and Smith (1973) demonstrated the teratogenic potential of alcohol, and they described the specific pattern of characteristics associated with in utero alcohol exposure. These investigators recognized that alcohol exposure in utero was a common occurrence and that the effects could be very severe and debilitating for the fetus. This condition, called fetal alcohol syndrome, is caused by in utero exposure to significant amounts of alcohol during gestation, with the most sensitive period of exposure being the first trimester of pregnancy, although significant exposure at any time during pregnancy can have adverse effects. It is generally accepted that women who take two alcoholic drinks daily are at risk for having babies with smaller birth size; however, with the intake of between four and six drinks per day, many additional clinical features become apparent (Jones, 1997).

Fetal alcohol syndrome is one of the more common causes of Pierre Robin sequence and cleft palate. It can also be associated with cleft lip, with or without cleft palate. The most striking features of children with fetal alcohol syndrome are small size at birth, microcephaly, short *palpebral fissures* (eye slits), short nose, flat philtrum, and thin upper lip. Congenital heart defects are relatively common, with the most common anomalies being *ventricular septal defect* (VSD), which is discontinuity of tissue that separates the lower chambers of the heart, and *atrial septal defect* (ASD), which is discontinuity in the tissue that separates the upper chambers of the heart.

Fetal alcohol syndrome is a common cause of mental retardation (Jones, 1986). The average intelligence quotient in this population has been estimated to be 63 (Jones, 1997). In addition to developmental disabilities, older children with fetal alcohol syndrome often have severe behavior problems with hyperactivity, distractibility, poor judgment, and difficulty interpreting social cues (Jones, 1997; Streissguth et al., 1991).

Genetics of Craniosynostosis

Craniosynostosis is the premature fusion of one or more cranial sutures. Although not as common as cleft lip or cleft palate, it is nonetheless a relatively common condition, with an incidence of 1 in 2000 to 1 in 2500 live births (Hunter & Rudd, 1976, 1977). Most cases are isolated, limited to the fusion of a single suture with no other associated anomalies, and these cases are usually sporadic without a genetic etiology. When craniosynostosis involves more than one suture or if there are associated congenital anomalies, the likelihood that there is an underlying syndrome or genetic etiology is greatly increased.

Craniosynostosis is a feature in over 150 syndromes (Cohen, 1979, 1991; Gorlin et al., 1990). Craniosynostosis syndromes include involvement of multiple cranial sutures and additional clinical features (Table 4–4). Most are inherited in an autosomal dominant manner. Recently, the genes that cause the common craniosynostosis syndromes have been

TABLE 4–4. Common craniosynostosis syndromes.[1]

Syndrome	Craniofacial Features	Gene (Chromosome)	Additional Anomalies
Crouzon syndrome	Coronal synostosis Shallow orbits Hypertelorism Exophthalmos	FGFR2 (10q26)	Occasional hydrocephalus Occasional hearing loss
Apert syndrome	Coronal synostosis Hypertelorism Beaked nose Occasional cleft palate Occasional upper airway obstruction	FGFR2 (10q26)	Syndactyly Mental retardation

Pfeiffer syndrome	Coronal synostosis
	Cloverleaf skull (type 2)
	Shallow orbits
	Hypertelorism
	Exophthalmos
		FGFR1
		(8p11.2- p11.1)
		
		FGFR2 (10q26)
			Broad toes and thumbs
			Mild syndactyly
			Hearing loss
			Mental retardation
			   (type 2 and type 3)
			Tracheal anomalies
			   (type 2 and type 3)

Saethre-Chotzen syndrome	Coronal synostosis
	Hypertelorism
	Ptosis
	Down slanting
	   palpebral fissures
	Dysplastic ears
	Occasional cleft
	   palate
		TWIST gene (7p21)	Broad thumbs and great
			   toes
			Mild syndactyly
			Occasional congenital
			   heart defect

[1]All of the listed disorders are autosomal dominant.

identified. Most fall within the category of what are called the fibroblast growth factor receptors. These receptors, which are located on the cell surface, bind the fibroblast growth factors, which help to regulate cell proliferation, differentiation, and migration (Robin, 1999; Wilkie, 1997).

The premature fusion of the cranial suture lines in craniosynostosis causes the skull to grow abnormally, resulting an abnormally shaped head. The resultant distortion of the skull depends on the sutures that are involved. If the sagittal suture is involved, the lateral growth of the skull will be prevented. Therefore, the growth occurs in an anterior-posterior (AP) direction, resulting in frontal bossing and *scaphacephaly*, where the skull is oblong from front to back. On the other hand, if the coronal suture is involved, the skull cannot expand in the AP direction, causing *brachycephaly*, which is a short skull. When multiple sutures are involved, there may be asymmetry of the skull, called *plagiocephaly. Dolichocephaly* is the long, narrow skull that is often seen with prematurity.

Children with isolated craniosynostosis have no associated malformations and have an excellent prognosis with regard to health, growth, and neurodevelopment. The prognosis for children who have a craniosynostosis syndrome is more guarded and depends on the specific syndrome diagnosed. If the cranium impairs brain development or there is an increase in intracranial pressure (ICP), mental retardation can result. Craniotomy and skull reshaping procedures are often required, both for normal brain development and function, and also to improve the aesthetics.

Craniosynostosis Syndromes

Saethre-Chotzen Syndrome

Saethre-Chotzen syndrome (Figure 4–8) is probably the most common craniosynostosis

syndrome, although many individuals with this disorder do not have craniosynostosis. The clinical features can be quite variable, but the most common presenting features are coronal synostosis, *ptosis* or drooping of the eyelids, midface hypoplasia, mild external ear anomalies, and mild digit anomalies, including mild syndactyly, mild brachydactyly or short fingers, and in some individuals broad thumbs and/or great toes with medial deviation of the great toes. A small number of individuals will have cleft palate or submucous cleft palate. Recently, it has been postulated that more severely affected individuals, especially those with developmental disabilities and/or cleft palate, have a complete or partial deletion of the TWIST gene, whereas more mildly affected individuals have point mutations of the gene (mutations involving one or a limited number of nucleotides) (Johnson et al., 1998; Robin, 1999).

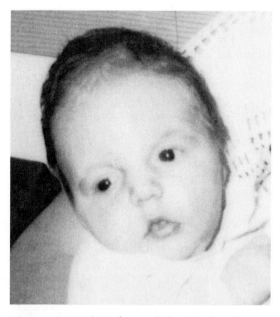

Figure 4–8. This infant male has Saethre-Chotzen syndrome. He has a depressed nasal bridge and downslanting palpebral fissures.

Intelligence in Saethre-Chotzen syndrome is usually normal, although there is an increased risk for developmental disabilities, including mental retardation. Most patients do not have significant speech or language difficulties, unless there are extenuating factors including cleft palate or mental retardation.

Crouzon Syndrome

Crouzon syndrome (Figure 4–9) is another common craniosynostosis syndrome. The major clinical characteristics are limited to cranial and facial involvement. The major features are craniosynostosis, usually involving the coronal sutures. The orbits are shallow, causing *exophthalmos*, or protrusion of the eyeballs. There is also hypertelorism, strabismus, and midface hypoplasia. Development is usually normal, but there is a higher incidence of mental retardation. Developmental disabilities can be related to brain anomalies identified in some pa-

tients including hydrocephalus and agenesis of the corpus callosum. Cleft palate and submucous cleft palate are seen in some patients, but these are uncommon findings (Jones, 1997; Robin, 1999).

Apert Syndrome

Individuals with Apert syndrome (Figure 4–10) tend to look remarkably like patients with Crouzon syndrome, with the exception that there are serious associated hand and foot anomalies. The cranial and facial involvement can be very similar to that seen in Crouzon syndrome, but the exophthalmos tends to be less pronounced, although the midface hypoplasia is similar (Cohen & Kreiborg, 1992; Jones, 1997). The nose is beaked, and strabismus is frequently seen. The palate is often narrow and cleft palate is seen more frequently in Apert syndrome than in Crouzon syndrome. The up-

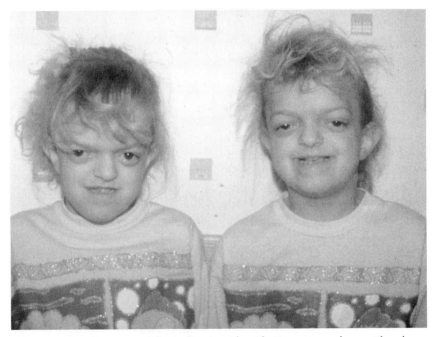

Figure 4–9. Monozyotic (identical) twin girls with Crouzon syndrome. They have shallow orbits with prominent eyes.

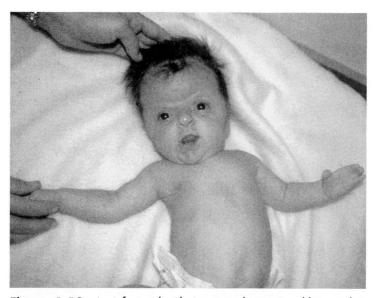

Figure 4–10. An infant girl with Apert syndrome. In addition to her craniosynostosis, she has syndactyly (webbing) of the fingers and toes of all four extremities.

per nasal and pharyngeal airway may be narrowed, causing respiratory obstruction and hyponasality in some patients. The main feature distinguishing these syndromes, however, is that individuals with Apert syndrome often have a mittenlike *syndactyly*, or webbing of the fingers of the fingers and toes. The webbing may be of soft tissue, but it often includes the bone as well.

Most patients with Apert syndrome have some degree of developmental disability. Although normal intelligence is found in some patients, many others have mild to moderate mental retardation. Speech disorders are common, with articulation defects presenting secondary to the small oral cavity, narrow palate, and hyponasality secondary to upper airway obstruction.

Pfeiffer Syndrome

Pfeiffer syndrome (Figure 4–11) is a genetically heterogeneous autosomal dominant cran-iosynostosis syndrome, with mutations being identified in two different fibroblast growth factor receptor genes. Most are new mutations, especially those with Pfeiffer syndrome type 2 or type 3. The severity and degree of craniofacial involvement and associated anomalies depends on the specific gene mutation (Plomp et al., 1998).

In most patients with classic Pfeiffer syndrome, or Pfieffer syndrome type 1, the common craniofacial features are coronal craniosynostosis, midface hypoplasia, shallow orbits with exophthalmos, and hypertelorism (Figure 4–11). Limb anomalies consist of broad thumbs and great toes with variable degrees of mild syndactyly. Hearing loss has also been reported (Robin, 1999). Cleft palate is seen on rare occasions and there is no association with cleft lip. Intelligence is usually normal.

In Pfeiffer syndrome type 2 and type 3, the clinical features are much more pronounced and severe. The craniosynostosis may involve multiple sutures, giving the skull a cloverleaf

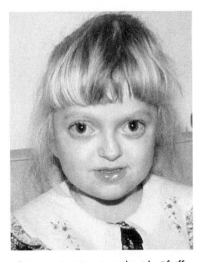

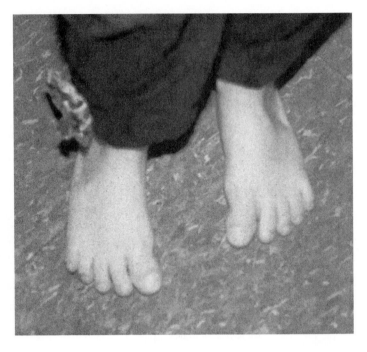

Figure 4–11. A girl with Pfeiffer syndrome. She has shallow orbits similar to those seen in Crouzon syndrome and also has broad and deviated great toes.

appearance, hence the term "cloverleaf skull." The exophthalmos is more pronounced and the midface hypoplasia more severe. Hearing loss is common. There can be severe airway compromise from tracheal anomalies and upper airway stenosis (Stone, Trevenen, Mitchell, & Rudd, 1990). Mental retardation is seen in almost all children with Pfeiffer syndrome type 2 and type 3 and is often severe. Death in early childhood is common, especially in Pfeiffer syndrome type 2, which is more likely to be associated with cloverleaf skull and more serious upper airway obstruction.

Miscellaneous Syndromes

Hemifacial Microsomia (Oculoauriculovertebral Dysplasia)

Hemifacial microsomia (Figure 4–12) is a condition with numerous names, most of which are descriptive. It is also known as oculoauriculovertebral dysplasia, facio-auriculo-vertebral spectrum, and there is a variant called the Goldenhar syndrome. This is a relatively common multiple anomaly disorder with a birth incidence of 1 in 3000 to 5000 live births (Jones, 1997). Most cases appear to be sporadic, but there are rare reports of more than one affected first-degree family member. Most cases have unilateral involvement, but in 30% of the cases, bilateral hemifacial microsomia can be demonstrated (Gorlin et al., 1990). The right side tends to be affected more often than the left side and boys are affected more frequently than girls (Jones, 1997).

The primary features of hemifacial microsomia include facial asymmetry due to unilateral hypoplasia. This causes malar, maxillary, and especially mandibular hypoplasia on the affected side. With the mandibular involvement, there is hypoplasia of the mandibular ramus and often dysplasia or aplasia of the temporo-

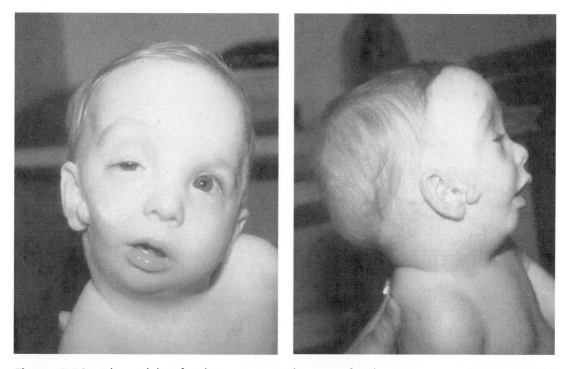

Figure 4–12. A boy with hemifacial microsomia. He has severe facial asymmetry exacerbated by cervical spine abnormalitites and fusion. The lateral view shows severe dysplasia of the right ear and an ear tag.

mandibular joint, limiting the excursion of the mandible and the opening of the mouth. There can also be weakness of cranial nerve VII on the affected side.

There is usually ear involvement on the affected side, ranging from mild aplasia to *anotia* with absence of the external auditory canal. Anomalies of the eyes are often noted, including *colobomas* of the upper eyelid, *epibulbar lipodermoids* (fatty tissue) of the eyes (distinguishing the Goldenhar syndrome), colobomas of the retina, and *microphthalmia* (Figure 4–12).

Brain anomalies that can be seen in this population include hydrocephalus, *encephalocele* (a congenital gap in the skull with herniation of brain tissue into the nose or palate), absence of the corpus callosum, and cell migration abnormalities. Vertebral anomalies are found in about 15% of cases, and usually involve the cervical vertebrae, although any segment of the spine may be affected. Heart defects also can be found with this syndrome and can be very serious, leading to significant morbidity. Some patients have also been found to have kidney abnormalities. Cleft lip and/or cleft palate are seen in about 15% of patients with hemifacial microsomia.

Although most patients have normal intelligence, learning disabilities are common in this population. Mental retardation may also be seen, and is more likely in patients with structural brain anomalies. Speech disorders are common, and contributing factors are orofacial clefts, cranial nerve VII weakness, inability to completely open the mouth, and, in some cases, cleft palate or unilateral velar paresis.

CHARGE Association

CHARGE association is a multiple congenital anomaly disorder that consists of statistically related malformations, although the etiology is not known. CHARGE is an acronym for *c*oloboma, *h*eart defect, choanal *a*tresia, *r*etarded growth and/or development, *g*enitourinary anomalies, and *e*ar anomalies and/or deafness. In order for an individual to have CHARGE association, at least four of the six clinical features must be present, and at least one of these features must be the presence of coloboma and/or choanal atresia (Pagon, Graham, Zonana, & Yong, 1981).

The colobomas usually affect the retina of the eye, and many children have significant visual impairment as a result. The heart defects are often very serious and life threatening. Genitourinary anomalies are usually related to *micropenis* (small penis) or *cryptorchidism* (undescended testicles) in males. External ear anomalies and deafness are very common as well. Brain anomalies also are very common and include abnormalities or absence of the pituitary gland that affect growth and genitourinary development. Although some individuals with CHARGE association have normal intelligence, mental retardation is seen in most patients and is often severe to profound. Cleft lip and/or cleft palate is also seen in many patients with CHARGE association (Blake et al., 1998).

Speech and language management depends on the identification of associated medical complications. Speech and language disorders related to clefts are often complicated by the coexistence of mental retardation and deafness.

Treacher Collins Syndrome

Although not a common disorder, Treacher Collins syndrome (Figure 4–13) is an autosomal dominant condition with variable expressivity. This variability can be seen within a family, making it difficult to predict outcome for offspring of affected individuals. The gene that

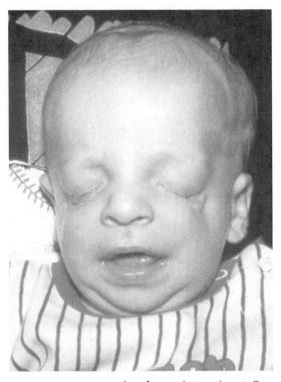

Figure 4–13. A male infant with Treacher Collins syndrome. He has micrognathia, severe hypoplasia of the zygomatic arches, and secondary low-set ears and downslanting palpebral fissures.

causes Treacher Collins syndrome has been mapped to the long arm of chromosome 5 (5q32-q33.3) (Dixon et al., 1992).

The classic features of Treacher Collins syndrome include downward slanting palpebral fissures, colobomas of the lower eyelids, microtia or small dysplastic ears, hypoplastic zygomatic arches, and macrostomia or large mouth (Figure 4–13). Conductive hearing loss is extremely common because of frequent middle-ear anomalies. There is also significant malar hypoplasia (Dixon, 1995). Treacher Collins syndrome usually includes Pierre Robin sequence, although most individuals with this condition do not have clefts, despite having pronounced micrognathia.

Intelligence is usually normal in this population. Speech disorders are common because of the hearing loss and micrognathia. The speech disorders are exacerbated when a cleft palate is present and there is also airway obstruction.

Beckwith-Wiedemann Syndrome

The Beckwith-Wiedemann syndrome (Figure 4–14) is a genetic disorder that has as its primary features prenatal and postnatal overgrowth, neonatal *hypoglycemia*, or low blood sugar, macroglossia or large tongue, and coarse facial features (Cohen, 1998). Often patients with Beckwith-Wiedemann syndrome have *hemihypertrophy* (Hoyme et al., 1998), where one side of the body grows faster than the other side, leading to asymmetry. Some individuals with this condition are also born with umbilical hernia or even an *omphalocele*, where part of the intestines are outside of the abdomen in the region of the umbilical cord. As noted, children with Beckwith-Wiedemann syndrome are usually born large for gestational age, some may even be more than 10 pounds at birth. They also are at risk for severe hypoglycemia, which can be life threatening and if blood sugar is low enough can result in seizures. Growth tends to be somewhat accelerated during early childhood. One very helpful diagnostic feature is the presence of macroglossia (Cohen, 1998). The tongue is sometimes large enough to interfere with normal breathing, leading to a Pierre Robin sequence (Figure 4–14). Rarely, a child with Beckwith-Wiedemann syndrome will have a cleft palate.

Children with Beckwith-Wiedemann syndrome have a significant risk to develop Wilms tumor, a malignant tumor of the kidney, and malignant tumors in the abdomen, including a liver tumor called hepatoblastoma (DeBaun, Siegel, & Choyke, 1998; DeBaun & Tucker, 1998; Hoyme et al., 1998; Schneid et al., 1997). The risk for developing such tumors is between 5% and 8%, with most cases occurring

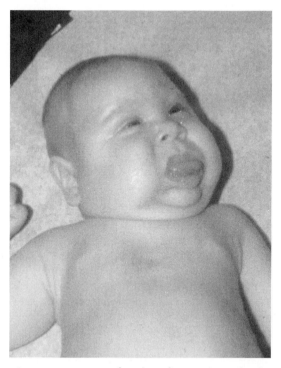

Figure 4–14. A female infant with Beckwith-Wiedemann syndrome. Note the macroglossia (large tongue), which can cause respiratory problems, eating difficulties, and speech problems.

before 8 years. For this reason, each child with Beckwith-Wiedemann syndrome is closely followed for the development of these tumors with renal and abdominal ultrasound examinations at least every 4 months.

The genetic etiology of Beckwith-Wiedemann syndrome appears to be complex. This is a genetically heterogeneous disorder, although the gene is located on the short arm of chromosome 11. Some children have been found to have a duplication of a portion of chromosome 11 (11p15.5) as the cause of their Beckwith-Wiedemann syndrome. For some individuals, the disorder is caused by inheriting both copies of chromosome 11 from the father (paternal disomy) with no maternal chromosome 11 contribution. In other cases, this is an autosomal dominant disorder (Cohen, 1998). Development in Beckwith-Wiedemann syndrome is usually normal. However, children with duplication of chromosome 11p15.5 usually have developmental delays or mental retardation. There is also a risk for developmental disabilities if neonatal hypoglycemia is prolonged. The large tongue may also contribute to obstructive respiratory problems, eating disorders, and abnormal cranial and dental growth and development, including *prognathism* (having a large mandible). For these reasons, some children with Beckwith-Wiedemann syndrome require surgical reduction of the tongue.

Language disorders may be associated with cognitive impairment and speech is usually affected by the macroglossia. Resonance can be affected not only by the history of cleft palate, but also by the size of the tongue, which can tend to block the transmission of acoustic energy in the oral cavity.

Summary

Patients who present with craniofacial anomalies should be seen for a complete genetics evaluation. This is important so that an appropriate diagnosis can be made and recurrence risks can be determined. Identification of a genetic syndrome is also important because it allows the physician to counsel the family regarding the natural course of the disorder and the potential medical, developmental, and communication problems that are associated with the syndrome. Armed with this knowledge, the family, in collaboration with the medical professionals from the craniofacial team, can plan appropriate medical, surgical, therapeutic, and educational interventions to achieve the best possible outcome.

References

Blake, K. D., Davenport, S. L., Hall, B. D., Hefner, M. A., Pagon, R. A., Williams, M. S., Lin, A. E., &

Graham, J. M., Jr. (1998). CHARGE association: An update and review for the primary pediatrician. *Clinical Pediatrics, 37*(3), 159–173.

Cary, J. C., Stevens, C. A., & Haskins, R. (1992). Craniofacial malformations and their syndromes: An overview for the speech and hearing practitioner. *Clinical Communication Disorders, 2*(4), 59–72.

Cohen, M. (1998). Perspectives in overgrowth syndromes. *American Journal of Medical Genetics, 79,* 234–237.

Cohen, M. M., Jr. (1979). Craniosynostosis and syndromes with craniosynostosis: Incidence, genetics, penetrance, variability, and new syndrome updating. *Birth Defects Original Article Series, 15*(5B), 13–63.

Cohen, M. M., Jr. (1991). Etiopathogenesis of craniosynostosis. *Neurosurgery Clinics of North America, 2*(3), 507–513.

Cohen, M. M., Jr., & Kreiborg, S. (1992). Upper and lower airway compromise in the Apert syndrome. *American Journal of Medical Genetics, 44*(1), 90–93.

D'Antonio, L. D., & Marsh, J. L. (1987). Abnormal carotid arteries in the velocardiofacial syndrome [Letter]. *Plastic and Reconstructive Surgery, 80*(3), 471–472.

DeBaun, M. R., Siegel, M. J., & Choyke, P. L. (1998). Nephromegaly in infancy and early childhood: A risk factor for Wilms tumor in Beckwith-Wiedemann syndrome [see Comments]. *Journal of Pediatrics, 132*(3, Pt. 1), 401–404.

DeBaun, M. R., & Tucker, M. A. (1998). Risk of cancer during the first four years of life in children from The Beckwith-Wiedemann Syndrome Registry [see Comments]. *Journal of Pediatrics, 132*(3, Pt. 1), 398–400.

Demczuk, S., & Aurias, A. (1995). DiGeorge syndrome and related syndromes associated with 22q11.2 deletions. A review. *Annales de Genetique, 38*(2), 59–76.

Dixon, M. J. (1995). Treacher Collins syndrome. *Journal of Medical Genetics, 32*(10), 806–808.

Dixon, M. J., Dixon, J., Raskova, D., Le Beau, M. M., Williamson, R., Klinger, K., & Landes, G. M. (1992). Genetic and physical mapping of the Treacher Collins syndrome locus: Refinement of the localization to chromosome 5q32-33.2. *Human Molecular Genetics, 1*(4), 249–253.

Finkelstein, Y., Zohar, Y., Nachmani, A., Talmi, Y. P., Lerner, M. A., Hauben, D. J., & Frydman, M.

(1993). The otolaryngologist and the patient with velocardiofacial syndrome. *Archives of Otolaryngology—Head and Neck Surgery, 119*(5), 563–569.

Fraser, F. C. (1970). The genetics of cleft lip and cleft palate. *American Journal of Human Genetics, 22*(3), 336–352.

Golding-Kushner, K. J., Weller, G., & Shprintzen, R. J. (1985). Velo-cardio-facial syndrome: Language and psychological profiles. *Journal of Craniofacial Genetics and Developmental Biology, 5*(3), 259–266.

Goodship, J., Platt, J., Smith, R., & Burn, J. (1991). A male with type I orofaciodigital syndrome. *Journal of Medical Genetics, 28*(10), 691–694.

Gorlin, R., Cohen, M. J., & Levin, L. (1990). *Syndromes of the head and neck* (3rd ed.). New York: Oxford University Press.

Heineman-de Boer, J. A., Van Haelst, M. J., Cordia-de Haan, M., & Beemer, F. A. (1999). Behavior problems and personality aspects of 40 children with velo-cardio-facial syndrome. *Genetic Counselling, 10*(1), 89–93.

Hoyme, H. E., Seaver, L. H., Jones, K. L., Procopio, F., Crooks, W., & Feingold, M. (1998). Isolated hemi-hyperplasia (hemihypertrophy): Report of a prospective multicenter study of the incidence of neoplasia and review. *American Journal of Human Genetics, 79*(4), 274–278.

Hunter, A. G., & Rudd, N. L. (1976). Craniosynostosis. I. Sagittal synostosis: Its genetics and associated clinical findings in 214 patients who lacked involvement of the coronal suture(s). *Teratology, 14*(2), 185–193.

Hunter, A. G., & Rudd, N. L. (1977). Craniosynostosis. II. Coronal synostosis: Its familial characteristics and associated clinical findings in 109 patients lacking bilateral polysyndactyly or syndactyly. *Teratology, 15*(3), 301–309.

Johnson, D., Horsley, S. W., Moloney, D. M., Oldridge, M., Twigg, S. R., Walsh, S., Barrow, M., Njolstad, P. R., Kunz, J., Ashworth, G. J., Wall, S. A., Kearney, L., & Wilkie, A. O. (1998). A comprehensive screen for TWIST mutations in patients with craniosynostosis identifies a new microdeletion syndrome of chromosome band 7p21.1 [see Comments]. *American Journal of Human Genetics, 63*(5), 1282–1293.

Jones, K. L. (1986). Fetal alcohol syndrome. *Pediatric Development, 8*(4), 122–126.

Jones, K. (1997). *Smith's recognizable patterns of human malformation*. (5th ed.). Philadelphia: W. B. Saunders Company.

Jones, K. L., & Smith, D. W. (1973). Recognition of the fetal alcohol syndrome in early infancy. *Lancet, 2*(7836), 999–1001.

Karayiorgou, M., Morris, M. A., Morrow, B., Shprintzen, R. J., Goldberg, R., Borrow, J., Gos, A., Nestadt, G., Wolyniec, P. S., Lasseter, V. K., & et al. (1995). Schizophrenia susceptibility associated with interstitial deletions of chromosome 22q11. *Proceedings of the National Academy of Sciences of the United States of America, 92*(17), 7612–7616.

Kok, L. L., & Solman, R. T. (1995). Velocardiofacial syndrome: Learning difficulties and intervention. *Journal of Medical Genetics, 32*(8), 612–618.

Lidral, A. C., Romitti, P. A., Basart, A. M., Doetschman, T., Leysens, N. J., Daack-Hirsch, S., Semina, E. V., Johnson, L. R., Machida, J., Burds, A., Parnell, T. J., Rubenstein, J. L., & Murray, J. C. (1998). Association of MSX1 and TGFB3 with nonsyndromic clefting in humans. *American Journal of Human Genetics, 63*(2), 557–568.

MacKenzie-Stepner, K., Witzel, M. A., Stringer, D. A., Lindsay, W. K., Munro, I. R., & Hughes, H. (1987). Abnormal carotid arteries in the velocardiofacial syndrome: A report of three cases. *Plastic and Reconstructive Surgery, 80*(3), 347–351.

Motzkin, B., Marion, R., Goldberg, R., Shprintzen, R., & Saenger, P. (1993). Variable phenotypes in velocardiofacial syndrome with chromosomal deletion. *Journal of Pediatrics, 123*(3), 406–410.

Murray, J. C. (1995). Face facts: Genes, environment, and clefts [Editorial; Comment]. *American Journal of Human Genetics, 57*(2), 227–232.

Murray, J. C., Nishimura, D. Y., Buetow, K. H., Ardinger, H. H., Spence, M. A., Sparkes, R. S., Falk, R. E., Falk, P. M., Gardner, R. J., Harkness, E. M., & et al. (1990). Linkage of an autosomal dominant clefting syndrome (Van der Woude) to loci on chromosome 1q. *American Journal of Human Genetics, 46*(3), 486–491.

Naiglin, L., Clayton, J., Gazagne, C., Dallongeville, F., Malecaze, F., & Calvas, P. (1999). Familial high myopia: Evidence of an autosomal dominant mode of inheritance and genetic heterogeneity. *Annales de Genetique, 42*(3), 140–146.

Nowak, C. B. (1998). Genetics and hearing loss: A review of Stickler syndrome. *Journal of Communication Disorders, 31*(5), 437–453, 453–454.

Pagon, R. A., Graham, J. M., Jr., Zonana, J., & Yong, S. L. (1981). Coloboma, congenital heart disease, and choanal atresia with multiple anomalies: CHARGE association. *Journal of Pediatrics, 99*(2), 223–227.

Plomp, A. S., Hamel, B. C., Cobben, J. M., Verloes, A., Offermans, J. P., Lajeunie, E., Fryns, J. P., & de Die-Smulders, C. E. (1998). Pfeiffer syndrome type 2: Further delineation and review of the literature. *American Journal of Medical Genetics, 75*(3), 245–251.

Robin, N. H. (1999). Molecular genetic advances in understanding craniosynostosis. *Plastic and Reconstructive Surgery, 103*(3), 1060–1070.

Robin, N. H., Opitz, J. M., & Muenke, M. (1996). Opitz G/BBB syndrome: Clinical comparisons of families linked to Xp22 and 22q, and a review of the literature. *American Journal of Medical Genetics, 62*(3), 305–317.

Ross, D. A., Witzel, M. A., Armstrong, D. C., & Thomson, H. G. (1996). Is pharyngoplasty a risk in velocardiofacial syndrome? An assessment of medially displaced carotid arteries. *Plastic and Reconstructive Surgery, 98*(7), 1182–1190.

Ryan, A. K., Goodship, J. A., Wilson, D. I., Philip, N., Levy, A., Seidel, H., Schuffenhauer, S., Oechsler, H., Belohradsky, B., Prieur, M., Aurias, A., Raymond, F. L., Clayton-Smith, J., Hatchwell, E., McKeown, C., Beemer, F. A., Dallapiccola, B., Novelli, G., Hurst, J. A., Ignatius, J., Green, A. J., Winter, R. M., Brueton, L., Brondum-Nielsen, K., Scambler, P. J., & et al. (1997). Spectrum of clinical features associated with interstitial chromosome 22q11 deletions: A European collaborative study [see Comments]. *Journal of Medical Genetics, 34*(10), 798–804.

Schneid, H., Vazquez, M. P., Vacher, C., Gourmelen, M., Cabrol, S., & Le Bouc, Y. (1997). The Beckwith-Wiedemann syndrome phenotype and the risk of cancer. *Medical and Pediatric Oncology, 28*(6), 411–415.

Shprintzen, R. J., Goldberg, R. B., Lewin, M. L., Sidoti, E. J., Berkman, M. D., Argamaso, R. V., & Young, D. (1978). A new syndrome involving cleft palate, cardiac anomalies, typical facies, and learning disabilities: Velo-cardio-facial syndrome. *Cleft Palate Journal, 15*(1), 56–62.

Snead, M. P., & Yates, J. R. (1999). Clinical and Molecular genetics of Stickler syndrome. *Journal of Medical Genetics, 36*(5), 353–359.

Spranger, J. (1998). The type XI collagenopathies. *Pediatric Radiology, 28*(10), 745–750.

Spranger, J., Benirschke, K., Hall, J. G., Lenz, W., Lowry, R. B., Opitz, J. M., Pinsky, L., Schwarzacher, H. G., & Smith, D. W. (1982). Errors of morphogenesis: Concepts and terms. Recommendations of an international working group. *Journal of Pediatrics, 100*(1), 160–165.

Stein, J., Mulliken, J. B., Stal, S., Gasser, D. L., Malcolm, S., Winter, R., Blanton, S. H., Amos, C., Seemanova, E., & Hecht, J. T. (1995). Nonsyndromic cleft lip with or without cleft palate: Evidence of linkage to BCL3 in 17 multigenerational families [see Comments] [published erratum appears in *American Journal of Human Genetics* 1996, *59*(3), 744]. *American Journal of Human Genetics, 57*(2), 257–272.

Stevens, C. A., Carey, J. C., & Shigeoka, A. O. (1990). Di George anomaly and velocardiofacial syndrome. *Pediatrics, 85*(4), 526–530.

Stone, P., Trevenen, C. L., Mitchell, I., & Rudd, N. (1990). Congenital tracheal stenosis in Pfeiffer syndrome. *Clinical Genetics, 38*(2), 145–148.

Streissguth, A. P., Aase, J. M., Clarren, S. K., Randels, S. P., LaDue, R. A., & Smith, D. F. (1991). Fetal alcohol syndrome in adolescents and adults [see Comments]. *JAMA, 265*(15), 1961–1967.

Swillen, A., Devriendt, K., Legius, E., Eyskens, B., Dumoulin, M., Gewillig, M., & Fryns, J. P. (1997). Intelligence and psychosocial adjustment in velocardiofacial syndrome: A study of 37 children and adolescents with VCFS. *Journal of Medical Genetics, 34*(6), 453–458.

Swillen, A., Devriendt, K., Legius, E., Prinzie, P., Vogels, A., Ghesquiere, P., & Fryns, J. P. (1999). The behavioural phenotype in velo-cardio-facial syndrome (VCFS): From infancy to adolescence. *Genetic Counseling, 10*(1), 79–88.

Tomaski, S. M., Zalzal, G. H., & Saal, H. M. (1995). Airway obstruction in Pierre Robin sequence. *Laryngoscope, 105*, 111–115.

Wilkie, A. O. (1997). Craniosynostosis: Genes and mechanisms. *Human Molecular Genetics, 6*(10), 1647–1656.

Winter, R. M., & Baraitser, M. (1996). *London dysmorphology database.* London: Oxford University Press.

Wyszynski, D. F., Beaty, T. H., & Maestri, N. E. (1996). Genetics of nonsyndromic oral clefts revisited. *Cleft Palate Craniofacial Journal, 33*(5), 406–417.

PART II

Problems Associated With Clefts and Craniofacial Anomalies

CHAPTER

Feeding Problems of Infants With Cleft Lip/Palate or Craniofacial Anomalies

Claire K. Miller, M.S.
Ann W. Kummer, Ph.D.

CONTENTS

The inability to feed efficiently can be an immediate problem for the infant born with cleft lip and/or palate. An opening in the lip and/or palate can have a profound effect on oral-motor mechanics, specifically in regard to the ability to generate the intraoral pressure necessary for effective sucking during infant feeding. Generally, the more extensive the cleft, the greater the chance for significant oral feeding problems and consequently poor volume of oral intake. The volume of intake must be sufficient for adequate weight gain prior to the surgical repair of lip/palatal clefts. Therefore, early identification of feeding problems and subsequent modifications in the feeding method must be made so that the infant can receive adequate nutrition for growth.

This chapter focuses upon the disruptions in the normal feeding process that occur secondary to clefts and craniofacial anomalies. Evaluation of feeding difficulties and the importance of individualizing modifications to the feeding method are discussed.

Function of Feeding

Feeding, which is accomplished entirely by sucking in early infancy, provides nourishment for normal growth and development. The feeding process provides satisfaction from hunger and helps the infant to maintain homeostasis. The reflexive activity of both nutritive and non-nutritive sucking helps the infant with state regulation. Feeding serves other important functions as well, including opportunities for sensory and motor stimulation, mother-infant bonding, and oral-motor skill development.

Feeding provides the infant with important sensory stimulation. The tactile input to the mouth initiates both the rooting and suck-swallow response in neurologically intact infants. The sensory input eliciting the sucking reflex represents the primary step in initiation of the suck-swallow-breathe synchrony central to the infant feeding process. The activity of feeding also serves as an important part of the bonding process between the caregiver and infant. The caregiver spends time holding and cuddling the infant during the feeding. In addition to the physical contact, there is mutual eye contact during feeding. The feeder learns to identify the infant's cues during feeding and respond appropriately. Mutual eye contact and the vocalizations of the parent help the infant to gain some of the prerequisite skills for communication development. The behaviors of both the caretaker and infant during feeding have been shown to contribute significantly to the overall success of the feeding interaction as well as the feeding performance (Meyer, et al., 1994).

The physical act of sucking during feeding increases overall oral movements and oral activity. Sucking requires the active use of the jaw, cheeks, lips, and tongue. The active movement of these oral structures during feeding helps to provide a basis for the movements that are later required for more mature feeding skills (Morris & Klein, 1987). The infant uses sucking to satiate hunger and quickly learns to use sucking for calming and self-regulation as well.

In summary, the early experience of feeding is the foundation of important developmental functions. The presence of a cleft has the potential to interrupt the normal feeding process, which can have significant implications in regard to a successful feeding outcome. Adequacy of nutrition, caregiver interaction patterns, and oral-motor development all have the potential to be affected.

Normal Anatomy and Physiology of Infant Feeding

Oral/Pharyngeal/Laryngeal Anatomy of the Infant

There are distinct differences in location and the size of the oral, pharyngeal, and laryngeal structures of the infant as compared to the adult. The anatomic relationships of these areas change significantly during the first several months of infancy as well as during the first 2 to 3 years of life (Figure 5–1). The infant's structures are smaller and are in close proximity. As the infant grows, the structures become larger and move apart. They become supported by increased amounts of connective tissue and by complex muscle control secondary to normal maturational development of the central nervous system (Bosma, 1985).

The small size and shape of the infant's oral cavity are ideal for sucking. The infant's tongue, which is relatively large, but only half the size of the adult tongue, fills the oral cavity. The infant's buccal pads are also relatively large and stabilize the lateral walls of the oral cavity. Because the infant has not yet developed teeth, the effective vertical dimension of the oral cavity is further reduced in size, causing the tongue to rest in a more anterior position than is typically seen in the adult. The tongue tip protrudes past the alveolar ridge and maintains contact with the lower lip. The temporomandibular joint does not allow much movement of jaw due to undeveloped connective tissue, causing the mouth opening to be smaller in the infant than in the adult. All of these oral characteristics facilitate early *suckling*, characterized by extension-retraction movements of the tongue, as well as the development of more mature up-down tongue movements that are characteristic of true sucking (Arvedson & Lefton-Greif, 1996; Morris & Klein, 1987).

The pharyngeal area in the newborn is also characterized by the closeness in proximity of the structures. The soft palate is relatively large and has a large area of contact with the tongue. The tongue base, soft palate, and pharyngeal walls are all in close approximation. The inferior border of the uvula and velum rest in front of the epiglottis.

The position of the infant's larynx, which is one third the adult size, is high in the hypopharynx, residing adjacent to cervical vertebrae C-1–C-3. In comparison, the larynx in the adult is located at the C-6–C-7 vertebral level. The high position of the infant larynx causes the epiglottis to pass superiorly to the free margin of the soft palate and project into the nasopharynx. The epiglottis is tubular, proportionally narrow, and more vertical in the infant as compared to the adult.

As the infant matures, the oral cavity gradually becomes larger with concurrent mandibular growth and dental eruption. The tongue begins to descend and move back into the mouth, the tip becoming positioned behind the alveolar ridge. The increased space facilitates the development of a range of oral-motor movements for feeding as well as for speech production. The pharynx begins to elongate and the larynx begins its gradual descent from C-3 to C-6, which is complete by age 3 (Sasaki, Levine, Laitman, Phil, & Crelin, 1977).

Physiology of Normal Infant Feeding

The feeding process itself is dependent on smooth synchronization of sucking, swallowing, and breathing. Sucking and swallowing occur in phases generally described as the oral, pharyngeal, and esophageal stages of swallowing.

Oral Phase of Swallowing

The oral phase of swallowing in infants is composed of rhythmic sucking, during which the oral structures work together to stabilize the nipple, create pressure gradients for fluid flow, and control the bolus prior to swallowing initiation. The presence of the rooting reflex aids in the search for the nipple and the subsequent lip seal around the nipple. The sucking reflex is initiated as the tongue elevates to squeeze the

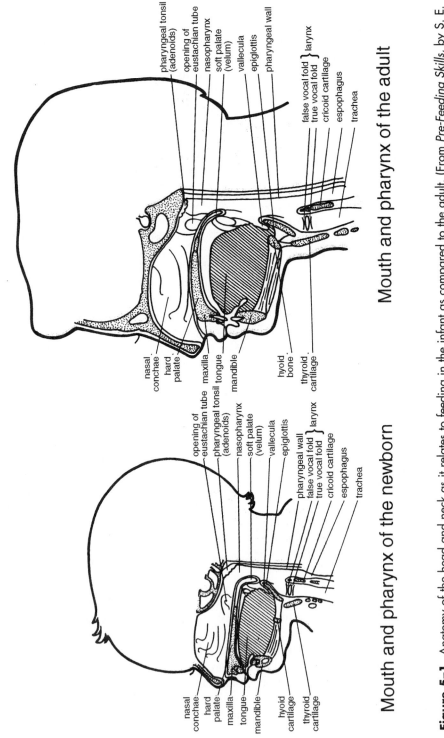
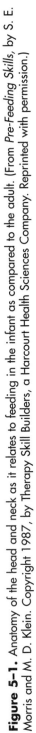

Mouth and pharynx of the adult

Mouth and pharynx of the newborn

Figure 5–1. Anatomy of the head and neck as it relates to feeding in the infant as compared to the adult. (From *Pre-Feeding Skills*, by S. E. Morris and M. D. Klein. Copyright 1987, by Therapy Skill Builders, a Harcourt Health Sciences Company. Reprinted with permission.)

nipple against the alveolar ridge and hard palate. The compression of the nipple against this bony surface creates positive pressure within the nipple and causes the release of a small amount of fluid. The infant then initiates sucking; a rhythmic forward-backward tongue motion. The tongue is cupped around the nipple and a depression in the center of the tongue forms a groove. As the tongue moves backward during sucking, the infant's jaw drops, thus enlarging the space in the oral cavity. This action generates negative pressure, resulting in suction or pulling of the milk from the nipple into the infant's oral cavity. Therefore, both nipple compression and the generation of negative pressure suction are important for normal feeding (Figure 5–2).

To achieve compression of the nipple against the bony roof of the mouth, the palate must be intact in the area of the nipple. To achieve suction in the oral cavity, there must be adequate lip closure around the nipple, and the oral cavity must be closed off posteriorly with the back

of the tongue against the soft palate. The hard palate, and to some extent the soft palate, serve to close off the nose from the mouth during feeding. Any opening in this cavity can reduce or eliminate the ability to create negative suction pressure.

Pharyngeal Phase of Swallowing

The pharyngeal phase of swallowing is initiated once the fluid bolus is channeled by the tongue into the pharynx. Because the pharynx serves as a conduit for food as well as respiratory air, precise coordination of breathing, sucking, and swallowing is necessary during the pharyngeal swallowing phase (Figure 5–3). There are significant differences in the pharyngeal phase of swallowing in infancy, due to the size and location of the pharyngeal and laryngeal structures in the first several months.

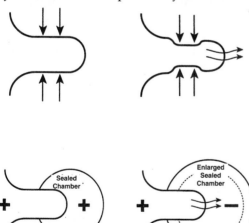

Figure 5–2. Comparison of positive pressure (compression) and negative pressure (suction) components during sucking (From *Feeding and Swallowing Disorders in Infancy*, by L. Wolf and R. Glass, 1992, p. 17. Therapy Skill Builders, a division of Communication Skill Builders, Inc., 3830 E. Bellevue, P.O. Box 42050. Copyright 1992 Therapy Skill Builders, Inc. Reprinted with permission.)

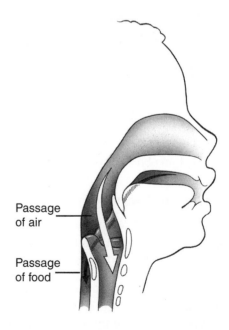

Figure 5–3. The pharynx as a conduit of food and air. (From *The Pediatric Airway: An Interdisciplinary Approach*, by C. M. Myer, R. T. Cotton, & S. R. Shott, 1995, p. 9. Philadelphia: J. B. Lippincott Company. Copyright 1995 J. B. Lippincott. Reprinted with permission.)

When the liquid reaches the posterior oral cavity, the posterior pharyngeal wall, velum, and tongue base work together to provide the driving force for bolus transfer through the pharynx. The velum elevates to close off the nasal cavity from the oral cavity by closing the velopharyngeal valve. The tongue base moves back as negative pressure builds in the pharynx. The bolus diverts around the epiglottis as the pharynx fills and contracts sequentially for swallowing (Newman, Cleveland, Blickman, Hillman, & Jaramillo, 1991). Throughout the sucking action, the infant continues to maintain nasal breathing. To facilitate this, the epiglottis is positioned around the back of the velum, which keeps the pharynx open and allows the nasal cavity to be in direct contact with the glottis for a continuous patent airway. However, at the time of swallow initiation, respiration ceases as the larynx closes by adduction of the true and false vocal folds, the forward and medial movement of the arytenoids, and the subsequent retroversion of the epiglottis (Koenig, Davies, & Thach, 1990; Mathew, 1991). Additional respiratory effort is necessary to support the work of feeding. The normal infant is able to tolerate the decreased ventilation during feeding; however, this may not be the case in infants presenting with borderline respiratory reserve (Mathew, 1988b; Mathew, Clark, Pronske, Luna-Solarzano, & Peterson, 1985).

Esophageal Phase of Swallowing

The bolus moves through the pharynx and into the esophagus, where the esophageal phase of swallowing is initiated. The upper part of the esophagus, commonly referred to as the *upper esophageal sphincter* (UES), is normally closed, but stretches open as the bolus travels through the hypopharynx and into the esophagus. The *lower esophageal sphincter* (LES) relaxes to allow the bolus to enter the stomach. After each swallow occurs, the velum drops down to the base of the tongue and in front of the epiglottis, the tongue returns to an anterior position, sucking and breathing resume, and both the upper and lower esophageal sphincters maintain a closed position.

The suck-swallow-breathe ratio during bottle feeding is generally considered to be 1:1:1. Some variations to this pattern occur during the initial rapid sucking phase, generally described as the initial 2 to 3 minutes of feeding, as compared to the slower sucking rates occurring during the subsequent intermittent sucking phase (Bu'Lock, Woolridge, & Baum, 1990; Mathew, 1991; Wolf & Glass, 1992).

Changes in the Swallowing Process With Growth

The swallowing process changes as the oral cavity enlarges, the pharynx elongates, and the hyoid, epiglottis, and larynx descend. The increased size of the oral cavity supports the development of more refined oral-motor skills, such as chewing and cup drinking. Neuromuscular maturation as well as increased cartilage and connective tissue are reflected in the mobility of the hyoid and larynx, which must become more active during the swallowing process for maintenance of airway protection when it is no longer facilitated by the proximity of structures. The hyoid and larynx must be mobile enough to elevate and provide sphincteric closure during swallowing (Bosma & Donner, 1980).

Craniofacial Anomalies and Pediatric Dysphagia

Any anatomical malformation in the oral cavity, pharynx, or larynx can cause or contribute to a feeding or swallowing problem. Anomalies that are associated with feeding problems include cleft lip and palate, *micrognathia* (small mandible), *macroglossia* (large tongue), pharyngeal *stenosis* (narrowing), laryngeal cleft, tracheoesophageal fistula, and vascular anomalies causing compression in the esophagus and/or airway. Cortical or cranial nerve involvement, as seen in some syndromes, may affect the neuromuscular coordination required for sucking and swallowing. Finally, conditions that can cause airway compromise, such as Pierre Robin sequence, midface retrusion, congenital heart or lung disease, or *choanal atresia* (congenital closure of the opening to the pharynx from the back of the nose) can interfere with the suck-swallow-breathe sequence. Of all of these anomalies, cleft palate is the most common.

Characteristics of Feeding Problems Due to Clefts

The feeding problems of infants who have a cleft will reflect the type and the severity of the cleft. The issues with feeding problems vary greatly depending on whether the cleft is of the lip and/or palate and if it is unilateral, bilateral, complete, or incomplete. Typically, the feeding problems include poor oral suction, poor intake with lengthy feeding times, nasal regurgitation, choking, gagging, and excessive air intake (Clarren, Anderson, & Wolf, 1987). These difficulties are due to the structural problems in the oral cavity, but in most cases, pharyngeal swallowing function is normal. Therefore, once the milk reaches the oropharynx, swallowing is initiated and coordinated with airway protection. Problems with maintaining airway protection during the pharyngeal phase of the swallow can occur when pharyngeal, esophageal, or central nervous system abnormalities occur in conjunction with the anatomic defect. Problems with airway protection can also occur when the timing of the oral phase of

swallowing is so disorganized that the integrity of airway protection is compromised.

Infants with a cleft of the lip usually do not have significant problems with feeding, especially if the cleft is unilateral. There may be some initial difficulty learning how to latch onto the nipple. However, once the nipple is placed intraorally, the infant's tongue and jaw movements should be sufficient to produce compression of the nipple against the intact part of the alveolus and palate. There may be some difficulty in achieving negative pressure suction, depending on how much the lip seal on the nipple is compromised.

Infants with a minimal cleft of the soft palate may be able to feed without special modifications. With a small, posterior cleft, the infant may actually occlude the cleft with the tongue during part of the sucking movement, so that negative pressure can be obtained normally.

Infants with a cleft of the hard and soft palate have more difficulty feeding for several reasons. Depending on the extent of the cleft, the infant may be unable to find a hard palatal surface to work against, making compression of the nipple impossible. This situation may result in the nipple being pushed into the area of the cleft if placement cannot be achieved against an area of hard palate. Another concern is that with an open cavity, the subsequent generation of suction is difficult and perhaps impossible to achieve. The extent of difficulty again depends on the size and location of the cleft. Posterior clefts may be occluded with the base of the tongue during the sucking movement. The more anterior the cleft is, the harder it is for the infant to achieve compression of the nipple and subsequent generation of negative pressure for efficient sucking.

The hard palate and the velum normally serve to separate the oral cavity from the nasal cavity during feeding. With an open palate, *nasal regurgitation,* which is reflux of milk into the nasopharynx and nasal cavity, will often occur. This can cause discomfort and disorganization with the coordination of breathing and feeding.

In addition, several secondary problems can occur due to the difficulty with oral feeding. These include poor weight gain, excessive energy expenditure during feeding, lengthy feeding times, discomfort with feeding, and stressful feeding interactions between the infant and caretaker (Carlisle, 1998).

Several studies have documented poor weight gain in the cleft palate population, especially during the first 6 months (Avedian & Ruberg, 1980; Jones, 1988; Lee, Nunn, & Wright, 1997). A full-term newborn infant will generally need 2 to 3 ounces of breast milk or formula per pound of body weight per day in order to gain weight appropriately (The Cleft Palate Foundation, 1998). Therefore, an infant who weighs 10 pounds will require between 20 and 30 ounces per day; a significant amount for an infant having feeding difficulty. As the infant gains weight, his or her daily intake should increase accordingly. If the infant has a cleft palate, however, it is harder to achieve compression of the nipple to generate the suction needed for efficient ingestion of the amount of formula required for continued growth. There is also frequent nasal regurgitation, which must be subtracted from total intake of formula.

The infant with a cleft may take much longer to feed than an infant without a cleft yet still not get enough to be satisfied during each feeding to gain weight. To complicate this problem, the infant must work much harder to feed, and therefore, expends more calories during the feeding process than the average infant. Most infants can complete a feeding within 20 to 30 minutes. If the infant takes 45 minutes or longer to feed, with clearly increased effort and relatively little intake, consultation with the pediatrician, as well as a nutritionist and feeding specialist, is indicated. Weight gain should

be monitored closely by the pediatrician, especially during the first few months.

Because air continues to flow in through the nose and then the mouth during feeding due to the open cleft, this may result in excessive intake of air. This can cause the infant to become bloated or have episodes of frequent "spit up." Excess air intake needs to be monitored closely by the caretaker as it is a potential source of discomfort for the infant, both during and after feeding.

A final concern is for the parents. Normally, the feeding process serves as a loving and bonding experience between the caregiver and the infant. However, feeding an infant with cleft palate can be very time-consuming for the caregivers and often results in a great deal of frustration. Fortunately, most feeding problems can be avoided or minimized with individualized feeding modifications.

Feeding Problems Due to Other Anomalies

Pierre Robin Sequence

Patients with a diagnosis of Pierre Robin sequence (mandibular hypoplasia, glossoptosis, and cleft palate) may have feeding problems due to the cleft palate as well as potential problems with the coordination of the suck-swallow-breathe triad (Lehman, Fishman, & Neiman, 1995; Shprintzen, 1992). Micrognathia is often associated with a wide U-shaped cleft of the palate. The tongue is posteriorly positioned in relation to the oral cavity, a condition generally referred to as *glossoptosis*. The presence of glossoptosis creates the potential for upper airway obstruction, which may be exacerbated by the respiratory effort of feeding. Episodic or chronic airway obstruction can occur during the infant's effort to maintain sequential chain swallowing sequences (Shprintzen & Singer, 1992).

Moebius Syndrome

Moebius syndrome involves specific cranial nerve damage with weakness affecting the oral musculature. The weakness in the lips limits the infant's ability to achieve and maintain an adequate seal on the nipple for sucking. Anterior loss of formula is a common finding during the clinical feeding evaluation. A chronic open-mouth posture with limited range of movement in the jaw and tongue has a profound effect on the oral-motor mechanics necessary for efficient sucking (Arvedson & Brodsky, 1993).

Hemifacial Microsomia

Hemifacial microsomia results in various degrees of both unilateral mandibular hypoplasia and facial weakness. This generally results in limitations to the range of motion in the jaw, lips, and tongue on one side. Utilization of the stronger side of the mouth during feeding presentations while providing stabilization to the weaker side may work when attempting to establish a compensatory feeding pattern (Arvedson & Brodsky, 1993).

Other Craniofacial Anomalies With Concomitant Congenital Anomalies

If the infant has other oral, tracheal, or laryngeal anomalies in addition to the cleft palate, feeding can become even more of a challenge. Micrognathia or a posterior tongue position associated with a variety of syndromes can result in problems with oral-motor mechanics and/or airway compromise and further affect the ability to coordinate breathing and feeding. A tracheoesophageal fistula can cause aspiration during feeding secondary to communication between the esophagus and trachea. Hypotonia, hypertonia, or generalized oral-motor dysfunction secondary to weakness or myopathy all can affect the infant's ability to

suck efficiently as well as to coordinate the suck-swallow-breathe triad.

General Feeding Modifications

Unfortunately, there is no single feeding method that will be successful for infants presenting with unilateral or bilateral cleft lip, cleft palate, or cleft lip and palate as well as other craniofacial abnormalities. The infant's performance during the initial feedings will dictate which feeding method and technique is feasible (Wolf & Glass, 1992). Individualized modifications should allow the infant to feed with relative ease as well as to obtain an adequate amount of nutrition in a reasonable amount of time.

Infants who present with feeding problems that are not easily resolved by a simple adjustment in feeding method postnatally will benefit from a clinical oral-motor/ feeding evaluation performed by a qualified speech pathologist or occupational therapist, or other feeding specialist. Such an evaluation can assess an infant's specific oral-motor strengths and weaknesses with the ultimate goals being:

- To maximize the infant's ability to orally fed for adequate nutrition and weight gain by matching feeding modifications to oral-motor skills.
- To facilitate the suck-swallow-breathe synchrony for safe and efficient feeding.

The Issue of Breast Feeding

Whether or not breast feeding will be possible is often one of the mother's first questions. Opinions regarding breast feeding when clefting is present vary across centers (Alexander-Doelle, 1997; Crossman, 1998; Danner, 1992; Darzi, Chowdri, & Bhat, 1996; Fisher, 1991; Kogo et al., 1997). As with other feeding methods, the success of breast feeding will depend on the placement of the cleft as well as its severity.

Breast feeding is usually not a problem for the infant who has a cleft lip only, since the infant should still be able to achieve adequate suction. Even with a cleft in the lip and alveolus, the breast tends to fill the opening by molding to the shape of the oral cavity. Upright positioning while attempting breast feeding is generally recommended. Supplemental bottle feeding or a complete switch to the bottle may be necessary if difficulties with breast feeding are immediately apparent.

Breast feeding the infant with a cleft palate is very difficult, however, and this can be a particular disappointment for many new mothers. Breast feeding a child with a cleft palate can be done, but to be successful it requires specialized modifications (Wolf & Glass, 1992). Monitoring weight gain closely during a trial period of breast feeding will provide objective evidence regarding its feasibility and definitive information as to whether a supplementary feeding method is needed.

If the mother wishes to try breast feeding, she should consult with a feeding specialist or lactation consultant who has experience with patients having special needs, particularly those with cleft lip or palate. If a trial of breast feeding proves unsuccessful and the mother still wishes to continue breast feeding, a supplemental nursing system may be an option. The supplemental nursing system utilizes a reservoir and tubing. The reservoir can be filled with formula or with milk that the mother has expressed. A thin tube, connected to the reservoir, is taped above the mother's breast and nipple. As the infant latches onto the breast for feeding, the mother supplements the breast milk with milk that is squeezed manually through the tube. The flow of milk needs to be simultaneous with the baby's efforts at sucking. With this method, the baby is supplemented at the breast, while maintaining the impor-

tant physical contact for infant and mother. In addition, this method stimulates the breast to continue to produce and maintain the milk supply. Drawbacks to the use of supplemental nursing systems include the potential for difficulty in maintaining the proper flow rate, as well as possible refusal of the baby to accept the tube during breast feeding attempts.

After attempting breast feeding with modifications, some mothers may find that bottle feeding is easier and more expedient using a modified bottle and/or a modified nipple. Breast milk can be used in lieu of formula and given via the modified bottle or nipple.

Use of Breast Milk

Most pediatricians and health care providers agree that breast milk is best for the newborn infant for several reasons. It contains the mother's antibodies against illnesses and therefore can provide the infant with some immunity. Early food allergies can also be avoided through the use of breast milk. Therefore, if the mother will need to use a modified bottle feeding method, she may prefer to use breast milk rather than formula (Oseid, 1979).

Breast Pumps

Breast milk can be expressed through the use of a variety of breast pumps. Breast pumps are available for purchase or for rental through local home health suppliers. There are several kinds of breast pumps, including manual pumps, battery-operated pumps, and electric pumps. The electric pumps tend to be more efficient and faster than the manual pumps. An electric pump that allows both breasts to be pumped at the same time is particularly useful because it can greatly reduce the amount of time required to express the milk. This is a definite advantage, especially if breast milk is used exclusively.

Breast pumps may be covered by the family's insurance plan, but this usually requires a signed prescription in the baby's name and a letter from the physician describing the special circumstances that make this equipment necessary.

Modified Nipples

If problems with feeding are immediately apparent, a variety of special bottles and nipples are available. Commonly used nipples and bottles are described in Table 5–1. When con-

TABLE 5–1. Commercially available bottles and nipples.

- **Mead-Johnson Cleft Lip/Palate Nurser:** This is a soft bottle that is easily squeezed and also has a soft cross-cut nipple. A standard nipple will also fit onto the Mead-Johnson bottle and works well for some infants. The caregiver can help to regulate the liquid by assistive squeezing. The use of either the cross-cut nipple or a standard nipple with a modified hole will depend on the oral-motor skills of each particular infant.

- **Ross Cleft Palate Nurser:** This bottle has a long, thin nipple that delivers milk to the back of the throat. The small diameter and length of this nipple does not facilitate tongue movements for sucking. The long length may cause gagging in some infants. Fluid flow is steady and rapid and can be difficult for infants who cannot tolerate a rapid flow rate. This could result in disorganization of airway protection and possible aspiration.

- **Lamb's Nipple:** This nipple is long, wide, and soft, with compression occurring between the lateral alveolar ridges. The shape of this nipple does not facilitate normal sucking movements. The hole may be too large for infants who cannot tolerate a rapid fluid flow. The length of the nipple may induce gagging in some infants. This nipple, although used widely in the past, has been found to have a high nitrate level and therefore is now not commonly used.

- **Haberman Feeder:** This feeding system is designed to allow release of milk through the infant's compressions alone. There is a valving component, which prevents rapid milk flow by opening only when the baby sucks. This valve is also designed to prevent excessive intake of air. The nipple has a slit, which allows flow control during feeding depending on the orientation of the slit in the infant's mouth. The flow can thus be easily regulated by the caregiver. This bottle is expensive in comparison with others.

- **Preemie Nipple:** This nipple is smaller, thinner, and softer than a standard nipple, making suction easier. This is a fast flow nipple, which should be used only by infants who have demonstrated tolerance for the increased respiratory effort associated with increased swallowing due to the fast fluid flow.

- **Obturator Nipple:** This may also be referred to as a Brophy nipple. This is a nipple with a flap above the nipple, which is intended to occlude the cleft and facilitate normal sucking. This is rarely recommended as it has the potential to obstruct the oral cavity, irritate the nasopharyngeal space, and cause sucking/swallowing disorganization.

- **Ascepto Feeder:** This is a small syringe with a rubber tube attachment. The tubing is placed intraorally in the cheek pocket with the milk subsequently being delivered by squeezing the syringe. The flow rate is typically rapid and hard to control, which may compromise the infant's ability to protect the airway. This device does not promote normal sucking movements.

- **Standard Amber Nipple:** This nipple has a narrow base and has been shown to be effective when used in conjunction with a squeeze bottle while feeding infants who have demonstrated the ability to develop some suction independently. A slight enlargement of the nipple hole may be necessary.

- **Nuk Nipple:** This is a wide-based nipple with a fast flow rate.

sidering what nipple to use for enhancement of sucking, there are four basic parameters to consider, including pliability, shape, size, and hole type and size (Mathew, 1988a). Table 5–2 compares the characteristics of the commonly used nipples. The type of nipple chosen must be in relation to a particular baby's type and extent of clefting as well as present oral-motor/feeding skills. The type of nipple will ideally maximize the baby's current oral-motor skills for feeding as determined by the initial feeding evaluation.

Pliability

When specialized nipples or bottles are required, they need to be designed to improve the ability to express milk with limited need for compression or for suction. However, the nipple chosen will need to be firm enough to provide an appropriate degree of proprioceptive input to facilitate sucking. The degree of pliability must match the infant's strength of sucking to support an appropriate flow rate. A soft nipple tends to have a higher flow rate than a firmer nipple and thus requires less suction. A "preemie" nipple is often used, as it is designed

to be very soft and pliable. Another option is to use a standard nipple that has been softened through boiling. A variety of specialized nipples and bottle systems such as the Mead-Johnson (Figure 5–4) and Haberman Feeder (Figure 5–5) are designed specifically for cleft palate infants. The degree of pliability and subsequent increase in flow rate must be considered in relation to the baby's ability to coordinate the suck-swallow-breathe sequence. Increased flow will be reflected in increased number of swallows and subsequently increased respiratory effort during feeding (Mathew, 1991).

Hole Type and Size

The size of the nipple hole, as well as the type of hole, determines flow rate. Two types of holes are found in nipples: standard holes and crosscuts. The holes are usually very small openings in nipples and the size can vary widely across different styles of nipples. A cross-cut opening is basically an "X" configuration. A standard nipple hole can be modified with a single-edged razor blade to a cross-cut. The size of the hole is generally considered to be indicative of flow rate during sucking

TABLE 5–2. Characteristics of commonly used nipples.

Nipple Type	Pliability	Flow Rate	Shape	Hole Type
Preemie	Soft	Fast	Traditional	Hole and cross-cut
Nuk style	Soft	Fast	Broad, flat	Hole on top surface of tip
Ross Cleft	Soft	Fast	Long, thin	Large hole
Standard	Medium	Low	Traditional	Hole and cross-cut, several holes
Mead-Johnson	Soft	Feeder regulated	Customized	Cross-cut
Haberman Feeding System	Soft	Feeder regulated	Customized	Slit

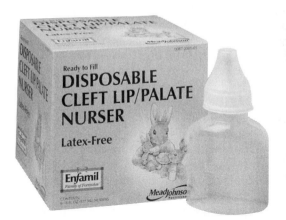

Figure 5–4. Mead-Johnson Cleft Palate Nurser. (Photo courtesy of the Mead-Johnson Company.)

(Mathew, 1990). The type of hole an infant should use is determined during an initial feeding assessment.

The cross-cut configuration allows the milk to flow only when the infant compresses the nipple to make the cross-cut open. This allows the infant to control the milk flow with the normal rhythm of sucking and swallowing and prevents the infant from getting too much liquid, which can cause choking. A nipple with a traditional hole should have an opening that is large enough so that, when the bottle is held upside down, the liquid drips out but does not run out rapidly. A very hot needle can be placed in a standard hole to increase the size of the hole, but this may result in an overly rapid flow of milk. This may result in difficulty coordinating swallowing and breathing with possible compromise of airway protection during feeding and a risk of aspiration.

Shape

Regardless of what nipple is used, the shape of the nipple needs to provide adequate contact between the nipple and the tongue for adequate compression. The shape also must sup-

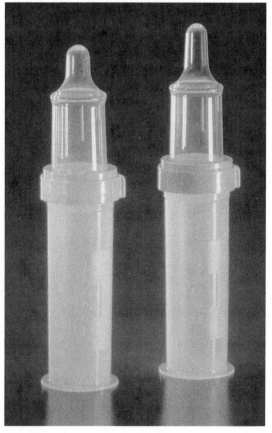

Figure 5–5. Haberman™ Feeder by Medela. (Photo courtesy of the Medela, Inc. Haberman Feeder and MiniHaberman Feeders are trademarks of Mandy Haberman.)

port the oral-motor patterns desired during sucking. Numerous nipple designs are available; however, nipple shapes basically fall into two categories: traditional, straight-shaped nipples and broad, flat nipples (Figure 5–6). The traditional nipple has a straight configuration, which gradually tapers to a flared base. The broad, flat nipples, sometimes referred to as "orthodontic nipples," have bulb-type ends that flare to a large, wide base. This style is perhaps best known as the "Nuk" nipple; however many manufacturers, including Gerber and Playtex, now make nipples shaped similarly to

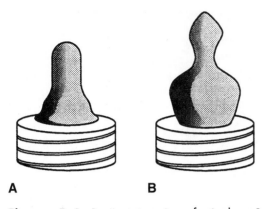

A   **B**

Figure 5–6. Basic categories of nipples. **A.** Round cross-section. **B.** Broad, flat, cross-section. (From *Feeding and Swallowing Disorders in Infancy,* by L. Wolf and R. Glass, 1992, p. 404. Therapy Skill Builders, a division of Communication Skill Builders, Inc., 3830 E. Bellevue, P.O. Box 42050. Copyright 1992 Therapy Skill Builders, Inc. Reprinted with permission.)

the original "Nuk" style. Such nipples are generally advantageous for infants with isolated cleft lip as they may conform to the cleft and prevent air leakage while sucking.

Nipple Size

Determining the appropriate size nipple to use should be based on the length needed to provide adequate contact between the nipple and tongue for effective tongue movements. Nipple length can vary substantially in regard to the type of base and the distance from the tip to the base. The amount of the nipple that is in the infant's mouth will vary more with nipples that have tapered bases. The strength of the infant's suck, the degree of lip closure around the nipple, and the control the feeder provides to maintain the nipple position are all factors that should be considered.

Modified Bottles

In considering the appropriate bottle, a soft plastic squeeze bottle or plastic bottle liner can

be used. Feeder-assisted squeezing for mild expression allows the infant to conserve energy and thus have less calorie expenditure during feeding. If a plastic liner is used, the caregiver can reduce the excess intake of air by pushing all the air out of the liner before beginning the feeding and by applying intermittent pressure to the liner to push milk out as the infant compresses the nipple (Barone & Tallman, 1998). The flow of milk can be difficult to modulate, which may make it more difficult for the infant to maintain organization of sucking, swallowing, and breathing.

A soft bottle, such as the Mead-Johnson cleft palate nurser or the Haberman Feeder, may allow for more precision in the amount of milk squeezed. The Mead-Johnson bottle is soft and easily held in the feeder's hand and requires the use of an assistive squeeze for release of the milk. The Haberman Feeder allows milk release from the infant's compression alone, and also allows for control of flow during feeding by changing the orientation of the nipple slit in the infant's mouth. The softness of the Haberman nipple also allows for assistive squeezing (Campbell & Tremouth, 1987).

Regardless of which device is used, the pressure applied to a squeeze bottle or plastic liner must be in rhythm with the infant's suck and swallow to ensure that the infant does not become discoordinated with the suck-swallow-breathe synchrony. The feeder must become skilled at providing the assistive squeeze in synchrony with the infant's sucking movements, allowing time for each swallow to take place. An inappropriately rapid rate will result in an increased rate of swallowing, which will decrease available breathing time. This may result in problems with maintaining an appropriate respiratory rate and may also result in discoordination of the suck-swallow-breathe synchrony with subsequent aspiration into the airway.

Overall, the device chosen must also allow the infant to receive an adequate amount of intake for nutrition and weight gain. It should be easy enough so that the infant can conserve energy and fast enough so that it does not cause lengthy feeding times and eventual frustration for the caregiver. Consistency of use is important, as is consistency of the feeder's method. The feeding system should allow the infant to experience some sucking for normal oral-motor development. Finally, the option chosen should be relatively inexpensive and readily available.

Specific Feeding Considerations and Techniques

Cleft Lip Only

Clefts of the lip may be unilateral or bilateral and may extend into the nares and alveolus. This will result in problems in achieving an adequate anterior lip seal on the nipple of the bottle or breast, which is needed to generate negative pressure during feeding.

Breast Feeding

Breast feeding often will work well in cases of cleft lip only, as the breast tends to conform to and fill in the cleft area. If necessary, the mother can assist with lip closure by gently holding the upper lip together while the baby sucks. Positioning should be as upright as possible to allow gravity to pull the liquid into the pharynx.

Bottle Feeding

Infants who present with a cleft lip only generally feed adequately; however, occasionally air leak from the cleft will interrupt the generation of negative pressure. The use of a soft, wide-based nipple as depicted in Figure 5–6 will close the area of cleft and allow suction generation.

Cleft Palate Only

A cleft of the palate can involve only the soft palate or can also extend into the hard palate. Whatever the case, there will be compromise in the infant's ability to seal the oral cavity and create negative pressure for suction.

Breast Feeding

Generally, infants with a narrow or posterior cleft (soft palate only) will be able to breast-feed without undue difficulty. The infant will likely be able to develop adequate suction to form and position the nipple for adequate compression (Wolf & Glass, 1992). Infants with a complete clefting of the soft and hard palate are much more likely to have a difficult time with breast-feeding due to the fact that they will simply be unable to create negative pressure for suction due to the large opening and lack of surface for the tongue to compress against.

Bottle Feeding

Generally the options for bottle feeding include a system whereby the feeder will assist with milk delivery by squeezing a soft, plastic bottle as well as modification of the nipple to assist with efficient delivery of fluid. Nipple modifications may include the use of a soft, cross-cut nipple with a wide base.

Cleft Lip and Palate

The infant presenting with a cleft of the lip and palate will generally have significant difficulty with all aspects of feeding due to the inability to achieve an anterior seal with the lips, inability to compress the nipple due to the open palate, and failure to generate negative pressure suction. Significant nasopharyngeal reflux of liquid secondary to the open nasopharynx will also be present.

Breast Feeding

Infants with a cleft lip and palate will have a large area of cleft, which has a direct impact on the baby's sucking mechanics overall. Breast feeding is highly unlikely in this group of infants. Unlike the infant with a posterior cleft, there is no effective means for positioning or compressing the nipple. The use of a supplemental nursing system, such as the Medela Supplemental Nursing System or the Lact-Aide, may offer some help in supporting breast feeding; however, the infant's growth and hydration status should be carefully monitored. Supplemental or exclusive transition to bottle feeding is highly likely.

Bottle Feeding

A variety of modified feeding devices, both nipples and bottles, that assist in delivery of milk will be necessary for the infant with cleft lip and palate. Assistive squeezing of the bottle by the feeder and the use of a soft nipple are often necessary. The feeder must control the flow of milk to give the infant time to swallow.

Pierre Robin Sequence and Micrognathia

The infant's ability to compress the nipple adequately is often decreased secondary to the presence of micrognathia and thus a retracted tongue position. The habitual position of the tongue does not allow for positioning beneath the nipple to allow for compressive action. If the infant has Pierre Robin sequence, which includes the typical U-shaped cleft palate, problems with generation of negative pressure also contribute to feeding difficulty. The presence of *glossoptosis* (posterior displacement of the tongue) creates an airway obstruction, which may be exacerbated by the increased respiratory effort required during feeding. A patent airway must be confirmed prior to attempts at oral feeding (Bath & Bull, 1997). Some patients may require placement of a nasopharyngeal (NP) airway to maintain a patent airway. Oral feedings can be done with the NP tube in place.

If medical clearance is given for oral feedings, prone positioning may help to position the tongue anteriorly and facilitate tongue movements during feeding. However, if the infant has a cleft palate, prone positioning is generally not helpful, as the infant will not be able to move the milk to the back of the mouth for the initiation of swallowing. Using a semi-reclined or standard feeding position will help to minimize gravitational pull on the tongue. Sidelying positioning may be an option with use of either the Haberman feeder or a Mead Johnson bottle. Success with feeding will need to be closely monitored with the possible need for supplemental feedings (Glass & Wolf, 1999).

Breast Feeding

The success of breast feeding in the infant with Pierre Robin sequence will depend on the degree of micrognathia, the status of the airway, and whether the infant has a cleft. In infants without clefts and with mild retrognathia, breast feeding may be an option. It should be noted, however, that breast feeding will probably be difficult. The retracted tongue position may cause inadequate compression of the milk ducts in the breast, which will lead to limited milk flow, and ultimately less milk production. If micrognathia, upper airway obstruction, and a velar cleft are present, breast feeding is unlikely to be successful due to the inability to position the nipple, increased respiratory effort during feeding, and reduced sucking mechanics (Wolf & Glass, 1992).

Bottle Feeding

Generally, the nipple that will work most effectively in feeding the infant with micrognathia and a retracted tongue will need to be long enough to provide adequate contact between the nipple and tongue without causing gagging. A narrow base or standard nipple will allow full insertion of the nipple into the infant's mouth. The nipple should compress easily and be used in conjunction with a bottle that allows assistive squeezing to assist with the flow of milk.

Oral-Motor Facilitation Techniques

Positioning the Infant

Optimal positioning is key to successful feeding (Morris & Klein, 1987). Proper positioning facilitates control of jaw, cheek, lip, and tongue movements for sucking/swallowing coordination. Feeding the infant in an upright position of at least 60 degrees so that gravity can work to assist in swallowing is often helpful (Wolf & Glass, 1992). The baby's head should be supported in a chin tuck position, with arms forward, trunk in midline, and the hips flexed. The use of this upright positioning can help to prevent nasal regurgitation. Placing the infant in a horizontal position increases the potential for nasal regurgitation, coughing, and sneezing. In addition, there may be flooding of the eustachian tube and reflux into the middle ear, causing middle ear effusion. The use of a bottle with an angled neck provides a downward flow of milk and simplifies feeding the infant in upright positioning.

Positioning the Nipple

Working with the baby during an initial feeding session to find the optimal intraoral position for the nipple is critical for feeding success. Studies have shown that the difference between success and failure of nipple placement for feeding effectiveness consists of only a few millimeters (Clarren et al., 1987). It is important to position the nipple under a shelf of bone to provide the stable base needed to achieve compression. The use of the proper size and shape of the nipple, based on the patient's cleft, will facilitate proper positioning intraorally.

Pacing Intake

The caregiver should carefully pace the flow rate by providing fluid in rhythm with the infant's movements and reactions. Identifying the infant's cues during feeding is a learning process for both the caregiver and the infant. Eye widening, change in facial expression, or a decrease in alertness are all signs the infant may give during feeding, which may signal stress responses or subtle avoidance in response to feeding. If the infant begins feeding rapidly and then shows signs of swallowing disorganization, such as coughing or choking, the feeder will need to make adjustments in the feeding process, such as slowing the pace of fluid presentation. If the infant begins to slow down or stop sucking during the feeding, this may be an indication that the infant has tired and needs a pause before continuing feeding. The infant may show signs of excessive air intake and need a pause in feeding to allow burping. The feeder must be able to deliver enough nutrition before the infant becomes tired; however, allowing enough time to facilitate safe feeding is central to overall feeding success. Consulting a dietitian about the use of a higher calorie formula preparation with a lower intake requirement will allow the infant to spend less time feeding and allow a slower pace of intake while still ingesting an adequate amount of calories for growth (Kovar, 1997).

Oral Facilitation

It may be necessary for the feeder to provide oral facilitation techniques such as jaw and cheek support to increase the infant's oral control during feeding. The need for such strategies can be determined during an oral-motor/feeding assessment. The type of bottle used can facilitate the use of strategies to increase oral control. For example, the use of a small diameter bottle, such as the infant volufeed, will allow the feeder to use hand and finger positioning

Case Report: Appropriate Positioning and Placement

Lydia was born with Pierre Robin sequence with the characteristic micrognathia, posteriorly displaced tongue, and wide U-shaped cleft palate. The potential for upper airway obstruction secondary to the posterior placement of the tongue was analyzed by continuous oxygen saturation monitoring and by a formal sleep study. The results of the sleep study were within normal limits and oxygen saturation levels were maintained, except during the mother's initial attempts at oral feedings. Lydia was described as a poor feeder with little sucking, frequent gasping, and oxygen desaturations. Despite the mother's efforts, Lydia's intake was only minimal (5–10 cc) before she would completely "shut down" and fall asleep, usually 10 minutes into the feeding.

A speech pathology oral-motor/feeding consultation was requested The results of the evaluation indicated normal oral reflexes with good rooting as well as the ability to initiate and sustain a rhythmical non-nutritive sucking pattern. Observation was then made of the mother as she demonstrated the methods she had been using while attempting oral feeding. The mother explained that she had already tried numerous nipples, including a variety of specialized nipples and bottles, without success. She was noted to position Lydia in a semireclined, cradle position as she offered her a standard nipple, which had been slit to assist with a faster milk delivery. She explained that she had been advised that the cleft would make sucking difficult and that she would need a nipple that would not require sucking. Upon presentation of the nipple, Lydia made a few tentative sucking attempts as the milk rapidly flowed from the nipple. She coughed, sputtered, and pulled away from the nipple. An oxygen desaturation event was documented. The mother attempted to place the nipple intraorally again and had difficulty placing the nipple onto the tongue body. She continued these attempts with the baby continuing to resist with intermittent oxygen desaturations. Lydia then fell asleep after struggling to accept an intake of only 10 cc. The remainder of the feeding was then presented via oral gavage. The mother agreed to allow the speech pathologist to try interventional feeding techniques during the next feeding time.

Interventional techniques that were recommended included the use of upright positioning as opposed to the semireclined cradle position. Being upright helped Lydia avoid further posterior displacement of her tongue during her efforts at feeding. Non-nutritive oral stimulation was then provided with Lydia in upright positioning to help increase alertness and to help facilitate and organize oral movements for feeding. The Haberman feeder was then presented intraorally. The longer size of this nipple made placement onto the tongue easier. In addition, there is no flow of liquid from the nipple prior to either active sucking or assistive squeezing, which allowed Lydia to become accustomed to the presence of the nipple without being flooded by formula. Once Lydia began to attempt sucking, a gentle assistive squeeze to deliver a small amount of formula was given in synchrony with her sucking attempts. Lydia was able to successfully transfer this small amount of formula without any clinical signs of swallowing dysfunction. A cycle of approximately eight assistive squeezes was completed before Lydia showed some disorganization by again pulling away from the nipple. After a brief pause, additional feeding trials revealed that Lydia could handle approximately five sequences of assistive squeeze for completion of suck-swallow before requiring a pause with repetition of the cycles for intake of approximately 30 cc. Gradually over a 3-week period, oral intake improved with toleration of longer cycles of assitive squeezing. Eventually the transition to complete oral feedings with maintenance of good oxygen saturation levels was accomplished.

for facilitation to the jaw and cheeks during feeding (Morris & Klein, 1987).

Preventing Excessive Air Intake

The caregiver may need to increase the frequency of burping as the infant with a cleft will take in an increased amount of air with the liquid. If the infant is sucking vigorously, the feeder may need to impose a pause in feeding for burping to prevent excessive air intake and subsequent discomfort. As a general rule of thumb, the infant should be burped every ounce to prevent the discomfort associated with the intake of air that inevitably will occur with each feeding.

Managing Nasal Regurgitation

Infants with a cleft palate often experience nasal regurgitation through the nose, and they may cough frequently during the feeding and seem to "choke." When nasal regurgitation occurs, the caregiver should stop feeding and allow the infant some time to cough or sneeze to clear the nasal passage. If nasal regurgitation occurs frequently during feeding, the caregiver should check positioning to assure the infant is in an upright position to allow gravity to assist with downward flow of liquid. If coughing occurs frequently in conjunction with the nasal regurgitation, the feeder should consider using a slower flow nipple. Using pacing to additionally slow the presentation of fluid may help the infant to become more organized in maintain-

ing synchrony of the sucking, swallowing, and breathing.

Consistency of Feeder Method

Consistency in how the baby is fed will contribute to overall feeding success. The baby should be fed in the same position, with the same nipple and bottle, as well as the same technique during each feeding. The feeder must learn how to easily position the baby, how much of an assistive squeeze is required, how long to keep feeding, how often to burp the baby, and how to read the baby's cues related to feeding. If several different nipples are intermittently tried as well as different bottles, with varying positions as well as different rates of assistive squeezing by a range of feeders, it is almost certain that feeding confusion and a poor feeding outcome will result. Fortunately, for the majority of infants, the normal maturation of the feeding process as well as increased experience with feeding will help gradually ease the process of oral intake in spite of variations in method which may occur.

Use of Feeding Obturators

A feeding obturator consists of an acrylic plate, which is inserted in the mouth and fits over the hard palate (see Chapter 19). It is retained in the crevices of the cleft and provides a seal between the mouth and the nasal cavity. This effectively closes the palatal defect and maintains a separation between the nasal cavity and oral cavity. The obturator can promote a more normal tongue position and it improves the infant's ability to achieve compression of the nipple against the plate. A pediatric dentist or prosthodontist is the professional who will construct the feeding appliance and check it frequently so that it can be modified periodically as the child grows. If the obturator is to be successful, it should be used within the first few days of life.

There are differing views regarding the use of palatal appliances to assist with feeding in infants with a cleft (Balluff & Udin, 1986; Choi, Kleinheinz, Joos, & Komposch, 1991; Delgado, Schaaf, & Emrich, 1992; Jones, Henderson, & Avery, 1982; Kamegai et al., 1988; Kogo et al., 1997; Osuji, 1995; Razek, 1980; Selley & Boxall, 1986; Sorathesn, 1989). Some craniofacial centers advocate the use of a palatal obturator or feeding appliance and recommend its use on a regular basis. There have been reports of increased weight gain in selected groups of infants who have been fitted with feeding appliances (Balluff & Udin, 1986). In other settings, infants are given a trial of oral feedings and are fitted with appliances only if significant feeding problems are demonstrated. In some settings, appliances are rarely recommended, as those professionals feel that, with modifications of the nipple or bottle, correct positioning, and appropriate feeding technique, the obturator simply is not necessary.

Disadvantages of the obturator include the expense and the difficulty of use. Because the infant has no teeth to stabilize the appliance, it may be hard to insert the appliance as well as keep it in place. Other disadvantages include the possibility of irritation to the oral tissues and the need for ongoing replacement to accommodate growth. Hygiene may also be a concern if the appliance is not properly cleaned prior to insertion into the infant's oral cavity. Others maintain that, although the obturator can assist during feeding by helping the infant achieve compression of the nipple, the generation of negative pressure does not always occur

(Choi et al., 1991). However, even without allowing suction, the opportunity to compress the nipple by providing a hard palatal surface is considered a distinct advantage by some (Crossman, 1998).

Oral Hygiene

With all infants, it is important to maintain good oral hygiene. Although the mouths of infants tend to be self-cleaning, it is particularly important to attend to the infant's oral hygiene if there is a cleft lip or palate. With an open cleft, fluid will often enter the cleft area and nose. In addition, even with an upright feeding position, some nasal regurgitation is to be expected. The fluid can mix with mucous secretions from the mouth and nose and form a hard crust, which can become infected, causing irritation and soreness. Therefore, after each feeding the caregiver should cleanse the areas surrounding the cleft. The pediatrician may recommend using a washcloth, a small piece of gauze moistened with water, or water with hydrogen peroxide to gently wipe the mucous membrane in the oral cavity, with particular attention to that area that surrounds the cleft.

The caregiver should be careful not to cause discomfort or injury during this process; therefore, the use of a syringe or cotton swab is usually not recommended. However, it should be remembered that the cleft is not a wound, and therefore, it is not sore to touch. Gentle cleansing of this area will not cause discomfort or irritation.

Feeding the Older Infant

Transitioning to a Cup

Most infants are ready for transition to the cup by about 8 or 9 months of age. Some normally developing infants show readiness even earlier, between 6 to 8 months of age (Lang, Lawrence,

& Orme, 1994). The initial response to the cup is generally sucking, with tongue protrusion and loss of liquid from the mouth. Gradually the infant will demonstrate increased oral skills for cup drinking and is able to take one or two sip-swallows as the cup is held by the caregiver. The use of a slightly thickened liquid to slow the liquid flow during initial training with cup drinking is often beneficial. Many types of infant cups are available, so different options can be tried until one is found that works well for the infant.

Most surgeons recommend weaning from the bottle to the cup prior to the palate repair. Immediately after the palate repair, sucking is discouraged because it can result in a breakdown of the repair. The palate repair is usually done around 9 to 10 months of age, so weaning to the cup should be done sometime before this age to avoid feeding problems postoperatively.

Introduction of Solid Foods

Solid foods can be introduced to the baby with cleft palate at about the same time as with any infant. Usually, spoon-feedings begin with rice cereals and strained foods at or around 4 to 6 months of age. The baby will respond to the spoon feedings at first by suckling. This may result in food being pushed into the nasal cavity. As the baby becomes more skilled in eating and begins to use more mature tongue patterns, this will occur less often. The feeder should use a slow rate of presentation while spoon-feeding to allow the baby to gradually learn how to direct the food around the area of the cleft. The feeder should watch the baby for cues to know when to present the next bite. These cues include leaning forward or opening the mouth in anticipation of the spoon. Leaving the spoon in the baby's mouth long enough to allow the baby to use his or her lips to clean the spoon will help to facilitate lip mobility. This is especially important following the surgery for cleft lip repair. Overly rapid

feeding or large spoonfuls may cause nasal regurgitation as well as disorganization of safe swallowing (Morris & Klein, 1987).

The transition to more textured foods, such as lumpy or bite-sized table foods, also can be introduced in the same sequence as for other children. Foods should initially be offered by spoon with the baby seated in an upright position to reduce nasal regurgitation. Allowing the baby to practice finger feeding with small pieces of soft solids, such as cookies, will give the baby practice with the tongue movement needed for mastication. If food is observed passing from the nose or becomes lodged in the area of the cleft, it should be removed gently with either a finger or a swab. As the baby's oral-motor skills become more proficient, the baby will learn how to efficiently manage transfer of solids for swallowing.

Until the palate is repaired, washing out the oral cavity by feeding the baby water after each meal is important for the maintenance of oral hygiene. In addition, foods that are acidic or spicy should be avoided prior to the palate repair as the lining of the nose is particularly sensitive to this kind of food.

Objective Studies for Assessment of Airway Protection During Feeding

When the feeding difficulties are significant, as characterized by clinical signs of airway compromise, further evaluation is needed. Clinical signs of feeding dysfunction and airway protection problems can include the inability to establish and maintain a coordinated suck-swallow-breathe sequence, coughing, choking, color change, increased respiratory rate, as well as oxygen desaturations during feedings. The infant may respond to feeding attempts with arching or refusal to accept the nipple. Objective studies of swallowing function need to be performed to assess the infant's ability to safely feed and may also give information regarding the effect of compensatory strategies to improve the infant's feeding performance.

Videofluoroscopic Swallowing Study (VSS)

A *videofluoroscopic swallowing study*, also referred to as a *modified barium swallow*, is generally performed by a radiologist in cooperation with a speech pathologist. The videofluoroscopic study allows an overall view of the oral, pharyngeal, and esophageal phases of swallowing as well as the interactions between the phases. Swallowing function, as well as the infant's ability to maintain airway protection during swallowing, is carefully assessed. The degree of nasopharyngeal reflux and the occurrence of aspiration can be documented. The infant's protective reaction to aspirated material can also be assessed. Compensatory strategies, such as positional adaptations, different nipples, and pacing of presentations, can be utilized to determine their effect on improving the feeding process (Kramer, 1985; Newman et al., 1991). Disadvantages to the videofluoroscopic study include radiation to the infant as well as the feeder during the study, the necessity of adding barium contrast to the formula (increases viscosity, unfamiliar taste), and the fact that the swallows viewed represent a relatively small sample of feeding overall.

Fiberoptic Endoscopic Evaluation of Swallowing (FEES)

Pediatric *fiberoptic endoscopic evaluation of swallowing* (FEES) involves the transnasal passage of an endoscope for viewing of the pharyngeal and laryngeal structures (Willging, 1995). The focus of this study is on assessing the integrity of airway protection during swallowing. FEES also provides information regarding sensory threshold in the pharynx and larynx (Aviv et al., 1998). Advantages of the FEES procedure

include the ability to clearly visualize pharyngeal and laryngeal structures as well as the spontaneous swallowing of secretions. Feeding can be assessed using the infant's customary bottle and nipple and the usual formula. Green food coloring is added to enhance visualization of the bolus during the study. Compensatory swallowing strategies can be tried during the FEES study without the time limitations of fluoroscopy. Disadvantages include the temporary loss of view that occurs as the velopharyngeal valve closes around the scope during swallowing. This is generally not a problem with single swallows as the structures quickly return to their resting position following the swallow, thus restoring the view. There is, however, a particular disadvantage while viewing the rapid chain swallowing sequences characteristic of early infancy as the view is obscured with more frequency.

Management of Severe Cases

Alternative Feeding Methods for Severe Cases

When the feeding problem is not easily resolved with modifications of the nipple or bottle, supplemental feeding through a *nasogastric (NG) tube* may be required for a period of time. *Orogastric feeding* could also be used. Oral-motor treatment strategies during this time period to improve oral-motor function for feeding should be provided, as appropriate. If the feeding problems persist for a period of time and cannot be adequately resolved with other measures, *gastrostomy (G) tube* feeding is then considered. This is particularly indicated if the infant presents with abnormal oral reflexes or shows poor ability to coordinate airway protection with swallowing during a videofluoroscopic or endoscopic swallowing study. A gastrostomy tube is inserted through a surgical procedure, and may remain in place for an extended period of time. Should the infant show considerable signs of progress in regard to feeding skill development and oral intake, the tube can be removed (Rudolph, 1994).

Interdisciplinary Feeding Team Evaluation

In more severe cases, an evaluation by a team of specialists may be indicated. Typically, an interdisciplinary feeding team consists of a core group of medical professionals that may include a gastroenterologist, nutritionist, nurse, speech pathologist, occupational therapist, behavioral psychologist, otolaryngologist, pulmonologist, and consulting radiologist. The composition of interdisciplinary teams varies among centers (Lefton-Greif & Arvedson, 1997; Rudolph, 1994). With the coordinated assessment of these specialists, management and long-term planning for treatment of complicated feeding problems can be made.

Summary

Whatever feeding method is chosen, it is important that the feeding process becomes relatively easy and efficient. The infant must receive adequate nutrition in a relatively short period of time and without undue effort. Weight gain should be monitored closely by the pediatrician. If there is any evidence of inadequate weight gain, the pediatrician may consider the need for assessment of feeding modifications as well as supplemental feedings if necessary.

It is important that the feeding process is made to be a pleasurable experience for both the infant and the caregiver. It should not be forgotten that the time spent in feeding usually serves as an important part of the bonding process as well as the foundation for early sensorimotor and developmental experiences.

References

Alexander-Doelle, A. (1997). Breastfeeding and cleft palates [see Comments]. *AWHONN Lifelines, 1*(4), 27.

Arvedson, J., & Brodsky, L. (Eds.). (1993). *Pediatric swallowing and feeding: Assessment and management.* San Diego, CA: Singular Publishing Group.

Arvedson, J. C., & Lefton-Greif, M. A. (1996). Anatomy, physiology, and development of feeding. *Seminars in Speech and Language, 17*(4), 261–268.

Avedian, L. V., & Ruberg, R. L. (1980). Impaired weight gain in cleft palate infants. *Cleft Palate Journal, 17*(1), 24–26.

Aviv, J. E., Kim, T., Thomson, J. E., Sunshine, S., Kaplan, S., & Close, L. G. (1998). Fiberoptic endoscopic evaluation of swallowing with sensory testing (FEESST) in healthy controls [see Comments]. *Dysphagia, 13*(2), 87–92.

Balluff, M. A., & Udin, R. D. (1986). Using a feeding appliance to aid the infant with a cleft palate. *Ear, Nose, and Throat Journal, 65*(7), 316–320.

Barone, C. M., & Tallman, L. L. (1998). Modification of Playtex nurser for cleft palate patients [see Comments]. *Journal of Craniofacial Surgery, 9*(3), 271–274.

Bath, A. P., & Bull, P. D. (1997). Management of upper airway obstruction in Pierre Robin sequence. *Journal of Laryngology and Otology, 111*(12), 1155–1157.

Bosma, J. D. (1985). Postnatal ontogeny of performances of the pharynx, larynx, and mouth. *American Review of Respiratory Disorders, 131,* S10–S15.

Bosma, J. D., & Donner, M. W. (1980). *Physiology of the pharynx.* Philadelphia: W. B. Saunders.

Bu'Lock, F., Woolridge, M. W., & Baum, J. D. (1990). Development of coordination of sucking, swallowing and breathing: Ultrasound study of term and preterm infants. *Developmental Medical Child Neurology, 32*(8), 669–678.

Campbell, A. N., & Tremouth, M. J. (1987). New feeder for infants with cleft palate [Letter]. *Archives of Diseases in Childhood, 62*(12), 1292.

Carlisle, D. (1998). Feeding babies with cleft lip and palate. *Nursing Times, 94*(4), 59–60.

Choi, B. H., Kleinheinz, J., Joos, U., & Komposch, G. (1991). Sucking efficiency of early orthopaedic plate and teats in infants with cleft lip and palate. *International Journal of Oral Maxillofacical Surgery, 20*(3), 167–169.

Clarren, S. K., Anderson, B., & Wolf, L. S. (1987). Feeding infants with cleft lip, cleft palate, or cleft lip and palate. *Cleft Palate Journal, 24*(3), 244–249.

The Cleft Palate Foundation. (1998). *Feeding an infant with a cleft*. Chapel Hill, NC: Author.

Crossman, K. (1998). Breastfeeding a baby with a cleft palate: A case report. *Journal of Human Lactation, 14*(1), 47–50.

Danner, S. C. (1992). Breastfeeding the infant with a cleft defect. *NAACOGS Clinical Issues in Perinatal Women's Health Nursing, 3*(4), 634–639.

Darzi, M. A., Chowdri, N. A., & Bhat, A. N. (1996). Breast feeding or spoon feeding after cleft lip repair: A prospective, randomised study [see Comments]. *British Journal of Plastic Surgery, 49*(1), 24–26.

Delgado, A. A., Schaaf, N. G., & Emrich, L. (1992). Trends in prosthodontic treatment of cleft palate patients at one institution: A twenty-one year review. *Cleft Palate Craniofacial Journal, 29*(5), 425–428.

Fisher, J. C. (1991). Feeding children who have cleft lip or palate. *Western Journal of Medicine, 154*(2), 207.

Glass, R. P., & Wolf, L. S. (1999). Feeding management of infants with cleft lip and palate and micrognathia. *Infants and Young Children, 12*(1), 70–81.

Jones, J. E., Henderson, L., & Avery, D. R. (1982). Use of a feeding obturator for infants with severe cleft lip and palate. *Special Care in Dentistry, 2*(3), 116–120.

Jones, W. B. (1988). Weight gain and feeding in the neonate with cleft: A three-center study. *Cleft Palate Journal, 25*(4), 379–384.

Kamegai, A., Matsuoka, Y., Shimamura, N., Muramatsu, Y., Tanabe, T., Kurenuma, S., Kimura, Y., Shibata, K., Naitoh, K., & Kitajima, T. (1988). The clinical use of Hotz-type orthopedic plate [in Japanese]. *Gifu Shika Gakkai Zasshi, 15*(2), 521–530.

Koenig, J. S., Davies, A. M., & Thach, B. T. (1990). Coordination of breathing, sucking, and swallowing during bottle feedings in human infants. *Journal of Applied Physiology, 69*, 1623–1629.

Kogo, M., Okada, G., Ishii, S., Shikata, M., Iida, S., & Matsuya, T. (1997). Breast feeding for cleft lip and palate patients, using the Hotz-type plate. *Cleft Palate Craniofacial Journal, 34*(4), 351–353.

Kovar, A. J. (1997). Nutrition assessment and management in pediatric dysphagia. *Seminars in Speech and Language, 18*(1), 39–49.

Kramer, S. S. (1985). Special swallowing problems in children. *Gastrointestinal Radiology, 10*, 241–250.

Lang, S., Lawrence, C. J., & Orme, R. L. (1994). Cup feeding: An alternative method of infant feeding. *Archives of Diseases in Childhood, 71*(4), 365–369.

Lee, J., Nunn, J., & Wright, C. (1997). Height and weight achievement in cleft lip and palate [corrected and republished article originally printed in *Archives of Diseases in Childhood* (1996) 75(4), 327–329] [see Comments]. *Archchives of Diseases in Childhood, 76*(1), 70–72.

Lefton-Greif, M. A., & Arvedson, J. C. (1997). Pediatric feeding/swallowing teams. *Seminars in Speech and Language, 18*(1), 5–11; Quiz 12.

Lehman, J. A., Fishman, J. R., & Neiman, G. S. (1995). Treatment of cleft palate associated with Robin sequence: Appraisal of risk factors. *Cleft Palate Craniofacial Journal, 32*(1), 25–29.

Mathew, O. P. (1988a). Nipple units for newborn infants: A functional comparison. *Pediatrics, 81*(5), 688–691.

Mathew, O. P. (1988b). Respiratory control during nipple feeding in preterm infants. *Pediatric Pulmonology, 5*(4), 220–224.

Mathew, O. P. (1990). Determinants of milk flow through nipple units. Role of hole size and nipple thickness [see Comments]. *American Journal of Diseases of Children, 144*(2), 222–224.

Mathew, O. P. (1991). Science of bottle feeding. *Journal of Pediatrics, 119*(4), 511–519.

Mathew, O. P., Clark, M. L., Pronske, M. L., Luna-Solarzano, H. G., & Peterson, M. D. (1985). Breathing pattern and ventilation during oral feeding in term newborn infants. *Journal of Pediatrics, 106*(5), 810–813.

Meyer, E. C., Coll, C. T., Lester, B. M., Boukydis, C. F., McDonough, S. M., & Oh, W. (1994). Family-based intervention improves maternal psychological well-being and feeding interaction of preterm infants. *Pediatrics, 93*(2), 241–246.

Myer, C. M., Cotton, R. T., & Shott, S. R. (1995). *The pediatric airway: An interdisciplinary approach.* Philadelphia: J. B. Lippincott.

Morris, S. E., & Klein, M. D. (1987). *Pre-feeding skills: A comprehensive resource for feeding development.* Tucson, AZ: Therapy Skill Builders.

Newman, L. A., Cleveland, R. H., Blickman, J. G., Hillman, R. E., & Jaramillo, D. (1991). Videofluoroscopic analysis of the infant swallow. *Investigative Radiology, 26*(10), 870–873.

Oseid, B. (1979). Breast-feeding and infant health. *Seminars in Perinatology, 3*(3), 249–254.

Osuji, O. O. (1995). Preparation of feeding obturators for infants with cleft lip and palate. *Journal of Clinical Pediatric Dentistry, 19*(3), 211–214.

Razek, M. K. (1980). Prosthetic feeding aids for infants with cleft lip and palate. *Journal of Prosthetic Dentistry, 44*(5), 556–561.

Rudolph, C. D. (1994). Feeding disorders in infants and children. *Journal of Pediatrics, 125*(6, Pt. 2), S116–S124.

Sasaki, C. T., Levine, P. A., Laitman, J. T., Phil, M., & Crelin, E. S. (1977). Postnatal descent of the epiglottis in man. *Archives of Otolaryngology, 103,* 169–171.

Selley, W. G., & Boxall, J. (1986). A new way to treat sucking and swallowing difficulties in babies. *Lancet, 1*(8491), 1182–1184.

Shprintzen, R. J. (1992). The implications of the diagnosis of Robin sequence. *Cleft Palate Craniofacial Journal, 29*(3), 205–209.

Shprintzen, R. J., & Singer, L. (1992). Upper airway obstruction and the Robin sequence. *International Anesthesiology Clinics of North America, 30*(4), 109–114.

Sorathesn, P. (1989). Obturators for cleft lip and cleft palate [in Thai]. *Journal of the Dental Association of Thailand, 39*(2), 66–74.

Willging, J. P. (1995). Endoscopic evaluation of swallowing in children. *International Journal of Pediatric Otorhinolaryngology, 32*(Suppl.), S107–S108.

Wolf, L. S., & Glass, R. P. (1992). *Feeding and swallowing disorders in infancy: Assessment and management.* Tucson, AZ: Therapy Skill Builders.

CHAPTER

6

Developmental Aspects: Language, Cognition, and Phonology

CONTENTS

Children with a history of cleft palate or craniofacial anomalies are at risk for delays in the acquisition of speech and language skills. For example, children with a cleft palate will be behind their unaffected peers in the acquisition of certain early developmental phonemes due to the open palate. This delay will persist until the palate is repaired and usually for some time postoperatively.

The articulation problems secondary to velopharyngeal dysfunction have been well documented in the literature. There seems to be a good understanding of how the abnormal structure and function of the velopharyngeal valve affect speech by causing obligatory errors (Trost-Cardamone, 1997). It is also easy to understand how the child may respond to these difficulties in speech production by developing compensatory productions.

Understanding how the physical characteristics of cleft lip and palate or other craniofacial anomalies affect language and cognition is much harder. Of course, significant difficulties with speech production may cause expressive language skills to appear delayed due to the shortened utterance length. In addition, abnormalities of the brain or neurological dysfunction secondary to a craniofacial syndrome can result in cognitive and language disorders. However, there are other more subtle factors that may affect language acquisition and cognition in this population, such as multiple hospitalizations, a lack of adequate stimulation, or even social isolation.

This chapter outlines what is known about the language development of children with a history of a cleft or craniofacial anomalies secondary to a syndrome. The specific language and learning problems that are seen in these populations are discussed. It is hoped that the reader will learn to be concerned about the development of the whole child, including the areas of language and learning, when evaluating a young patient from these populations. Developmental aspects are critically important

to recognize and remediate in order for the child to become an integrated member of our society.

Developmental and Language Problems Associated With Clefts and Craniofacial Syndromes

Language refers to the symbolic system that is agreed upon by a community and used to convey a meaning or a message during communication. *Receptive language* is the ability to understand a message that is received and *expressive language* is the ability to generate and transmit a message. Although language is not innate in humans, humans have the innate ability to learn to communicate through spoken or *verbal language*. The ability to learn is dependent on the individual's cognitive abilities. In fact, *cognition* refers to the ability to engage in conscious intellectual activities, such as thinking, reasoning, imagining, or learning.

Developmental Problems

There is relatively little information in the literature on the developmental status of children with a repaired cleft or children with craniofacial anomalies. This may be due to the fact that, given the heterogeneous nature of these populations, it is difficult to determine what is "typical" for these children. In an early report, Starr, Chinski, Canter, and Meier (1977) reported that young children with a history of cleft performed essentially normally on either the Mental Development Index or the Psychomotor Index of the Bayley Scales of Infant Development (Bayley, 1969) at 6 months and 12 months. At 12 months and 24 months, however, there was more passivity in their response to stimuli. Fox, Lynch, and Brookshire (1978) used several developmental screening instruments to assess children with cleft palate who were between 2 months to 33 months.

They found a lag of 1 to 3 months on all measures. Because individuals with cleft palate only are at risk for developmental problems due to other factors, this is really not surprising.

Nieman and Savage (1997) studied the development of infants and toddlers with cleft lip and palate through a caregiver report. Their results showed "at-risk/delayed development" behaviors in the 5-month-olds with clefts, particularly those with cleft palate. At 13 months (which is usually after the palate repair) and again at 24 months, these children performed like the normative group. This was found again at 36 months, with the exception of "at-risk/delayed development" in the area of expressive language.

Language Problems

Some early research found that, in the cleft population, verbal performance scores were lower than nonverbal performance on standardized tests (Estes & Morris, 1970; Lamb, Wilson, & Leeper, 1973; Ruess, 1965; Wirls, 1971). In a more recent study, Broen, Devers, Doyle, Prouty, and Moller (1998) also found lower verbal performance than nonverbal performance in the cleft population. These differences were attributed to the hearing status of the children and the presence of velopharyngeal dysfunction. Two studies have shown no verbal-performance differences in the cleft population (Leeper, Pannbacker, & Roginski, 1980; McWilliams & Matthews, 1979).

Several early studies reported immature syntactic development, short utterance length, and overall delays in expressive language in children with a repaired cleft as compared to their unaffected peers (Horn, 1972; Morris, 1962; Smith & McWilliams, 1968; Spriestersbach, Darley, & Morris, 1958; Whitcomb, Ochsner, & Wayte, 1976). Others have found the linguistic abilities of children with repaired clefts to be within the normal range (Buescher & Paynter, 1973; Saxman & Bless, 1973). If there are delays

in early language development, there is also evidence to suggest that these delays disappear with time (Musgrave, McWilliams, & Matthews, 1975; Shames & Rubin, 1979; Zimmerman & Canfield, 1968). This may be due to the resolution of middle-ear disease or velopharyngeal dysfunction.

In a series of reports, Long and Dalston (1982a, 1982b, 1983) compared the prelinguistic behaviors of children with a history of cleft lip and palate with the performance of their unaffected peers. In the first study, Long and Dalston (1982a) evaluated the gestural communication of 12-month-old children. Their results showed that, even at an early age, children with history of cleft establish a need to communicate and a nonverbal means to do so in a normal way. However, in another study, Long and Dalston (1982b) found significant differences between a cleft group and noncleft group in the amount of vocalization behavior paired with gestures, suggesting difficulty with the prerequisites for sound production and verbalization at an early age. In the third study in their series, Long and Dalston (1983) found no significant difference between the two groups on measures of comprehension skills.

Chapman, Graham, Gooch, and Visconti (1998) studied the conversational skills of preschool and school-aged children with history of cleft lip and palate. When compared to their same-aged peers, there was no significant difference between the groups in the level of conversational participation. When individual child comparisons were done, however, the children with a history of cleft revealed less assertive profiles of conversational participation, particularly at the preschool level. The authors suggested that craniofacial team evaluations should include examination of conversational competency, particularly for children who are demonstrating difficulty with other aspects of speech, language, or social development.

Although language problems may not be significant in the isolated cleft lip and palate population, language disorders are common when the cleft is associated with a syndrome. For example, one of the features of Velocardiofacial syndrome (VCF) is language delay. In a recent study, Scherer, D'Antonio, and Kalbfleisch (1999) found that children with VCF showed severe limitations in speech sound inventories and early vocabulary development, even when compared to children with cleft lip and palate or isolated cleft palate.

In describing the language characteristics of children with a history of cleft or craniofacial anomalies, it is important to point out that these populations are not homogenous groups. In fact, these populations are extremely heterogeneous with respect to many factors, such as parental attitudes and involvement; environmental factors; contributing medical factors, such as hearing loss; the history of surgeries and hospitalizations; and the treatment history and treatment outcomes. These populations, particularly the cleft populations, are more dissimilar than similar. When language deficits occur, this makes it harder to determine specific etiology.

Despite the dissimilarities among individuals within these populations and the multiple factors that can influence language learning, there are some commonalties in these populations that place the child at risk for language delay. When we refer back to the basic prerequisites for normal language learning, even at a glance it is easy to guess why some children with craniofacial anomalies, including clefts, are at risk for language delays or even disorders.

Factors That Affect the Development of Language and Cognition

Language development and cognition are dependent on some basic prerequisites. These prerequisites include intelligence, environmental stimulation and experiences with the environment, sensory perception, motivation, and attending skills. Normal anatomy and physiology of the speech mechanism is also important for expressive language production. This section describes the need for these prerequisites and how these areas are affected by clefts or craniofacial anomalies.

Intelligence

The most important requirement for language learning is intelligence because it affects the ability to learn. Since language skills must be learned indirectly through exposure to the environment, the child must have the ability to learn to perceive, comprehend, assimilate, analyze, imitate, and then generate language.

Intelligence and brain development have a direct impact on the rate of acquisition of all developmental milestones. When intelligence is significantly below normal, there are usually generalized developmental delays that affect function in all aspects of development, including language and speech. For example, if a child is 3 years old but is cognitively functioning at the 12-month level, then language skills would be expected to be commensurate with developmental age rather than chronological age. Intelligence and cognitive function are totally dependent on the structure of the brain and the function of the central nervous system. Therefore, normal brain structure and function, and the resultant intelligence and cognition, are necessary requirements for the development of language and also for speech.

Considering intelligence, research has not shown a marked difference between children with a history of cleft and those with no congenital anomaly. Therefore, the presence of a cleft does not forebode an abnormal intellect. Some studies have shown minor differences in intellectual function in children with history of cleft in the early years of development, however. McWilliams (1970) and McWilliams, Morris, and Shelton (1990) used the term "intellectual depression" rather than "intellectual impairment" to describe the abilities of children with a history of cleft. This distinction was made to suggest that the status of intellectual function is probably due to a variety of factors, not just inherent intellectual ability.

Based on a review of the available research, McWilliams et al. (1990) concluded that children with history of cleft and no other anomalies are not at great risk for cognitive or developmental problems. However, children with a history of cleft palate only (CPO), especially those who have other congenital anomalies, appear to be at significant risk for developmental and intellectual deficits (Broder, Richman, & Matheson, 1998; Goodstein, 1961; Lewis, 1961; Richman, 1980; Richman, Eliason, & Lindgren, 1988; Strauss & Broder, 1993). These children are more likely to exhibit mental retardation or neurological dysfunction, sensorineural hearing loss, speech difficulties due to velopharyngeal dysfunction or malocclusion, attention deficits, frequent hospitalizations, and even social isolation (Elfenbein, Waziri, & Morris, 1981; Peterson, 1973). For instance, McWilliams and Matthews (1979) found that in a population of 108 children with history of isolated cleft palate and other anomalies, 51% had a full-scale IQ of 89 or below and 37% had IQs of 69 or below. This increased risk for cognitive and developmental problems is due to the fact that, when there has been an isolated cleft palate with other anomalies, there is a strong possibility that the cleft is part of a syndrome that includes mental retardation as a phenotypic feature.

There are many craniofacial syndromes, some that include clefts and some that do not, that include mental retardation or neurolinguistic deficits as a phenotypic feature. In describing various complex craniofacial disorders, Shprintzen (1998) listed the following conditions as ones that include mental retardation: Apert syndrome, BBB (Opitz) syndrome, Beckwith-Wiedemann syndrome, Carpenter syndrome, CHARGE Association, Down syndrome, Cornelia de Lange syndrome, Fetal Alcohol, Fetal Hydantoin, Holoprosencephaly Sequence, Noonan syndrome, Otopalatodigi-

tal syndrome, Rubinstein-Taybi syndrome, Shprintzen-Goldberg I syndrome, Shprintzen-Goldberg II syndrome, Weaver syndrome and Williams syndrome. Some syndromes and conditions do not have mental retardation or neurological dysfunction as typical phenotypic features, but have the potential for causing impairment in intellectual or neurological function. For example, in craniofrontonasal dysplasia, intellect is generally normal unless there are also midline defects of the brain. In Crouzon syndrome, hydrocephalus with increased intracranial pressure may occur due to the craniosynostosis. If left untreated, this can have a permanent effect on intelligence and cognitive function. Many of these syndromes and conditions include language disorder as a component of the phenotypic spectrum, in part due to the mental retardation.

Learning disabilities are also commonly found in individuals with craniofacial syndromes and these learning problems can also affect language. For example, it is well documented that the presence of learning disabilities is one of the most common characteristics of individuals with Velocardiofacial syndrome (Golding-Kushner, Weller, & Shprintzen, 1985; Kok & Solman, 1995; Motzkin, Marion, Goldberg, Shprintzen, & Saenger, 1993; Shprintzen, 1998; Shprintzen et al., 1978; Swillen et al., 1999; Vantrappen et al., 1999). Although intellectual ability may test within normal limits in the early years, the intelligence score tends to deteriorate in later years due to the individual's significant difficulty with abstract thinking. Mathematics and reading comprehension are the most severely affected due to this difficulty with abstraction.

Environmental Stimulation and Experiences With the Environment

Environmental stimulation and experience with the environment are important factors in language development. Children who live in a language-rich environment are likely to develop language skills faster and have a more extensive vocabulary than children with little language stimulation. If we consider the fact that young children are learning language for the first time, in a sense, it is like learning a foreign language. It is common knowledge that the more one is exposed to a foreign language, the faster and more completely that language is learned. Therefore, it is no surprise that the extent of language stimulation in initial language learning is a determining factor in the speed of language acquisition.

Young children have very "plastic" brains for language learning, particularly those under the age of 5 and before the myelination process has been completed. Children can learn language much faster than an adult, and most children can learn two languages almost as fast as one if they live in a bilingual environment. Given the capabilities of the young child's brain, it is easy to underestimate what the child is capable of learning. Most children under the age of 3 would know the word "apple" because it has been named for them in the presence of the object or the picture. However, very few children at this age know the word "artichoke." This is not because this word is harder to say or to learn. Instead, it is because very few children are exposed to an artichoke in a situation in which it is named.

In addition to being exposed to a great deal of language, children must have experiences with the environment before words about the environment are meaningful to them. For example, the word "hot" is a word that most very young children understand, but not because the word was defined or explained to them. Instead, they have experienced the feeling of hot in the environment while the word was used to describe that feeling. If a parent says, "Be careful, the stove is hot" and the child touches the stove anyway, the word and the experience are quickly associated. It is only when the word is associated with its perceptual aspects that the word begins to carry meaning.

Children with a history of cleft or craniofacial anomalies are usually not different in their opportunities to live in a stimulating environment. In one study, the language input of their mothers was found to be similar to the input of mothers of noncleft children (Chapman & Hardin, 1991).

In some cases, children with history of cleft or craniofacial anomaly may actually have an advantage over their noncleft peers. This is due to the fact that most of these children are followed by a cleft palate or craniofacial anomaly team and the speech pathologist on the team will usually counsel the parents on methods of language stimulation in the home. Some parents are so concerned about the child's development due to the anomalies, that they become very diligent in working on language stimulation. Another advantage these children may have is that many qualify for enrollment in an early intervention program, most of which are geared toward the development of language skills.

Although some affected children may have some advantages in early stimulation, others are not as fortunate. Children with significant anomalies and serious medical conditions may undergo many surgical procedures and frequent hospitalizations in the early years. Unfortunately, a hospital room is usually not a language-rich environment. Additionally, due to the compromised medical condition, and possibly due to the child's appearance, the severely affected child may not have as many opportunities to interact with others as their unaffected or less affected peers. This social isolation can negatively affect language learning.

Sensory Deprivation

It is through sensory perception that we learn about the world around us and develop a method to communicate with each other about that world. The need for adequate auditory skills for normal speech and language development is well understood. Severe hearing loss or deafness affects the child's ability to perceive and thus imitate speech sounds. It also affects the child's ability to hear words and associate those words with the meaning. A child who is deaf or severely hearing impaired will have difficulty learning the syntax of language or perceiving the changes in meaning with alterations in intonation and stress. As a result, verbal communication is extremely difficult, if not impossible, to acquire without hearing. Even partial hearing loss can affect the acquisition of oral language skills. Speech can be difficult to develop as a result of the inability to adequately perceive high-frequency, low-intensity sounds. Resonance can be affected by the inability to monitor and therefore modulate velopharyngeal function. Language development can be affected by even mild, fluctuating conductive hearing loss. Just as it is when the television is turned down too low, these children are able to hear only with effort and concentration. However, making that constant effort is exhausting and the child may respond by giving up and tuning out. Consequently, less language is heard, perceived, analyzed, and learned.

Although the need for hearing in language development is fairly obvious, the need for vision is also very important. Most of the way we categorize the world is through visual (not auditory or tactile) perception. Based on visual perceptual features, children learn the meaning of such diverse words as "big," "tree," "fast," "red," "truck," "empty," "run," and so on. The meaning of words is often learned by associating what is heard with the visual perceptual features of the object or action.

The process of learning the meaning of words is complex, and requires categorization based on certain perceptual features. Children learn to categorize and code substantive words (nouns, verbs, and adjectives) by both perceptual and functional features. For example, the word "chair" is a simple word that is usually acquired well before the second birthday. Yet, the child must go through a series of steps to try to place appropriate objects in the category that we call "chair." First, the child may attempt to code the object that he sees in the environment by perceptual features. If so, he could determine that all objects with four legs fit into the category that is called "chair." This feature alone does not work, however, as tables also have four legs. To resolve this, the child might need to code the word by functional features in addition to the perceptual features. Thus, the word "chair" might be coded as an object with four legs and is something on which you can sit. This still does not work all the time, because a couch (or do we say "sofa"?) is also an object that has four legs and is something to sit on. Now the child has to determine the one feature that works for all objects that are called "chair." The child finally realizes that a chair is something that people sit on, but only one person can sit on it at a time. Aha! The child is finally able to understand the word "chair" and to use the word appropriately after this process is complete.

Once a category is determined for the word, children continue to make mistakes in using the word. These mistakes are those of either overinclusion or underinclusion in the category. For example, the word "dog" is often the first animal that a child is able to name. In the early stages of language development, the child might include all animals with a tail, a snout, and four legs into the category called "dog." If shown a picture of a cow, the child might name it as a dog. On the other hand, the child may underinclude objects. For example, the child may include only the family dog in the dog category, or a Chihuahua or St. Bernard may be excluded from the category because one looks more like a mouse and the other looks more like a sheep.

The process of semantic development, as just described, requires normal sensory perception, including both auditory and visual perception. Children with a history of cleft palate are at high risk for chronic middle-ear effusion and conductive hearing loss due to eustachian tube malfunction. Some authors have suggested that the presence of hearing loss seems to be the primary reason that some children with history of cleft function at a lower level on verbal performance measures than their noncleft peers (Broen et al., 1998; Jocelyn, Penko, & Rode, 1996; Kritzinger, Louw, & Hugo, 1996; Lamb et al., 1973). Additional support for hearing loss as a factor comes from the studies that show that these differences in intelligence between children with history of cleft and their unaffected peers tend to disappear with age (Musgrave et al., 1975). This suggests that the depression in intellectual function is related to a temporary condition, such as a fluctuating conductive hearing loss due to chronic middle-ear effusion. The literature is equivocal about the long-term effect of chronic otitis media with fluctuating conductive hearing on language development (Paradise, 1998). A review of these studies leads one to believe that middle-ear disease may have some subtle effects on the development of language skills, especially if it is chronic. However, these effects seem to be erased with the resolution of the disease through time or with the insertion of pressure equalizing (PE) tubes.

Many craniofacial syndromes include conductive hearing loss secondary to chronic otitis media, and some include congenital sensorineural hearing loss as a phenotypic feature. For example, a primary phenotypic feature of Waardenburg syndrome is congenital sensorineural hearing loss that is usually severe and bilateral. Sensorineural hearing loss can also be found in Hemifacial Microsomia (also known as Goldenhar syndrome, Facio-Auriculo-Vertebral Malformation Sequence and

Oculo-Auriculo-Vertebral Dysplasia), CHARGE Association, Stickler syndrome, Treacher Collins syndrome, Turner syndrome, and others. Of course, hearing loss can have a significant impact on language development and can also be the cause of the depression in measures of intelligence in individuals with history of cleft, particularly in the early years.

Visual impairment is a feature in some craniofacial syndromes, such as Stickler's syndrome (which includes myopia). Fortunately, it is uncommon for the visual impairment in craniofacial syndromes to be significant enough to affect the process of visual coding of words for language. When blindness is presented however, vocabulary development will certainly be affected.

Motivation Problems

The next prerequisite for language development is motivation. Although a new skill can be learned passively, the skill will be acquired much more rapidly if there is a need and desire to learn the skill. This general principal holds true for language learning. Children must be motivated to talk in order to learn to talk. In most cases, young children have a great deal of motivation to talk since, by talking, they are able to communicate their wants and needs. However, if the parent, caregiver, or older sibling gives the child everything that is needed and also anticipates the child's wants, then a simple gestural system is sufficient and the child has no need to learn to talk. This can be a particular concern when children are hospitalized because all of their needs are taken care of and the hospital staff has little time for requiring the child to verbalize his or her requests.

During most of the first 2 years, a gestural system of reaching and pointing with grunting works well. This fulfills the child's communication needs since at this stage, communication is about the "here and now" and most of what the child needs to communicate is "Look at that" or "I want that." At this early age, the child does not need to tell the parent about what happened during his day. It is only when the child wants to communicate more that this system is no longer effective. With the increase in the need to communicate, there is a corresponding increase in the motivation to communicate. It is at this point that language development will pick up, assuming that everything else is normal.

For the most part, children with a history of cleft are no different from their unaffected peers in communicating their needs through gestures during the first year. The child begins to use verbal language and discontinue the use of gestures because verbal language is usually a more effective form of communication. However, if the child has difficulty with speech sound production and as a result, the parents and caregivers are unable to understand the child's speech, verbal language becomes an ineffective means of communication. Therefore, children with a history of cleft or other anomalies may revert back to using gestures out of necessity. Unless they are able to produce enough speech sounds so that verbal language is clear most of the time, gestures will continue to be used, at least to augment the speech. Because of this difficulty with speech sound production and the need to communicate as effectively as possible, some children will even economize in the length of their utterances. On the surface, this appears to be an expressive language disorder due to the telegraphic nature of the speech. Instead, it is often a compensatory strategy because shorter utterances are easier to produce clearly and easier for the listener to understand.

The family's response to their child with anomalies can also affect the child's motivation to learn to talk. Some families (including parents, older siblings, aunts, uncles, and grandparents) react by catering to the child's every need. They feel sorry for what the child has to go through and so they may react by overprotecting the child. Although this may be understandable at times, it can have a detrimental effect on the child's need to communicate to express his or her needs.

Attentional Deficits

The final prerequisite for this discussion is the ability to attend to the environment. Children who are abnormally active or are very distractible may have difficulty attending to the language in the environment. When there are significant attentional difficulties, the stimulation from the environment may not be adequately perceived or processed and language learning will be affected. Another problem is that hyperactive children are less likely to want to participate in language enriching activities, such as reading a book, listening to a story, or playing a game. They may also have difficulty learning other language-based skills, such as reading, for the same reason.

Attentional difficulties are a primary characteristic of *Attention Deficit-Hyperactivity Disorder* (ADHD). ADHD refers to a cluster of behavioral characteristics that involve impaired attention, impulsivity, and hyperactivity. It has been estimated that 3 to 5% of elementary school-aged children have this disorder, making it the most prevalent psychiatric disorder of childhood (American Psychiatric Association, 1994). ADHD is five to nine times more prevalent in boys than in girls (Sanberg, Rutter, & Taylor, 1980).

Although this disorder is usually diagnosed in children with no apparent history of a neurological lesion or infarct, the same characteristics are commonly seen in individuals with documented brain damage or neurological deficits (Max et al., 1998; Niemann, Ruff, & Kramer, 1996). In fact, this disorder used to be described as "minimal brain dysfunction" in children. Children with craniofacial syndromes that include neurological dysfunction are at significant risk for difficulties with attention and concentration. As an example, attentional deficits and difficulty with concentration are typical problems with Velocardiofacial syndrome (Heineman-de Boer, Van Haelst, Cordia-de Haan, & Beemer, 1999; Swillen et al., 1997; Swillen et al., 1999).

Children with attention deficit-hyperactivity disorder are prone to learning disabilites (Cantwell & Baker, 1991; Cherkes-Julkowski, 1998; Sidoti, Marsh, Marty-Grames, & Noetzel, 1996; Tirosh, Berger, Cohn-Ophir, Davidovitch, & Cohen, 1998). Because attentional deficits, distractibility and excessively high activity levels are not compatible with learning, it is not surprising that children with these behavioral characteristics are often found to have corresponding language disorders as well. In fact, a great deal of recent research has shown a high prevalence of language impairment in children with ADHD (Cantwell & Baker, 1991; Cherkes-Julkowski, 1998; Damico, Damico, & Armstrong, 1999; Fergusson & Horwood, 1992; Love & Thompson, 1988; Purvis & Tannock, 1997; Tirosh et al., 1998; Tirosh & Cohen, 1998; Wright, 1982). One study found that 30% of children with speech and language impairments had ADHD (Beitchman, Hood, Rochon, & Peterson, 1989).

Abnormal Anatomy and Physiology

The above prerequisites are important for receptive and expressive language learning. For oral expressive language and for speech, there are physical prerequisites that are also important. The subsystems of speech production require normal structure, from the lungs up through the entire vocal tract. There must be normal function for respiration, phonation, resonance, and articulation. Normal neurological function is also critically important. Anything

that affects the physical ability to produce sounds and to sequence sounds for connected speech can affect articulation and the production of oral expressive language. In fact, if the child is unable to sequence sounds easily for words, the child will not be able to sequence words together for sentences and shortened utterances may be used as a compensatory strategy. If the child shortens the utterance and concentrates on the important words, this can increase intelligibility. Of course, short utterance length and telegraphic speech will present as an expressive language disorder. Grunwell and Russell (1988) have pointed out that there is a close relationship between linguistic development and articulatory constraints. Therefore, expressive language skills cannot be fully developed if restrained by difficulty with articulation production.

Individuals with a history of cleft or craniofacial anomalies often have difficulties with the physical production of individual sounds. These difficulties may be due to velopharyngeal dysfunction, dental malocclusion, or other oral anomalies that make speech production a challenge. Because of the difficulty in speech sound production, greater effort is required to produce speech. As a result, individuals with defective articulation, especially if the intelligibility is poor, may not talk as much as those with less defective articulation. In fact, immature development of syntax and shortened sentence length have been reported in several studies of speakers with a history of cleft (Horn, 1972; Whitcomb et al., 1976). Comparing adults with repaired cleft with 20 unaffected adults, Pannbacker (1975) found significant correlations between the intelligibility of speech and measures of expressive language, such as mean length of response and number of words in the longest utterance. Of course, short utterance length and telegraphic speech may be due not only to the difficulty in producing speech, but may also be used as an active compensatory strategy to increase intelligibility. Therefore, when sentence structure is short and telegraphic in individuals with severely defective articulation, it is highly possible that the physical constraints in production are the cause of the apparent expressive language delay.

Phonological Development With a History of Cleft Palate

Before the Palate Repair

Early sound production is critical for normal speech and language development because it forms the basis for phonetic and linguistic development. By associating the physical movement of sound production with the auditory results through a tactile-kinesthetic-auditory feedback loop, infants are able to learn to produce sounds volitionally. Infants with cleft palate, however, have an inadequate sound production mechanism and they frequently have an impaired auditory system due to chronic otitis media. Because of these two factors alone, they are at risk for delays in phonological development (O'Gara & Logemann, 1988). Early palate repair and consistent otologic care can help to mitigate these risk factors.

The speech sounds that are developed by the infant with a cleft palate are influenced by his or her response to the structural anomaly during phonological development (Harding & Grunwell, 1996). O'Gara and Logemann (1988) suggested that, when structural constraints restrict phonemic development in the prelinguistic period, atypical or compensatory productions can occur even prior to the onset of meaningful speech. Chapman (1991) observed that infants with an unrepaired cleft palate demonstrate the use of nasal phonemes, glides, and the glottal fricative /h/ in spontaneous vocalizations, rather than the stop-plosives (p, b, t, d, k, g) that are typical of a normal babbling pattern. Russell (1991)

found a predominance of glottal stops during the babble stage of development. Certainly, infants with unrepaired clefts will have less variety in speech sound production than their nonaffected peers, at least until the palate is repaired. Some authors have reported that the presence of an unrepaired cleft palate can not only influence the infant's early phonological development, but that the predominant babble patterns also persist into early speech (Estrem & Broen, 1989; Hardin, 1991; O'Gara, Logemann, & Rademaker, 1994).

After the Palate Repair

Once the palate is repaired, usually around 10 months of age, most children will have an adequate structure for speech sound production. However, they will have missed the developmental stage (usually around 6 months) where stop plosives are usually produced and practiced through normal babbling. How quickly children with repaired clefts are able to acquire oral sounds and "catch up" with their unaffected peers has been a subject of several investigations.

One factor that may affect the acquisition of articulation skills is the age of palate repair. Dorf and Curtin (1990) reported significantly fewer compensatory articulation errors in the speech of their patients with cleft palate when the palatoplasty was accomplished by 12 months of age as compared to children with later repairs. Other authors have also suggested that children who undergo early palate repair demonstrate better overall speech than those with a later repair (Grobbelaar, Hudson, Fernandes, & Lentin, 1995; McWilliams et al., 1990; O'Gara & Logemann, 1988; Peterson-Falzone, 1996).

Although early articulatory patterns persist for some time after palate repair, several investigators have found that, within the first few years, glottal productions gradually decrease and the oral productions increase. As a result, the speech of those with a successful palate repair may gradually become similar to the noncleft peers by the age of 4 or 5 (Chapman, 1993; Chapman & Hardin, 1992; O'Gara & Logemann, 1988; O'Gara et al., 1994).

As the child's expressive language increases, there is a need for a wider range of consonants for intelligibility. If the child has significant velopharyngeal dysfunction, this limits the range of normal English consonants that can be produced. In this situation, many children increase their consonant repertoire by developing active, compensatory articulation productions, where articulation is primarily produced in the pharynx or larynx. Harding and Grunwell (1996) reported that, around 30 months of age, the nasal fricative became prevalent in the speech of their patients with repaired clefts. This may be due to the fact that at this point in phonological development, there is a definite need for a fricative-plosive contrast, and a normal fricative may be difficult to produce if there is velopharyngeal dysfunction. Once acquired and habituated, compensatory productions usually persist, even if the velopharyngeal dysfunction is corrected. Speech therapy is then required for a correction in production.

Summary

Early research showed differences in the language skills of children with a repaired cleft as compared to unaffected children. Unfortunately, these studies usually included children with all types of clefts, including isolated clefts of the palate. This inclusion can affect the results as it has been found that children with isolated cleft palate are at greater risk for a syndrome with mental retardation or neurological involvement. In future studies, the type of cleft should be considered in the analysis. It may also be that the differences in

language development that were found in early reports are less relevant today because in recent years, there has been a greater emphasis on early language stimulation and prophylactic otologic management.

Based on the existing research and the known prerequisites for language learning, it might be concluded that, when language deficits occur in the cleft population, they are relatively minor. In addition, language may not be a primary deficit, but may occur secondary to other factors (McWilliams et al., 1990). These factors include a fluctuating conductive hearing loss or speech production difficulties as a result of velopharyngeal dysfunction or malocclusion. The research has shown that, when language deficits occur, they tend to improve with time and the child usually catches up with his or her noncleft peers. It is important to remember that children with a history of cleft are at risk for language deficits, but these are usually minor and can often be prevented with early intervention. Language deficits in many craniofacial syndromes, which often includes isolated cleft palate, have more complex etiologies than in the cleft-only population. These individuals should be carefully observed and evaluated for language deficits at an early age, so that intervention can be initiated as soon as possible if needed.

In considering phonological development, infants with cleft palate necessarily acquire certain consonants, specifically stop plosives, at a later time than their unaffected peers. The rate of this development varies and is somewhat affected by the age at the time of palate repair and the passage of time. If the palate is repaired before 12 months, most children eventually catch up in phonological development, unless they have velopharyngeal dysfunction. Certainly stimulation offered in the environment can also speed up the process. Even though the prognosis for normal speech development is fairly good once the palate is repaired, the child remains at risk for persistent articulation errors, compensatory productions, and abnormal resonance due to velopharyngeal dysfunction. Therefore, phonological development should be carefully monitored throughout preschool years.

References

American Psychiatric Association. (1994). Diagnostic and statistical manual of mental disorders (4th ed.). Washington, DC: Author.

Bayley, N. (1969). *Bayley scales of infant development*. New York: Psychological Corporation.

Beitchman, J. H., Hood, J., Rochon, J., & Peterson, M. (1989). Empirical classification of speech/language impairments in children: II. Behavioral characteristics. *Journal of the American Academy of Child and Adolescent Psychiatry, 28,* 118–123.

Broder, H. L., Richman, L. C., & Matheson, P. B. (1998). Learning disability, school achievement, and grade retention among children with cleft: A two-center study [see Comments]. *Cleft Palate Craniofacial Journal, 35*(2), 127–131.

Broen, P. A., Devers, M. C., Doyle, S. S., Prouty, J. M., & Moller, K. T. (1998). Acquisition of linguistic and cognitive skills by children with cleft palate. *Journal of Speech Language and Hearing Research, 41*(3), 676–687.

Buescher, N., & Paynter, E. (1973). *Linguistic abilities of children with palatal clefts*. Paper presented at the Annual Meeting of the American Cleft Palate Association. Oklahoma City, OK.

Cantwell, D. P., & Baker, L. (1991). Association between attention deficit-hyperactivity disorder and learning disorders. *Journal of Learning Disabilities, 24*(2), 88–95.

Chapman, K. L. (1991). Vocalizations of toddlers with cleft lip and palate. *Cleft Palate Craniofacial Journal, 28*(2), 172–178.

Chapman, K. L. (1993). Phonologic processes in children with cleft palate. *Cleft Palate Craniofacial Journal, 30*(1), 64–72.

Chapman, K. L., Graham, K. T., Gooch, J., & Visconti, C. (1998). Conversational skills of preschool and school-aged children with cleft lip and palate. *Cleft Palate Craniofacial Journal, 35*(6), 503–516.

Chapman, K. L., & Hardin, M. A. (1991). Language input of mothers interacting with their young children with cleft lip and palate. *Cleft Palate Craniofacial Journal, 28*(1), 78–85; Discussion 85–86.

Chapman, K. L., & Hardin, M. A. (1992). Phonetic and phonological skills of two-year-olds with cleft palate. *Cleft Palate Craniofacial Journal, 29*(5), 435–443.

Cherkes-Julkowski, M. (1998). Learning disability, attention-deficit disorder, and language impairment as outcomes of prematurity: A longitudinal descriptive study. *Journal of Learning Disabilities, 31*(3), 294–306.

Damico, J. S., Damico, S. K., & Armstrong, M. B. (1999). Attention-deficit hyperactivity disorder and communication disorders: Issues and clinical practices. *Child and Adolescents Psychiatry Clinics of North America, 8*(1), 37–60, vi.

Dorf, D. S., & Curtin, J. W. (1990). Early cleft repair and speech outcome: A ten year experience. In J. Bardach & H. L. Morris (Eds.), *Multidisciplinary management of cleft lip and palate* (pp. 341–348). Philadelphia: W.B. Saunders.

Elfenbein, J. L., Waziri, M., & Morris, H. L. (1981). Verbal communication skills of six children with craniofacial anomalies. *Cleft Palate Journal, 18*(1), 59–64.

Estes, R. E., & Morris, H. L. (1970). Relationships among intelligence, speech proficiency, and hearing sensitivity in children with cleft palates. *Cleft Palate Journal, 7,* 763–773.

Estrem, T., & Broen, P. A. (1989). Early speech production of children with cleft palate. *Journal of Speech and Hearing Research, 32*(1), 12–23.

Fergusson, D. M., & Horwood, L. J. (1992). Attention deficit and reading achievement. *Journal of Child Psychology and Psychiatry and Allied Disciplines, 33*(2), 375–385.

Fox, D., Lynch, J., & Brookshire, B. (1978). Selected developmental factors of cleft palate children between two and thirty-three months of age. *Cleft Palate Journal, 15*(3), 239–245.

Golding-Kushner, K. J., Weller, G., & Shprintzen, R. J. (1985). Velo-cardio-facial syndrome: Language and psychological profiles. *Journal of Craniofacial Genetics and Developmental Biology, 5*(3), 259–266.

Goodstein, L. D. (1961). Intellectual impairment in children with cleft palates. *Journal of Speech and Hearing Research, 4,* 287.

Grobbelaar, A. O., Hudson, D. A., Fernandes, D. B., & Lentin, R. (1995). Speech results after repair of the cleft soft palate. *Plastic and Reconstructive Surgery, 95*(7), 1150–1154.

Grunwell, P., & Russell, V. J. (1988). Phonological development in children with cleft palate. *Clinical Linguistics and Phonetics, 2,* 75–95.

Hardin, M. A. (1991). Cleft palate: Intervention. *Clinics in Communication Disorders, 1*(3), 12–18.

Harding, A., & Grunwell, P. (1996). Characteristics of cleft palate speech. *European Journal of Disorders of Communication, 31,* 331–357.

Heineman-de Boer, J. A., Van Haelst, M. J., Cordia-de Haan, M., & Beemer, F. A. (1999). Behavior problems and personality aspects of 40 children with velo-cardio-facial syndrome. *Genetic Counseling, 10*(1), 89–93.

Horn, L. (1972). Language development of the cleft palate child. *Journal of South African Speech and Hearing Association, 19*(1), 17–29.

Jocelyn, L. J., Penko, M. A., & Rode, H. L. (1996). Cognition, communication, and hearing in young children with cleft lip and palate and in control children: A longitudinal study. *Pediatrics, 97*(4), 529–534.

Kok, L. L., & Solman, R. T. (1995). Velocardiofacial syndrome: Learning difficulties and intervention. *Journal of Medical Genetics, 32*(8), 612–618.

Kritzinger, A., Louw, B., & Hugo, R. (1996). Early communication functioning of infants with cleft lip and palate. *South African Journal of Communication Disorders, 43,* 77–84.

Lamb, M., Wilson, F., & Leeper, H. (1973). The intellectual function of cleft palate children compared on the basis of cleft type and sex. *Cleft Palate Journal, 10,* 367.

Leeper, H. A., Jr., Pannbacker, M., & Roginski, J. (1980). Oral language characteristics of adult cleft-palate speakers compared on the basis of cleft type and sex. *Journal of Communication Disorders, 13*(2), 133–146.

Lewis, R. (1961, April). *A survey of intelligence of cleft lip and cleft palate children in Ontario.* Presented at the 19th Annual Meeting of the American Association of Cleft Palate Rehabilitation, Montreal, Canada.

Long, N. V., & Dalston, R. M. (1982a). Gestural communication in twelve-month-old cleft lip and palate children. *Cleft Palate Journal, 19*(1), 57–61.

Long, N. V., & Dalston, R. M. (1982b). Paired gestural and vocal behavior in one-year-old cleft lip and palate children. *Journal of Speech and Hearing Disorders, 47*(4), 403–406.

Long, N. V., & Dalston, R. M. (1983). Comprehension abilities of one-year-old infants with cleft lip and palate. *Cleft Palate Journal, 20*(4), 303–306.

Love, A. J., & Thompson, M. G. (1988). Language disorders and attention deficit disorders in young children referred for psychiatric services: Analysis of prevalence and a conceptual synthesis. *American Journal of Orthopsychiatry, 58*(1), 52–64.

Max, J. E., Arndt, S., Castillo, C. S., Bokura, H., Robin, D. A., Lindgren, S. D., Smith, W. L., Jr., Sato, Y., & Mattheis, P. J. (1998). Attention-deficit hyperactivity symptomatology after traumatic brain injury: A prospective study. *Journal of the American Academy of Child Adolescent Psychiatry, 37*(8), 841–847.

McWilliams, B. J. (1970). Psychosocial development and modification. *ASHA Reports, 5,* 165.

McWilliams, B. J., & Matthews, H. P. (1979). A comparison of intelligence and social maturity in children with unilateral complete clefts and those with isolated cleft palates. *Cleft Palate Journal, 16,* 363.

McWilliams, B. J., Morris, H. L., & Shelton, R. L. (1990). Language disorders. In B. J. McWilliams, H. L. Morris, & R. L. Shelton (Eds.), *Cleft palate speech* (Vol. 2, pp. 236–246). Philadelphia: B.C. Decker.

Morris, H. L. (1962). Communication skills of children with cleft lip and palate. *Journal of Speech and Hearing Research, 5,* 79.

Motzkin, B., Marion, R., Goldberg, R., Shprintzen, R., & Saenger, P. (1993). Variable phenotypes in velocardiofacial syndrome with chromosomal deletion. *Journal of Pediatrics, 123*(3), 406–410.

Musgrave, R. H., McWilliams, B. J., & Matthews, H. P. (1975). A review of the results of two different surgical procedures for the repair of clefts of the soft palate only. *Cleft Palate Journal, 12,* 281–290.

Neiman, G. S., & Savage, H. E. (1997). Development of infants and toddlers with clefts from birth to three years of age. *Cleft Palate Craniofacial Journal, 34*(3), 218–225.

Niemann, H., Ruff, R. M., & Kramer, J. H. (1996). An attempt towards differentiating attentional deficits in traumatic brain injury. *Neuropsychological Review, 6*(1), 11–46.

O'Gara, M. M., & Logemann, J. A. (1988). Phonetic analyses of the speech development of babies with cleft palate. *Cleft Palate Journal, 25*(2), 122–134.

O'Gara, M. M., Logemann, J. A., & Rademaker, A. W. (1994). Phonetic features by babies with unilateral cleft lip and palate. *Cleft Palate Craniofacial Journal, 31*(6), 446–451.

Pannbacker, M. (1975). Oral language skills of adult cleft palate speakers. *Cleft Palate Journal, 12*(1), 95–106.

Paradise, J. L. (1998). Otitis media and child development: Should we worry? *Pediatric Infectious Disease Journal, 17*(11), 1076–1083; Discussion 1099–1100.

Peterson, S. J. (1973). Speech pathology in craniofacial malformations other than cleft lip and palate. *Asha Reports, 8*, 11–131.

Peterson-Falzone, S. J. (1996). The relationship between timing of cleft palate surgery and speech outcome: What have we learned, and where do we stand in the 1990s? *Seminars in Orthodontics, 2*(3), 185–191.

Purvis, K. L., & Tannock, R. (1997). Language abilities in children with attention deficit hyperactivity disorder, reading disabilities, and normal controls. *Journal of Abnormal Child Psychology, 25*(2), 133–144.

Richman, L. C. (1980). Cognitive patterns and learning disabilities of cleft palate children with verbal deficits. *Journal of Speech and Hearing Research, 23*(2), 447–456.

Richman, L. C., Eliason, M. J., & Lindgren, S. D. (1988). Reading disability in children with clefts. *Cleft Palate Journal, 25*(1), 21–25.

Ruess, A. L. (1965). A comparative study of cleft palate children and their siblings. *Journal of Clinical Psychology, 21*, 354.

Russell, V. J. (1991). *Speech development in children with cleft lip and palate* [Unpublished Ph.D. Thesis]. Leicester Polytechnic, Leicester, UK.

Sanberg, S. T., Rutter, M., & Taylor, E. (1980). Hyperkinetic disorder and conduct problem children in primary school population: Some epidemiological considerations. *Journal of Child Psychology and Psychiatry, 21*, 293–311.

Saxman, J., & Bless, D. (1973, April). *Patterns of language development in cleft palate children aged three to eight years.* Paper presented at the Annual Meeting of the American Cleft Palate Association, Oklahoma City, OK.

Scherer, N. J., D'Antonio, L. L., & Kalbfleisch, J. H. (1999). Early speech and language development in children with velocardiofacial syndrome. *American Journal of Medical Genetics, 88*(6), 714–723.

Shames, G., & Rubin, H. (1979). Psycholinguistic measures of language and speech. In K. R. Bzoch (Ed.), *Communicative disorders related to cleft lip and palate* (p. 202). Boston: Little, Brown.

Shprintzen, R. J. (1998). Complex craniofacial disorders. In S. E. Gerber (Ed.), *Etiology and prevention of communicative disorders* (Vol. 2, pp. 147–199). San Diego, CA: Singular Publishing Group.

Shprintzen, R. J., Goldberg, R. B., Lewin, M. L., Sidoti, E. J., Berkman, M. D., Argamaso, R. V., & Young, D. (1978). A new syndrome involving cleft palate, cardiac anomalies, typical facies, and learning disabilities: Velo-cardio-facial syndrome. *Cleft Palate Journal, 15*(1), 56–62.

Sidoti, E. J., Jr., Marsh, J. L., Marty-Grames, L., & Noetzel, M. J. (1996). Long-term studies of metopic synostosis: Frequency of cognitive impairment and behavioral disturbances. *Plastic and Reconstructive Surgery, 97*(2), 276–281.

Smith, R. M., & McWilliams, B. J. (1968). Psycholinguistic abilities of children with clefts. *Cleft Palate Journal, 5*, 238–249.

Spriestersbach, D. C., Darley, F., & Morris, H. L. (1958). Language skills in children with cleft palate. *Journal of Speech and Hearing Research, 1*, 279–285.

Starr, P., Chinski, R., Canter, H., & Meier, J. (1977). Mental, motor, and social behavior of infants with cleft lip and/or palate. *Cleft Palate Journal, 14*, 140.

Strauss, R. P., & Broder, H. (1993). Children with cleft lip/palate and mental retardation: A subpopulation of cleft-craniofacial team patients. *Cleft Palate Craniofacial Journal, 30*(6), 548–556.

Swillen, A., Devriendt, K., Legius, E., Eyskens, B., Dumoulin, M., Gewillig, M., & Fryns, J. P. (1997). Intelligence and psychosocial adjustment in velocardiofacial syndrome: A study of 37 children and adolescents with VCFS. *Journal of Medical Genetics, 34*(6), 453–458.

Swillen, A., Devriendt, K., Legius, E., Prinzie, P., Vogels, A., Ghesquiere, P., & Fryns, J. P. (1999). The behavioural phenotype in velo-cardio-facial syndrome (VCFS): From infancy to adolescence. *Genetic Counseling, 10*(1), 79–88.

Tirosh, E., Berger, J., Cohen-Ophir, M., Davidovitch, M., & Cohen, A. (1998). Learning disabilities with and without attention-deficit hyperactivity disorder: Parents' and teachers' perspectives. *Journal of Child Neurology, 13*(6), 270–276.

Tirosh, E., & Cohen, A. (1998). Language deficit with attention-deficit disorder: A prevalent comorbidity. *Journal of Child Neurology, 13*(10), 493–497.

Trost-Cardamone, J. E. (1997). Diagnosis of specific cleft palate speech error patterns for planning therapy of physical management needs. In K. R. Bzoch (Ed.), *Communicative disorders related to cleft lip and palate* (Vol. 4, pp. 313–330). Austin, TX: Pro-Ed.

Vantrappen, G., Devriendt, K., Swillen, A., Rommel, N., Vogels, A., Eyskens, B., Gewillig, M., Feenstra, L., & Fryns, J. P. (1999). Presenting symptoms and clinical features in 130 patients with the velo-cardio-facial syndrome. The Leuven experience. *Genetic Counseling, 10*(1), 3–9.

Whitcomb, L., Ochsner, G., & Wayte, R. (1976). A comparison of expressive language skills of cleft palate and non-cleft palate children: A preliminary investigation. *Journal of the Oklahoma Speech and Hearing Association, 3*, 25–28.

Wirls, C. J. (1971). Psychosocial aspects of cleft lip and palate. In W. C. Grabb, S. W. Rosenstein, & K. Bzoch (Eds.), *Cleft lip and palate* (p. 119). Boston: Little, Brown.

Wright, G. F. (1982). Attention deficit disorder. *Journal of School Health, 52*(2), 119–120.

Zimmerman, J., & Canfield, W. (1968). Language and speech development. In R. Stark (Ed.), *Cleft palate: A multidiscipline approach* (p. 220). New York: Harper and Row.

CHAPTER

7

Velopharyngeal Dysfunction (VPD) and Resonance Disorders

CONTENTS

The velopharyngeal valve is critically important for normal speech production. When this valve does not function normally, there is a significant effect on resonance and various aspects of speech. The size, shape, and configuration of the cavities of the vocal tract also have a significant effect on the resulting resonance and even on the intelligibility of speech.

The purpose of this chapter is to acquaint the reader with common abnormalities of the velopharyngeal valve and the vocal tract, and how these abnormalities can affect speech and resonance. This chapter discusses the types of velopharyngeal dysfunction and their causes. The effects of velopharyngeal dysfunction on resonance and also on articulation are described. Finally, resonance disorders, including and in addition to hypernasality, will be discussed with their various etiologies.

Velopharyngeal Dysfunction: Terminology

The literature is replete with inconsistencies in the use of terminology for disorders of the velopharyngeal valve. Some authors and clinicians use the common terms (velopharyngeal inadequacy, velopharyngeal insufficiency, velopharyngeal incompetence, and velopharyngeal dysfunction) interchangeably; others use these terms in a specific way to suggest etiology. Unfortunately, the careless or incorrect use of terminology can be dangerous if etiology is assumed from a term's use. For this reason, the careful use of terminology is important so that clear communication can occur between evaluating and treating professionals.

Some authors have proposed a taxonomy for velopharyngeal disorders based on etiology (Loney & Bloem, 1987; Trost, 1981; Trost-Cardamone, 1989). According to the classification system suggested by Trost-Cardamone (1981, 1989), the term *velopharyngeal inadequacy (VPI)* can be used as the general term for all types of velopharyngeal dysfunction. The term

velopharyngeal insufficiency (VPI) is used to describe an anatomical or structural defect that precludes adequate velopharyngeal closure. On the other hand, *velopharyngeal incompetence (VPI)* is used to refer to a neuromotor or physiological disorder that results in poor movement of the velopharyngeal structures. Finally, *velopharyngeal mislearning* refers to inadequate velopharyngeal closure secondary to faulty learning of appropriate articulation patterns. Although Loney and Bloem (1987) suggested a different use of this terminology, the classification system described by Trost-Cardamone seems to be the most widely accepted and has been adopted by many authors and clinicians in the field. Conveniently, all of these terms are abbreviated with "VPI."

Another general term that has gained wide acceptance is *velopharyngeal dysfunction (VPD)* (D'Antonio, Muntz, Province, & Marsh, 1988; Folkins, 1988; Jones, 1991; Loney & Bloem, 1987; Marsh, 1991; Morris, 1992; Netsell, 1988; Penfold, 1997; Witt et al., 1997). This term avoids any confusion regarding etiology. It also makes intuitive sense since it is the opposite of "velopharyngeal function," which is frequently discussed.

In this text, the terminology proposed by Trost-Cardamone will be used when etiology is known. However, the term "velopharyngeal dysfunction" is primarily used as the generic term.

Velopharyngeal Insufficiency (VPI)

As noted above, velopharyngeal insufficiency refers to a structural defect that causes the velum to be short relative to the posterior pharyngeal wall. For velopharyngeal contact to be made, the velum must be of sufficient length, once elevation and stretching have occurred, to span the depth of the velopharynx. There are many causes of discrepancies between the length of the velum and the needed length for firm velopharyngeal contact. These causes will be described.

History of Cleft Palate or Submucous Cleft

Velopharyngeal insufficiency occurs most commonly in individuals with a history of cleft palate. Despite surgical repair of the cleft, approximately 20% of these patients will demonstrate velopharyngeal insufficiency due to either inadequate velar length following the repair or velopharyngeal incompetence due to poor muscle function.

Individuals with a submucous cleft palate often have characteristics of velopharyngeal insufficiency, although the vast majority of these patients will have normal speech, even through adulthood (Chen, Wu, & Noordhoff, 1994; McWilliams, 1991). Obvious characteristics of a submucous cleft include a hypoplastic or bifid uvula; a bluish zona pellucida; visible diastasis of the soft palate musculature in the midline; or notching of the posterior border of the hard palate as noted through palpation. Some abnormalities, such as hypoplastic musculus uvulae muscles, can only be seen on the nasal surface of the velum, and therefore, must be detected through nasopharyngoscopy or operative dissection. This is called an occult submucous cleft and it can also cause incomplete closure of the velum against the pharyngeal wall. Regardless of whether the submucous cleft is overt or occult, the defect in the velum is typically in the midline, and this is usually where the velopharyngeal gap will be as well.

Short Velum or Deep Pharynx

Velopharyngeal insufficiency is sometimes noted when, despite normal velar morphology, the velum appears short relative to the posterior pharyngeal wall (Figure 7–1). When the velum cannot stretch enough to meet the posterior pharyngeal wall during speech, complete velopharyngeal closure cannot be achieved. In some cases, this is due to a congenitally short velum. In other cases, it is due

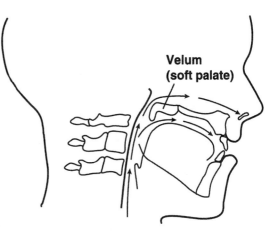

Figure 7–1. Velopharyngeal insufficiency. In this case, the velum is too short to achieve velopharyngeal closure during speech.

to a deep pharynx secondary to cranial base abnormalities (Haapanen, Heliovaara, & Ranta, 1991; Peterson-Falzone, 1985).

Status Post Adenoidectomy

A well-known and well-documented risk of an adenoidectomy is postoperative velopharyngeal insufficiency, causing hypernasality (Andreassen, Leeper, & MacRae, 1991; Blum & Neel, 1983; Croft, Shprintzen, & Ruben, 1981; Donnelly, 1994; Eufinger, Eggeling, & Immenkamp, 1994; Fernandes, Grobbelaar, Hudson, & Lentin, 1996; Kummer, Myer, Smith, & Shott, 1993; Parton & Jones, 1998; Ren, Isberg, & Henningsson, 1995; Robinson, 1992; Seid, 1990; Witzel, Rich, Margar-Bacal, & Cox, 1986). This is due to the fact that young children with a prominent adenoid pad usually achieve velo-adenoidal closure rather than velopharyngeal closure (Figure 7–2). Removal of the adenoids results in a deeper nasopharynx and a greater distance for the velum to stretch in order to achieve closure. For more information regarding adenoids, please see Chapter 8.

Temporary hypernasality following adenoidectomy can occur in individuals with no

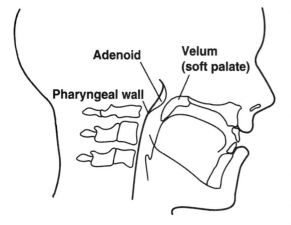

Figure 7–2. Position of the adenoid in the pharynx. The adenoid pad can help with closure in many cases. In many young children, there is velo-adenoidal closure rather than velopharyngeal closure.

velar defect. However, certain compensations occur in the velopharyngeal mechanism to adapt to the changes in the pharyngeal dimension. These compensations include an increase in velar mobility, an increase in velar height during closure, an increase in velar stretch, and increased movement of the pharyngeal walls (Neiman & Simpson, 1975). Therefore, postoperative hypernasality in individuals with normal velar morphology is typically short lived, lasting from a few hours to no more than 6 weeks. It usually resolves totally once these adaptations are made.

The incidence of permanent velopharyngeal insufficiency following adenoidectomy has been estimated to be approximately 1 out of 1500 procedures (Donnelly, 1994). This problem is more likely to occur if closure was achieved against the adenoid pad or was tenuous from the start. The primary etiological factor, however, is an underlying congenital abnormality of the velum that becomes apparent with removal of the adenoids. Although velar abnormalities are usually ruled out prior to performing an adenoidectomy, many patients with velopharyngeal insufficiency following adenoidectomy are found to have either obvious risk factors or subtle findings through nasopharyngoscopy that, in retrospect, would have been suggestive of velar abnormality (Parton & Jones, 1998; Schmaman, Jordaan, & Jammine, 1998). Certainly, individuals with a history of cleft palate or submucous cleft are at a much greater risk for velopharyngeal insufficiency following adenoidectomy due to tenuous velopharyngeal closure preoperatively and the lack of reserve muscle mass to stretch postoperatively (Parton & Jones, 1998). Therefore, adenoidectomy is usually contraindicated for individuals with a history of cleft or submucous cleft. If, however, the adenoid pad is so large that it causes airway obstruction or blocks the opening to the eustachian tube on one or both sides, a conservative adenoidectomy would be done. In this case, only a small portion of the adenoid pad or only the lateral borders would be removed.

Adenoid Atrophy

Individuals with a history of cleft palate or with a submucous cleft may demonstrate normal resonance and no evidence of velopharyngeal dysfunction during the preschool and early school years. However, they may begin to show signs of incomplete velopharyngeal closure when they reach adolescence. When this occurs, it is usually because there was tenuous, although effective, velopharyngeal closure against the adenoid pad, resulting in normal velopharyngeal function. With the onset of puberty, there is often significant, and sometimes sudden, atrophy of the adenoid tissue. As a result, there is an increase in the distance between the velum and posterior pharyngeal wall. If the velum is normal with no scarring from a cleft repair or no submucous cleft, it eventually stretches to accommodate the difference in the depth of the pharynx. Therefore, normal velopharyngeal closure is maintained.

However, if there is a h istory of cleft or there is a submucous cleft, the velum may not be capable of stretching and lengthening. As a result, velopharyngeal insufficiency occurs following the involution of the adenoid tissue (Handelman & Osborne, 1976; Mason & Warren, 1980; Morris, Wroblewski, Brown, & Van Demark, 1990; Shapiro, 1980; Siegel-Sadewitz & Shprintzen, 1986).

Irregular Adenoids

Although it is not commonly recognized, irregular adenoids can cause velopharyngeal insufficiency in some cases (Ren, et al., 1989). Enlarged adenoids are usually associated with hyponasality because they can block the entrance to the nasal cavity. Even when the adenoid pad is large, however, velopharyngeal insufficiency can occur if the surface of the adenoid has a deep indentation or cleft, as shown in Figure 7–3A. During attempts at closure, the velum is unable to achieve a tight seal against the adenoid as a result of this adenoid irregularity. This usually results in a small velopharyngeal (actually velo-adenoidal) opening, as can be seen in Figure 7–3B. Since the opening is usually small, it rarely causes hypernasality. In fact, there may be hyponasality if the adenoid tissue is large. However, this opening will cause nasal air emission. Ironically, irregular adenoids commonly occur after adenoidectomy. Since the entire adenoid capsule cannot be removed during adenoidectomy, some regrowth of the tissue often occurs. As it regrows, irregularities in the surface are often found.

Post Maxillary Advancement

Orthognathic surgery includes operations that involve the bones of the upper jaw (the maxilla) and the lower jaw (the mandible). This type of surgery can affect both speech and resonance, because it alters the occlusal relationship and can reduce the effectiveness of the

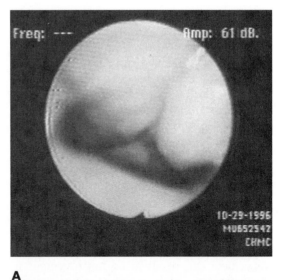

A

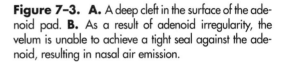

B

Figure 7–3. A. A deep cleft in the surface of the adenoid pad. **B.** As a result of adenoid irregularity, the velum is unable to achieve a tight seal against the adenoid, resulting in nasal air emission.

velopharyngeal valve. For additional information on this type of surgery, please see Chapter 20.

One type of orthognathic surgery, the Le Fort I maxillary advancement procedure, is commonly done with individuals who have a history of cleft palate. Its purpose is to correct midface deficiency by downfracturing the maxilla, and then bringing it forward to overlap the mandible. This is intended to normalize the occlusion and the facial profile. This procedure results in a dramatic improvement in facial aesthetics. In addition, the normalization of occlusion often results in improved articulation, particularly of sibilant sounds (Kummer, Strife, Grau, Creaghead, & Lee, 1989; McCarthy, Coccaro, & Schwartz, 1979). If there is nasal obstruction or hyponasality due to nasal airway resistance, maxillary advancement can result in an improvement in these problems by increasing the nasal cavity space (Dalston & Vig, 1984).

Although maxillary advancement can improve aesthetics, articulation, the nasal airway, and hyponasality, it can have a negative effect on velopharyngeal function. With this procedure, the anterior movement of the maxilla results in movement of the posterior border of the hard palate, with its soft palate attachments. This results in an increase in the pharyngeal depth. If there is only tenuous velopharyngeal closure preoperatively or if the velum is scarred due to a previous velar repair, it may not be able to stretch adequately following the surgery to span the entire pharyngeal depth.

The exact risk of velopharyngeal insufficiency following maxillary advancement is not known, but it is not a common occurrence in individuals who have no history of cleft palate or velar abnormality. In fact, the velopharyngeal mechanism normally makes the same types of adaptations following maxillary advancement as it does following normal adenoid atrophy or adenoidectomy (Kummer et al., 1989). Therefore, most patients will not experience a long-term problem with velopharyngeal function postoperatively.

Those at greatest risk for hypernasality following maxillary advancement are the individuals who often can benefit the most from the procedure: particularly patients with a history of cleft palate and resulting midface retrusion (Haapanen, Kalland, Heliovaara, Hukki, & Ranta, 1997; Kummer et al., 1989; Maegawa, Sells, & David, 1998; Mason, Turvey, & Waren, 1980; McCarthy et al., 1979; Okazaki et al., 1993; Watzke, Turvey, Warren, & Dalston, 1990). The effect on velopharyngeal function, and thus resonance, appears to be somewhat related to the amount of advancement, so that those with the greatest maxillary movement are at greatest risk for velopharyngeal dysfunction (Maegawa et al., 1998). If speech and velopharyngeal function deteriorate after maxillary advancement, a pharyngeal flap is usually the treatment procedure of choice, given the fact that the deficit is in the anterior-posterior dimension (Maegawa et al., 1998).

Oral Cavity Tumors

Oral cavity tumors occur in both children and in adults. In children, the most common tumor is a *hemangioma*, which is a congenital anomaly in which a proliferation of blood vessels results in a large mass. In adults, malignant tumors of the oral cavity are often seen. When a tumor or growth interferes with function or becomes life-threatening, it is usually resected. Resections of areas of the oral cavity can affect the integrity of the separation of the nasal and oral cavities and the function of the velopharyngeal valve (Bodin, Lind, & Arnander, 1994; Brown, Zuydam, Jones, Rogers, & Vaughan, 1997; Fee, Gilmer, & Goffinet, 1988; Myers & Aramany, 1977; Rintala, 1987; Yoshida, Michi, Yamashita, & Ohno, 1993). This is particularly a concern if tissue is taken from the hard palate, velum, or pharyngeal walls. If radiation is used as treatment, it can cause shrinkage of the structures and further impair the function of the velopharyngeal valve.

Hypertrophic Tonsils

Due to the position of the tonsils in the oral cavity, they usually do not have an effect on speech. There are some exceptions however. The role of tonsils in speech production is further discussed in Chapter 8.

Hypertrophic tonsils, on rare occasions, can cause mechanical interference with the function of the velopharyngeal valve. If one tonsil is much larger than the other, it will often push the velum upward on that side. Due to the pulling and stretching of the velum on that side, the uvula will deviate and appear to point to the large tonsil. Large tonsils can restrict the medial movement of the lateral pharyngeal walls, thus affecting velopharyngeal closure. If both of the tonsils are very large so that they are almost touching in midline, this will restrict the transmission of sound and air pressure into the oral cavity.

There may also be an association between large tonsils and decreased velopharyngeal activity for speech sounds articulated in the back of the mouth. Large tonsils can force the tongue to move forward and can interfere with the articulation of velar sounds (k, g). Henningsson and Isberg (1988) have suggested that large tonsils can also affect velopharyngeal activity for these sounds.

The most dramatic effect of hypertrophic tonsils on velopharyngeal function occurs when a tonsil is so large that the upper pole of the tonsil projects into the pharynx as is illustrated in Figure 7–4A. If it is positioned between the velum and posterior pharyngeal wall, it prevents the velum from achieving an adequate velopharyngeal seal during speech, as can be seen in Figure 7–4B (Kummer et al., 1993; MacKenzie-Stepner, Witzel, Stringer, & Laskin, 1987; Misra, Gill, & Lal, 1981; Peterson-Falzone, 1985; Shprintzen, Sher, & Croft, 1987). This results in a small velopharyngeal gap, which usually causes nasal air emission. The tonsil in the pharynx can also obstruct sound transmission into both the oral and nasal

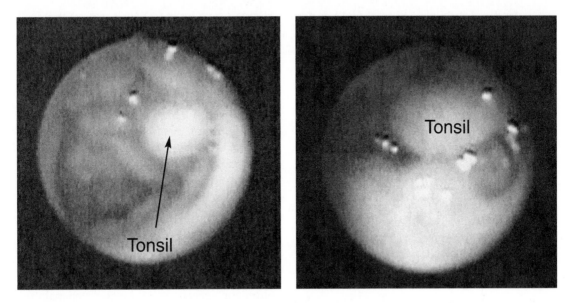

A   **B**

Figure 7–4. A. Large tonsil on the right that can be seen in the nasopharynx from above through nasopharyngoscopy. **B.** Tonsil can be seen between the velum and posterior pharyngeal wall during velopharyngeal closure. During closure, a small opening remains, just to the left of the tonsil. There is a bubble in this area due to nasal air emission.

Case Report: Enlarged Tonsils

Ellen was a 9-year-old child with a history of normal speech and language development. She had never had speech therapy. However, over about a 2-year period, her speech had gradually become "nasal" and hard to understand. The parents reported that Ellen had also begun to snore loudly at night.

On examination, Ellen was noted to have an open mouth posture with an anterior tongue position at rest. An evaluation of her speech revealed normal articulation, but nasal emission during the production of pressure-sensitive phonemes. Resonance was characterized by hyponasality and a cul-de-sac quality.

An intraoral examination revealed the cause of the speech characteristics. The right tonsil was very large (grade 4+) and extended medially beyond the point of the midline of the oral cavity. The left tonsil was grade 1+ in size. A nasopharyngoscopy assessment showed the tonsil to be in the nasopharynx and between the velum and posterior pharyngeal wall during velopharyngeal closure. Because of the position of the tonsil, complete velopharyngeal closure could not be achieved, resulting in nasal air emission. The large tonsil in the pharynx interfered with the transmission of sound energy into the nasal cavity during the production of nasal sounds, thus causing hyponasality. The size of the tonsil also blocked the sound energy from entering the oral cavity during the production of oral sounds. This was the cause of the cul-de-sac resonance.

Given these findings, the obvious treatment was a tonsillectomy. Once this was done, resonance returned to normal and nasal air emission was eliminated. Ellen was able to maintain a closed-mouth posture and snoring was no longer noted at night

cavities, causing a mixture of hyponasality and cul-de-sac resonance. Tonsillectomy is obviously indicated to eliminate these characteristics.

Velopharyngeal Incompetence (VPI)

Velopharyngeal incompetence refers to a physiological deficiency, that results in poor movement of the velopharyngeal structures. Velopharyngeal incompetence may cause poor elevation of the velum and inadequate "knee action" during speech (Figure 7–5). Lateral pharyngeal wall motion may also be very poor so that there is minimal medial movement to assist with closure. There are many causes of velopharyngeal incompetence, as will be discussed below.

Abnormal Muscle Insertion

Velopharyngeal incompetence can occur following a cleft palate repair due to poor muscle function. Even though the surgeon may attempt to dissect the levator veli palatini muscle and repair its orientation, it does not guarantee that this muscle will function normally. When there is a submucous cleft palate that extends through the velum, the levator veli palatini muscle is inserted into the hard palate, rendering it useless in elevating the velum for speech. If the levator veli palatini muscles are not appropriately inserted to form the levator sling, then the velum will not elevate enough during speech to achieve velopharyngeal closure. On lateral videofluoroscopy, the velum will appear to be well be-

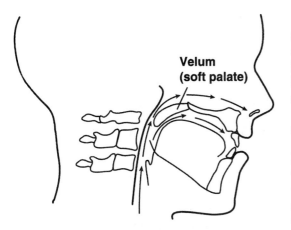

Figure 7–5. Velopharyngeal incompetence. In this case, the velum does not move well enough to achieve velopharyngeal closure during speech.

low the level of the hard palate during speech and the velar eminence will not be significant.

Poor Lateral Pharyngeal Wall Movement

Poor lateral pharyngeal wall movement may contribute to velopharyngeal incompetence. It should be noted, however, that when lateral wall motion is limited, it may not be the result of a physiological defect. Instead, limited movement of the lateral walls may be a normal finding if the primary pattern of closure is the coronal pattern (Finkelstein, Talmi, Nachmani, Hauben, & Zohar, 1992; Shprintzen, Rakof, Skolnick, & Lavorato, 1977; Siegel-Sadewitz & Shprintzen, 1982; Skolnick, Shprintzen, McCall, & Rakoff, 1975; Witzel & Posnick, 1989). Extensive lateral wall motion is noted only in the sagittal pattern, which is the least common pattern found in both normal and abnormal speakers (Witzel & Posnick, 1989). Therefore, although poor lateral pharyngeal wall movement may contribute to a velopharyngeal opening, by itself it is not an abnormal finding.

Although posterior pharyngeal wall motion is noted in some speakers, its contribution to the closure of the velopharyngeal valve is minimal in comparison. Therefore, the observation of a lack of posterior pharyngeal wall motion in an abnormal speaker is not particularly significant.

Oral-Motor Dysfunction

Dysarthria is one form of oral-motor dysfunction that can cause velopharyngeal incompetence and, thus, hypernasality. *Dysarthria* is characterized by abnormalities of strength, range of motion, speed, accuracy, and tonicity of the speech muscles due to central and/or peripheral nervous system impairment. As a result, speech is very slow, slurred, and characterized by inaccurate movement of the articulators. Dysarthria affects all the subsystems of speech, including respiration, phonation, resonance, and articulation.

Dysarthria causes poor motor movement of the anterior articulators, such as the tongue, the lips, and the jaws; and it also affects the movement of the posterior articulators, which are the velopharyngeal structures. As a result, hypernasality secondary to velopharyngeal incompetence is one of the primary characteristics of dysarthria (Yorkston, Beukelman, & Traynor, 1988). Other common characteristics of velopharyngeal incompetence due to dysarthria include weak consonants and short utterance length as a result of the loss of air pressure nasally.

Dysarthria with hypernasality has been associated with a variety of neurological causes. It can be secondary to either upper or lower motor neuron lesions. Some of the causes include cerebral palsy (Ansel & Kent, 1992; Neilson & O'Dwyer, 1981; Platt, Andrews, & Howie, 1980; Platt, Andrews, Young, & Quinn, 1980), myasthenia gravis (Hagstrom, Parsons, Landa, & Robson, 1979; Wolski, 1967), myotonic dystrophy (Hillarp, Ekberg, Jacobsson, Nylander, & Aberg, 1994; Salomonson, Kawamoto, & Wilson, 1988), neurofibromatosis (Pollack & Shprintzen, 1981), and cerebral or brainstem tumors (Lefaivre, Cohen, Riski, & Burstein, 1997; Van Mourik, Catsman-Berrevoets, Yousef-Bak, Paquier, & van Dongen, 1998). Dysarthria with hypernasality has been associated with mental retardation or developmental delay (Bradley, 1979; Heller, Gens, Moe, & Lewin, 1974; Kline & Hutchinson, 1980; Peterson-Falzone, 1985) and it can also occur secondary to acquired neurological damage due to traumatic brain injury (TBI) (Theodoros, Murdoch, Stokes, & Chenery, 1993; Upton & Berger, 1995; Workinger & Netsell, 1992) or cerebral vascular accident (CVA) (Thompson & Murdoch, 1995). Any disorder that causes cerebral, cerebellar or brainstem damage potentially can cause dysarthria with hypernasality.

Apraxia of speech (AOS) is another oral-motor disorder that can cause velopharyngeal incompetence. *Apraxia of speech*, also called *verbal apraxia* or *dyspraxia*, is characterized by difficulty executing volitional oral movements and difficulty in sequencing oral movements for connected speech. Apraxia of speech can result in an inability to adequately coordinate velopharyngeal movement with the other subsystems of speech (respiration, phonation, and articulation) (Bradley, 1997; McWilliams, Morris, & Shelton, 1990b; Trost-Cardamone, 1989). In addition, there may be difficulty coordinating and sequencing the upward movement of the velum for oral sounds with the downward movement of the velum for nasal sounds, as is needed in connected speech. At times, the velum may elevate for closure, but drop down before it is appropriate. The velum may appear to pulse up and down during connected speech, rather than staying up throughout the production of oral sounds. At other times, the timing of closure may be affected by poor coordination so that closure does not occur until after the initiation of phonation when it is too late (Warren, Dalston, & Mayo, 1993; Warren, Dalston, Trier, & Holder, 1985). Velopharyngeal incompetence as a result of apraxia of speech is usually very

inconsistent. The speaker may produced both correct and incorrect productions of each phoneme, even within a single utterance. All errors, including those of resonance, will tend to increase in severity with an increase in utterance length and phonemic complexity.

Cranial Nerve Defects

Individuals with either congenital or acquired lower motor neuron damage may demonstrate specific velopharyngeal paralysis or paresis (weakness) of the velum or pharyngeal musculature (Rousseaux, Lesoin, & Quint, 1987). This can occur with involvement of the glossopharyngeal nerve (CN IX), the vagus nerve (CN X), or the hypoglossal nerve (CN XII). The paralysis or paresis is usually unilateral and can occur in the absence of other oral-motor deficits. When the vagus nerve (CN X) is involved, there may also be unilateral involvement of the larynx and vocal fold on the same side.

With unilateral paralysis or paresis, one side of the velum will elevate normally during speech and may achieve closure. On the affected side, however, the velum will hang down during speech and a velopharyngeal opening will occur on that side of the midline. When this is observed from an intraoral perspective, the velum can be seem to droop on the affected side and the uvula will point to the side with better movement. Unilateral paralysis or paresis is commonly observed in individuals with hemifacial microsomia (Luce, McGibbon, & Hoopes, 1977).

Velar Fatigue in Wind Instrument Players

Playing a wind instrument requires a large amount of intraoral air pressure and a certain amount of velopharyngeal strength and stamina to maintain closure with that amount of pressure. Velopharyngeal dysfunction, second-

Case Report: Hypernasality Secondary to Dysarthria

Brandon was a 20-year-old college student when he had a cerebral hemorrhage secondary to an arterial venous (AV) malformation. This affected his speech, swallowing, the movement of the right side of the body, his walking, and vision. Fortunately, there was no cognitive loss. Brandon had received speech therapy for characteristics of dysarthria.

Brandon was referred to our VPI Clinic because one of the primary concerns was hypernasality. He had already tried a prosthetic device, but it was not effective and caused other problems. At the time of the evaluation, Brandon was found to have normal articulatory placement, but characteristics of dysarthria including slow rate, imprecise movements, difficulty with initiation of movements for sound production, and labored movement. Articulation was affected by weak consonants due to significant nasal air emission. In addition, there was poor breath support, short utterance length, glottal fry, aphonia at the ends of utterances, and severe hypernasality.

Nasopharyngoscopy (a nasal endoscopic procedure) showed inconsistent velar elevation with occasional touch closure of the velum against the posterior pharyngeal wall at midline. The velum was noted to tire easily, however, and drop down inappropriately. There was also poor lateral pharyngeal wall motion.

Because prosthetic treatment had been tried unsuccessfully, it was decided to try surgical intervention, specifically a pharyngeal flap. The goals of the surgery were to improve the quality and clarity of speech while decreasing the effort required to produce speech.

Brandon was seen 6 weeks postoperatively for a reassessment. At that time, he demonstrated significantly improved speech. The hypernasality was reduced to a mild degree and there was only slight nasal air emission. Of most significance was the increase in oral pressure and, thus, speech sound clarity. In addition, utterance length was longer and Brandon no longer needed to take frequent breaths to replenish breath support because there was less loss of air pressure for speech. In fact, Brandon was able to count to 23 on one breath rather than to 4 as he had preoperatively.

Although the pharyngeal flap did not result in a total correction of speech, it did result in significant improvement in the quality and clarity of speech. It also made speech less effortful. Brandon and his family were very pleased with the result.

ary to stress on the mechanism, has been reported in wind instrument musicians who do not have velopharyngeal dysfunction in speech (Dibbell, Ewanowski, & Carter, 1979; Gordon, Astrachan, & Yanagisawa, 1994; Peterson-Falzone, 1985; Shanks, 1990). Velopharyngeal incompetence can occur due to velar fatigue if the strength and stamina are not adequate and cannot be maintained over a period of time. When this occurs only in certain circumstances, such as when playing a wind instrument, or if it occurs suddenly, the person should be monitored over a period of time because this may be the first symptom of a progressive neurological disorder and may be a precursor to hypernasality in speech.

Velopharyngeal Mislearning

Velopharyngeal mislearning can cause abnormal resonance and nasal air emission with speech. With velopharyngeal mislearning, resonance and speech may sound similar to that of individuals with true velopharyngeal dysfunction. However, these individuals do not have a primary velopharyngeal disorder, and therefore, they are not candidates for surgical or prosthetic intervention. Instead, speech therapy is usually successful in correcting or at least improving these functional speech characteristics.

Faulty Articulation

Some children develop articulation patterns that include a *posterior nasal fricative*. With this production, the velum is down and air pressure through the velopharyngeal opening creates a friction sound with audible nasal air emission. This production is typically used as a substitution for sibilant sounds, particularly s/z. Because the nasal air emission occurs only on certain speech sounds, it is called *phoneme-specific nasal air emission* (PSNAE). In this case, the nasal air emission is the result of faulty articulation and is not due to an anatomical or physiological cause.

Articulation patterns can affect resonance in other ways. If the tongue position is high in the back of the mouth or if the tongue is retracted, the transmission of sound energy into the oral cavity is restricted and the quality of the resonance will be affected (McDonald & Baker, 1951; Falk & Kopp, 1968; McWilliams et al., 1990b). Limited mouth opening can have a similar effect because it reduces the size of the oral cavity space during speech and restricts oral resonance. The same effect occurs when the size of the oral cavity is small due to the history of a cleft (Falk & Kopp, 1968). Low volume and reduced respiratory effort can give the perception of increased hypernasality. Finally, oral inactivity resulting in poor movement of the articulators can cause characteristics of velopharyngeal dysfunction. This is due to the fact that, when there is poor movement of the anterior articulators, it usually results in poor movement of the posterior articulators, which are the velopharyngeal structures.

Habituated Speech Patterns

Characteristics of velopharyngeal dysfunction can continue, even after surgical correction of the cause. This is because the individual has already learned and habituated speech patterns of articulation prior to the correction. In addition, the auditory feedback loop that monitors resonance can cause hypernasality to persist, because it was the "normal" sound of the speech before surgical correction. Since changing structure does not change function, speech therapy is usually required to change those patterns once the structural defects have been corrected. Postoperative speech therapy is important to help the individual to learn to make the best use of the new structure and to correct articulation errors that occur as a result of the history of velopharyngeal dysfunction.

Lack of Auditory Feedback

Individuals with severe hearing loss or deafness usually demonstrate abnormal resonance. There may be hypernasality, hyponasality, or a combination of the two. The velopharyngeal valve may close inappropriately on nasal phonemes and open on oral phonemes. This is usually not due to a structural or physiological abnormality. Instead, it is the result of a lack of auditory feedback, which makes it impossible to regulate and modulate velopharyngeal function. Because velopharyngeal movement is not felt and is controlled primarily by auditory feedback, resonance is negatively affected. As a result, the speech patterns that are learned include velopharyngeal dysfunction (Abdullah, 1988; Fletcher & Daly, 1976; Ysunza & Vazquez, 1993).

Conversion Disorder

Although it is rare, velopharyngeal incompetence resulting in hypernasality can occur as a conversion disorder, or learned reaction to a certain event. This has been reported following tonsillectomy (Gibb & Stewart, 1975). The tonsils reside in the oral cavity and their removal usually does not cause velopharyngeal dysfunction. However, tonsillectomy can be a very painful procedure and patients can experience a severe psychological reaction to the surgery. In our center, we recently treated a patient with severe velopharyngeal incompetence following tonsillectomy. Nasopharyngoscopy showed very little velopharyngeal movement during speech and velopharyngeal closure did not occur, even with swallowing. It was apparent through nasopharyngoscopy that the tongue base was being held in an anterior position. It was hypothesized that this occurred initially to avoid pain during velopharyngeal movement, and then became habituated after the pain resolved. Therefore, it was treated as a conversion disorder. In fact, after 4 weeks of speech therapy, speech and swallowing returned to normal. A lesson to be learned from this case, and others like it, is that, even when severe velopharyngeal incompetence is noted perceptually and through nasopharyngoscopy, it reflects only what the individual is currently doing with the velopharyngeal mechanism. It does not reflect what the individual is capable of doing.

Effect of Velopharyngeal Dysfunction on Speech

Velopharyngeal dysfunction can affect speech and resonance in many ways. Because velopharyngeal closure is important for the production of most speech sounds, disruption in the function of this valve can result in hypernasality, nasal air emission, weak or omitted consonants, short utterance length, compen-satory articulation productions, and even dysphonia. The same speech characteristics can be found if there is oral-nasal coupling due to a palatal opening or a fistula. The characteristics of velopharyngeal dysfunction or palatal opening are described further in the following sections.

Hypernasality

Hypernasality is a resonance disorder that occurs when there is abnormal coupling of the oral and nasal cavities during speech. The resultant quality of speech is often described as muffled, characterized by mumbling, or just "nasal." It is important to note that hypernasality refers to abnormal resonance of sound. Therefore, hypernasality is always associated with speech sounds that are phonated and does not affect voiceless consonants, because these phonemes are not associated with voicing and thus sound (Cassassolles et al., 1995).

Hypernasality is particularly perceptible on vowels, because vowels are voiced and relatively long in duration. Andrews and Rutherford (1972) have shown that the perception of hypernasality is greater on high vowels than on low vowels and this is also seen with the acoustic correlates of hypernasality. It might be assumed that the high position of the tongue in the oral cavity during the production of high vowels reduces oral resonance, resulting in this perception of increased hypernasality. The consonant context of a vowel may also affect the perception of hypernasality on that vowel. If the vowel is bordered by nasal consonants or nasalized consonants, the vowel will be perceived as more hypernasal than if it is bordered by oral consonants.

Nasalization of voiced phonemes is common when there is mild-to-moderate hypernasality. It makes sense that when the velopharyngeal valve remains open during the attempted production of a voiced plosive, for example, that the acoustic product will be the nasal cognate of that sound. In fact, the voiced plosives will sound as if they are substituted by their nasal cognates (m/b, n/d, and ng/g). In this case, placement of the phoneme is preserved, but manner is necessarily changed from oral to nasal due to the open velopharyngeal port. Nasalization can also occur on other oral sounds and even as a substitute for voiceless sounds in severe cases. As a result, there may be a predominate use of the nasal sounds (m, n, and ng) throughout connected speech.

Hypernasality is best perceived in connected speech, because that is that the best way to appreciate the resonance on vowels and voiced consonants. Hypernasality will often increase with an increase in connected speech due to the additional demands on the velopharyngeal mechanism and the oral-motor system. Rapid rate and muscular fatigue can further affect the timing and effectiveness of the function of the velopharyngeal valve, resulting in an increase in the perception of hypernasality

The severity of the hypernasality is often determined by the size of the opening. In general, hypernasality is associated with a moderate-to-large sized opening into the nasal cavity. (Small openings generally cause nasal air emission rather than hypernasality.) The severity of the hypernasality is also affected by the movement, coordination, and timing of the velopharyngeal valve and by the articulation. All of these factors affect the quality and intelligibility of the speech.

The most common cause of hypernasality is velopharyngeal dysfunction. This may be due to velopharyngeal insufficiency (where there is a structural defect) or velopharyngeal incompetence (where there is inadequate movement of the velopharyngeal structures). An open palate, due to a cleft or a large oronasal fistula, can also result in inappropriate or excessive nasal resonance with speech. Figure 7–6 shows a very large palatal fistula that would definitely cause hypernasality. Finally,

velopharyngeal. mislearning can result in characteristics of hypernasality.

A final note is that hypernasality should not be confused with a "nasal twang," which has been described as a characteristic of certain dialects. Although this quality may seem hypernasal from a perceptual analysis, the nasal twang is probably not due to an open velopharyngeal port. In fact, Yanagisawa and colleagues (Yanagisawa, Estill, Mambrino, & Talkin, 1991; Yanagisawa, Kmucha, & Estill, 1990) have shown that there are both acoustic and physiological differences between hypernasality and a nasal twang. They concluded from their studies that the nasal twang quality is the result of constriction of the pharynx, rather than an open velopharyngeal valve. Therefore, dialectical differences should not be confused with true hypernasality.

Nasal Air Emission

Nasal air emission refers to the inappropriate release of the air pressure through the nasal

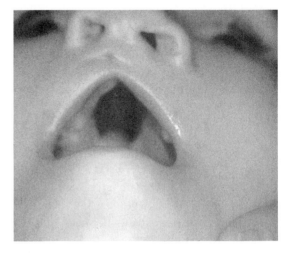

Figure 7–6. A very large palatal fistula that would cause significant hypernasality. A fistula of this size is a very unusual finding.

cavity during speech production. It is usually audible and presents as a high-frequency, low-intensity sound. Nasal air emission only occurs on consonants, particularly pressure-sensitive phonemes (plosives, fricatives, and affricates). It does not occur during the production of vowels or semivowels because for these phonemes, there is no need to build up air pressure. It should be noted that, although nasal air emission often occurs with hypernasality and has the same cause as hypernasality, it is not the same as hypernasality. Hypernasality is associated with the sound that is created through phonation and it is a disorder of resonance. On the other hand, nasal air emission is associated with air pressure and airflow, and thus affects articulation.

Nasal air emission can occur as the result of a leak in the velopharyngeal valve when there is an attempt to build up intraoral air pressure for consonants. This can be the result of velopharyngeal insufficiency, velopharyngeal incompetence, or even mislearning. It can also occur with an oronasal fistula.

Nasal air emission typically is a very soft sound and is due to air going through a fairly large opening. Two other forms of nasal air emission can result in a louder, more distracting sound. These include the nasal rustle, which is due to a form of turbulence, and a nasal snort.

A *nasal rustle*, as described by Mason and Grandstaff (1971), is a fricative sound that occurs as air pressure is forced through a partially opened velopharyngeal valve. The partial restriction causes the airflow to become turbulent as it passes through the valve; therefore, the resulting sound is also referred to as *nasal turbulence*. Warren, Wood, and Bradley (1969) noted that nasal turbulence can also occur when airway resistance is high. Therefore, a narrow velopharyngeal opening, nasal obstruction, or even temporary nasal congestion can cause the nasal air emission to become turbulent, thus resulting in a nasal rustle.

A nasal rustle typically occurs due to a small velopharyngeal opening (Kummer, Curtis,

Wiggs, Lee, & Strife, 1992; Kummer et al., 1989). In fact, smaller openings often result in a louder distortion due to the degree of airflow restriction. This restriction of the airflow causes turbulence and results in bubbling of secretions above the opening. This bubbling can be seen with the help of barium on videofluoroscopy, but it is best seen through nasopharyngoscopy.

The nasal rustle is heard as a bubbly sound at the back of the nose. (In fact, it is similar to the sound of blowing the nose.) It can be very loud and distracting and can mask the sound of the consonant, thus affecting the quality and intelligibility of speech. Voiceless fricatives are more often distorted by nasal air emission or a nasal rustle because they are associated with more air pressure than their voiced counterparts when the vocal folds attenuate the air pressure somewhat.

The *nasal snort* is another form of nasal air emission. It is produced by a forcible emission of air pressure through the nose during consonant production. This results in a noisy, sneezelike sound. The nasal snort is typically associated with the production of the /s/ sound, but can also be associated with other sibilant sounds (sh, ch, j). It is most common with the production of /s/ blends. A nasal snort often occurs concurrently with a nasal grimace. Nasal snorting may occur with other forms of nasal air emission or may be noted inconsistently in speech without evidence of additional nasal air emission.

A *nasal grimace* is a muscle contraction in the face around the area of the nose that occurs during speech. The grimace is typically noted either above the nasal bridge in the area between the eyes or around the nares when there is nasal air emission. Just as muscle contractions can be noted in the face when a person is trying to lift something heavy, the nasal grimace is also an overflow muscle reaction that occurs with extreme effort to achieve velopharyngeal closure.

Phoneme-specific nasal air emission (PSNAE) is the release of air pressure that occurs on certain phonemes only and does not occur on other oral sounds. This has been called "phoneme-specific velopharyngeal insufficiency" in the past. This term is very misleading, however, and is actually a misnomer, because the nasal air emission in this case occurs in the absence of velopharyngeal insufficiency. In fact, phoneme-specific nasal air emission is the result of faulty articulation due to mislearning, rather than velopharyngeal dysfunction. It occurs most commonly on sibilant sounds, particularly /s/, and tends to occur when the individual uses posterior nasal fricatives as a substitution for these sounds. (See Posterior Nasal Fricative in this chapter.) Nasal air emission always occurs with the use of posterior nasal fricatives due to the fact that the velum is down with this production. Changing articulatory placement will result in elimination of the nasal air emission if the cause is truly phoneme-specific nasal air emission.

Weak or Omitted Consonants

When air pressure is leaked through the velopharyngeal valve or an oronasal fistula, it causes a reduction in the air pressure that is available in the oral cavity for the production of consonants. As a result, consonants may be weak in intensity and pressure, or may be omitted completely (Baken, 1987; McWilliams et al., 1990b). There is usually a direct inverse correlation between the amount of nasal air emission and the pressure for production of oral consonants. Therefore, the greater the nasal air emission, the weaker the consonants will become.

As could be expected, pressure-sensitive consonants are affected primarily by the reduction of air pressure. The weak consonants, in addition to the nasal air emission or hypernasality, cause the speech to sound muffled and indistinct. The loss of air pressure can also affect utterance length as frequent breaths are required to replace air pressure.

Short Utterance Length

Utterance length is determined, at least in part, by the supply of breath pressure that is available for speech. When velopharyngeal dysfunction causes a leak of air pressure, it shortens the supply of oral air pressure for connected speech. This results in the need to increase respiratory effort to compensate for the loss of breath pressure. In fact, there are data to show that individuals with a large velopharyngeal opening attempt to raise intraoral pressure by increasing airflow rate during consonant production. As a result, they may produce respiratory volumes that are twice that of normals (Warren et al., 1969). This increased effort makes speech physically difficult and can cause the individual to become fatigued. There is also a need to take breaths more frequently during utterances to replenish the air pressure that is lost. This causes utterance length to be short and connected speech to be choppy.

When utterance length is affected by the loss of air pressure, it is usually associated with a large velopharyngeal or palatal opening. If the gap is small, there is usually sufficient intraoral air pressure for normal phrasing of utterances.

Altered Rate and Speech Segment Durations

Speech segment durations have been shown to be abnormal in individuals with velopharyngeal dysfunction (Forner, 1983). Forner used spectrograms to measure segment durations of utterances produced by children with and without a history of cleft palate and velopharyngeal dysfunction. This investigator found that both syllable and sentence durations were longer when produced by those children with a history of cleft. In addition, subjects with hypernasality had longer voice onset times than those with normal or less disordered speech. These findings suggest that coordinating speech production in the presence of a malfunctioning velopharyngeal valve is very difficult and thus it affects the overall rate of speech.

Compensatory and Obligatory Articulation Productions

Speech characteristics, such as hypernasality, nasal air emission, weak consonants, and short utterance length, are the direct result of velopharyngeal dysfunction or a palatal opening. Therefore, these characteristics have been described as *passive speech characteristics* (Harding & Grunwell, 1996, 1998) or *obligatory errors* (Trost-Cardamone, 1990) because they are the product of structural abnormality or dysfunction. The nasalization of oral consonants, resulting in the substitution of nasal phonemes for oral phonemes, is the only obligatory error that changes articulation production. In contrast, articulation productions that are not the direct result of velopharyngeal dysfunction, but rather are the individual's response to this dysfunction are considered *active speech characteristics* (Harding & Grunwell, 1996, 1998) or *compensatory errors* (Trost-Cardamone, 1990). Using the terminology of Trost-Cardamone, a distinction between obligatory errors and compensatory errors is important to make because the compensatory characteristics are under the patient's control and, therefore, can respond to speech therapy. Obligatory errors are the result of the status of the velopharyngeal mechanism and therefore, require surgical or prosthetic intervention for correction.

Compensatory articulation productions are often developed by the individual as a response to inadequate intraoral air pressure for normal articulation. When the compensatory productions are used, the manner of production is usually maintained. However, the place of articulation is altered and moved posteriorly to the pharynx or larynx. This allows the individual to take advantage of the air pressure that is available in the pharynx before it is lost through the velopharyngeal valve. The most common compensatory productions include glottal stops, pharyngeal stops, and pharyngeal fricatives. However, other compensatory articulation productions have also been described (Trost, 1981). Mid-dorsum palatal stops (palatal-dorsal productions) are also common in this population, but this production is usually due to malocclusion and crowding of the oral cavity rather than velopharyngeal dysfunction. The various types of obligatory and compensatory articulation productions are described further in the following sections. For an excellent tutorial on the various types of compensatory productions, please refer to the videotape by Trost-Cardamone (1987).

Nasalization of Oral Consonants

The *nasalization of oral phonemes* is an obligatory error due to an open velopharyngeal valve. Nasalized phonemes are usually associated with the presence of hypernasality and are the result of a moderate to large velopharyngeal opening. The nasalization of voiced plosives is an obligatory error as the nasal cognate of voiced plosives is a nasal phoneme. Therefore, when the velopharyngeal valve remains open during production of a voiced plosive, the acoustic product will be the nasal sound. In fact, the voiced plosives will sound as if they are substituted by their nasal cognates (m/b, n/d, and ng/g). In this case, placement of the phoneme is preserved, but manner is necessarily changed from oral to nasal due to the open velopharyngeal port. The production of /m/ and /n/ as a substitution of other sounds can also be noted in cases of severe velopharyngeal dysfunction.

Glottal Stop

A *glottal stop (glottal plosive)* is a consonant stop that is produced at the level of the glottis.

The production begins with the forceful adduction of the vocal folds and the build-up of air pressure under the glottis. The ventricular folds, often called the false vocal folds, often approximate with the forceful closure of the true folds. The vocal folds are then suddenly opened, releasing the air pressure to produce the sound. The acoustic product is essentially a grunt sound. Glottal stops can be confused with a simple consonant omission. It should be remembered that glottal stops are produced with a quick sound and rapid voice onset time. This can often be seen by increased laryngeal activity in the throat area. If the phoneme is completely omitted, the voice onset is smooth with the initiation of the vowel and the vowel duration is longer.

Glottal stops are typically substituted for plosive sounds, but they may also be substituted for fricatives and affricates, especially if the individual has not yet developed the fricative manner in his or her phonemic repertoire. A glottal stop is usually perceived as a voiced phoneme because this production results in rapid voice onset for the vowel.

Henningsson and Isberg (1986) found that limited or no velopharyngeal movement may be associated with glottal stop substitutions. Through videofluoroscopy or nasopharyngoscopy, glottal stops often appear to be associated with a significant velopharyngeal opening. It is important to note, however, that this does not reflect the individual's ability to achieve velopharyngeal closure when oral phonemes are attempted.

Glottal stops are often coarticulated with other phonemes. A *coarticulation* is an abnormal consonant production characterized by one manner of production with simultaneous valving at two places of production (Trost-Cardamone, 1997). When this occurs, it appears as if the person is producing the sound correctly with appropriate placement. Although the oral placement may be normal, the individual is actually initiating the plosive production at the level of the glottis. For example, the patient may have normal bilabial closure for the production of a /b/ sound, while the plosive portion of the phoneme is actually produced at the glottis as a glottal stop.

Pharyngeal Plosive

The *pharyngeal plosive (pharyngeal stop)* is a consonant that is produced with the back of the tongue against the pharyngeal wall. During production of this sound, the dorsum of the tongue is convex in configuration and low in the oral cavity tongue. The entire tongue moves posteriorly in order to articulate against the posterior pharyngeal wall and use the air pressure that is in the pharynx before it is lost through the velopharyngeal valve. An increase in pharyngeal activity can often be noted by observing the throat area. Due to the difficulty of producing this phoneme, it is not coarticulated and there is often a longer duration between the consonant and the following vowel than is typically noted with other consonants.

Pharyngeal plosives can be voiced or unvoiced. Although they can be substituted for other consonants, they are typically substituted only for the velar plosives (k, g). It is more common for glottal stops to be substituted for other sounds, probably because glottal stops are much easier to produce and can be coarticulated.

Pharyngeal Fricative

A *pharyngeal fricative* is another consonant that uses the back of the tongue and pharynx. It is produced when the tongue is retracted so that the base of the tongue approximates, but does not touch, the pharyngeal wall. A friction sound occurs as the air pressure is forced through the narrow opening that is created between the base of the tongue and pharyngeal wall.

Pharyngeal fricatives can be substituted for fricatives and affricates, and are usually substituted for the sibilant sounds (s, z, sh, zh, ch, and j). Pharyngeal fricatives can be voiced or unvoiced, although the unvoiced version is most commonly noted. A pharyngeal fricative can sound similar to a lateral lisp, particularly to an inexperienced listener. It is important to make the right judgment as to which sound is being produced because this judgment will have a significant impact on the recommendations for treatment. This is done by determining whether the location of the friction is oral or pharyngeal through certain diagnostic procedures. The procedure for making this distinction is discussed in Chapter 12.

A laryngeal fricative has also been described in the literature (Kawano, Isshiki, Harita, & Tanokuchi, 1985). It is probable that this is a slight variation of the pharyngeal fricative, and therefore, it will not be discussed separately in this text.

Pharyngeal Affricate

A *pharyngeal affricate* has the same initial placement as a pharyngeal plosive. However, as with other affricates, it combines the manner of a plosive and a fricative. Therefore, the pharyngeal affricate is the combination of either a pharyngeal plosive or a glottal stop and a pharyngeal fricative. As with the other pharyngeal compensatory productions, an increase in pharyngeal activity can be noted in the throat area during speech. Pharyngeal affricates are not co-articulated with other placements.

Pharyngeal affricates typically are substituted for the other affricates (ch and j), although they can also be noted to be substituted for the other sibilant sounds (s, z, sh, and zh). They can be unvoiced or voiced. Pharyngeal affricates can sometimes be difficult to distinguish from pharyngeal fricatives, especially in connected speech.

Velar Fricative

The *velar fricative* is produced with the back of the tongue in the same position as for the production of a /y/ sound. With the back of the tongue elevated and positioned under the velum, a small space is created. The velar frica-

tive is produced as air is forced through that small opening.

The velar fricative may be substituted for any fricative sound, but is most commonly substituted for sibilants. It can be voiced or voiceless. This production is sometimes difficult to distinguish from a pharyngeal fricative, but with good diagnostic technique, the source of the friction sound can be located.

Posterior Nasal Fricative

A *posterior nasal fricative* can be seen radiographically or through nasopharyngoscopy as incomplete closure of the velopharyngeal valve. As a result, it is accompanied by nasal air emission. The posterior nasal fricative has been described as a compensatory articulation production characterized by audible nasal emission and friction (Trost, 1981). Although it may be a compensatory articulation production as a result of velopharyngeal dysfunction, it is often merely a learned articulation gesture that results in phoneme-specific nasal air emission. The posterior nasal fricative may be used as a substitution for any of the pressure-sensitive phonemes, but it is typically used for sibilants, particularly /s/.

Use of /h/ for Voiceless Plosives

Voiceless plosives require a build-up of intra-oral air pressure and sudden release for production. If there is significantly reduced oral air pressure during production, the acoustic product may be that of an /h/, since the aspiration is the only perceptible distinctive feature (Harding & Grunwell, 1998). This may be compensatory and part of the use of a pattern of glottal and pharyngeal articulation.

Nasal Sniff

The *nasal sniff* is not a common compensatory articulation production, but it does occur. In this case, the phoneme is produced by a forcible inspiration through the nose. In a sense, this is the opposite of nasal emission. The nasal sniff is usually substituted for sibilant sounds, particularly the /s/. Due to the difficulty in coordinating the inspiration and expiration during articulation with this sound, it typically occurs only in the final word position, rather than in all word positions.

Generalized Backing

It has long been recognized that some patients with velopharyngeal dysfunction will articulate with generalized *backing of phonemes* or palatalized articulation (Ainoda, Yamashita, & Tsukada, 1985; Powers, 1962). This occurs when the patient produces most phonemes with the back of the tongue and with the velum or with the posterior pharyngeal wall. This posterior articulation occurs so that the individual can take advantage of the air pressure that is in this area before too much is lost through the velopharyngeal port. It is also common in individuals with a palatal fistula because posterior articulation may avoid the air loss through the fistula. In addition to making use of the air pressure in the pharynx, posterior articulation serves another function. It has been shown through radiographic studies that, with posterior articulation, the tongue can push the velum upward to assist with closure. Therefore, this also may be a compensatory strategy for velopharyngeal incompetence (Brooks, Shelton, & Youngstrom, 1965; McWilliams et al., 1990b).

Posterior articulation can be used for all oral sounds. Even posterior nasal sounds are sometimes used for anterior sounds. In particular, the /ng/ sound is commonly substituted for the /l/ and /n/ sounds. Other anterior sounds may also be substituted by this posterior nasal sound (Trost-Cardamone, 1997).

Mid-Dorsum Palatal Stop (Palatal-Dorsals)

The *mid-dorsum palatal stop*, also called a *palatal-dorsal production*, is a stop consonant that is produced with the dorsum of the tongue against the middle of the hard palate. This production is substituted for the lingual-alveolar sounds (t, d, n, l) and often for the velar sounds (k, g). In some cases, a palatal-dorsal placement will also be used for the production of sibilant sounds (s, z, sh, zh, ch, and j). Because the place of production is between that for lingual-alveolars and velars, the boundaries to distinguish the two placements are lost and the acoustic product sounds like a cross between the two placements.

The mid-dorsum palatal stop is a compensatory error that occurs commonly in individuals with a history of cleft lip and palate. It does not seem to occur as a compensation for velopharyngeal dysfunction, however. Instead, it is often a compensation for anterior crowding in the oral cavity due to a Class III malocclusion or anterior crossbite. In these cases, the tongue is in the normal position in the mandible, but the maxillary teeth are inside the mandibular teeth. As a result, the alveolar ridge is well behind the position of the tongue tip. In fact, the alveolar ridge is often just above the dorsum of the tongue, making the mid-dorsum palatal stop a natural articulation production. This compensatory error can also be seen in individuals with macroglossia, where the tongue tip protrudes past the incisors so that the dorsum of the tongue is under the alveolar ridge. When there is a mid-palatal fistula, the individual may use this placement to prevent nasal emission through the opening.

Breathiness

A breathy vocal quality may be used as a strategy to compensate for velopharyngeal dysfunction. Releasing the air pressure at the level of the glottis reduces the amount of air pressure that can and will be lost through the velopharyngeal valve. Therefore, this compensatory maneuver can be especially effective in improving the quality of speech in the short term. Breathiness can also mask the sound of the nasal air emission and hypernasality.

Dysphonia

Dysphonia refers to voice disorder that results in an alteration in the normal phonatory quality of the voice. It can be characterized by breathiness, hoarseness, low intensity, and glottal fry. The most common cause of dysphonia in children is vocal nodules (Boone & McFarlane, 1988). *Vocal nodules* are bilateral, circumscribed enlargements on the vocal folds that are the result of abuse, overuse, or misuse of the voice.

Children with a history of cleft palate or velopharyngeal dysfunction have an increased risk for dysphonia for several reasons (D'Antonio et al., 1988; Hess, 1959; McWilliams, Bluestone, & Musgrave, 1969; McWilliams, Lavorato, & Bluestone, 1973). Dysphonia may be secondary to congenital abnormalities of the laryngeal structures in association with congenital malformation syndromes. It may also be due to hyperfunction of the vocal folds or the use of certain compensatory articulation productions.

Speakers with impaired velopharyngeal valving are at risk for hyperfunctional voice disorders, especially if the velopharyngeal opening is small or inconsistent. When the opening is small or inconsistent, the individual will often respond by increasing respiratory and muscular effort in an attempt to close the velopharyngeal port. Initially, the vocal fold pathology from this strain may include thickening and edema of the vocal folds. Ultimately, the strain and tension in the vocal tract can lead to the formation of vocal nodules. In patients with velopharyngeal dysfunction, vocal nodules may also develop secondary to the use of compensatory articulation productions, particularly glottal stops. Since glottal stops are produced by quickly and forcibly adducting the vocal folds, damage to the vocal fold edges is not surprising. In fact, the development of vocal nodules is common in individuals who use glottal stops.

Once vocal nodules develop, their location interferes with the ability of the folds to approximate during phonation. Through laryngoscopy, an examiner might note that because the nodules prevent complete vocal fold closure, a posterior glottal chink is apparent in the area behind the nodules. This chink affects the phonatory quality of the voice and causes the voice to become very breathy. As the nodules harden, these growths can change the shape, mass, viscosity, and stiffness of the folds. As a result, the folds do not vibrate smoothly or evenly, which causes hoarseness and glottal fry during phonation.

When there is very mild or inconsistent nasal air emission, speech therapy is often done on a trial basis. However, McWilliams and colleagues (McWilliams et al., 1990b) have suggested that aggressive speech therapy to improve velopharyngeal function can cause compensatory laryngeal valving and result in vocal fold pathology. Therefore, the speech pathologist should be cautioned to watch for strain in the vocal tract during therapy. In addition, the speech pathologist should consider referral for surgical intervention for velopharyngeal dysfunction, if therapy is not successful in a reasonably short time. Surgical correction of mild velopharyngeal dysfunction can eliminate the strain in the vocal tract, and in many cases, this is enough so that the vocal nodules gradually disappear without surgical intervention.

A soft voice or low phonatory intensity has also been described as a common finding with velopharyngeal dysfunction (McWilliams, Morris, & Shelton, 1990a). This may be the result of a lack of adequate oral acoustic energy in combination with the absorption of sound energy by the pharyngeal tissues, resulting in a damping effect (Bernthal & Beukelman, 1977). As previously noted, low intensity and breathiness may also be used as a compensatory strategy to mask the hypernasality and nasal air emission.

Severity and Consistency of Velopharyngeal Dysfunction

The severity of velopharyngeal dysfunction can vary from a very small pinhole-sized opening to a very large opening that includes the entire velopharyngeal port. The size of the opening can be estimated through aerodynamic instrumentation or nasometry, or the opening can be viewed directly through videofluoroscopy or nasopharyngoscopy. Although the size of the velopharyngeal opening and thus the severity of velopharyngeal dysfunction can be determined through instrumentation, this information does not correlate well with the severity of the speech disorder and the effect on intelligibility (Warren et al., 1969). The lack of a one-to-one correlation is due to several factors, including nasal airway resistance and the use of compensatory articulation productions.

Effects of Articulation and Phonation on Severity

One factor that affects the intelligibility of speech and judgments of severity is the status of articulation. If the individual has developed good articulation skills and has preserved the appropriate place of articulation, the overall intelligibility of speech will probably be better than that of another person with the same opening who has poor articulation skill and compensates by backing of phonemes. The status of the individual's articulation skills, unrelated to the velopharyngeal dysfunction, also affects the judgment of severity. If the person has articulation errors related to malocclusion, oral-motor dysfunction, or just delayed acquisition, these errors impact the intelligibility of speech and the judgment of severity.

The quality of phonation is another factor that affects severity. The use of a breathy voice may reduce the amount of nasal emission and may mask hypernasality so that it is less detectable. On the other hand, low volume and other dysphonic characteristics, such as hoarseness and glottal fry, can have a negative effect on the overall intelligibility of the speech. If vocal effort is increased, there may be a corresponding increase in velopharyngeal function and a decrease in the velopharyngeal orifice area (Mc-

Henry, 1997). In some cases, this decrease can improve the perception of hypernasality.

Effects of a Small Velopharyngeal Opening on Severity

If the effects of articulation and phonation are factored out or if both are normal, there still would be a poor correlation between the size of the velopharyngeal opening and the severity of the speech. This has to do with the effect of the transmission of air pressure and sound through various sized openings. In normal speech, as the air pressure travels from the lungs and through the glottis, it continues to travel in a superior direction until it is blocked by the velopharyngeal valve. At that point, the air pressure is redirected in an anterior direction to enter the oral cavity. Because the air pressure is not redirected anteriorly until it reaches the velopharyngeal valve, the same amount of air pressure will hit the valve, regardless of whether there is an opening or not and regardless of the size of the opening.

If there is a small velopharyngeal opening, air pressure is forced through the small opening during speech. This causes friction and bubbling of secretions on the top of the valve. Perceptually, this is recognized as nasal turbulence or a nasal rustle. With a small opening, there is usually normal oral resonance and adequate air pressure for consonants. Therefore, the consonants will not be weak in intensity or substituted by compensatory productions. Utterance length should also be normal. Overall, when the velopharyngeal gap is small, a nasal rustle (nasal turbulence) may be the predominate, or the only, characteristic of velopharyngeal dysfunction.

At first glance, it may seem that the speech would be mildly affected by a small, inconsistent velopharyngeal gap. However, the nasal rustle is a very loud and distracting form of nasal emission. It is loud enough to mask the oral sound that is being articulated. Therefore, the nasal rustle can actually have a significant effect on both the quality and the intelligibility of speech, causing speech to be judged as more severely affected.

Individuals who demonstrate a small, yet consistent velopharyngeal gap have been termed the *almost-but-not-quite* (ABNQ) group by Morris (1984). These individuals are generally not stimulable for improvement through auditory discrimination training or articulation therapy. This is because an underlying structural or physiological disorder precludes complete velopharyngeal closure. Therefore, surgical or prosthetic management is more appropriate. Correction is definitely indicated, even though the opening is small, because this size of opening often results in more severely affected speech than a larger opening.

Effects of a Moderate-Sized Velopharyngeal Opening on Severity

If there is a moderate-sized velopharyngeal opening, there will be more nasal air emission than with a small opening. As a result, the air pressure loss can be heard as nasal air emission that is soft in intensity and not very distracting. Very little friction is associated with this sound and there will be less bubbling of secretions. However, because more air pressure is lost through the nasal cavity with the size of opening, less air pressure is available for articulation. Therefore, the consonants may be mildly weak in intensity and pressure. The individual may also have some compensatory articulation errors. Resonance may be mildly to moderately hypernasal.

Effects of a Large Velopharyngeal Opening on Severity

When the velopharyngeal gap is large, air pressure is released through the opening without resistance. The release of air pressure without

friction can be very soft and therefore not very audible. What is noticeable, however, is the hypernasality. With a large opening, the sound energy that is traveling in a superior direction through the pharynx will continue to travel superiorly right through the velopharyngeal valve. As a result, moderate-to-severe hypernasality will be noted. Because there is a significant amount of nasal air emission, the consonants will be very weak in intensity and most oral sounds will be nasalized or substituted by compensatory productions. Utterance length will be short due to the significant loss of air pressure through the velopharyngeal valve with each utterance.

Consistency of Closure

Throughout speech production, velopharyngeal closure attempts may be inconsistent in their success, particularly if the opening is small. Morris (1984) termed this subgroup of individuals the *sometimes-but-not-always* (SBNA) group. Individuals in this group may be able to achieve total closure with effort. However, just as it is difficult to carry a 50-pound weight for long, it is difficult for these individuals to continue to exert enough effort to maintain that closure for a prolonged period of time. Closure may be complete for single words or short utterances, but break down with the motoric demands of connected speech. Speech may be best at the beginning of the day, but become noticeably worse as the day goes on and the individual becomes fatigued.

Inconsistencies in closure may also be noted between various speech sounds. Complete closure might be obtained for certain sounds, such as plosives, but not for other sounds, such as fricatives. Finally, velopharyngeal closure may be inconsistent due to oral-motor dysfunction, particularly due to the sequencing and coordination problems that are characteristic of apraxia of speech.

Whenever there is inconsistent velopharyngeal closure, the examiner can surmise that complete closure can be achieved during speech production, but cannot be maintained as appropriate throughout the utterance. In this case, the examiner must determine if the person can learn to improve the consistency of velopharyngeal closure through speech therapy, without having to exert an unreasonable amount of effort.

Speech therapy is sometimes appropriate for individuals who demonstrate inconsistent velopharyngeal closure. If the person can learn to improve the consistency of closure through articulation therapy and auditory discrimination, surgery may not be necessary. This is particularly true if there is phoneme-specific nasal air emission (PSNAE), or the opening is small in addition to inconsistent. However, it is unreasonable to expect the individual to exert extra effort to achieve closure at all times. When speech becomes hard work, it is very tiring and the effort cannot be maintained. In those cases, surgical or prosthetic intervention should be considered.

Other Resonance Disorders

Resonance is the quality of the voice that results from sound vibrations in the pharynx, oral cavity, and nasal cavity. The relative balance of sound vibration in these anatomical cavities determines whether the quality of the speech and voice is perceived as normal or as deviant due to a type of "nasality." Anything that disrupts the transmission of sound or the normal balance of oral and nasal resonance can cause a resonance disorder.

Resonance disorders, particularly hypernasality, are often labeled as "voice disorders" (Riski & Verdolini, 1999). By definition, however, a voice disorder is characterized by an abnormality in the vibration of the vocal folds, which causes disordered phonatory quality.

Although resonance contributes to overall "voice quality," hypernasality and other resonance disorders are not laryngeal in origin. Instead, they are the result of abnormal vibration of vocal sound in the cavities of the vocal tract. Therefore, classifying these abnormalities as "resonance disorders" is more appropriate.

There are various types of resonance disorders, depending on the function of the velopharyngeal valve, the size and shape of the resonating cavities, and the presence of blockage in the vocal tract. Hypernasality was already discussed on page 157 of this chapter. Therefore, other types of resonance disorders and their potential causes are discussed in the following sections.

Hyponasality and Denasality

Hyponasality occurs when there is a reduction in normal nasal resonance during speech. This can be due to blockage in the nasopharynx or blockage in the nasal cavity. Hyponasality particularly affects the production of the nasal consonants (m, n, ng). When nasal resonance is reduced for nasal consonants, these consonants sound similar to their oral phoneme cognates (b, d, g). Hyponasality can also affect the quality of vowels if it is severe and there is a blockage of the entrance to the oral cavity. The term *denasality* is typically used to refer to total nasal airway obstruction and the resultant effect on resonance. The causes of denasality are the same as for hyponasality, but there is a difference in severity. Because it is impossible to know if there is total blockage of the nasal cavity through a perceptual assessment alone, the term "hyponasality" should be used because it is appropriate for all cases of inadequate nasal resonance.

The cause of hyponasality is almost always obstruction somewhere in the nasopharynx or nasal cavity. This obstruction may be due to swelling of the nasal passages secondary to allergic rhinitis or the common cold. In this case, medication and time relieve the symptoms. Hyponasality can also be due to adenoid hypertrophy, which is a common cause in the pediatric population. Adenoidectomy is often done to alleviate this symptom and the accompanying upper airway obstruction. Hyponasality also can be due to hypertrophic tonsils that intrude into the pharynx (Kummer et al., 1993). Characteristics of hyponasality also can be noted as a result of apraxia of speech. This is due to a difficulty in lowering the velum rapidly enough for nasal phonemes once it is in a raised position for oral sounds.

Hyponasality is very common in individuals with a history of cleft palate, and may actually be more common than hypernasality in adolescents and adults in this population. This can be due to a variety of factors. If velopharyngeal dysfunction causes hypernasality, it is usually corrected in the preschool or early school years so that hypernasality is no longer present as the individual enters adolescence. However, because the surgical procedures that are designed to correct velopharyngeal dysfunction narrow or reduce the size of the nasopharyngeal space, hyponasality is often a complication of the surgery (de Serres et al., 1999; Hall, Golding-Kushner, Argamaso, & Strauch, 1991; Thurston, Larson, Shanks, Bennett, & Parsons, 1980; Witt, Myckatyn, & Marsh, 1998). For example, when a pharyngeal flap procedure is done, the flap serves as a static obturator and closes the middle section of the nasopharynx. If the flap is too wide, the lateral ports are not able to open sufficiently for normal nasal breathing and normal nasal resonance. A pharyngeal implant for velopharyngeal dysfunction can also reduce the size and patency of the nasopharyngeal portal, thus causing hyponasality. The upper airway and nasal resonance can even be affected by a sphincteroplasty, which restricts the lateral edges of the pharyngeal port but leaves an opening in the midline. Anything that reduces the size of the nasopharynx can result in a chronic open mouth posture and mouth breathing, loud snoring at night, and even sleep apnea. When these symptoms of upper airway obstruction occur, hyponasality is almost always noted. The characteristics of upper airway obstruction, including hyponasality, can improve gradually with time if the cause is the secondary surgery. If the symptoms persist and include sleep apnea, surgical revision is usually indicated. On the other hand, mild hyponasality may be considered a necessary side effect of the secondary surgery and may not be corrected if it is not causing sleep apnea, especially since mild hyponasality does not usually affect speech intelligibility.

Hyponasality is also common in individuals with repaired clefts of the palate and no history of secondary palatal surgery (Riski, 1995). This can be due to a deviated septum, choanal stenosis or atresia, or a stenotic naris. Maxillary retrusion can also cause hyponasality due to the restriction that it causes of the pharyngeal airway and nasal cavity space. Maxillary retrusion with midface deficiency is common in individuals with a history of cleft lip and palate. It is also a phenotypic feature of several craniofacial syndromes, such as Crouzon syndrome, Apert syndrome, and Pfeiffer syndrome. When patients undergo maxillary advancement, the airway, and thus hyponasality, often improves (Dalston, 1996; Maegawa et al., 1998; McCarthy et al., 1979).

Because the cause of reduced nasal resonance is almost always obstruction somewhere in the nasal cavity or pharynx, further evaluation and treatment should be done by a physician. Speech therapy is indicated only if the hyponasality is inconsistent and is due to timing errors as a result of apraxia of speech.

Cul-de-Sac Resonance

Cul-de-sac resonance occurs when the transmission of acoustic energy is trapped in a blind pouch with only an entrance and no outlet. The speech is perceived as muffled and has been described as "potato-in-the-mouth" speech (Finkelstein, Bar-Ziv, Nachmani, Berger, & Ophir, 1993). Essentially, the sound is stuck in a cavity with no direct means of escape.

A form of cul-de-sac resonance can be simulated by producing a series of nasal phonemes (i.e. ma, ma, ma, ma, ma) or simulating hypernasality and then pinching the nose. As the sound resonates in the nasal cavity for the nasal phonemes, it normally is emitted through the nares. However, when the nose is closed, the sound energy is trapped in the nasal cavity and results in cul-de-sac resonance. It should be noted that pinching the nose during the production of nasal phonemes does not result in oral resonance. This is because the blockage is at the front of the nasal cavity and not in the area of the velopharyngeal valve.

The cause of cul-de-sac resonance can vary, but it is usually due to an area of blockage somewhere in the vocal tract. For example, it can occur in individuals with very large tonsils that block the entrance to the oral cavity (Kummer et al., 1993; Shprintzen et al., 1987). As a result, the sound energy is trapped and vibration occurs primarily in the oropharynx. Another cause of cul-de-sac resonance is a combination of velopharyngeal dysfunction and anterior blockage of the nasal cavity. This blockage could be due to a deviated septum, nasal polyps, or stenotic nares. In this situation, the sound energy resonates in the nasal cavity, but is not released through the nares.

Because cul-de-sac resonance is due to a structural abnormality, particularly a blockage of one of the resonating cavities, this type of resonance disorder requires medical or surgical intervention to eliminate the cause.

Mixed Resonance

Hypernasality and hyponasality are not mutually exclusive and can occur together in mixed resonance. *Mixed resonance*, with a combination of hypernasality and hyponasality, can occur when there is velopharyngeal insufficiency in addition to significant nasal airway or nasal cavity blockage. In this case, hypernasality may be the predominate characteristic of connected speech, but hyponasality is noted during the production of nasal consonants. Mixed resonance can also occur in individuals with oral-motor disorders, due to inappropriate timing of the upward or downward movement of the velum for speech (Netsell, 1969).

In addition to mixed resonance, some individuals demonstrate hyponasality and nasal air emission (which has the same cause as hypernasality). Dalston and colleagues (Dalston, Warren, & Dalston, 1991) reported that some of their hyponasal patients had high nasalance scores on the Nasometer due to a degree of nasal air emission. A common cause for this combination is enlarged, yet irregular adenoid tissue. During the production of oral sounds, the velum closes against the adenoid pad, but a tight velopharyngeal seal cannot be obtained due to a cleft or "divot" in the adenoid tissue. As a result, there is nasal air emission. On the other hand, when the velum goes down for the production of nasal sounds, the adenoid pad is large enough that it obstructs the transmission of sound into the nasal cavity, thus causing hyponasality.

Summary

The velopharyngeal valve is responsible for regulating the transmission of sound energy from the oral to the nasal cavities during speech. Malfunction of this valve can have a significant effect on resonance and the quality of speech. Velopharyngeal dysfunction is a common problem for individuals with a history of cleft palate. It can also occur due to a variety of other causes. When the velopharyngeal valve does not close completely, quickly, and in coordination with the other subsystems of speech, abnormal resonance and articulation can be the result. The speech pathologist needs to be knowledgeable about the effects of velopharyngeal dysfunction on speech so that these problems can be managed appropriately.

Resonance is affected not only by the function of the velopharyngeal valve, but also by the size, shape, and structure of the resonating cavities. Abnormalities in these cavities, particularly in the form of blockage, can cause a variety of resonance disorders. Although these disorders are not always treated by the speech pathologist, they should be correctly diagnosed by the speech pathologist so that recommendations for appropriate treatment can be made.

References

Abdullah, S. (1988). A study of the results of speech language and hearing assessment of three groups of repaired cleft palate children and adults. *Annals of the Academy of Medicine of Singapore, 17*(3), 388–391.

Ainoda, N., Yamashita, K., & Tsukada, S. (1985). Articulation at age 4 in children with early repair of cleft palate. *Annals of Plastic Surgery, 15*(5), 415–422.

Andreassen, M. L., Leeper, H. A., & MacRae, D. L. (1991). Changes in vocal resonance and nasalization following adenoidectomy in normal children: Preliminary findings. *Journal of Otolaryngology, 20*(4), 237–242.

Andrews, J. R., & Rutherford, D. (1972). Contribution of nasally emitted sound to the perception of hypernasality of vowels. *Cleft Palate Journal, 9,* 147–156.

Ansel, B. M., & Kent, R. D. (1992). Acoustic-phonetic contrasts and intelligibility in the dysarthria associated with mixed cerebral palsy. *Journal of Speech and Hearing Research, 35*(2), 296–308.

Baken, R. J. (1987). *Clinical measurement of speech and voice.* Boston: College-Hill Press.

Bernthal, J. E., & Beukelman, D. R. (1977). The effect of changes in velopharyngeal orifice area on vowel intensity. *Cleft Palate Journal, 14*(1), 63–77.

Blum, D. J., & Neel, H. B. D. (1983). Current thinking on tonsillectomy and adenoidectomy. *Comprehensive Therapy, 9*(12), 48–56.

Bodin, I. K., Lind, M. G., & Arnander, C. (1994). Free radial forearm flap reconstruction in surgery of the oral cavity and pharynx: Surgical complications, impairment of speech and swallowing. *Clinics in Otolaryngology, 19*(1), 28–34.

Boone, D. R., & McFarlane, S. (1988). *The voice and voice therapy* (4th ed.). Englewood Cliffs, NJ: Prentice-Hall.

Bradley, D. P. (1979). Congenital and acquired palatopharyngeal insufficiency. In K. R. Bzoch (Ed.), *Communicative disorders related to cleft lip and palate* (Vol. 2, pp. 77–89). Boston: Little, Brown and Company.

Bradley, D. P. (1997). Congenital and acquired velopharyngeal inadequacy. In K. R. Bzoch (Ed.), *Communicative disorders related to cleft lip and palate* (Vol. 4, pp. 23–243). Austin, TX: Pro-Ed.

Brooks, A. R., Shelton, R. L., & Youngstrom, K. A. (1965). Compensatory tongue-palate-posterior pharyngeal wall relationships in cleft palate. *Journal of Speech and Hearing Disorders, 30,* 166.

Brown, J. S., Zuydam, A. C., Jones, D. C., Rogers, S. N., & Vaughan, E. D. (1997). Functional outcome in soft palate reconstruction using a radial forearm free flap in conjunction with a superiorly based pharyngeal flap. *Head and Neck, 19*(6), 524–534.

Cassassolles, S., Paulus, C., Ajacques, J. C., Berger-Vachon, C., Laurent, M., & Perrin, E. (1995). Acoustic characterization of velar insufficiency in young children. *Revue de Stomatologie et de Chirurgie Maxillofaciale, 96*(1), 13–20.

Chen, K. T., Wu, J., & Noordhoff, S. M. (1994). Submucous cleft palate. *Chang Keng I Hsueh, 17*(2), 131–137.

Croft, C. B., Shprintzen, R. J., & Ruben, R. J. (1981). Hypernasal speech following adenotonsillectomy. *Otolaryngology—Head and Neck Surgery, 89*(2), 179–188.

Dalston, R. M. (1996). Velopharyngeal impairment in the orthodontic population. *Seminars in Orthodontics, 2*(3), 220–227.

Dalston, R. M., & Vig, P. S. (1984). Effects of orthognathic surgery on speech: A prospective study. *American Journal of Orthodontics, 86*(4), 291–298.

Dalston, R. M., Warren, D. W., & Dalston, E. T. (1991). A preliminary investigation concerning the use of nasometry in identifying patients with hyponasality and/or nasal airway impairment. *Journal of Speech and Hearing Research, 34*(1), 11–18.

D'Antonio, L. L., Muntz, H. R., Province, M. A., & Marsh, J. L. (1988). Laryngeal/voice findings in patients with velopharyngeal dysfunction. *Laryngoscope, 98*(4), 432–438.

de Serres, L. M., Deleyiannis, F. W., Eblen, L. E., Gruss, J. S., Richardson, M. A., & Sie, K. C. (1999). Results with sphincter pharyngoplasty and pharyngeal flap. *International Journal of Pediatratic Otorhinolaryngology, 48*(1), 17–25.

Dibbell, D. G., Ewanowski, S., & Carter, W. L. (1979). Successful correction of velopharyngeal stress incompetence in musicians playing wind instruments. *Plastic and Reconstructive Surgery, 64*(5), 662–664.

Donnelly, M. J. (1994). Hypernasality following adenoid removal. *Irish Journal of Medical Science, 163*(5), 225–227.

Eufinger, H., Eggeling, V., & Immenkamp, E. (1994). Velopharyngoplasty with or without tonsillectomy and/or adenotomy—A retrospective evaluation of speech characteristics in 143 patients. *Journal of Craniomaxillofacial Surgery, 22*(1), 37–42.

Falk, M. L., & Kopp, G. A. (1968). Tongue position and hypernasality in cleft palate speech. *Cleft Palate Journal, 5*(3), 228–237.

Fee, W. E., Jr., Gilmer, P. A., & Goffinet, D. R. (1988). Surgical management of recurrent nasopharyngeal carcinoma after radiation failure at the primary site. *Laryngoscope, 98*(11), 1220–1226.

Fernandes, D. B., Grobbelaar, A. O., Hudson, D. A., & Lentin, R. (1996). Velopharyngeal incompetence after adenotonsillectomy in non-cleft patients. *British Journal of Oral and Maxillofacial Surgery, 34*(5), 364–367.

Finkelstein, Y., Bar-Ziv, J., Nachmani, A., Berger, G., & Ophir, D. (1993). Peritonsillar abscess as a cause of transient velopharyngeal insufficiency. *Cleft Palate Craniofacial Journal, 30*(4), 421–428.

Finkelstein, Y., Talmi, Y. P., Nachmani, A., Hauben, D. J., & Zohar, Y. (1992). On the variability of velopharyngeal valve anatomy and function: A combined peroral and nasendoscopic study. *Plastic and Reconstructive Surgery, 89*(4), 631–639.

Fletcher, S. G., & Daly, D. A. (1976). Nasalance in utterances of hearing-impaired speakers. *Journal of Communication Disorders, 9*(1), 63–73.

Folkins, J. W. (1988). Velopharyngeal nomenclature: Incompetence, inadequacy, insufficiency, and dysfunction. *Cleft Palate Journal, 25*(4), 413–416.

Forner, L. L. (1983). Speech segment durations produced by five and six year old speakers with and without cleft palates. *Cleft Palate Journal, 20*(3), 185–198.

Gibb, A. G., & Stewart, I. A. (1975). Hypernasality following tonsil dissection—Hysterical aetiology. *Journal of Laryngology and Otology, 89*(7), 779–781.

Gordon, N. A., Astrachan, D., & Yanagisawa, E. (1994). Videoendoscopic diagnosis and correction of velopharyngeal stress incompetence in a bassoonist. *Annals of Otology, Rhinology, and Laryngology, 103*(8, Pt. 1), 595–600.

Haapanen, M. L., Heliovaara, A., & Ranta, R. (1991). Hypernasality and the nasopharyngeal space. A cephalometric study. *Journal of Craniomaxillofacial Surgery, 19*(2), 77–80.

Haapanen, M. L., Kalland, M., Heliovaara, A., Hukki, J., & Ranta, R. (1997). Velopharyngeal function in cleft patients undergoing maxillary advancement. *Folia Phoniatrica et Logopedica, 49*(1), 42–47.

Hagstrom, W. J., Parsons, R. W., Landa, S. J., & Robson, M. C. (1979). Familial velopharyngeal incompetence caused by myasthenia gravis. *Annals of Plastic Surgery, 3*(6), 555–557.

Hall, C. D., Golding-Kushner, K. J., Argamaso, R. V., & Strauch, B. (1991). Pharyngeal flap surgery in adults. *Cleft Palate Craniofacial Journal, 28*(2), 179–182; Discussion 182–183.

Handelman, C. S., & Osborne, G. (1976). Growth of the nasopharynx and adenoid development from one to eighteeen years. *Angle Orthodontist, 46*(3), 243–259.

Harding, A., & Grunwell, P. (1996). Characteristics of cleft palate speech. *European Journal of Disorders of Communication, 31*(4), 331–357.

Harding, A., & Grunwell, P. (1998). Active versus passive cleft-type speech characteristics. *International Journal of Language and Communication Disorders, 33*(3), 329–352.

Heller, J. C., Gens, G. W., Moe, D. G., & Lewin, M. L. (1974). Velopharyngeal insufficiency in patients with neurologic, emotional, and mental disorders.

Journal of Speech and Hearing Disorders, 39(3), 350–359.

Henningsson, G. E., & Isberg, A. M. (1986). Velopharyngeal movement patterns in patients alternating between oral and glottal articulation: A clinical and cineradiographical study. *Cleft Palate Journal, 23*(1), 1–9.

Henningsson, G., & Isberg, A. (1988). Influence of tonsils on velopharyngeal movements in children with craniofacial anomalies and hypernasality. *American Journal of Orthodontics and Dentofacial Orthopedics, 94*(3), 253–261.

Hess, D. A. (1959). Pitch, intensity and cleft palate voice quality. *Journal of Speech and Hearing Research, 2*, 113.

Hillarp, B., Ekberg, O., Jacobsson, S., Nylander, G., & Aberg, M. (1994). Myotonic dystrophy revealed at videoradiography of deglutition and speech in adult patients with velopharyngeal insufficiency: Presentation of four cases. *Cleft Palate Craniofacial Journal, 31*(2), 125–133.

Jones, D. L. (1991). Velopharyngeal function and dysfunction. *Clinics in Communication Disorders, 1*(3), 19–25.

Kawano, M., Isshiki, N., Harita, Y., & Tanokuchi, F. (1985). Laryngeal fricative in cleft palate speech. *Acta Otolaryngologica, 419*(Suppl.), 180–187.

Kline, L. S., & Hutchinson, J. M. (1980). Acoustic and perceptual evaluation of hypernasality of mentally retarded persons. *American Journal of Mental Deficiency, 85*(2), 153–160.

Kummer, A. W., Curtis, C., Wiggs, M., Lee, L., & Strife, J. L. (1992). Comparison of velopharyngeal gap size in patients with hypernasality, hypernasality and nasal emission, or nasal turbulence (rustle) as the primary speech characteristic. *Cleft Palate Craniofacial Journal, 29*(2), 152–156.

Kummer, A. W., Myer, C. M. I., Smith, M. E., & Shott, S. R. (1993). Changes in nasal resonance secondary to adenotonsillectomy. *American Journal of Otolaryngology, 14*(4), 285–290.

Kummer, A. W., Strife, J. L., Grau, W. H., Creaghead, N. A., & Lee, L. (1989). The effects of Le Fort I osteotomy with maxillary movement on articulation, resonance, and velopharyngeal function. *Cleft Palate Journal, 26*(3), 193–199; Discussion 199–200.

Lefaivre, J. F., Cohen, S. R., Riski, J. E., & Burstein, F. D. (1997). Velopharyngeal incompetence as the presenting symptom of malignant brainstem tumor. *Cleft Palate Craniofacial Journal, 34*(2), 154–158.

Loney, R. W., & Bloem, T. J. (1987). Velopharyngeal dysfunction: Recommendations for use of nomenclature. *Cleft Palate Journal, 24*(4), 334–335.

Luce, E. A., McGibbon, B., & Hoopes, J. E. (1977). Velopharyngeal insufficiency in hemifacial microsomia. *Plastic and Reconstructive Surgery, 60*(4), 602–606.

MacKenzie-Stepner, K., Witzel, M. A., Stringer, D. A., & Laskin, R. (1987). Velopharyngeal insufficiency due to hypertrophic tonsils. A report of two cases. *International Journal of Pediatric Otorhinolaryngology, 14*(1), 57–63.

Maegawa, J., Sells, R. K., & David, D. J. (1998). Speech changes after maxillary advancement in 40 cleft lip and palate patients. *Journal of Craniofacial Surgery, 9*(2), 177–182; Discussion 183–184.

Marsh, J. L. (1991). Cleft palate and velopharyngeal dysfunction. *Clinics in Communication Disorders, 1*(3), 29–34.

Mason, R. M., & Grandstaff, H. L. (1971). Evaluating the velopharyngeal mechanism in hypernasal speakers. *Language, Speech, and Hearing Services in the Schools, 2*(4), 53–61.

Mason, R., Turvey, T. A., & Warren, D. W. (1980). Speech considerations with maxillary advancement procedures. *Journal of Oral Surgery, 38*(10), 752–758.

Mason, R. M., & Warren, D. W. (1980). Adenoid involution and developing hypernasality in cleft palate. *Journal of Speech and Hearing Disorders, 45*(4), 469–480.

McCarthy, J. G., Coccaro, P. J., & Schwartz, M. D. (1979). Velopharyngeal function following maxillary advancement. *Plastic and Reconstructive Surgery, 64*(2), 180–189.

McDonald, E. T., & Baker H. (1951). Cleft palate speech: An integration of research and clinical observation. *Journal of Speech and Hearing Disorders, 16*, 9–20.

McHenry, M. A. (1997). The effect of increased vocal effort on estimated velopharyngeal orifice area. *American Journal of Speech-Language Pathology, 6*(4), 55–61.

McWilliams, B. J. (1991). Submucous clefts of the palate: How likely are they to be symptomatic? *Cleft Palate Craniofacial Journal, 28*(3), 247–249; Discussion 250–251.

McWilliams, B. J., Bluestone, C. D., & Musgrave, R. H. (1969). Diagnostic implications of vocal cord nodules in children with cleft palate. *Laryngoscope, 79*(12), 2072–2080.

McWilliams, B. J., Lavorato, A. S., & Bluestone, C. D. (1973). Vocal cord abnormalities in children with velopharyngeal valving problems. *Laryngoscope, 83,* 1745.

McWilliams, B. J., Morris, H. L., & Shelton, R. L. (1990a). Disorders of phonation and resonance. In B. J. McWilliams, H. L. Morris, & R. L. Shelton (Eds.), *Cleft palate speech* (Vol. 2, pp. 247–268). Philadelphia: B.C. Decker.

McWilliams, B. J., Morris, H. L., & Shelton, R. L. (1990b). The nature of the velopharyngeal mechanism. In B. J. McWilliams, H. L. Morris, & R. L. Shelton (Eds.), *Cleft palate speech* (Vol. 2, pp. 197–235). Philadelphia: B.C. Decker.

Misra, U. C., Gill, R. S., & Lal, M. (1981). Tonsil transposition into posterior pharyngeal wall in palato-pharyngeal incompetence. *Journal of Laryngology and Otology, 95*(7), 713–716.

Morris, H. L. (1984). Types of velopharyngeal incompetence. In H. Winitz (Ed.), *Treating articulation disorders: For clinicians by clinicians* (p. 211). Baltimore: University Park Press.

Morris, H. L. (1992). Some questions and answers about velopharyngeal dysfunction during speech. *American Journal of Speech-Language Pathology, 1*(3), 26–28.

Morris, H. L., Wroblewski, S. K., Brown, C. K., & Van Demark, D. R. (1990). Velar-pharyngeal status in cleft palate patients with expected adenoidal involution. *Annals of Otology, Rhinology, and Laryngology, 99*(6, Pt. 1), 432–437.

Myers, E. N., & Aramany, M. A. (1977). Rehabilitation of the oral cavity following resection of the hard and soft palate. *Transactions of the American Academy of Ophthalmology and Otolaryngology, 84*(5), 941–951.

Neilson, P. D., & O'Dwyer, N. J. (1981). Pathophysiology of dysarthria in cerebral palsy. *Journal of Neurolology, Neurosurgery, and Psychiatry, 44*(11), 1013–1019.

Neiman, G. S., & Simpson, R. K. (1975). A roentgencephalometric investigation of the effect of adenoid removal upon selected measures of velopharyngeal function. *Cleft Palate Journal, 12,* 377–389.

Netsell, R. (1969). Evaluation of velopharyngeal function in dysarthria. *Journal of Speech and Hearing Disorders, 34*(2), 113–122.

Netsell, R. (1988). Velopharyngeal dysfunction. In D. Yoder & R. Kent (Eds.), *Decision-making in speech-language pathology* (pp. 150–151). Toronto: B. C. Decker.

Okazaki, K., Satoh, K., Kato, M., Iwanami, M., Ohokubo, F., & Kobayashi, K. (1993). Speech and velopharyngeal function following maxillary advancement in patients with cleft lip and palate. *Annals of Plastic Surgery, 30*(4), 304–311.

Parton, M. J., & Jones, A. S. (1998). Hypernasality following adenoidectomy: A significant and avoidable complication. *Clinical Otolaryngology, 23*(1), 18–19.

Penfold, C. N. (1997). Management of velopharyngeal dysfunction [Letter; comment]. *British Journal of Oral and Maxillofacial Surgery, 35*(6), 454.

Peterson-Falzone, S. J. (1985). Velopharyngeal inadequacy in the absence of overt cleft palate. *Journal of Craniofacial Genetics and Developmental Biology Supplement, 1,* 97–124.

Platt, L. J., Andrews, G., & Howie, P. M. (1980). Dysarthria of adult cerebral palsy: II. Phonemic analysis of articulation errors. *Journal of Speech and Hearing Research, 23*(1), 41–55.

Platt, L. J., Andrews, G., Young, M., & Quinn, P. T. (1980). Dysarthria of adult cerebral palsy: I. Intelligibility and articulatory impairment. *Journal of Speech and Hearing Research, 23*(1), 28–40.

Pollack, M. A., & Shprintzen, R. J. (1981). Velopharyngeal insufficiency in neurofibromatosis. *International Journal of Pediatric Otorhinolaryngology, 3*(3), 257–262.

Powers, G. R. (1962). Cinefluorographic investigation of articulatory movements of selected individuals with cleft palates. *Journal of Speech and Hearing Research, 5,* 59.

Ren, Y. F., Isberg, A., & Henningsson, G. (1995). Velopharyngeal incompetence and persistent hypernasality after adenoidectomy in children without palatal defect. *Cleft Palate Craniofacial Journal, 32*(6), 476–482.

Rintala, A. E. (1987). Solitary metastatic melanoma of the soft palate. *Annals of Plastic Surgery, 19*(5), 463–465.

Riski, J. E. (1995). Speech assessment of adolescents. *Cleft Palate Craniofacial Journal, 32*(2), 109–113.

Riski, J. E., & Verdolini, K. (1999). Is hypernasality a voice disorder? *Asha, 41*(1), 10–11.

Robinson, J. H. (1992). Association between adenoidectomy, velopharyngeal incompetence, and submucous cleft [Letter]. *Cleft Palate Craniofacial Journal, 29*(4), 385.

Rousseaux, M., Lesoin, F., & Quint, S. (1987). Unilateral pseudobulbar syndrome with limited capsulothalamic infarction. *European Neurology, 27*(4), 227–230.

Salomonson, J., Kawamoto, H., & Wilson, L. (1988). Velopharyngeal incompetence as the presenting symptom of myotonic dystrophy. *Cleft Palate Journal, 25*(3), 296–300.

Schmaman, L., Jordaan, H., & Jammine, G. H. (1998). Risk factors for permanent hypernasality after adenoidectomy. *South African Medical Journal, 88*(3), 266–269.

Seid, A. B. (1990). Velopharyngeal insufficiency versus adenoidectomy for obstructive apnea: A quandary [Clinical conference]. *Cleft Palate Journal, 27*(2), 200–202.

Shanks, J. C. (1990). Velopharyngeal incompetence manifested initially in playing a musical instrument. *Journal of Voice, 4*(2), 169–171.

Shapiro, R. S. (1980). Velopharyngeal insufficiency starting at puberty without adenoidectomy. *International Journal of Pediatric Otorhinolaryngology, 2*(3), 255–260.

Shprintzen, R. J., Rakof, S. J., Skolnick, M. L., & Lavorato, A. S. (1977). Incongruous movements of the velum and lateral pharyngeal walls. *Cleft Palate Journal, 14*(2), 148–157.

Shprintzen, R. J., Sher, A. E., & Croft, C. B. (1987). Hypernasal speech caused by tonsillar hypertrophy. *International Journal of Pediatric Otorhinolaryngology, 14*(1), 45–56.

Siegel-Sadewitz, V. L., & Shprintzen, R. J. (1982). Nasopharyngoscopy of the normal velopharyngeal sphincter: An experiment of biofeedback. *Cleft Palate Journal, 19*(3), 194–200.

Siegel-Sadewitz, V. L., & Shprintzen, R. J. (1986). Changes in velopharyngeal valving with age. *International Journal of Pediatric Otorhinolaryngology, 11*(2), 171–182.

Skolnick, M. L., Shprintzen, R. J., McCall, G. N., & Rakoff, S. (1975). Patterns of velopharyngeal closure in subjects with repaired cleft palate and normal speech: A multi-view videofluoroscopic analysis. *Cleft Palate Journal, 12*, 369–376.

Theodoros, D., Murdoch, B. E., Stokes, P. D., & Chenery, H. J. (1993). Hypernasality in dysarthric speakers following severe closed head injury: A perceptual and instrumental analysis. *Brain Injury, 7*(1), 59–69.

Thompson, E. C., & Murdoch, B. E. (1995). Disorders of nasality in subjects with upper motor neuron type dysarthria following cerebrovascular accident. *Journal of Communication Disorders, 28*(3), 261–276.

Thurston, J. B., Larson, D. L., Shanks, J. C., Bennett, J. E., & Parsons, R. W. (1980). Nasal obstruction as a complication of pharyngeal flap surgery. *Cleft Palate Journal, 17*(2), 148–154.

Trost, J. E. (1981). Articulatory additions to the classical description of the speech of persons with cleft palate. *Cleft Palate Journal, 18*(3), 193–203.

Trost-Cardamone, J. E. (1987). *Cleft palate misarticulations: A teaching tape* [Videotape]. California State University, Northridge, CA: Instructional Media Center.

Trost-Cardamone, J. E. (1989). Coming to terms with VPI: A response to Loney and Bloem. *Cleft Palate Journal, 26*(1), 68–70.

Trost-Cardamone, J. E. (1990). Speech in the first year of life: A perspective on early acquisition. In D. E. Kernahan & S. W. Rosenstein (Eds.), *Cleft lip and palate: A system of management* (pp. 91–103). Baltimore: Williams & Wilkins.

Trost-Cardamone, J. E. (1997). Diagnosis of specific cleft palate speech error patterns for planning therapy of physical management needs. In K. R. Bzoch (Ed.), *Communicative disorders related to cleft lip and palate* (Vol. 4, pp. 313–330). Austin, TX: Pro-Ed.

Upton, L. G., & Berger, M. K. (1995). Use of pharyngoplasty to improve resonance in adult closed-head injury patients: Report of cases [see Comments]. *Journal of Oral and Maxillofacial Surgery, 53*(6), 717–719.

Van Mourik, M., Catsman-Berrevoets, C. E., Yousef-Bak, E., Paquier, P. F., & van Dongen, H. R. (1998). Dysarthria in children with cerebellar or brainstem tumors. *Pediatric Neurology, 18*(5), 411–414.

Warren, D. W., Dalston, R. M., & Mayo, R. (1993). Hypernasality in the presence of "adequate" velopharyngeal closure. *Cleft Palate Craniofacial Journal, 30*(2), 150–154.

Warren, D. W., Dalston, R. M., Trier, W. C., & Holder, M. B. (1985). A pressure-flow technique for quantifying temporal patterns of palatopharyngeal closure. *Cleft Palate Journal, 22*(1), 11–19.

Warren, D. W., Wood, M. T., & Bradley, D. P. (1969). Respiratory volumes in normal and cleft palate speech. *Cleft Palate Journal, 6,* 449–460.

Watzke, I., Turvey, T. A., Warren, D. W., & Dalston, R. (1990). Alterations in velopharyngeal function after maxillary advancement in cleft palate patients. *Journal of Oral and Maxillofacial Surgery, 48*(7), 685–689.

Witt, P. D., Myckatyn, T., & Marsh, J. L. (1998). Salvaging the failed pharyngoplasty: Intervention outcome. *Cleft Palate Craniofacial Journal, 35*(5), 447–453.

Witt, P. D., O'Daniel, T. G., Marsh, J. L., Grames, L. M., Muntz, H. R., & Pilgram, T. K. (1997). Surgical management of velopharyngeal dysfunction: Outcome analysis of autogenous posterior pharyngeal wall augmentation. *Plastic and Reconstructive Surgery, 99*(5), 1287–1296; Discussion 1297–1300.

Witzel, M. A., & Posnick, J. C. (1989). Patterns and location of velopharyngeal valving problems: Atypical findings on video nasopharyngoscopy. *Cleft Palate Journal, 26*(1), 63–67.

Witzel, M. A., Rich, R. H., Margar-Bacal, F., & Cox, C. (1986). Velopharyngeal insufficiency after ade-noidectomy: An 8-year review. *International Journal of Pediatric Otorhinolaryngology, 11*(1), 15–20.

Wolski, W. (1967). Hypernasality as the presenting symptom of myasthenia gravis. *Journal of Speech and Hearing Disorders, 32*(1), 36–38.

Workinger, M. S., & Netsell, R. (1992). Restoration of intelligible speech 13 years post-head injury. *Brain Injury, 6*(2), 183–187.

Yanagisawa, E., Estill, J., Mambrino, L., & Talkin, D. (1991). Supraglottic contributions to pitch raising. Videoendoscopic study with spectroanalysis. *Annals of Otology, Rhinology, and Laryngology, 100*(1), 19–30.

Yanagisawa, E., Kmucha, S. T., & Estill, J. (1990). Role of the soft palate in laryngeal functions and selected voice qualities. Simultaneous velolaryngeal videoendoscopy [Published Erratum appears in *Annals of Otology, Rhinology, Laryngology, 99*(6, Pt. 1), 431] [see Comments]. *Annals of Otology, Rhinology, and Laryngology, 99*(1), 18–28.

Yorkston, K. M., Beukelman, D. R., & Traynor, C. D. (1988). Articulatory adequacy in dysarthric speakers: A comparison of judging formats. *Journal of Communication Disorders, 21*(4), 351–361.

Yoshida, H., Michi, K., Yamashita, Y., & Ohno, K. (1993). A comparison of surgical and prosthetic treatment for speech disorders attributable to surgically acquired soft palate defects. *Journal of Oral and Maxillofacial Surgery, 51*(4), 361–365.

Ysunza, A., & Vazquez, M. C. (1993). Velopharyngeal sphincter physiology in deaf individuals. *Cleft Palate Craniofacial Journal, 30*(2), 141–143.

CHAPTER

8

Facial and Oral Anomalies: Effects on Speech and Resonance

J. Paul Willging, M.D.
Ann W. Kummer, Ph.D.

CONTENTS

Craniofacial disorders can have a great impact on the function of head and neck structures. The typical disease processes that exist in the general population are often found with an increased prevalence in this specific group of patients. Structural as well as physiologic abnormalities join to create special problems for the patient with abnormalities of the craniofacial skeleton.

The Ear

Patients born with craniofacial anomalies may have associated malformations of the external or middle ear. Abnormalities of the inner ear are less commonly encountered, but can occur. These malformations can affect aesthetics and can cause hearing loss that can ultimately affect the ability to communicate.

Anatomy of the Ear

The *external ear* is comprised of the pinna and the external auditory canal. The *pinna* is the delicate cartilaginous framework surrounding the external auditory canal (Figure 8–1A). It functions to direct sound energy into the *external auditory canal*, which is a skin-lined canal leading to the eardrum.

The *middle ear* is a hollow space within the temporal bone. The *mastoid cavity* connects to the middle ear space posteriorly and is comprised of a collection of air cells within the temporal bone. Both the middle ear and *mastoid cavities*, which are in the temporal bone behind the ear, are lined with a mucous membrane. The *tympanic membrane*, also called the *eardrum*, is considered part of the middle ear. The tympanic membrane transmits sound energy through the ossicles to the inner ear. The three tiny bones in the middle ear are called the *ossicles* and they include the malleus, incus, and stapes. The *malleus* (hammer) is firmly attached to the tympanic membrane. The *incus* (anvil) has an articulation with the malleus and the stapes. The

stapes acts as a piston to create pressure waves within the fluid-filled cochlea. The tympanic membrane and ossicles act to amplify the sound energy and efficiently introduce this energy into the liquid environment of the cochlea.

The *inner ear* consists of the cochlea and semicircular canals. The *cochlea* is composed of a bony spiral tube that is shaped as a snail's shell. Within this bony tube are delicate membranes separating the canal into three separate fluid-filled spaces. The *organ of corti* is the site where mechanical energy introduced into the cochlea is converted into electrical stimulation conducted by the auditory nerves to the auditory cortex, which provides an awareness of sound. Inner and outer *hair cells* (sensory cells with hairlike properties) of the cochlea may be damaged by a variety of mechanisms leading to sensorineural hearing loss. A second function of the inner ear is balance. The *semicircular canals* are the loop-shaped tubular parts of the inner ear that provide a sense of spatial orientation. They are oriented in three planes at right angles to one another. They provide a sense of spatial orientation. The *saccule* and *utricle* are additional sensory organs within the inner ear that provide a sensation of acceleration. Hair cells within these organs have small calcium carbonate granules that respond to gravity and acceleration forces to create the sense of motion.

Malformations of the External Ear

Patients with craniofacial anomalies, especially those with syndromes, often have *microtia*, which is a malformation of the pinna (Brent, 1999) (Figure 8–1B). The more severely malformed the pinna is, the greater the chances are for significant problems within the middle ear or involving the ossicles (Kountakis, Helidonis, & Jahrsdoerfer, 1995).

When there is microtia of the external ear, it is not uncommon to also find aural atresia. *Aural atresia*, also called *auditory atresia*, refers

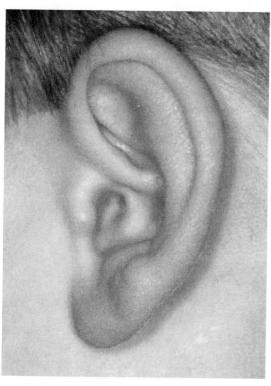

A

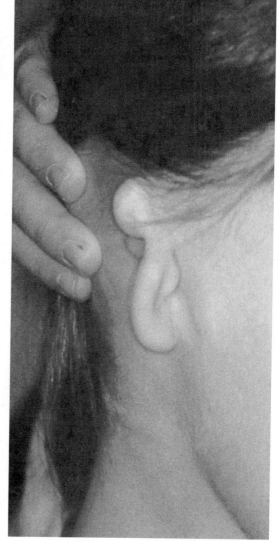

B

Figure 8–1. A. A normal pinna. The pinna is composed of fibroelastic cartilage covered by a thin layer of skin. The delicate folding of the cartilage provides the normal shape of the ear. **B.** A case of microtia. Microtia is the result of abnormal development of the external ear. The more severe the external deformity, the more likely the middle ear cannot be reconstructed despite their development from different sites of origin.

to the congenital abnormality of closure of the external auditory canal. The external auditory canal and tympanic membrane may be very small, or may fail to develop entirely, as in Treacher-Collins syndrome, hemifacial microsomia or Nager syndrome. This results in a *conductive hearing loss* because the sound energy cannot travel directly through the external auditory canal to the tympanic membrane and therefore, cannot reach the inner ear.

Children with bilateral aural atresia require bone-conducting hearing aids. These attach firmly to the bone of the skull and directly vibrate the end organ within the cochlea. Children with unilateral aural atresia generally do not require a hearing aid if their hearing is normal in the unaffected ear. It is of interest that children with aural atresia rarely experience ear infections. The explanation for this is not known.

Reconstruction of the auditory canal, tympanic membrane, and ossicular chain can be done in the early school years. Patients with bilateral aural atresia benefit from reconstruction with an improvement in hearing. Patients with unilateral atresia are often reconstructed, but the benefits are less easily quantifiable. The risk of this surgical procedure lies in the potential damage to the CN VII (Jahrsdoerfer & Lambert, 1998), which is the facial nerve. This is the main nerve that controls motion on each side of the face. Damage to the nerve can cause paralysis of one side of the face. The paralysis may be complete or partial, temporary or permanent, depending on the degree of injury to the nerve. Computed tomography scans of the temporal bone can be used in predicting the course of the facial nerve in atretic ears, but these scans are not always of value. A rating scale has been developed to predict the outcome of the surgical correction of the external auditory canal and tympanic membrane. It is based on the overall development of the middle ear space, the size and position of the ossicles, the presence of the stapes, and the position of the facial nerve.

Malformations of the Middle Ear

When malformations are found in the external ear, there are often malformations or anomalies of the middle ear structures as well. This may include abnormal formation of the ossicles, as can be found in Crouzon, Apert, and Goldenhar syndromes. In some cases, there is fusion of the ossicles to the surrounding bone. When the ossicles are abnormally formed or fused, this affects the transmission of the sound to the inner ear, causing a conductive hearing loss.

In many cases, surgical correction is possible for abnormalities of the external auditory canal, the tympanic membrane, or the ossicles (Jahrsadoerfer, Yeakley, Aguilar, Cole, & Gray, 1992). In addition, hearing aids allow correction of most kinds of conductive hearing loss. Cochlear implants are offered as a means to treat sensorineural hearing loss in patients who derive no benefit from conventional hearing aids.

Eustachian Tube Dysfunction and Middle Ear Disease

Otitis Media

The middle ear and mastoid cavities must have the air within them replenished at regular intervals to prevent problems from developing. This is accomplished by the function of the eustachian tube.

The *eustachian tube* connects the middle ear with the nasopharynx. This tube is closed at rest, and opens when the tensor veli palatini muscle, which is attached directly to the cartilage of the eustachian tube, contracts in the act of swallowing. As the eustachian tube opens, it allows for middle ear ventilation and the equalization of middle ear pressure with the environment. When the eustachian tube fails to function normally, fluids tend to develop within the middle ear space due to the negative pressure, resulting in *middle ear effusion*. If the eustachian tube begins to function, the fluids will be absorbed by the lymphatics in the middle ear mucosa, and the normal condition will be restored. If the eustachian tube continues to malfunction however, the middle ear effusion will persist and may become infected. Bacteria can ascend the eustachian tube and grow in this effusion, leading to acute *otitis media*.

Acute otitis media is a common disease process in children. Half of children under the age of 3 have had at least one episode of otitis. The children frequently have high fever and severe ear pain. As a result, they are often inconsolable. Occasionally, the tympanic membrane ruptures due to the increased pressure produced by the inflammatory process in the middle ear, and the toxic effect of the bacterial infection (Figure 8–2).

Causes of Eustachian Tube Dysfunction

All young children, even those without ear anomalies, are at risk for middle ear disease. This is due to the fact that, in children, the eustachian tubes are oriented in such a way that the tensor veli palatini muscles, which open the tube, are directed at an unfavorable angle for this function. In addition, the eustachian tubes lie in a horizontal plane between the nasopharynx and the middle ear, which impairs middle ear drainage and allows for reflux of secretions from the pharynx into the tube. Both of these anatomic relationships predispose children to an increased tendency for ear infections. As growth and development occur, the skull base flexes upon itself, moving the origin of the eustachian tube musculature into a more favorable orientation for the opening of the tube. The palate also drops over time in relation to the ear, resulting in a 45° angulation of the eustachian tube up to the middle ear. This angulation prevents some of the reflux of nasopharyngeal secretions into the eustachian tube and thereby minimizes the incidence of infections (Figure 8–3).

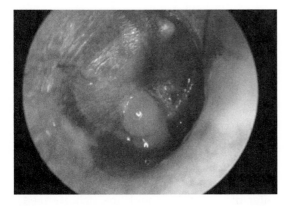

Figure 8–2. Acute otitis media treated with a myringotomy. The infected middle ear fluid can be seen exuding from the hole created in the eardrum.

In addition to the normal risk for middle ear disease in the early years, patients with craniofacial anomalies are at increased risk for recurrent otitis media or persistent middle ear effusions. A cleft palate or any abnormality that affects the soft palate, and therefore the tensor veli palatini muscle, may have an adverse affect on eustachian tube function, and therefore the middle ear (Bluestone, Beery, Cantekin, & Paradise, 1975; Bluestone, Paradise, Beery, & Wittel, 1972; Doyle, Cantekin, & Bluestone, 1980; Durr & Shapiro, 1989; Heller, Gens, Croft, & Moe, 1978; Paradise, 1976; Paradise et al., 1974; Paradise & Bluestone, 1974; Trujillo, 1994).

Effects and Complications of Otitis Media

In addition to causing discomfort and pain, there is a potential for complications to develop as a result of acute otitis media. Therefore, frequent ear infections are a cause of concern.

Otitis media causes a conductive hearing loss because of the diminished mobility of the tympanic membrane in vibrating against the ossicles in the middle ear. The extent of the conductive hearing loss is variable, ranging from 5–55 decibels according to the physical nature of the effusion. It is unlikely that mild hearing loss will "cause" speech and language difficulties, but it is likely that diminished hearing can aggravate an underlying tendency for the development of articulation errors and can disrupt speech and language acquisition (Hubbard, Paradise, McWilliams, Elster, & Taylor, 1985). Auditory stimulation is particularly important during the first year of life. During this time, the neurons in the auditory brainstem are maturing, and the neural connections are being formed (Sininger, Doyle, & Moore, 1999). If sensory input to the auditory nervous system is interrupted during early development, this can have a deleterious effect on speech and language learning (Rvachew, Slawinski, Williams, & Green, 1999). Hearing must always be eval-

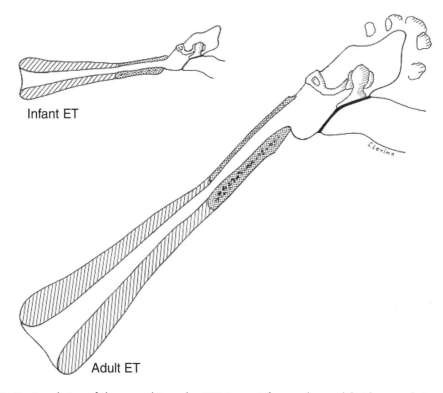

Infant ET

Adult ET

Figure 8–3. Angulation of the eustachian tube (ET) in an infant and an adult. The angulation of the eustachian tube changes with growth and development. In the young child, the eustachian tube ascends up to the middle ear at a 10° angle. In the adult, this angle changes to 45°. The orientation of the musculature around the eustachian tube also changes over time, improving the ability to ventilate the middle ear with age.

uated in the presence of speech and language difficulties to ensure normal auditory function prior to initiation of therapeutic intervention for speech and language disorders.

One serious potential complication of otitis media is *mastoiditis*, which is an infection within the temporal bone that begins to erode bone, leading to potentially life-threatening complications. Mastoiditis is essentially a closed-space abscess that has the ability to erode bone.

The infection often extends laterally behind the ear, causing the ear to protrude from the side of the head. It could also erode medially, causing meningitis or brain abscess.

Another potential complication of repeated ear infections may cause sensorineural hearing loss. The toxins produced by the bacteria may enter the cochlea through the delicate membranes in the middle ear. With repeated exposure to these toxins, the hair cells of the cochlea may be damaged, leading to a permanent hearing loss.

Treatment of Otitis Media

Acute otitis media is treated with oral antibiotics with rapid resolution of the child's ear symptoms. The antibiotic will sterilize the middle ear effusion but will not make the fluid resolve. The treatment for recurrent acute otitis media includes multiple courses of antibiotics. However, the potential for the development of antibiotic-resistant bacteria increases with the number of antibiotics prescribed and the total duration of antibiotic treatment.

After an ear infection has been eradicated, the middle ear effusion may persist for a period of time. While the fluid is in the middle ear space, a mild conductive hearing loss will be present. Once the eustachian tube begins to function normally, allowing a return to normal middle ear pressure, the fluid in the middle ear will be absorbed.

The middle ear fluid will persist in children after the infection has been resolved for about 1 month in 40% of patients, up to 2 months in 20% of patients, and about 3 months in 5% of patients (Teele, Klein, & Rosner, 1980). With fluid present in the middle ear, antibiotics may help prevent additional infections from developing but will have no effect in speeding the resolution of the effusion. Chronic antibiotic use in the treatment of noninfected middle ear effusion has been one of the major factors in the development of antibiotic resistant bacteria. The middle ear effusion will resolve when the normal aeration function of the eustachian tube has been re-established.

Surgical intervention is recommended if the child has had six or more episodes of otitis, or the child has had a middle ear effusion that persists for 3 months or longer and is associated with a conductive hearing loss. Recurrent acute otitis media and persistent middle ear effusions are treated with a myringotomy and

insertion of ventilation tubes. A *myringotomy* is a small, surgical incision that is made in the tympanic membrane to allow for drainage of middle ear fluid. *Ventilation tubes,* also called *pressure equalizing (PE) tubes* (Figure 8–4), are surgically inserted in the eardrum to provide an alternate route for air to enter the middle ear if the eustachian tube is nonfunctional. Ventilation tubes do not correct the underlying problems related to recurrent otitis media. Instead, they bypass the eustachian tube until growth and development have progressed to the point where normal eustachian tube function can be achieved. If normal pressures can be established in the middle ear, the effusion will resolve and not recur, and the irritative effect of the effusion on the mucosa will reverse, leading to a normal middle ear system. The conductive hearing loss due to the effusion will also disappear, returning hearing to normal.

Ventilation tubes typically remain in the eardrum for a length of time determined by their size. The longer the flanges of the tube, the longer their retention. The tubes will generally be extruding within 1 to 2 years. As the tube is expelled, the tympanic membrane heals. Ventilation tubes are generally required only once in the majority (80%) of patients requiring their placement. If recurring ear infections are again encountered after the ventilation tubes have extruded, another set of tubes can be inserted.

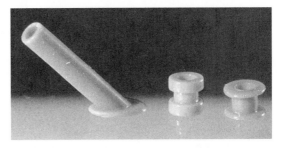

Figure 8–4. Examples of types of pressure equalizing (PE) tubes.

An adenoidectomy is often considered in conjunction with the second set of tubes. The *adenoid* is lymphoid tissue (similar to the tissue found in tonsils) that resides on the skull base in the nasopharynx. The eustachian tubes open on either side of the nasopharynx with the adenoid lying between these openings. If the adenoid is enlarged, or if the adenoid is frequently infected, mucosal edema or the adenoid tissue itself may obstruct the eustachian tube openings, contributing to continued middle ear pathology. An adenoidectomy may be beneficial in establishing improved eustachian tube function (Gates, Avery, Prihoda, & Cooper, 1987).

In patients with craniofacial anomalies, given their increased risk, a particularly aggressive approach to the management of recurrent ear infections is required. This includes early insertion of ventilation tubes. In fact, those children who have a cleft lip and palate often have PE tubes inserted prophylactically at the time of the lip repair. Children with craniofacial anomalies should have their hearing tested by 6 months of age, and repeat testing performed as necessary. Following palatoplasty, eustachian tube function usually improves and the incidence of ear infections decreases. The incidence rates of recurrent otitis media among children with a history of a cleft palate never reach that of a child born with a normal palate, but approach it over time.

Malformations of the Inner Ear

Structural malformations of the inner ear arise from abnormal development of the otic capsule within the temporal bone. Abnormalities of the inner ear are uncommon, but may be associated with craniofacial anomalies, especially with certain syndromes. Inner ear abnormalities typically cause a *sensorineural hearing loss*, which is a problem with the creation of nerve impulses within the inner ear or the transmission of the nerve impulse through the brainstem to the auditory cortex.

The Nose

Anatomy of the Nose

The function of the nose is threefold. It filters inspired air of gross contaminants, it warms the air, and it humidifies the air to the saturation point. These functions are enhanced by the turbulent airflow created as the inspired air impacts the intranasal structures. The nasal septum separates the nasal cavity into two halves. It lies in the midline and is cartilaginous anteriorly and bony posteriorly. The turbinates are bones that are covered with mucosa and are attached to the lateral walls of the nasal cavity. The turbinates create small eddies of air currents, which maximize contact of the inspired air with the nasal mucosa. The nasal mucosa demonstrates a period of vascular engorgement followed by a period of decongestion. The engorgement of the nasal lining promotes humidification and warming of the inspired air. The mucous blanket covering the nasal mucosa traps particulate contaminants. This nasal cycle alternates between sides every 90 minutes. The sinuses are air-filled spaces that are found in the cheeks and between the eyes. These structures are shown in Figure 8–5 as they would be seen through computed tomography.

Malformations of the Nose

Anomalies of the nose range from severe external deformities (facial clefting) to abnormalities of the nasal base (cleft lip and palate) to internal derangement (deviated nasal septum). A deviated nasal septum may occur as a result of a cleft palate, where there is inadequate structural support for the cartilaginous septum to remain in the midline. The septum generally deflects into the cleft side of the nose. A deviated septum may also occur as a result of birth trauma, when the nose of the neonate is forced against the pelvis during delivery, causing the septum to slip off the maxillary crest.

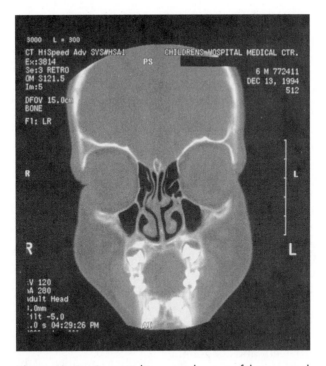

Figure 8–5. Computed tomography scan of the nose and paranasal sinuses. This scan shows the nasal cavities separated by the nasal septum. The turbinates are the small bones arising from the lateral aspect of the nasal cavity. The sinuses are air-filled spaces that are found in the cheeks and between the eyes.

In addition to obstructing the nasal passages to airflow, a significantly deviated septum may affect nasal resonance during speech. Hyponasality may result due to the decrease transmission of sound energy through the nasal cavity. Cul-de-sac resonance may result in severe cases if the sound energy vibrates in a completely obstructed nasal cavity.

Anomalies can also be noted in the front and back openings of the nasal cavity. The nasal cavity opens anteriorly through the nares and posteriorly through the choanae. The choanal openings communicate with the nasopharynx. The anterior nasal openings can be narrowed by overgrowth of the maxilla, an anomaly known as *piriform aperture stenosis* (Brown, Myer, & Manning, 1989). The posterior choanae may be narrowed in a condition known as *choanal stenosis* or completely blocked, as in *choanal atresia*. These abnormalities can be either unilateral or bilateral.

Neonates are obligate nasal breathers. Neonates with bilateral choanal atresia will attempt nasal respiration, and when it is unsuccessful, they become fussy and eventually begin to cry. The infants breathe well while crying, but as they settle down, they again attempt nasal respiration unsuccessfully, only to repeat the process. Without early surgical intervention, this cyclical cyanosis can lead to death from exhaustion. Choanal atresia occurs more commonly in females and has an incidence of 1:8000 births. It is associated with other congenital abnormalities in 50% of patients.

Facial Structures

Maxilla

Maxillary retrusion (also known as *midface deficiency*) is a common anomaly, especially in individuals with repaired cleft lip and palate. It is characterized by a small upper jaw (maxilla) relative to the lower jaw (mandible). This is due to the inherent deficiency in the maxilla from the cleft and the possible restriction in maxillary growth with the surgical repair. With maxillary retrusion, there is usually at least an anterior crossbite and often a *Class III malocclusion*, where the maxilla is retrusive relative to the mandible.

In normal occlusion, the maxillary teeth overlap the mandibular teeth and the tongue resides in the mandible. The tongue tip has sufficient room for movement, including elevation, within the oral cavity. When there is maxillary retrusion, however, the tongue tip may be anterior to the alveolar ridge and anterior to the maxillary teeth. When this is the case, the production of anterior sounds, such as sibilants, will be distorted by the anterior tongue position. This causes a frontal lisp as an obligatory error, because it is due to the structure of the mouth. If the individual attempts to compensate for the anterior position of the tongue relative to the teeth, the tongue will be retracted. As the tongue moves backward, the dorsum moves upward and articulates against the alveolar ridge or palate. This causes a mid-dorsum palatal stop (palatal-dorsal) production as a compensatory error. When this position is used for the production of sibilant sounds (s, z, sh, ch, and j), a lateral lisp distortion is the result.

Maxillary retrusion can also affect lingual-alveolar sounds (t, d, n, l), causing a palatal-dorsal production. In severe cases, it affects the production of bilabial and labio-dental sounds. If it is too far for the lower lip to move back to articulate against the upper teeth for labio-dental sounds, the individual may learn to compensate by reversing this production. In this case, the upper lip articulates against the lower incisors. Although this causes little acoustic distortion, it does appear different and, therefore, can be visually distracting.

Facial Nerve

Facial paralysis may occur as a result of an injury (surgical or traumatic), infection (*Bell's palsy*) (Peitersen, 1992), or due to congenital abnormalities of the nerve or associated muscles. The paralysis may be partial, as in hemifacial microsomia, or may be complete and bilateral, as in Moebius syndrome. Facial paralysis can result in masklike facies. A lack of facial expression can inhibit lip movement for feeding and speech. Facial paralysis can affect the ability to produce bilabial and even labio-dental sounds. The individual may learn to compensate by producing these sounds with the tongue tip. Some individuals become very adept in producing the sound in a way that is acoustically similar to the labial sound.

The Oral Cavity

The oral cavity extends from the lips anteriorly to the faucial pillars posteriorly. Anomalies of the oral cavity are common and can have a significant effect on speech. Dental anomalies are discussed in Chapter 9 and therefore, are not covered in this chapter.

Lips

The lips are paired structures. They function in articulation, eating, and preventing *sialorrhea* (drooling). A common problem following a cleft lip repair is a short upper lip. The lip is deficient in tissue because of the cleft, and also secondary to the contractile effects of the scar from the cleft lip repair. If the premaxilla is protrusive, the relative shortening of the lip is further increased, resulting in the appearance of a protrusive lower lip. Even if the upper lip is of normal length, a protrusive premaxilla may make it appear to be short and can interfere with normal bilabial closure.

When the upper lip is short, there may be difficulties in the production of bilabial sounds, because total lip closure is difficult to accomplish. As a result, the individual may compensate by producing bilabial sounds with a labiodental placement. This can result in a remarkably similar sound to the bilabial sound so that most listeners do not notice a distortion. However, this production looks different and can be distracting to the listener.

There may be additional anomalies of the upper lip following repair of a cleft lip. There may be a mismatch of the vermilion border, asymmetry of the lip, or a flattening of cupid's bow. The obicularis oris muscle must be approximated during the lip repair, or a discontinuity of these muscle bundles may be apparent over time. These anomalies are cosmetic and do not affect speech.

Mouth

Congenital abnormalities of the size and shape of the mouth can occur, especially with some syndromes. The suffix "*stomia*" is used for the word "mouth." This is not to be confused with the suffix "*somia*," which refers to body. *Macrostomia* refers to an excessively large mouth opening. When this occurs, one corner of the mouth may extend into the cheek, making the mouth opening on that particular side large and distorted in appearance. This is particularly common with Hemifacial microsomia. On the other hand, *microstomia* refers to a small mouth opening. Microstomia more often results from acquired injuries, such as electrical burns sustained after a child chews on an electrical cord resulting in an orofacial burn. Severe contractures of the mouth are possible second-

ary to scarring.

Macrostomia does not usually cause speech problems. On the other hand, if the microstomia is severe enough to affect mouth opening, it can potentially affect articulation. This is due to the fact that a small mouth opening restricts the effective oral cavity space and therefore, tongue movement. It can also affect resonance, because the sound energy is inhibited from exiting through the oral cavity.

Tongue

Abnormalities of the tongue are associated with certain syndromes. The tongue may be very large in a condition called *macroglossia*. This is one of the main characteristics of Beckwith-Wiedemann syndrome (Figure 8–6). When this occurs, the tongue does not fit the oral cavity space, and therefore, it protrudes past the alveolar ridge. This often results in an open-mouth posture. As the dentition develops, an anterior open bite may occur due to the position of the tongue in the area where the

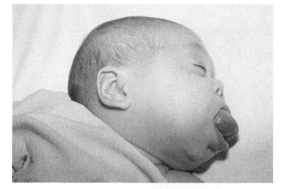

Figure 8–6. Macroglossia secondary to Beckwith-Wiedemann syndrome. Beckwith-Wiedemann syndrome is a congenital disorder characterized by macroglossia, omphalocele, hypoglycemia, and abnormalities of the kidneys, pancreas, and adrenal cortex. This photo demonstrates macroglossia with severe discrepancy between the size of the oral cavity and the size of the tongue.

teeth should be. The chronic open-mouth posture can also contribute to excessive drooling. Macroglossia can affect the production of tongue tip sounds and can cause either a frontal or lateral distortion of sibilants. It can also contribute to the use of palatal-dorsal articulation, especially if the tongue tip rests anterior to the alveolar ridge. The opposite problem of macroglossia is *microglossia*, which is a small tongue, especially in relation to the oral cavity space. This may cause difficulty with tongue tip sounds, but it often has no detrimental effect on speech.

Other lingual (tongue) anomalies include a *lobulated tongue*. In this case, the tongue may appear to have multiple lobes, with fissures between each lobe. This is common in oral-facial-digital (OFD) syndrome. This condition may or may not affect lingual mobility. However, if mobility is affected, speech will be affected as well.

Finally, a discussion of lingual anomalies would not be complete without a mention of ankyloglossia. *Ankyloglossia*, commonly referred to as *"tongue-tie,"* is a condition where the lingual frenulum is short and attaches to the anterior tongue tip (Figure 8–7). The attachment may be right at the tip of the tongue, rather than a third of the way back, as is normally seen. When the attachment is too far forward, tongue tip protrusion results in an indentation in the tip of the tongue, making a heart shape. With ankyloglossia, lingual movement can be somewhat restricted, particularly for eating (Kern, 1991). This can affect the person's ability to move a bolus in the mouth in preparation for swallowing, particularly if the bolus is in the *buccal sulcus* (area between the teeth and cheeks).

Ankyloglossia has less effect on speech, because very little tongue tip excursion is needed for normal speech production. In fact, the most the tongue needs to protrude is against the back of the maxillary incisors for a /th/ sound, and the most it has to elevate is to the alveolar ridge for the /l/ sound. Since ankyloglossia rarely causes problems with speech, unless there is also oral-motor dysfunction, frenulectomy is usually not indicated for speech purposes. However, it may be indicated for feeding purposes and to improve aesthetics.

Palate

Palatal arch anomalies are common, particularly in individuals with a history of cleft palate, and also in patients with other craniofacial syndromes. These anomalies include abnormalities in the height, width, and configuration of the palatal arch. The palatal vault may be low and flat due to collapsed lateral palatal segments or it may be very high and narrow, causing crowding of the teeth and tongue. A narrow, high-arched palate is often seen in children who have had an endotracheal tube at birth.

Whenever the palatal arch is low, flat, or narrow, it restricts the oral cavity space, which may cause the tongue to protrude. As the tongue protrudes, the tongue tip is in an abnormal position for tongue tip articulation. As a result, distortion of speech is inevitable. The obligatory error would be a frontal lisp or fronting of anterior sounds. The compensatory error would be a palatal-dorsal placement due to the articu-

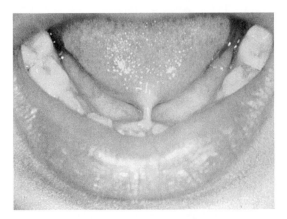

Figure 8–7. Ankyloglossia. Ankyloglossia is a condition involving the attachment of the lingual frenulum to the anterior tongue tip. It may impede normal tongue mobility for feeding, but usually does not require intervention for speech purposes.

lation of the dorsum of the tongue against the palate as the tongue is retracted. When this placement is used for sibilant sounds, it typically results in a lateral distortion or lateral lisp.

A *palatal fistula*, also called an *oronasal fistula*, is a hole or opening in the palate that goes all the way through to the nasal cavity. It is important to make a distinction between a fistula that is "intentional" versus one that is "unintentional" (Folk, D'Antonio, & Hardesty, 1997). A fistula can occur as an unintentional postoperative complication of a cleft repair due to a lack of adequate healing. The most common site for a breakdown of the mucoperiosteum, resulting in an unintentional fistula, is at the junction of the hard and soft palate. On the other hand, an anterior fistula in the alveolus or the area of the incisive foramen is often left open intentionally by the surgeon, especially when there was a bilateral cleft lip and palate. The fistula is later closed with an alveolar bone graft.

Depending on its size and location, a fistula can cause nasal air emission and even hypernasality. A small fistula is usually not symptomatic for speech since during speech, the airflow courses under rather than perpendicular to the opening. A small fistula that is asymptomatic can become symptomatic, however, with maxillary expansion because this can make it larger. If the fistula is above the tongue tip, there may be nasal air emission on lingual-alveolar sounds as the tongue tip elevates, thus pushing the airstream into the fistula. A moderate size fistula can cause consistent nasal air emission on all sounds, particularly anterior sounds. Only a very large fistula will cause hypernasality. A fistula can result in nasal regurgitation of fluids and can even cause food to become stuck in the opening and nasal cavity.

If the fistula is symptomatic for speech, it should be covered prosthetically or surgically closed. If a patient demonstrates inadequate velopharyngeal movement and a symptomatic fistula, the fistula should be covered prior to considering intervention for the velopharyngeal dysfunction. Research has shown that an open fistula can affect levator veli palatini muscle movement, and thus velopharyngeal function (Isberg & Henningsson, 1987; Tachimura, Hara, Koh, & Wada, 1997). The only way to determine the potential for velopharyngeal function is to close the fistula and thus the anterior leak in the system. If velopharyngeal dysfunction persists after closure of the fistula, surgical correction of the velopharyngeal dysfunction will also be needed to normalize the speech and resonance.

Tonsils and Adenoids

Function of the Tonsils and Adenoids

The tonsils surround the opening to the oropharynx. The *faucial tonsils* are located on either side of the mouth posteriorly within the anterior and posterior faucial pillars. The *lingual tonsils* are located at the base of the tongue, and the *pharyngeal tonsil*, also know as the adenoid, is located in the nasopharynx. This collection of lymphoid tissue is known as *Waldeyer's ring*. This lymphoid tissue is most important during the first 2 years of life. Foreign materials entering the body through the nose and mouth pass over this specialized tissue. Antigens adhere to the specialized lining of this tissue where it is incorporated into the substance of the tonsil to be presented to the immune system. This is one of the body's surveillance systems whereby antibodies can be developed to ward off infections (Brodsky, Moore, Stanievich, & Ogra, 1988). Over time, the tonsil and adenoid tissue tends to atrophy. Generally by the age of 16, the tissue persists as only small remnants. Should surgical intervention be required to remove adenotonsillar tissue, there is much redundancy in the system so that no alteration in immunity would be expected after their removal. The entire gastrointestinal tract is lined with the same types of tissue as the tonsils and adenoid, and a similar function is maintained through this system.

Adenotonsillar Hypertrophy

Adenotonsillar hypertrophy is the enlargement of the tonsil and adenoid tissue to the point where the airway is compromised. The etiology for this overgrowth of tissue is undetermined, but is surmised to be secondary to chronic stimulation from infection or allergic sources.

When the tonsil and adenoid tissue are enlarged, airway obstruction may develop. For example, large adenoids can obstruct the pharyngeal airway or even the choanal opening into the nose (Figure 8–8). When this occurs, it may result in stertorous respiration, chronic mouth breathing, loud snoring, and even sleep apnea. In observing the child sleep, the work of breathing is noted to be increased. In addition, the child may appear to be very restless, constantly tossing and turning throughout the night to find a position where breathing can occur with decreased effort. The marginal airway is compromised further by the generalized hypotonia associated with deep sleep. This hypotonia causes collapse of the hypopharyngeal structures. The tongue base also retrodisplaces, causing further compromise of the airway. An *obstructive sleep apnea* (OSA) event is a period where the child is exerting muscular forces to inspire but is unsuccessful in moving air into the lungs. When observed in children, this is significant and requires attention. *Polysomnography* (a sleep study) may be beneficial if questions arise as to the extent of the sleep disturbances such that appropriate treatment can be initiated.

When there is chronic upper airway obstruction due to adenotonsillar hypertrophy, the patient may show evidence of this obstruction in the face. *Adenoid facies* is characterized by an open-mouth posture, anterior tongue position, the mandible in a forward or downward position, facial elongation, suborbital coloring and puffy eyes, and the appearance of pinched nostrils. These characteristics are all the result of upper airway obstruction and the effects of the difficulty in nasal breathing.

Adenotonsillar hypertrophy may be relative and may occur with "normal" size tonsils and adenoid tissue. For example, patients with midface hypoplasia, as in Crouzon, Apert, and Down syndromes, may have an adenoid pad situated in a relatively small nasopharynx, creating the obstructive symptoms. A similar problem may develop in patients with retrognathia, as in Treacher Collins syndrome or Pierre Robin sequence, where a narrow oropharyngeal inlet and glossoptosis combine to increase the likelihood of obstruction.

Adenotonsillectomy

The treatment of adenotonsillar hypertrophy with upper airway obstruction is an *adenotonsillectomy*, which is a surgical procedure where both the tonsil and adenoid tissue are removed. When a tonsillectomy is done, the tonsils are

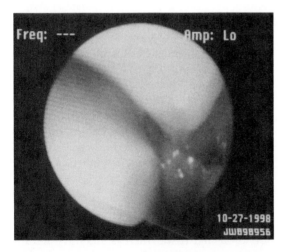

Figure 8–8. Adenoid tissue blocking the choana. The adenoid is a collection of lymphoid tissue in the nasopharynx. It has the capacity to enlarge and block nasal respiration. At times the adenoid tissue can grow into the posterior aspect of the nose, completely blocking the posterior choanae.

removed in their entirety. The capsule deep to the tonsil is removed with the specimen. With adenoidectomy however, the capsule deep to the adenoid pad is left in place, as it is protecting the underlying bone of the skull base. Because the capsule is left in place, it is possible to have some regrowth of the adenoid over time.

Although upper airway obstruction is an indication for adenotonsillectomy, the most common indicator for the removal of the tonsils and adenoids is recurrent infection. If a patient has four to six episodes of tonsillitis in a year, has had three or more infections in each of the preceding years, or has missed an excessive amount of school or work secondary to repeated infections, adenotonsillectomy is warranted. If complications of tonsillar hypertrophy, such as peritonsillar abscess, develop, tonsillectomy is also considered.

Lingual Tonsil Hypertrophy

Lingual tonsil hypertrophy is not common, but it can occur and may cause airway obstruction and problems with speech and resonance (Figure 8–9). If the airway is affected, the tongue may be forced into an anterior position in order to open the airway. This can cause fronting of anterior consonants during speech. The lingual tonsil may also block transmission of sound energy into the oral cavity, causing cul-de-sac resonance. The lingual tonsils rarely are large enough to require removal however.

Tonsils and Adenoids: The Effects on Speech

Tonsillar Hypertrophy

The size of the tonsils is graded on a scale of 1–4: 1+ tonsils are contained within the tonsillar pillars; 2+ tonsils extend minimally beyond the tonsillar pillars; 3+ tonsils obstruct the oropharyngeal inlet to a moderated degree; and 4+ tonsils touch in the midline. Figure 8–10

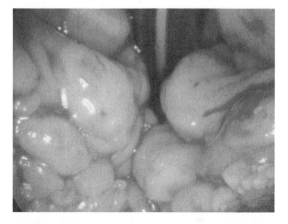

Figure 8–9. Lingual tonsils. Lingual tonsils are located at the base of the tongue. They can enlarge to the point that the airway is partially obstructed, leading to breathing difficulties. The larynx cannot be seen in this photograph due to the enlargement of the lingual tonsils. The vallecula is completely filled with lingual tonsil tissue.

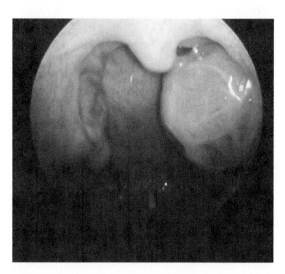

Figure 8–10. A large tonsil on the patient's left side. Asymmetric tonsils are a cause of concern, as a tumor may be causing the abnormal growth pattern. In this example, the left tonsil is a grade 4 while the right tonsil is a grade 1.

shows an excessively large tonsil on the patient's left side. If one or both of the tonsils are excessively large (grade 3+ or larger), they fill the oropharynx and can actually intrude into the nasopharynx. This can affect speech and resonance in several ways. The blockage of the entrance to the oral cavity can cause a cul-de-sac quality. If the tonsils also block the transmission of sound into the nasal cavity, this will cause hyponasality. If the tonsil is large enough to intrude into the area of the velopharyngeal port, it can prevent a tight seal during velopharyngeal closure, resulting in velopharyngeal insufficiency (Kummer, Billmire, & Myer, 1993; MacKenzie-Stepner, Witzel, Stringer, & Laskin, 1987; Shprintzen, Sher, & Croft, 1987). With large tonsils, it is possible for a single patient to demonstrate a mixture of hyponasality, cul-de-sac resonance, and nasal air emission. Even peritonsillar abscess has been associated with hypernasality in rare cases (Finkelstein, Bar-Ziv, Nachmani, Berger, & Ophir, 1993).

Hypertrophic tonsils can also affect the oral airway and indirectly affect articulation. When there is obstruction of the oral cavity, the tongue will often compensate by moving down and forward in order to open the airway. When the tongue is always in an anterior position, this can affect articulation. There may be fronting of sibilants and even lingual-alveolar sounds may be produced with an anterior tongue posture.

Tonsillectomy

The removal of the tonsils can result in alteration of oropharyngeal anatomy. Despite this change, tonsillectomy usually either has no effect on speech or has a positive effect by eliminating a source of blockage at the entry to the oral cavity. Hypernasality has been reported following tonsillectomy alone (Gibb & Stewart, 1975; Haapanen, Ignatius, Rihkanen, & Ertama, 1994), although it occurs very rarely. We have seen one case in our clinic. In our case and the case reported by Gibb and Stewart (1975), the hypernasality was secondary to a

conversion reaction to the pain of the procedure. Fortunately, this is easy to correct with only a few speech therapy sessions in most cases.

Adenoid Hypertrophy

Young children, particularly those who are prepubescent, are at increased risk for adenoid hypertrophy. When the adenoids are very large, they can obstruct the opening to the eustachian tube and disrupt middle ear function, leading to middle ear disease. As noted previously, chronic middle ear effusion can disrupt speech and language development.

Hyponasality is another very common symptom of adenoid hypertrophy. Hyponasality is caused by a lack of adequate nasal resonance during speech. If the adenoids block the choana or entry to the nasal cavity, this prevents the sound energy from being transmitted into the nasal cavity for normal nasal resonance. This results in an unpleasant vocal quality, affects the ability of the patient to produce nasal sounds (m, n, ng), and can affect the overall quality and intelligibility of speech.

When hyponasality occurs due to adenoid hypertrophy, or any other cause of blockage, speech therapy is not indicated for correction. Instead, adenoidectomy or surgical removal of the obstruction is required for correction of the resonance.

On lateral X rays, the adenoid tissue appears rounded and smooth. This is because the fact that the X-ray beam goes through all parts and projects an image of the sum of the parts. When the adenoids are viewed directly through nasopharyngoscopy, however, it becomes obvious to the examiner that this tissue is often very irregular on its surface, especially if there is adenoid regrowth after adenoidectomy. In fact, the adenoids are often lobulated and there may be deep clefts or fissures in the adenoid tissue. When the velum closes against the adenoid pad, as is common in young children, the irregularities on the surface can prevent an airtight seal of the velopharyngeal valve . Although the remaining opening is usually not large enough to cause hypernasality, it will cause some nasal air emission.

When irregular adenoid tissue precludes complete velopharyngeal closure, treatment options must be carefully considered. Standard treatment options, such as a pharyngeal flap, sphincteroplasty, or even a prosthetic device, are not appropriate in this case. In fact, these options potentially could cause unnecessary upper airway obstruction. Because irregular adenoid tissue is the cause of nasal air emission, smoothing the adenoid tissue with a laser or partial adenoidectomy could be considered. On the other hand, a wait-and-see approach should be strongly considered prior to surgical intervention, as adenoid atrophy may resolve the problem naturally.

Adenoidectomy

Temporary velopharyngeal insufficiency following adenoidectomy is not uncommon. Due to their location in the pharynx, the adenoid pads assist in velopharyngeal closure in young children. Preschool children usually have *velo-adenoidal closure* rather than velopharyngeal closure (Figure 8–11). When this tissue is suddenly removed, the patient must alter his or her normal method of closing the nasopharynx during speech. The soft palate must extend farther posteriorly, or the lateral walls must extend farther medially, or both to effect closure. Most patients are able to accomplish this task within a few days or weeks.

Hypernasality following adenoidectomy is always a risk (Donnelly, 1994; Fernandes, Grobbelaar, Hudson, & Lentin, 1996; Kavanagh & Beckford, 1988; Parton & Jones, 1998; Ren et al., 1995; Schmaman, Jordann, & Jammine, 1998; Witzel, Rich, Margar-Bacal, & Cox, 1986), although the risk is minimal and has been estimated to be between 1:1500 and at 1:3000. These studies include patients who were identified with an occult submucous cleft following the surgery. There are several risk factors for hypernasality due to velopharyngeal insufficiency following adenoidectomy. These include a fam-

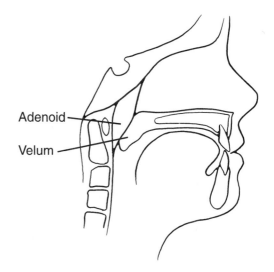

Figure 8–11. The adenoid pad assists in velopharyngeal closure in children. The sudden removal of adenoid tissue during adenoidectomy requires compensation of soft palate motion to maintain proper velopharyngeal closure. If any abnormality exists in the architecture or neurological function of the palate, this compensation may not be successful which leads to nasal air escape.

ily history of hypernasality or palatal clefting, a repaired cleft palate, a submucous cleft, and a history of nasal regurgitation or sucking difficulties as an infant. In addition, individuals with oral-motor dysfunction or other neuromuscular problems can also be considered at risk with this procedure.

When hypernasality does occur after adenotonsillectomy, the maximum improvement in resonance usually occurs within about a month to 6 weeks postoperatively. Therefore, a referral to a speech pathologist and an assessment of velopharyngeal function should be considered if the hypernasality perists beyond 6 to 8 weeks. If it persists beyond 3 months, it is unlikely to resolve spontaneously. Surgical repair would be required to correct the velopharyngeal dysfunction.

A preoperative speech assessment is recommended for patients when there is a question of hypernasality or tenuous velopharyngeal closure preoperatively or when there are any of the stigmata that would suggest the possibility of a submucous cleft. An adenoidectomy is usually contraindicated when a submucous cleft is identified. When in doubt, an instrumental assessment, such as nasopharyngoscopy, is particularly important so that the velopharyngeal mechanism can be visualized for potential abnormalities. In addition, a preoperative assessment should include objective measures, such as aerodynamic or nasometric scores, so that objective data are available for postoperative comparison if necessary. This information also could help the physician assess the potential effects of the surgery, determine what course of action should be taken, and what the parents or patient should know prior to the procedure.

Treatment of Upper Airway Obstruction

Tracheostomy

A *tracheostomy* is a surgical procedure that is done to relieve conditions that cause life-threatening airway obstruction. The tracheostomy procedure is done by making a vertical incision in the midline of the neck overlying the trachea. The trachea is incised vertically, usually through the third and fourth rings, creating an opening in the anterior wall of the trachea. A tracheostomy tube is then inserted into the tracheal opening, and the edges of the opening are sutured to the skin in the neck. The *stoma* is the opening through which the patient can breathe.

Tracheostomy is often indicated for certain congenital anomalies, such as subglottic stenosis, tracheal stenosis, or laryngeal web. Infants born with Pierre Robin sequence are often candidates for tracheostomy due to the airway problems that occur as a result of the small mandible and glossoptosis. Tracheostomy is also indicated for patients who cannot adequately raise their secretions from their airway and, therefore, need frequent suctioning. This includes patients who are unconscious, those with a paralysis that precludes coughing, and those with significant chest pain, which inhibits coughing.

Uvulopalatopharyngoplasty (UPPP)

In the pediatric population, upper airway obstruction is primarily caused by adenotonsillar hypertrophy. Therefore, adenotonsillectomy is the obvious choice for treatment. In teenagers and adults, however, the tonsils and adenoids are very small and therefore are not likely to cause obstruction. When older patients demonstrate obstructive sleep apnea, it is often secondary to redundant mucosa of the soft palate and posterior pharyngeal wall causing the oropharyngeal inlet to be small. In these cases, the treatment of the obstruction is a surgical procedure called a *uvulopalatopharyngoplasty* (UPPP) (Blythe, Henrich, & Pillsbury, 1995; Croft & Golding-Wood, 1990; Fairbanks, 1990; Isberg & Henningsson, 1987; Kavey, Whyte, Blitzer, & Gidro-Frank, 1990; Yanagisawa & Weaver, 1997). As part of the UPPP, the remaining tonsil tissue is removed and the anterior and posterior tonsillar pillars are sewn together to open the oropharyngeal inlet. The free margin of the soft palate is resected along with the uvula, and the soft palate is oversewn. Although snoring is usually markedly improved as a result of this procedure, the overall effect on the sleep apnea is often disappointing. Fortunately, if done properly, this procedure does not seem to have a negative effect on resonance (Rihkanen & Soini, 1992; Salas-Provance & Kuehn, 1990).

Continuous Positive Airway Pressure (CPAP)

Frequently, *continuous positive airway pressure* (CPAP) is required for long-term resolution of the obstructive apnea. The CPAP equipment consists of a face mask and an air pressure generator. The patient wears the mask over the nose during sleep, and a certain level of continuous positive air pressure, usually in the range of 6 to 20 cm water, is delivered to the pharynx through the nose. This forces the airway open and prevents pharyngeal collapse during respiration. Although CPAP is effective in overcoming the effects of obstructive sleep apnea, long-term tolerance of wearing the machine every night leads to a high degree of noncompliance over time.

Summary

The ears, the nose, and the oral cavity are essential organs for verbal communication. Congenital anomalies of these structures can therefore interfere with the development of articulation and language and the production of normal speech and resonance. Speech-language pathologists, whether working directly with craniofacial anomalies or not, need to form a partnership with otolaryngologists to adequately diagnose these disorders and treat them appropriately.

Case Report: Upper Airway Obstruction, Hypernasality, and CPAP

Tam was a Vietnamese male born with bilateral complete cleft lip and palate. The cleft lip was closed in Vietnam, but the palate was left unrepaired. When Tam entered the United States at the age of 21, the palate was still open and he did not speak any English. Soon after arriving in this country, the palate was repaired and a pharyngeal flap (to correct velopharyngeal dysfunction) was done. Although the prognosis for correcting speech is very guarded when the palate is closed that late, Tam exceeded all expectations. He received several months of speech therapy following his surgery and he quickly developed oral production of speech sounds and also learned English.

Tam was seen for an evaluation in VPI Clinic several years later at the age of 27. At that time, articulation was normal for the production of all speech sounds. However, Tam's accent had a negative effect on the intelligibility of his speech. Resonance was found to be mildly hypernasal, but very acceptable. There was barely audible nasal air emission during the production of pressure-sensitive phonemes. At the same time, Tam reported difficulty with nasal breathing and significant snoring at night, which was the primary reason for his return.

A nasopharyngoscopy (endoscopy) assessment showed the cause of these symptoms. Although the pharyngeal flap was an appropriate width and in good position, the lateral ports (for breathing on either side of the flap) were small for normal nasal breathing. During speech, the right port closed completely, but the left port remained partially open. Therefore, it was determined that the narrow ports restricted nasal breathing, particularly during sleep, but the open left port caused the hypernasality during speech.

With this combination of symptoms, determining the appropriate treatment is a big challenge. If the left port was narrowed further for speech, it would increase the airway problems. On the other hand, opening the ports to improve nasal breathing would increase the hypernasality. Therefore, it was decided that the current balance of the needs for speech and breathing was the best that could be achieved. However, because nasal obstruction was a concern at night, a sleep study was done. This confirmed sleep apnea so CPAP was recommended to be used at night. With this option, the flap could be left intact for speech, yet the airway was forced open at night for sleep. Parenthetically, Tam was also referred to an "English as a Second Language" program for accent reduction.

References

Bluestone, C. D., Beery, Q. C., Cantekin, E. I., & Paradise, J. L. (1975). Eustachian tube ventilatory function in relation to cleft palate. *Annals of Otology, Rhinology, and Laryngology, 84*(3, Pt. 1), 333–338.

Bluestone, C. D., Paradise, J. L., Beery, Q. C., & Wittel, R. (1972). Certain effects of cleft palate repair on eustachian tube function. *Cleft Palate Journal, 9*, 183–193.

Blythe, W. R., Henrich, D. E., & Pillsbury, H. C. (1995). Outpatient uvuloplasty: An inexpensive, single-staged procedure for the relief of symptomatic snoring. *Otolaryngology—Head and Neck Surgery, 113*(1), 1–4.

Brent, B. (1999). The pediatrician's role in caring for patients with congenital microtia and atresia. *Pediatric Annals, 28*(2), 374–383.

Brodsky, L., Moore, L., Stanievich, J., & Ogra, P. (1988). The immunology of tonsils in children: The effect of bacterial load on the presence of B- and T-cell subsets. *Laryngoscope, 98*(1), 93-98.

Brown, O. E., Myer, C. M., III, & Manning, S. C. (1989). Congenital nasal pyriform aperture stenosis. *Laryngoscope, 99*(1), 86–91.

Croft, C. B., & Golding-Wood, D. G. (1990). Uses and complications of uvulopalatopharyngoplasty. *Journal of Laryngology and Otology, 104*(11), 871–875.

Donnelly, M. J. (1994). Hypernasality following adenoid removal. *Irish Journal of Medical Science, 163*(5), 225–227.

Doyle, W. J., Cantekin, E. I., & Bluestone, C. D. (1980). Eustachian tube function in cleft palate children. *Annals of Otology, Rhinology, and Laryngology Supplement, 89*(3, Pt. 2), 34–40.

Durr, D. G., & Shapiro, R. S. (1989). Otologic manifestations in congenital velopharyngeal insufficiency. *American Journal of Diseases of Children, 143*(1), 75–77.

Fairbanks, D. N. (1990). Uvulopalatopharyngoplasty complications and avoidance strategies. *Otolaryngology—Head and Neck Surgery, 102*(3), 239–245.

Fernandes, D. B., Grobbelaar, A. O., Hudson, D. A., & Lentin, R. (1996). Velopharyngeal incompetence after adenotonsillectomy in non-cleft patients. *British Journal of Oral and Maxillofacial Surgery, 34*(5), 364–367.

Finkelstein, Y., Bar-Ziv, J., Nachmani, A., Berger, G., & Ophir, D. (1993). Peritonsillar abscess as a cause of transient velopharyngeal insufficiency. *Cleft Palate Craniofacial Journal, 30*(4), 421–428.

Folk, S. N., D'Antonio, L. L., & Hardesty, R. A. (1997). Secondary cleft deformities. *Clinics in Plastic Surgery, 24*(3), 599–611.

Gates, G., Avery, C., Prihoda, T., & Cooper, J. J. (1987, December 3). Effectiveness of adenoidectomy and tympanostomy tubes in the treatment of chronic otitis media with effusion. *New England Journal of Medicine, 317*, 1444–1451.

Gibb, A. G., & Stewart, I. A. (1975). Hypernasality following tonsil dissection—Hysterical aetiology. *Journal of Laryngology and Otology, 89*(7), 779–781.

Haapanen, M. L., Ignatius, J., Rihkanen, H., & Ertama, L. (1994). Velopharyngeal insufficiency following palatine tonsillectomy. *European Archives of Oto-Rhino-Laryngology, 251*(3), 186–189.

Heller, J. C., Gens, G. W., Croft, C. B., & Moe, D. G. (1978). Conductive hearing loss in patients with velopharyngeal insufficiency. *Cleft Palate Journal, 15*(3), 246–253.

Hollinshead, W. H. (1982). *The ear, anatomy for surgeons: The head and neck* (Vol. 1, 3rd ed., pp. 159–221). New York: Harper and Row.

Hubbard, T. W., Paradise, J. L., McWilliams, B. J., Elster, B. A., & Taylor, F. H. (1985). Consequences of unremitting middle ear disease in early life: Otologic, audiologic, and developmental findings in children with cleft palate. *New England Journal of Medicine, 312*(24), 1529–1534.

Isberg, A., & Henningsson, G. (1987). Influence of palatal fistulas on velopharyngeal movements: A cineradiographic study. *Plastic and Reconstructive Surgery, 79*(4), 525–1530.

Jahrsdoerfer, R., & Lambert, P. (1998, May). Facial nerve injury in congenital aural atresia surgery. *American Journal of Otology, 19*, 283–287.

Jahrsdoerfer, R., Yeakley, J., Aguilar, E., Cole, R., & Gray, L. (1992). Grading system for the selection of patients with congenital aural atresia. *American Journal of Otology, 13*(1), 6–12.

Kavanagh, K. T., & Beckford, N. S. (1988). Adenotonsillectomy in children: Indications and contraindications. *Southern Medical Journal, 81*(4), 507–514.

Kavey, N. B., Whyte, J., Blitzer, A., & Gidro-Frank, S. (1990). Postsurgical evaluation of uvulopalatopharyngoplasty: Two case reports. *Sleep, 13*(1), 79–84.

Kern, I. (1991, July 1). Tongue tie [see Comments]. *Medical Journal of Australia, 155*, 33–34.

Kountakis, S., Helidonis, E., & Jahrsdoerfer, R. (1995). Microtia grade as an indicator of middle ear development in aural atresia. *Archives of Otolaryngology—Head and Neck Surgery, 121*(8), 885–886.

Kummer, A. W., Billmire, D. A., & Myer, C. M. D. (1993). Hypertrophic tonsils: The effect on resonance and velopharyngeal closure. *Plastic and Reconstructive Surgery, 91*(4), 608–611.

MacKenzie-Stepner, K., Witzel, M. A., Stringer, D. A., & Laskin, R. (1987). Velopharyngeal insufficiency due to hypertrophic tonsils. A report of two cases. *International Journal of Pediatric Otorhinolaryngology, 14*(1), 57–63.

Paradise, J. L. (1976). Management of middle ear effusions in infants with cleft palate. *Annals of Otology, Rhinology, and Laryngology, 85*(2, Suppl. 25, Pt. 2), 285–288.

Paradise, J. L., Alberti, P. W., Bluestone, C. D., Cheek, D. B., Lis, E. F., & Stool, S. E. (1974). Pediatric and otologic aspects of clinical research in cleft palate. *Clinics in Pediatrics (Phila), 13*(7), 587–593.

Paradise, J. L., & Bluestone, C. D. (1974). Early treatment of the universal otitis media of infants with cleft palate. *Pediatrics, 53*(1), 48–54.

Parton, M. J., & Jones, A. S. (1998). Hypernasality following adenoidectomy: A significant and avoidable complication. *Clinics in Otolaryngology, 23*(1), 18–19.

Peitersen, E. (1992). Natural history of Bell's palsy. *Acta Oto-Laryngologica. 492*(Suppl.), 122–124.

Ren, Y. F., Isberg, A., & Henningsson, G. (1995). Velopharyngeal incompetence and persistent hypernasality after adenoidectomy in children without palatal defect. *Cleft Palate Craniofacial Journal, 32*(6), 476–482.

Rihkanen, H., & Soini, I. (1992). Changes in voice characteristics after uvulopalatopharyngoplasty. *European Archives of Otorhinolaryngology, 249*(6), 322–324.

Rvachew, S., Slawinski, E., Williams, M., & Green, C. (1999). The impact of early onset otitis media on babbling and early language development. *Journal of the Acoustical Society of America, 105*(1), 467–475.

Salas-Provance, M. B., & Kuehn, D. P. (1990). Speech status following uvulopalatopharyngoplasty [see Comments]. *Chest, 97*(1), 111–117.

Schmaman, L., Jordaan, H., & Jammine, G. H. (1998). Risk factors for permanent hypernasality after adenoidectomy. *South Africa Medical Journal, 88*(3), 266–269.

Shprintzen, R. J., Sher, A. E., & Croft, C. B. (1987). Hypernasal speech caused by tonsillar hypertrophy. *International Journal of Pediatric Otorhinolaryngology, 14*(1), 45–56.

Sininger, Y., Doyle, K., & Moore, J. (1999). The case for early identification of hearing loss in children. Auditory system development, experimental auditory deprivation, and development of speech perception and hearing. *Pediatric Clinics of North America, 46*(2), 1–14.

Tachimura, T., Hara, H., Koh, H., & Wada, T. (1997). Effect of temporary closure of oronasal fistulae on levator veli palatini muscle activity. *Cleft Palate Craniofacial Journal, 34*(6), 505–511.

Teele, D., Klein, J., & Rosner, B. (1980). Epidemiology of otitis media in children. *Annals of Otology, Rhinology, and Laryngology, 89*(3, Suppl.), 5–6.

Trujillo, L. (1994). Prevention of conductive hearing loss in cleft palate patients. *Folia Phoniatrica et Logopedica, 46*(3), 123–126.

Witzel, M. A., Rich, R. H., Margar-Bacal, F., & Cox, C. (1986). Velopharyngeal insufficiency after adenoidectomy: An 8-year review. *International Journal of Pediatric Otorhinolaryngology, 11*(1), 15–20.

Yanagisawa, E., & Weaver, E. M. (1997). An unusual appearance of velopharyngeal closure in a post-uvulopalatopharyngoplasty patient. *Ear Nose and Throat Journal, 76*(1), 14–15.

CHAPTER

9

Dental Anomalies Associated With Cleft Lip and Palate

Richard Campbell, D.M.D., M.S.
Murray Dock, D.D.S., M.S.D.

With contributions from Ann W. Kummer, Ph.D.

CONTENTS

Dental problems in children with cleft lip and palate or craniofacial syndromes can be quite complex. These problems frequently require dental specialists to coordinate treatment with other health care providers in order to properly manage the patient (Jacobson & Rosenstein, 1970; Mouradian, Omnell, & Williams, 1999; Tindlund & Holmefjord, 1997; Vig, 1980). The specialists involved usually include a pediatric dentist, an orthodontist, an oral maxillofacial surgeon, and a prosthodontist (Turvey, Vig, & Fonseca, 1996; Vig & Turvey, 1985). Together, they monitor and treat problems of the developing dentition, occlusion, and facial growth of the cleft lip/palate patient (Strauss, 1998, 1999). As dental professionals reconstruct the oral environment, the speech pathologist can correct functional modifications in speech that may have developed due to abnormal structure. Close cooperation between the dental specialists and the speech pathologist leads to a more holistic management of the structural and functional effects of dental and speech abnormalities.

A brief review of the dentition and its effect on speech production follows. Oral anatomy was covered in Chapter 1 and will not be repeated in this chapter.

Dentition

The dentition can be visualized as two arches of teeth, a maxillary and a mandibular arch. Each arch consists of a right and left half, so that the teeth in the arch are paired, one of each on either side (Figure 9–1).

There are two sets of teeth. The first set is known as the primary or *deciduous* teeth (Figure 9–2). They are sometimes referred to as deciduous because they are shed and replaced by the second set of teeth. The second set is known as the secondary, permanent, or *succedaneous* teeth. To be strictly correct, the permanent molars have no primary precursors and so they are not truly succedaneous.

Many terms are used to describe the positions of the teeth in the arch (Figure 9–1). The dental midline is at the apex of the arch where the left and right halves join. The direction toward the midline is *mesial*. The direction away from the midline is *distal*. The outer part of the arch that touches the lip is *labial*. The part of the arch that is posterior to the canine teeth is frequently referred to as *buccal,* for the buccinator muscle that moves the cheeks. The inner part of the upper and lower arch that is in contact with the tongue is referred to as *lingual*. Many clinicians refer to the inner part of the upper arch as *palatal*, because of its proximity to the surface of the hard palate.

Number and Types of Teeth

In the deciduous dentition there are 20 teeth, 10 in each arch. In one arch, starting from the midline and moving distally, the pairs are: the central incisors, the lateral incisors, the canines (cuspids), the primary first molars, and the primary second molars (Figure 9–2).

In the permanent dentition there are 32 teeth, 16 in each arch (see Figure 9–1). In one arch, starting from the midline and proceeding to the distal, the pairs are: the central incisors, the lateral incisors, the canines (cuspids), the first premolars (first bicuspids), the second premolars (second bicuspids), the first molars (6-year molars), the second molars (12-year molars) and last the third molars (wisdom teeth). In addition to these anatomical names, the primary teeth are often lettered A through T, and the permanent teeth are numbered 1 through 32.

The incisor teeth are somewhat shovel shaped, their biting surfaces are thin knifelike edges. The remaining teeth have rounded points for chewing. The points are known as *cusps*. Canines have one point or cusp. Premolars typically have two cusps, although they may sometimes have three. Cusps are arranged in rows, one to the outside (buccal or labial) and one to the inside (palatal or lingual). Upper

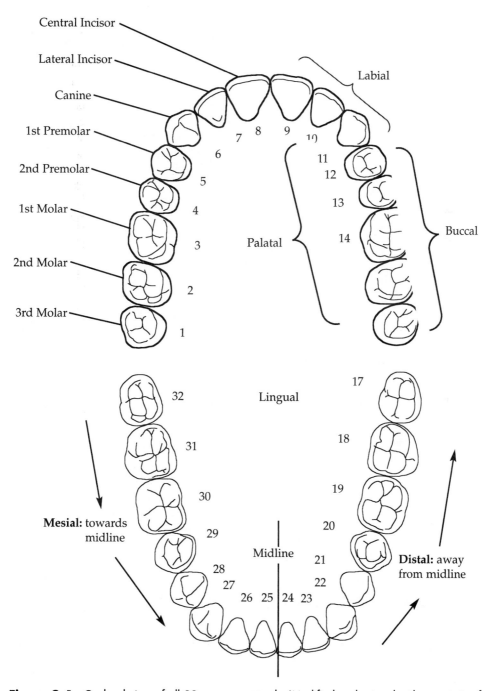

Figure 9–1. Occlusal view of all 32 permanent teeth. (Modified and printed with permission from LifeART Super Anatomy 6 Collection. Baltimore, MD: Lippincott Williams & Wilkins.)

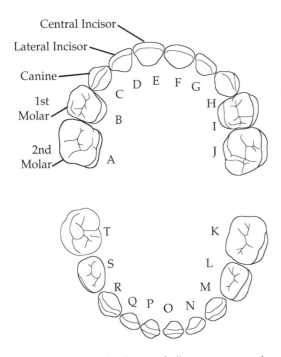

Central Incisor
Lateral Incisor
Canine
1st Molar
2nd Molar

Figure 9–2. Occlusal view of all 20 primary teeth. (Modified and printed with permission from Life Art Super Anatomy Collection. Baltimore; MD: Lippencott, Williams & Wilkins.)

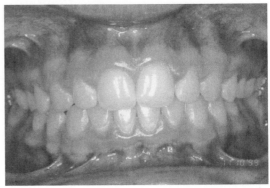

Figure 9–3. Normal overlap of the upper teeth over the lower teeth.

molars have four cusps, two buccal and two palatal (or linugal). Lower molars have four or five cusps, two or three buccal and two lingual. This buccal cusp to lingual cusp arrangement creates a valley between the cusps, called the *central fossa*. Variations in the shapes of teeth and the number of cusps do occur, but are usually of only academic interest to the clinician.

Occlusion and Molar Relationship

Dental occlusion is the manner in which the teeth fit together, or the bite. In normal occlusion, the upper arch overlaps the lower arch, so that the cusps of one arch fit into the fossae of the opposing arch (Figure 9–3).

The anterior-posterior relationship of the mesiobuccal cusp of the upper molar to the buccal groove of the lower molar is used to classify the type of occlusion. First described by Angle, the *Angle Classification System* differentiates normal occlusion and three types of malocclusion. Brilliant in its simplicity, it remains in widespread use today (Table 9–1) (Katz, 1992; Proffit & Fields, 2000).

Incisor Relationship

Overjet is the horizontal relationship of the upper to the lower incisors (Figure 9–4). It is typically measured in millimeters from the labial surface of the lower incisor to the labial surface of the upper incisor, with the teeth in occlusion. A normal amount of overjet is about 2 mm, with upper incisors and lower incisors in light contact. If the upper incisors are displaced anteriorly, with overjet greater than 2 mm, then *labioversion* is said to occur. Maxillary incisors that are labioverted protrude out toward the lips and in severe cases may prevent lip closure.

Labioversion affects speech by interfering with lip closure. This may alter the production of bilabial sounds. Patients may attempt to compensate for this by using a labio-dental placement as a substitute for bilabial articulation.

Underjet refers to a reversal of the normal incisor position, so that the upper incisors would

TABLE 9–1. Angle's classification of occlusion and skeletal relationships.

Dental Classification	Example	Skeletal Classification	Example
Class I occlusion The mesiobuccal cusp of the upper molar occludes in the buccal groove of the lower molar. The remaining teeth are arranged upon a smoothly curving line.	Mesial Buccal Cusp Mesial Buccal Cusp	**Class I—Normal**	
Class I malocclusion Normal relationship of the molars, but line of occlusion incorrect because of malposed teeth, rotations, or other causes.		**Class I—Normal**	(same as above)
Class II malocclusion Lower molar distally positioned relative to upper molar; line of occlusion not specified.		**Class II— Mandibular Retrusion and/or Maxillary Protrusion**	
Class III malocclusion Lower molar mesially positioned relative to upper molar, line of occlusion not specified.		**Class III— Mandibular Protrusion and/or Maxillary Retrusion**	

be lingual to the lower incisors (Figure 9–5). This is also called *linguoversion* or *anterior crossbite,* and implies that most of the incisors are involved. Underjet can be measured in millimeters. Maxillary incisors that are linguoverted can interfere with tongue tip movement, which alters the production of sibilants and lingual-alveolar sounds.

Overbite refers to the vertical overlap of the upper and lower incisors (Figure 9–6). It also may be measured in millimeters, though it is often reported as a percentage of coverage of the lower incisors by the upper incisors. Normal overbite is approximately 2 mm or about 25%. Greater amounts are associated with deep overbite, or *deepbite.* In some in-

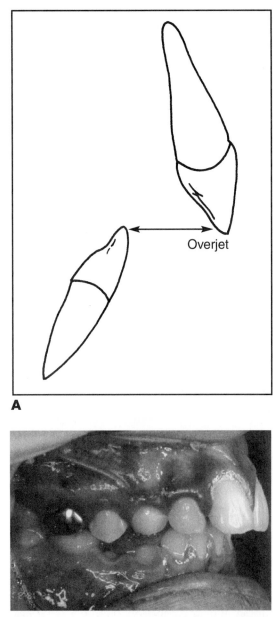

A

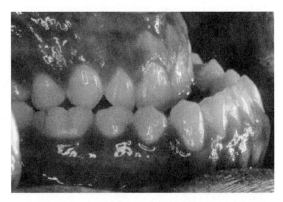

Figure 9–5. Underjet: The upper incisors are lingual to the lower incisors in this case of severe underjet.

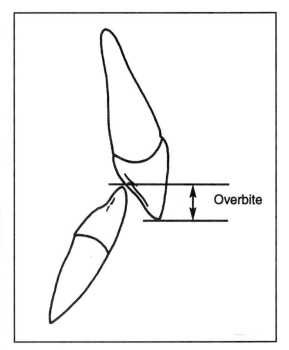

Figure 9–6. Overbite. An overbite is measured as the vertical overlap of the incisors, from the incisal edges. Often expressed as a percentage of overbite, in this instance the upper incisor overlaps the lower incisor approximately 50%, which may be expressed as 50% overbite.

B

Figure 9–4. A. Overjet. Overjet is the horizontal overlap of the incisors. Normal values average 2 mm. **B.** Larger values indicate increased overjet, usually from incisor protrusion.

stances, the upper teeth completely overlap the lower, which is 100% overbite. If the lower incisors are in contact with the palate, this too is considered a 100% overbite. Deep overbite is usually associated with crowding and restricted tongue movement, which may alter the production of sibilants and lingual-alveolar sounds.

Diastema

A *diastema* is a space or opening between the teeth, usually the upper central incisors. A diastema usually does not affect speech (Figure 9–7).

Skeletal Relationships

The Angle classification applies only to tooth relationships. It does not account for the influence of the relationship of the upper jaw to the lower jaw on tooth position or facial profile. Consequently, the Angle system must be supplemented to describe skeletal relationships. Angle's concept of the upper molar to lower molar relationship has been applied to describe the upper jaw to lower jaw relationship. The jaw relationships may be referred to as: Class I,

Class II, and Class III (see Table 9-1). Often the jaw relationship mirrors the dental relationship.

Cephalometric radiographs are lateral skull films, taken with the patient's head held in a standardized position (Figure 9–8). *Cephalometric analyses* are used to measure the jaw relationship and the soft tissue profile of the forehead, nose, lips, and chin (Figure 9–9). An abnormal skeletal relationship may result from the upper jaw, the lower jaw, or both being out of normal position relative to the base of the skull.

Dental Development and Stages of Cleft Lip and Palate Treatment

Treatment of dental problems in children with a history of cleft lip and palate is timed to follow the normal stages of dental development. For instance, maxillary expansion to correct crossbite may be coordinated with the eruption of specific teeth, because it also serves to pre-

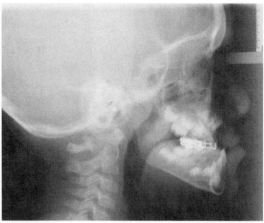

Figure 9–8. Cephalometric X ray. A cephalometric X ray is a lateral skull film, made with a cephalostat, a device with ear rods and a nasal bridge rest to allow reproducible head positioning. This allows comparisons from one X ray to another of the same patient taken at different times, as in longitudinal growth studies.

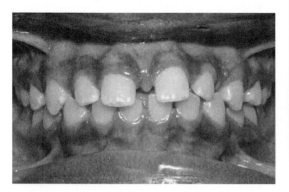

Figure 9–7. Diastema. A diastema is a space or opening between any of the teeth. Clinicians commonly use the term diastema to indicate the space between the maxillary central incisors, as seen in this case.

pare the patient for secondary alveolar bone grafting (Table 9–2). Some interventions may be done to coincide with growth spurts as in mixed dentition treatment. Others may be delayed until the completion of growth, such as combined orthodontic and orthognathic surgical treatment (Vig & Turvey, 1985).

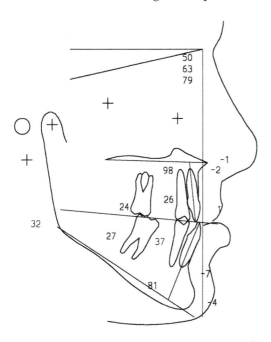

Figure 9–9. Cephalometric tracing. A tracing of a cephalometric X ray is made so that measurement can be drawn without damaging the film. A set of measurements is called an analysis, and is frequently named after its founder as in the Steiner Analysis, or the McNamara Analysis. This particular depiction is the COGS Analysis or Cephalometric Analysis for Orthognathic Surgery devised by Burstone. Image was generated by Dentofacial Planner.

Infant Stage

Most infants are born without any erupted teeth. The infant stage, therefore, involves the eruption of the primary teeth and lasts until 12 months of age. Occasionally a tooth may be present at birth and should be examined by a pediatric dentist to evaluate its stability in the arch. Most often, these teeth are not supernumerary and every attempt should be made to retain them when possible.

The eruption sequence for the primary teeth, as well as the permanent teeth is fairly predictable (Table 9–3); however there is considerable variation from one individual to another in chronological timing. For primary teeth, a variation in eruption of 6 months on either side of the expected eruption is no cause for alarm. The lower primary incisors are usually the first teeth to erupt, at around 8 months of age. The remaining incisors are close behind, completing their eruption by 10 to 13 months of age. The canines erupt between 19 and 20 months, followed by the first molars at 16 months, and finally the second molars by 27 to 29 months (Proffit & Fields, 2000).

Treatment for an infant with a cleft lip and palate typically consists of two stages: lip clo-

TABLE 9–2. Stages of dental development and treatment in cleft lip and palate.

Infant stage	0–12 months	Maxillary orthopedics if indicated, lip repair, palate repair
Primary dentition	1–6 years	Correction of crossbites affecting mandibular posture
Early mixed dentition	6–9 years	Maxillary expansion for bone graft, as indicated
Late mixed dentition	9–12 years	Incisor alignment and maxillary expansion for bone graft if not done earlier
Adolescent dentition	12–18 years	Orthodontics, orthognathic surgery often required. Prosthodontics if needed.

TABLE 9–3. Tooth eruption for primary and permanent dentitions.

	Maxillary	*Mandibular*
Primary Tooth		
Central	10 mo.	8 mo.
Lateral	11 mo.	13 mo.
Canine	19 mo.	20 mo.
1st Molar	16 mo.	16 mo.
2nd Molar	29 mo.	27 mo.
Permanent Tooth		
Central	7.25 yr.	6.25 yr.
Lateral	8.25 yr.	7.50 yr.
Canine	11.50 yr.	10.50 yr.
1st Premolar	10.25 yr.	10.50 yr.
2nd Premolar	11.00 yr.	11.25 yr.
1st Molar	6.25 yr.	6.00 yr.
2nd Molar	12.50 yr.	12.00 yr.
3rd Molar	20.00 yr.	20.00 yr.

sure and then palate closure. In the first stage, at about 12 weeks of age, the surgeon closes the lip. This facilitates feeding and the improvement in the infant's appearance helps with the parents' psychosocial adjustment. At the second stage, between 9 to 12 months of age, the cleft of the palate is closed.

The surgeon and dentist may need to adjust their treatment approach according to the size of the cleft and whether the cleft is unilateral or bilateral. In the case of a small unilateral or bilateral cleft of the lip, the lip can be closed without any need for manipulation of the alveolar segments. In the case of a large unilateral cleft (Figure 9–10), many surgeons prefer to have the interalveolar gap reduced prior to lip closure. Bilateral clefts of the lip and palate are more challenging (Figure 9–11). Not only are there two clefts to deal with but there is often a protruding premaxillary segment (King, Workman, & Latham, 1979; Liao, Huang, Liou, Lin, & Ko, 1998). Additionally, the posterior alveolar segments often will be

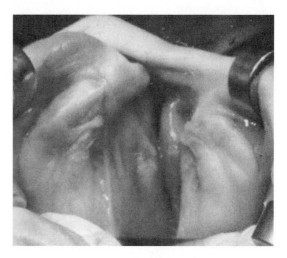

Figure 9–10. The occlusal view of the palate of a newborn with unilateral cleft lip and palate. The greater segment is on the left in the photograph and the lesser segment is on the right.

narrow. Treatment is usually directed at retracting the protruding premaxillary segment while widening the narrow lateral segments.

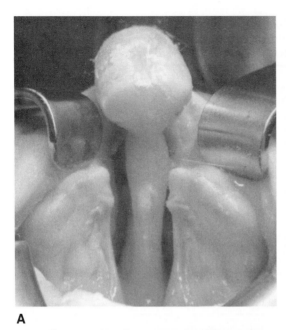

A

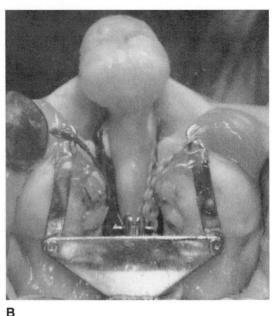

B

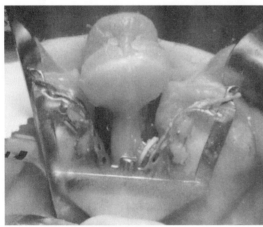

Figure 9–11. A. The occlusal view of the palate of an infant with bilateral cleft lip and palate. The premaxillary segment is at the top middle of the photograph and the two lateral segments are on either side, left or right and posterior to the premaxillary segment in the photograph. **B.** A pin-retained appliance used to reposition the segments. **C.** The maxillary segment retracted and the lateral segment widened.

C

There are numerous ways to accomplish alignment of the alveolar segments in both unilateral and bilateral clefts of the palate. Regardless of which technique is chosen, the process is referred to as *palatal orthopedics* or *infant oral orthopedics* (Figure 9–12). The techniques include, from least invasive to most invasive: taping of the lip (Figure 9–13); elastic straps over the lip and attached to a bonnet; passive molding appliances with or without taping; lip adhesion (temporary surgical closure) prior to lip repair; and pin retained active intraoral appliances (Figueroa, Reisberg, Polley, & Cohen, 1996; Jacobson & Rosenstein, 1984; Jacobson & Rosenstein, 1986; Latham, 1980; Latham, Kusy, & Georgiade, 1976; Millard & Latham, 1990; Monroe, Griffith, Rosenstein, & Jacobson, 1983; Reisberg, Figueroa, & Gold,

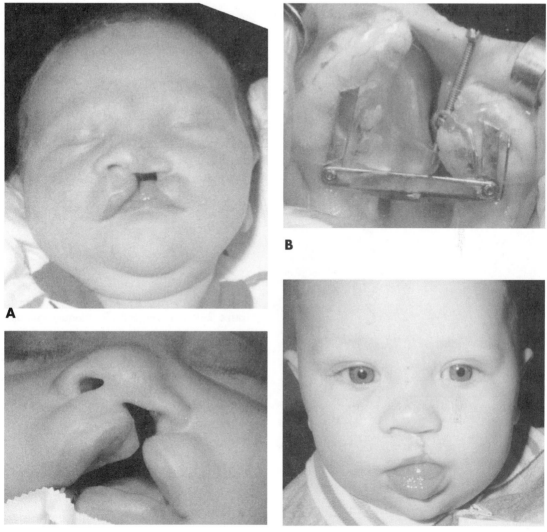

Figure 9–12. Pin-retained intraoral appliance. **A.** A wide unilateral cleft lip and palate. **B.** In cases of wide clefts, some surgeons prefer to have the width of the cleft between greater and lesser segments reduced with an appliance. In such instances the pediatric dentist usually manages the placement and activation of the appliance. **C.** The appliance gives a closer approximation of the lip segments. **D.** The closer approximation of the segments allows for lip closure with less tension than by other means.

1988). Each method has advantages and disadvantages (Table 9–4). The choice of one method over another will vary, depending on the individual needs of the patient, the experience of the practitioners, and the overall philosophy regarding palatal orthopedics at a particular treatment center. Palatal orthopedic methods are controversial and remain a lively

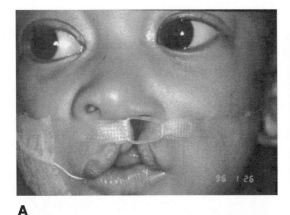

A

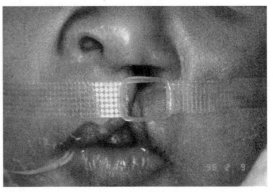

B

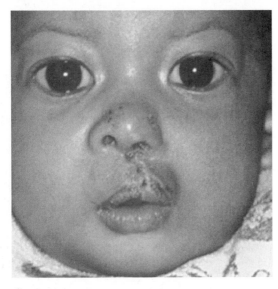

C

Figure 9–13. Taping of the lip. Narrow separations of the lip may be approximated by extra-oral taping, in this case with an additional elastic, making surgical closure less difficult. **A.** Beginning of taping shows separation of lip. **B.** After a few weeks, the lip segments are approximated. **C.** In this view, taken very shortly after lip closure, one can appreciate that there is little tension across the now joined lip segments.

topic of debate among practitioners. Indeed, some authors disparage any repositioning of the palatal segments. These authors also suggest that these procedures may result in decreased midfacial growth (Berkowitz, 1996; Ross, Hubert, & Chojnacka, 1977). Hopefully, further research will elucidate the appropriate application of each method (Millard, Latham, Huifen, Spiro, & Morovic, 1999).

The cleft condition affects not only the lip and alveolus, but the nose as well. As of this writing, a few treatment centers are showing promising results with repositioning of the nasal septum and ala, often termed *nasal molding* (Cutting et al., 1998; Grayson, Cutting, & Wood, 1993). In unilateral clefts, this usually involves an intraoral/nasal appliance combined with taping to reposition the distorted ala and septum of the nose prior to lip closure. In bilateral clefts, attempts are made to lengthen the columella of the nose, again with an intraoral/nasal appliance and various struts of wire

TABLE 9–4. Methods of unilateral cleft lip and palate closure.

Method	Advantages	Disadvantages
Surgical only	Quick, no pre-op manipulations required.	Limited to smaller clefts. No control of segment position post-op.
Taping	Noninvasive, no dental impressions required.	Parent cooperation essential. Skin irritation common. No control of segments.
Passive molding plates with or without taping.	Allows some repositioning of segments. Serves as retainers, aids feeding.	Dental impressions required. Parents cooperation a must. Denture adhesives often used.
Lip adhesion	Decreases size of intra-alveolar gap. Allows tension-free closure.	Requires additional surgery. Surgeon must perform final closure through scar tissue. No post-op segment control.
Pin retained active appliance	Greater control of segments. Effective at reducing wide clefts. Allows tension-free lip closure.	Requires dental impressions, OR visit for placement, parent cooperation. Long-term effects on maxillary growth unknown.

or acrylic. Quite often, taping is required (Grayson et al., 1993).

Some centers also perform primary *alveolar bone grafting* in the infant stage. An attempt to bridge the gap between the bony segments of the alveolus is made by placing bone formation-inducing material, such as split thickness rib or cancellous bone from the hip, into the cleft site (Hathaway, Eppley, Hennon, Nelson, & Sadove, 1999; Hathaway, Eppley, Nelson, & Sadove, 1999). The goal is to unify the alveolar segments into a continuous arch, thus consolidating the maxilla into one piece. Primary grafting is intended to stabilize the arch, thereby preventing future crossbite, as well as to create bone, which will provide a path for the eruption of teeth near the cleft (Rosenstein, Dado, Kernahan, Griffith, & Grasseschi, 1991; Rosenstein et al., 1982). Unfortunately, results are mixed; some infants will gain the desired arch unity and sufficient bone for tooth eruption, but many do not.

Markedly decreased growth of the midface is another undesirable effect that has been associated with primary alveolar bone grafting. Centers debate differences in surgical technique, timing, and so on as the causes of success or failure. In particular, much attention has been focused on the amount of gingival, nasal, and oral mucosa that is manipulated by the surgeon in closing the infant alveolar cleft. This procedure is often called *gingivoperiosteoplasty*, particularly in reference to closing the cleft of the alveolus with raised gingival flaps at the same time as the palatal closure (Millard et al., 1999). Success rates are low and secondary alveolar bone grafting procedures may be required (Dado, Rosenstein, Alder, & Kernahan, 1997; Millard et al., 1999; Santiago et al., 1998).

After the lip and palate are closed, the infant enjoys a reprieve from dental and surgical intervention for a few years until the primary dentition erupts.

Primary Dentition (1–6 Years)

The primary dentition is usually complete by 24 to 30 months of age with 10 teeth in the upper arch and 10 in the lower arch. Ideally, there should be spacing between all of the primary teeth. This may be upsetting to some parents, but spacing of the primary teeth is necessary to allow room for the larger permanent teeth that will replace them. Thus, a child with little or no spacing between the primary teeth is at risk for significant crowding of the permanent teeth (Ngan, Alkire, & Fields, 1999). Children with repaired cleft lip and palate often demonstrate maxillary retrusion, attributed to surgical scarring, as well as a maxilla that is smaller than normal in every dimension. Therefore, it is not unusual to see crowding associated with the primary teeth in this population (Semb & Shaw, 1996).

There may be several dental abnormalities in the primary dentition at this stage. The area of the cleft may be missing a primary lateral incisor. Conversely, a *supernumerary tooth* (extra tooth) may be located near the cleft site. They may appear either palatally or labially, but are not often directly in the cleft due to its deficit of tissue. Malformations of these teeth are common (Poyry, 1996). Crossbite in the cleft area is also very common due to the altered anatomy of the palate. The maxilla in unilateral clefts consists of two segments, a *lesser segment* on the cleft side (cleft segment) and a *greater segment* on the noncleft side (noncleft segment) (see Figure 9–10). The greater and lesser segments are not joined at the site of the cleft, and as a result, they can be displaced by lip pressure; thus it is common to find crossbite on the affected side. In bilateral clefts, there are three maxillary segments, one premaxillary segment, and two lateral segments. The lateral segments may be displaced medially, which frequently results in a bilateral crossbite. The premaxillary segment may be protrusive (see Figure 9–11).

Clinicians have long been aware that children with a repaired cleft lip and palate frequently appear to have relatively normal upper to lower jaw relationships in the primary dentition but that this does not last into adolescence (Figure 9–14) (Grayson, Bookstein, McCarthy, & Mueeddin, 1987). Although the cleft maxilla is smaller than those of unaffected children, the mandible also is normally smaller at this stage of development. Thus, maxillary position may appear to be relatively normal in the primary dentition stage because mandibular growth has not yet begun. During the adolescent growth spurt, however, the mandible increases to its normal size. Unfortunately, as the mandible grows, the maxilla appears more and more retrusive, thereby exposing its deficiency (Berkowitz, 1996).

Children with clefts are at risk for periodontal disease localized to teeth near the cleft; therefore, every effort to establish proper oral hygiene measures at home should be made (Cooper, Long, Long, & Pepek, 1979; Gaggl, Schultes, Karcher, & Mossbock, 1999; Schultes, Gaggl, & Karcher, 1999; Teja, Persson, & Omnell, 1992). Few conditions require orthodontic intervention in the primary dentition. However, any crossbite that causes a functional shift of the mandible, that is, a reposturing of the mandible to achieve a more comfortable bite, will need to be addressed as soon as feasible. Left untreated, such posturing may cause overgrowth of one *condyle* (jaw joint), resulting in an asymmetry of the mandible. This will appear as a chin that is deviated to the nonaffected side (Proffit & Fields, 2000). In children with clefts, a significant narrowing of the maxillary segments is sometimes addressed in the primary dentition, especially if a crossbite or crowding of the primary teeth occurs.

Treatment for crossbite in the primary dentition usually involves some form of maxillary expansion. Maxillary expansion may be started at 4 to 5 years of age in a cooperative child. Either one of two appliances is usually chosen for maxillary expansion. One appliance, the *quad helix*, consists of orthodontic bands on the most posterior molars, and frequently the primary canines as well (Figure 9–15B) (Tindlund, Rygh, & Boe, 1993). The bands are connected

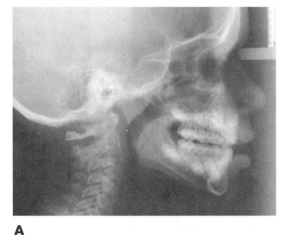

A

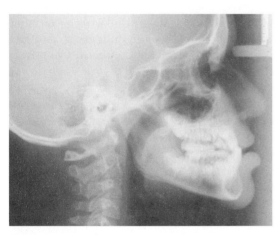

B

Figure 9–14. Normal occlusion in early dentition that changes in adolescence. **A.** The jaw and dental relationships are good in the early mixed dentition cephalogram of a patient with unilateral cleft lip and palate. This patient exhibits a nearly Class I occlusion and midfacial retrusion is not obvious. **B.** Unfortunately because of the mandibular growth spurt of adolescence, the relationships have changed for the worse. The patient now has a dental and skeletal Class III malocclusion with underbite and underjet, manifestations of the lack of midfacial growth often seen in cleft lip and palate patients.

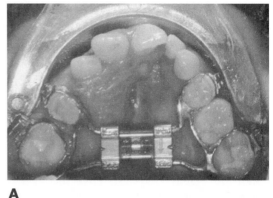

A

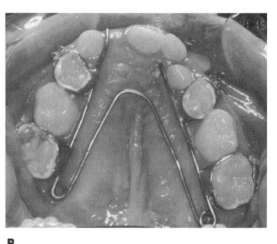

B

Figure 9–15. Appliances used for maxillary expansion. **A.** The rapid palatal expander (RPE) consists of a jackscrew mechanism that is activated with a key by the parents. **B.** The quad helix consists of a palatal spring that has four helices. Both appliances are versatile in that they can be modified to fit the individual needs of the patient. For instance, the quad helix shown in **B** actually has only two helices. The anterior helices were not used in this case due to the constricted space of the anterior palate. Both appliances are bulky and may interfere, at least temporarily, with articulation while in use.

by a palatal spring that has two posterior loops, each adjacent to a molar, and two anterior loops. These four loops or helices give the quad helix its name. Some clinicians prefer to not include the helices and the resulting W-shaped palatal spring is called a *W-arch*. The other appliance frequently used to correct crossbite is a *rapid palatal expander,* or RPE. It consists of two or four orthodontic bands connected by a jackscrew in the middle of the palate (Figure 9–15A). Turning the screw creates the necessary force to widen the arch. The rapid palatal expander is capable of delivering very heavy forces so it must be used with caution in the primary dentition. The goal for either the quad helix or the rapid palatal expander is to create adequate width of the maxilla. Because children with clefts may also have an anterior crossbite, some clinicians may wish to correct incisor position at this time (Vadiakas & Viazis, 1992). This is rarely necessary with primary incisors and should be reserved for the permanent incisors and then preferably at a stage of nearly completed root development.

Maxillary expansion can be accomplished within a few months in most cases. Children with repaired palatal clefts must have a fixed lingual upper arch wire to maintain the maxillary expansion. Without proper retention, the scar tissue of palatal repair exerts a strong tendency toward relapse into crossbite.

In children with repaired cleft palate, maxillary expansion may achieve crossbite correction but often at the expense of widening any pre-existing oral-antral fistula, or even opening a new fistula. Widening the narrow arch of the cleft palate separates the greater and lesser segments, resulting in tightly stretched tissue over the deficient or absent bone of the palate. Without proper bony support, palatal tissue necrosis may occur, which causes the fistula to manifest. These fistulae may be temporarily obturated with acrylic added to arch wires or with removable acrylic plates. Definitive repair is usually accomplished later with an alveolar bone graft (Proffit & White, 1991).

Early Mixed Dentition (6–9 Years)

Malpositioned permanent incisors are often the most noticeable sign that children with a repaired cleft lip and palate are entering the early mixed dentition stage. The permanent lower central incisors usually erupt first, followed by the upper central incisors and lower lateral incisors, and finally the upper lateral incisors. The permanent first molars usually erupt shortly after the lower central incisors, but it is not uncommon for them to erupt first.

In children who have had unilateral or bilateral clefts, it is common for the now erupting upper incisors to be misaligned (Figure 9–16). Although unaesthetic, these crowded incisors should not be corrected with orthodontics at this stage. The crowns of these teeth may be visible but the root formation remains very much incomplete. As a general rule, it takes at least 3 years after crown eruption before root formation is complete. The pressure from orthodontic appliances at this stage can damage forming roots, frequently resulting in roots of less than half their normal length. Consequently, correct-

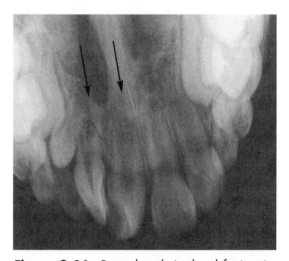

Figure 9–16. Rotated teeth in the cleft site. An occlusal X ray demonstrating that teeth in the line of the cleft are frequently malpositioned or rotated about the long axis of the roots. In this view, the maxillary right central and lateral incisors (arrows) are rotated approximately 90° each, so that the lingual surfaces of their crowns are facing each other. By comparison the maxillary left central and lateral incisors are nearly normal with almost no rotation (the right side of this view). Note there is also a supernumerary tooth distal to the rotated incisors.

ing anterior malalignment is not advised until after completion of root formation to avoid a poor long-term prognosis for these teeth (Figueroa, Polley, & Cohen, 1993).

During the mixed dentition stage, the interosseous sutures of the maxilla are beginning to fuse together but the mandible is beginning its growth spurt. The incidence of crossbite increases as the jaw discrepancy increases (see Figure 9–14). If the patient requires maxillary advancement, a *reverse pull headgear* may be an option. This is also an excellent time to correct any crossbite that may exist, using the crossbite appliance as anchorage for the face mask (Rygh & Tindlund, 1982; Tindlund, 1989; Tindlund, Rygh, & Boe, 1993). A typical quad helix or rapid palatal expander with labial hooks for face-mask attachment is used (Figure 9–17). Treatment is usually timed before the age of 8 to take advantage of remaining maxillary growth before suture fusion begins. Face-mask treatment requires 12 to 14 hours of wear per day to show midface improvement (Tindlund, 1994).

Another consideration of the early mixed dentition is the eruption of the lateral incisor, if present, and the need for an alveolar bone graft (Figure 9–18). As with primary bone grafting, a secondary alveolar bone graft is meant to introduce bone matrix inducing material into the alveolar cleft site. The introduced bone stimulates new bone formation in the cleft site. When successful, the introduced bone replaces the missing alveolar ridge, which provides bone for normal eruption of the permanent teeth and also serves as the missing nasal floor and piriform (nasal) rim. Frequently, illiac crestal (hip) bone is used, although other sources of bone such as the tibia, cranium, anterior chin, freeze-dried cadaver bone, and artificial substitutes, such as hydroxy apatite, have been used (Cohen, Figueroa, Haviv, Schafer, & Aduss, 1991). Secondary alveolar bone grafting is highly predictable in unilateral clefts when the greater and lesser segments are stabilized properly, approaching 95% success rates (Cohen, Figueroa, & Aduss, 1989; Cohen, Polley, & Figueroa, 1993; Kindelan & Roberts-Harry,

1999; Trotman, Papillon, Ross, McNamara, & Johnston, 1997; Vargervik, 1983). In repairing bilateral clefts, many clinicians prefer to graft one side at a time. Success rates with this technique approach 90% (Trotman et al., 1997; Turvey, Vig, Moriarty, & Hoke, 1984). Simultaneous grafting of the bilateral cleft has a greater chance for failure, with success rates dropping to 70% (Shashua & Omnell, 2000).

It is important for the clinician to note whether the lateral incisor is well formed and suitable to be used as a fully functioning tooth (Shashua & Omnell, 2000; Solis, Figueroa, Cohen, Polley, & Evans, 1998). As a tooth erupts, it carries its periodontal ligament and bony attachment with it. Without adequate bone, the erupting tooth will have a periodontal defect. This compromises not only the lateral incisor but other teeth adjacent to the defect as well. If the lateral incisor is usable it is best for it to erupt through bone. Thus, when the lateral incisor is beginning to reach one half to two thirds of normal root length, the maxilla should be prepared for secondary alveolar bone grafting. Maxillary expansion will usually be required, if not accomplished earlier. In cases in which the maxillary lateral incisor is missing or unusable, many clinicians prefer to delay bone grafting until the maxillary canine is ready to erupt, usually around age 11 to 13. Delaying expansion when possible has the benefit of not overwhelming the child with constant orthodontic treatment. Some clinicians argue, however, that delaying the bone graft until the time of canine eruption creates a defect around the central incisor. More studies are needed to evaluate the long-term outcome of periodontal health as it relates to early versus late grafting (Teja et al., 1992).

Late Mixed Dentition (9–12 Years)

Once the permanent incisors and first molars have erupted, visible changes in the dentition are not noticeable for 2 to 3 years. Midface retrusion, if present, may become more noticeable during this stage (see Figure 9–14). Late

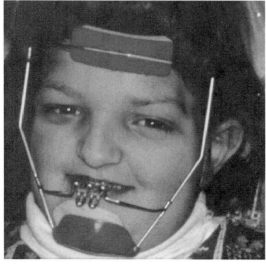

A

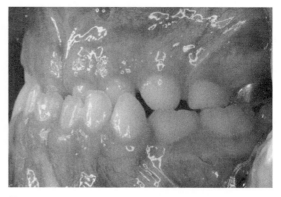

B

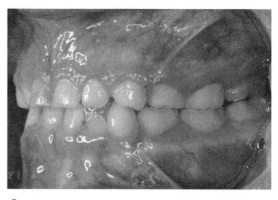

C

Figure 9–17. Removable reverse pull headgear, also known as a Delaire facial mask, can be used in cooperative children to correct midfacial retrusion. **A.** An appliance attached to the teeth engages the elastic bands on the facemask to generate an anterior force on the teeth, which is transmitted to the maxilla and its surrounding interosseous sutures. **B.** Underbite due to maxillary deficiency is an indication for this device, as in shown in this photograph before treatment. **C.** The correction achievable with the facial mask is readily apparent as normal overbite and overjet seen in the same patient as B.

mixed dentition treatment may involve maxillary expansion for alveolar bone grafting, if not done earlier, and is now timed around the eruption of the maxillary canine. Root formation of the incisors may have progressed to the point that they may now be aligned orthodontically. This may be begun 1 to 3 months (Vig, 1999) after bone grafting, which provides sufficient bone to move the incisors into, especially in bilateral clefts (Semb & Ramstad, 1999). Missing teeth may be replaced by adding artificial teeth to the orthodontic appliances, at least as a temporary measure.

Late mixed dentition treatment may also involve problems common to children without clefts. These may include space maintenance for prematurely lost primary teeth, controlling moderate to severe crowding problems through selective tooth extraction, or correction of jaw position with dentofacial orthopedic measures, such as headgear or functional appliances. The limitation of decreased maxillary growth in children with repaired clefts must be kept in consideration when prescribing any of these treatment modalities. Most clinicians will attempt to accomplish interceptive orthodontic treatment in a 12- to 18-month period, so that the child may have a rest from orthodontic treatment until the permanent dentition completely erupts. Realistic assessment of the risks

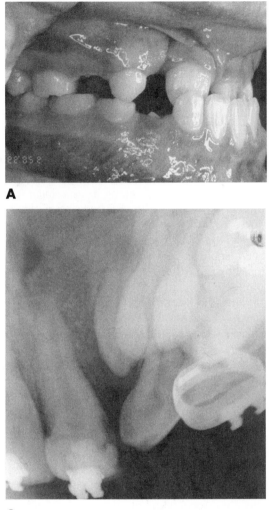

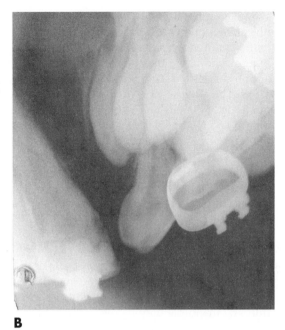

A

B

C

Figure 9-18. A patient needing an alveor bone graft. **A.** One can see the notching of the alveolus between the primary canine and the permanent lateral incisor. The anterior crossbite and narrowness of the maxilla will be corrected orthodontically prior to the bone graft. This gives the surgeon better access to the cleft and allows the lateral incisor to erupt through normal bone, thereby avoiding periodontal defects. **B.** In the occlusal radiograph, one can see the developing lateral incisor and the deficiency of alveolar bone. This is an indication for alveolar bone grafting. **C.** One can appreciate the new bone that formed after grafting.

and benefits of treatment in the late mixed dentition need to be considered before initiating treatment. The child with cleft lip and palate is likely to require orthodontic treatment in the permanent dentition and it is well known that tooth eruption is frequently delayed in children with clefts (McNamara, Foley, Garvey, & Kavanagh, 1999). Every attempt should be made to delay or combine treatment as much as possible to avoid "orthodontic fatigue" in the patient (Cooper et al., 1979). Much of orthodontic treatment depends on the coopera-

tion of the child, and cooperation will not be forthcoming in the child who is "burned out" or simply tired of orthodontic treatment (Cooper et al., 1979; Proffit & White, 1991).

Adolescent Dentition (12–18 Years)

Hopefully, by the time of eruption of the permanent dentition, crossbites have been corrected, alveolar bony defects are repaired, the incisors are well aligned, crowding has been managed, and the child has experienced good maxillary growth (Vargervik, 1981). Unfortunately, this is not always the case (Friede et al., 1986). For many children with clefts, the maxilla remains hypoplastic in all dimensions; vertical, sagittal, and transverse (Gaggl, Schultes, & Karcher, 1999). The adolescent growth spurt may have made these deficits more noticeable due to the mandible's relatively normal growth as well as the growth of the nose (Ishii & Vargervik, 1996). This discrepancy, an underdeveloped maxilla and normal mandible, often leads to one of two possible jaw relationships, a Class III with deep underbite or a Class I with anterior openbite.

If a severe anterior crossbite persists during growth, the mandibular incisors may over-erupt, causing a deep underbite. Because the maxilla is smaller than normal, the middle portion of the face is simply not as long as ideal, thus the mandible may be overclosed, further contributing to deepbite. Conversely, in some patients with relatively normal occlusion, mandibular growth may have been directed inferiorly and posteriorly. This allows the teeth to remain in a more normal occlusion but results in a longer facial profile and possible open bite (Trotman & Ross, 1993). Fortunately, these two phenomena appear to be occurring less often now, because improvements in surgical techniques have led to less detrimental effects on maxillary growth. Thus, adolescent treatment in about 80% of children with a repaired cleft may involve orthodontics alone (Figure 9–19). The remaining 20% often require orthodontics as well as orthognathic surgery to align the dental arches (Figure 9–20) (Figueroa et al., 1993; Proffit & White, 1991). These percentages vary from one treatment center to another.

Orthognathic surgery, which is surgery of the bones of the jaws, frequently involves a maxillary Le Fort I osteotomy to reposition the maxilla anteriorly (Figure 9–20). Orthodontic treatment, in preparation for surgery, intentionally worsens the discrepancy between the upper and lower teeth in order to create sufficient space for maximum jaw repositioning. When facial growth is complete, replacement of miss-

ing teeth with dental prostheses, such as bridgework or *dental implants,* may be necessary. Dental implants are cylindrical pieces of titanium that can take the place of a missing tooth's root and are able to support crowns (Kearns, Perrott, Sharma, Kaban, & Vargervik, 1997). The coordinated involvement of the surgeon, orthodontist, and prosthodontist is required for a successful outcome (Vig & Turvey, 1985).

A recent development in orthognathic surgical treatment is *distraction osteogenesis* (Figure 9–21). This involves making a *corticotomy* (cut in bone) in the middle of a bone, then slowly distracting the cut ends apart with a mechanical device. New osteoid is able to regenerate between the cut ends and in time becomes normal bone, obviating the need for bone grafts. Pioneered in mandibular applications by Molina and Monasterio in Mexico and McCarthy in the United States, when indicated, it is a very effective treatment option (Berkowitz, 1996). Distraction osteogenesis is especially effective in correcting severe discrepancies that are not amenable to standard surgical techniques. Rigid external distraction osteogenesis for the midface was introduced by Polley and Figueroa (Figueroa & Polley, 1999; Figueroa, Polley, & Ko, 1999; Polley & Figueroa, 1997, 1998), although internal appliances are appearing as well (Cohen, 1999). Orthodontists and surgeons work closely together to determine the final occlusion with these techniques (Motohashi & Kuroda, 1999). The field is rapidly changing, indications and treatment timing are still being developed, and new devices and their variants are being introduced at a rapid pace. At present, distraction osteogenesis is primarily being used to reduce or correct severe facial deformities.

Last, an adolescent who has had orthodontics and orthognathic surgery is likely to require prosthodontic replacement of missing teeth. This is frequently accomplished with fixed crowns and bridges, dental implants, or less commonly with removable prostheses such as dentures or partials (Mazaheri, 1979).

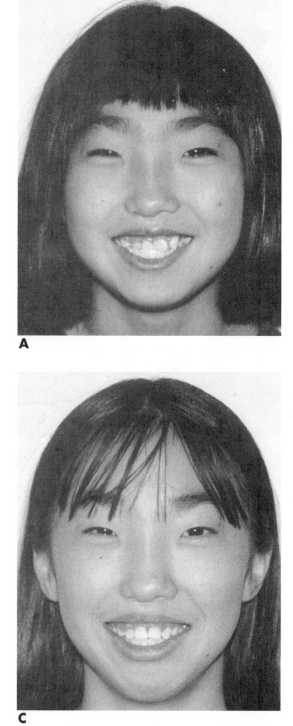

A

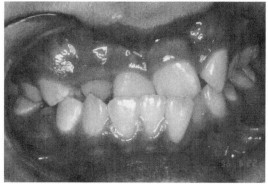

B

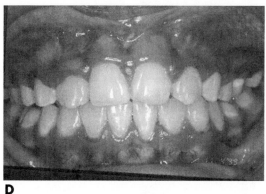

D

C

Figure 9–19. Adolescent treatment with orthodontics only. **A.** This patient with right unilateral cleft lip and palate exhibits only mild midfacial retrusion. **B.** The anterior crossbite of this patient, was judged to be amenable to orthodontic treatment alone. Orthognathic surgery was not considered to be necessary. **C.** After adolescent growth and orthodontic treatment the facial proportions remain well balanced. **D.** The post-treatment occlusal result was excellent. One lateral incisor was missing, the remaining lateral incisor was extracted, and the canines were substituted for the lateral incisors.

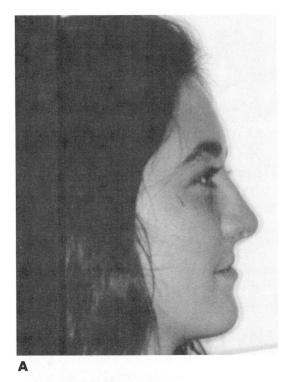

A

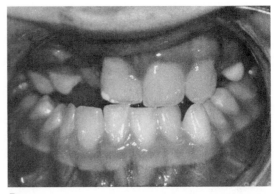

B

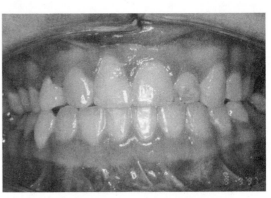

D

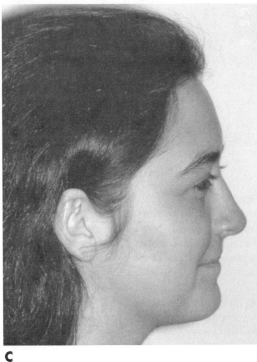

C

Figure 9-20. Adolescent dentition treatment involving orthodontics and orthognathic surgery. **A.** This patient with unilateral right cleft lip and palate was judged to need orthodontics and orthognathic surgery to correct her moderate midfacial retrusion and **B.** her malocclusion with anterior and posterior crossbite and missing right lateral incisor. **C.** After orthodontic preparation she underwent a LeFort I maxillary osteotomy to advance the upper jaw and teeth, as well as malar implants to augment the cheeks. She has an improved profile and upper lip position and **D.** a very much improved occlusal result. Extraction of multiple teeth to correct only her malocclusion without maxillary advancement surgery would have lessened her lip support and given her an "aged" or edentulous appearance.

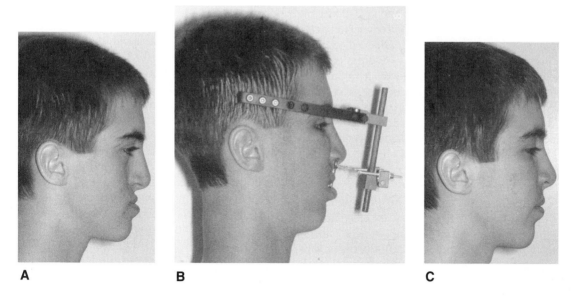

A **B** **C**

Figure 9–21. Rigid external distraction osteogenesis. **A.** This patient with bilateral cleft lip and palate exhibits midfacial retrusion that is far beyond the limits of conventional orthognathic surgery. **B.** He elected to undergo the rigid external distraction procedure of Polley and Figueroa. Following maxillary LeFort I osteotomy the rigid framework is attached to the skull with scalp pins and the maxilla is pulled forward or "distracted" with a screw mechanism over about an 8-week period. **C.** Following stabilization the headframe is removed, and the improvement in facial profile can be readily seen.

Dental Abnormalities and Their Effects on Speech

An abnormal dentition often affects speech because most consonants are produced in the anterior portion of the oral cavity (Shprintzen, Siegel-Sadewitz, Amato, & Goldberg, 1985). When abnormalities of the dentition inhibit the function of the tongue and lips, articulation will be defective (Shprintzen et al., 1985).

Two kinds of articulation errors may result from dental abnormalities: obligatory errors and compensatory errors (Trost-Cardamone, 1997). *Obligatory errors* are errors of distortion that occur due to structural abnormalities that interfere with normal tongue and lip positioning during speech. *Compensatory errors* are errors of distortion or substitution due to a modification in placement of normal tongue and lip position to compensate for the structural abnormalities.

Abnormalities in the dentition primarily affect the articulation of sibilant phonemes (s, z, sh, zh, ch, j), since these sounds are produced partly by the teeth. Dental abnormalities may also affect labio-dental phonemes (f, v), lingual-alveolar phonemes (t, d, n, l), and bilabial sounds (p, b, m). Vowels and posterior consonants are not affected by dental or occlusal anomalies. Dental abnormalities have the greatest effect on speech if they are present before or during speech development. The learned sound pattern may reflect a means to compensate for the structural restraints of the abnormality. Dental abnormalities have the least effect on speech if they occur after the development of normal speech, which is why the loss of teeth, as in an edentulous person, may cause little problem with speech.

Abnormalities of the teeth and jaws occur frequently in children with repaired cleft lip, cleft palate, or craniofacial anomalies. The more common occurrences include missing teeth, supernumerary teeth, rotated teeth, crowding, anterior crossbite, Class III malocclusion, open bite, and protruding premaxilla (Proffit & White, 1991). Each of these anomalies has the potential to cause a distortion of speech.

Missing Teeth

Congenitally missing teeth are a frequent finding in patients with history of cleft lip and palate (Figure 9–22). A tooth is often absent from the cleft alveolus, and occasionally, multiple teeth are missing. When present, teeth in the area of the cleft may be smaller than normal, misshapen, or malformed. The tooth most frequently missing from the cleft site is a maxillary lateral incisor or a canine. Missing teeth may cause an opening in the dental arch. The tongue may protrude through an anterior opening, producing a frontal lisp on sibilants. If the opening is lateral, the tongue may deviate to that opening, resulting in a lateral lisp on sibilants. When this occurs, the airstream is emitted on the side opposite the opening.

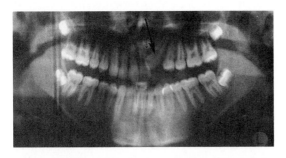

Figure 9–22. A panoramic X ray demonstrating a permanent tooth missing from the cleft site. The upper left lateral incisor, tooth #10, as in this case, is frequently missing (arrow), and the upper left canine has moved into its place.

Rotated Teeth

Rotations of teeth that erupt in the cleft site are common (see Figure 9–16). Central incisors and lateral incisors, if present, are most often affected. Additionally, the central incisor may be about 10% smaller than usual. Also, the central and lateral incisors may be fused at the roots. Fortunately, this is more commonly found in the primary than in the permanent dentition. Rotated or malformed teeth affect speech by diverting the airstream. Rotated teeth within the tongue tip area may cause a lateral lisp to occur. Patients who attempt to compensate for the position and interference of a rotated tooth may also develop a lateral distortion if the tongue is retracted to avoid the tooth and the dorsum is therefore elevated.

Supernumerary or Ectopic Teeth

When there has been a cleft, extra or supernumerary teeth may occur in the line of the cleft (Figure 9–23). These often remain unerupted, although they will occasionally erupt partially or even completely. If erupted, a supernumerary tooth may be displaced palatally or labially. A similar problem occurs with an *ectopic tooth*, which is a normal tooth that erupts into an abnormal position. Depending on its placement, the ectopic or supernumerary tooth may interfere with tongue movement, causing distortion of lingual-alveolar sounds or even interdental sounds (Bloomer, 1971). Sibilants can be affected by the diversion of the airstream laterally, causing a lateral lisp. If the tooth is in the area of the alveolar ridge, the patient may learn to compensate by using the dorsum of the tongue for articulation, resulting in distortion of tongue-tip sounds.

Crossbite

A dental abnormality that frequently occurs in children with a history of cleft lip and palate is *crossbite*. In crossbite, the normal overlap of the

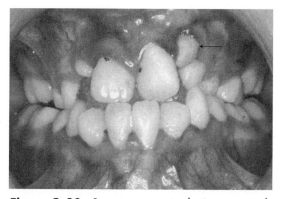

Figure 9–23. Supernumerary teeth. An extra tooth may occur in the line of the cleft, as in this case of a supernumerary primary incisor, distal and superior to the patient's maxillary left central incisor (arrow).

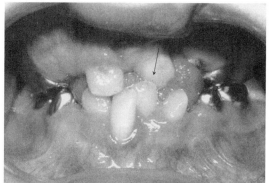

Figure 9–24. Single tooth crossbite. A crossbite involving only one tooth may be referred to as a single tooth crossbite. Often a maxillary central or lateral incisor is involved, as in this case of the upper left central incisor being displaced lingually to the lower left central incisor (arrow).

upper teeth to the lower teeth is reversed, so that the lower teeth overlap the upper teeth buccally. A crossbite may involve only one upper and one lower tooth, called a *single tooth crossbite* (Figure 9–24). When multitooth crossbites occur they are described by their position in the dental arch, either anterior or posterior. An *anterior crossbite* may involve any or all of the anterior teeth: the central incisors, lateral incisors, or canines (Figure 9–25). Anterior crossbites are commonly seen in patients with dental or skeletal Class III malocclusion. *Posterior crossbite* involves any combination of teeth distal (posterior) to the canines and usually occurs because the maxilla is too narrow. Often, a multiple tooth crossbite involves a combination of anterior as well as posterior teeth. When a posterior crossbite is limited to one side of the arch, the crossbite is referred to as being unilateral (Figure 9–26). When both the right and left posterior sides are involved, the crossbite is referred to as being bilateral (Figure 9–27A). When mild, a bilateral crossbite may produce a shift of the mandible to one side, which gives the clinical appearance of a unilateral crossbite. A more severe bilateral posterior crossbite rarely produces such a shift of the mandible. Careful examination of the pa-

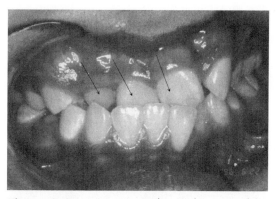

Figure 9–25. Anterior crossbite. When most of the incisors are involved in crossbite, an anterior crossbite is said to have occurred, as in this patient with anterior crossbite of both of the maxillary central incisors and the maxillary right cuspid (arrows).

tient's occlusion as the teeth first contact during closure helps to distinguish bilateral crossbite with mandibular shift from a true unilateral crossbite. A *buccal crossbite* occurs when one or more maxillary teeth are positioned buccally such that the maxillary lingual cusps reside buccal to the mandibular cusps. The relatively rare *Brodie crossbite* occurs when the lingual cusps of all the maxillary posterior teeth are buccal to the mandibular teeth.

A crossbite can affect speech in several ways. An anterior crossbite may interfere with tongue tip movement, causing distortion of sibilants or lingual-alveolar sounds. The anterior crossbite may cause a frontal lisp as an obligatory error if the tongue remains in normal position in the mandible. It can also cause a compensatory error if the tongue is retracted to compensate for crowding of the anterior part of the oral cavity. This causes the dorsum to elevate and articulate with the palate, resulting in a mid-dorsum palatal placement (palatal-dorsal production). This production can be substituted for lingual-alveolar sounds (t, d, n, l) and a mid-dorsum placement can also cause a lateral lisp on sibilants (s, z, zh, sh, ch, j). An anterior crossbite may interfere with labio-dental placement sounds (f, v), resulting in a reverse placement so that the upper lip articulates with the mandibular incisors. A posterior crossbite can result in distortion of speech because the teeth will often open during articulation to compensate for the lack of adequate oral cavity space. Complete crossbite can result in the distortion of many sounds, particularly tongue tip sounds, due to the very limited space for normal tongue movement (Figure 9–27B).

Protruding Premaxilla

Infants affected by bilateral cleft lip and palate often have a protruding premaxilla at birth. This condition has been attributed to an overgrowth of the premaxilla, which is untethered by the lat-

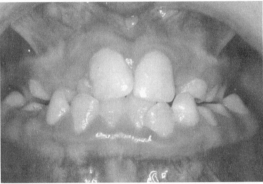

A

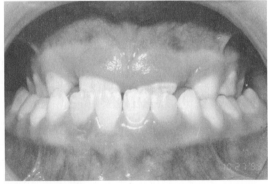

B

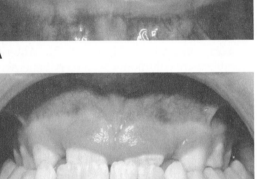

Figure 9–26. Unilateral posterior crossbite. The posterior teeth of the patient's maxillary left side are lingual to the mandibular teeth (arrows). This is referred to as a posterior crossbite. It may also be called a unilateral posterior crossbite.

Figure 9–27. Bilateral crossbite. **A.** The maxillary posterior teeth on both sides are lingual to the mandibular teeth. **B.** When all of the maxillary teeth fit inside the mandibular teeth, a total crossbite exists.

eral palatal segments. Past treatment included surgical removal of the premaxilla, but this had deleterious effects on midfacial growth (Monroe, Griffith, McKinney, Rosenstein, & Jacobson, 1970). Fortunately, the procedure has been abandoned. The lateral segments, lacking sufficient palatal shelf resistance, are displaced medially so that there is no room for the premaxilla to fit in its normal position. Untreated, the premaxilla remains protrusive due to lack of space.

When the premaxilla is in an anterior position, the position of the alveolar ridge relative to the tongue tip may be altered, causing a mild distortion of sibilants (Bloomer, 1971). A protruding premaxilla can particularly interfere with lip closure for production of bilabial sounds (p, b, m). Labio-dental placement may be used as a substitute, and although this results in little distortion in speech, it is visually distracting because of abnormal lip placement.

Open Bite

Open bite occurs when one or more maxillary teeth fail to occlude with the opposing mandibular teeth (Figure 9–28). Open bites primarily affect the anterior dentition (anterior open bite) and less commonly the posterior dentition (lateral open bite). Causes of open bite include missing teeth, digit or pacifier sucking habits, and skeletal discrepancies. Open bites will be sealed by the tongue on swallowing, which is often confused as tongue thrust (Proffit & Fields, 2000). An open bite has the same potential effect on speech production as missing teeth, but the effect is usually more pronounced. An anterior open bite is most likely to affect the production of sibilant sounds, particularly the fricatives (s, z, sh, zh), but often the affricates (ch, j) as well. With an anterior open bite, there is a tendency for the tongue to seek the opening so that the sounds are produced

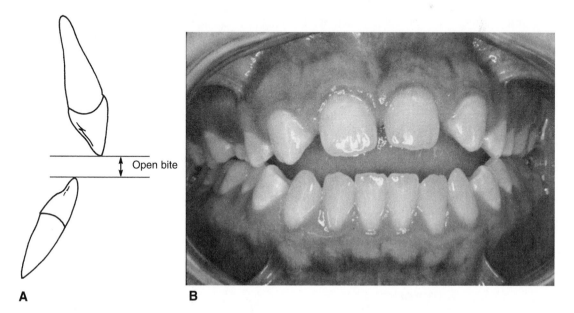

A   **B**

Figure 9–28. Open bite. **A.** The anterior teeth are not in contact. **B.** Open bite is often attributed to tongue thrust, but little evidence exists to support that cause. Open bite is difficult to treat, often involving orthognathic surgery in conjunction with orthodontics.

interdentally, resulting in a frontal lisp. Even if the tongue remains in the normal position, the acoustic product may lack appropriate sibilance (Bloomer, 1971). A lateral open bite is less likely to affect speech because it is away from the tongue tip and is lateral to the direction of the airstream. If the tongue tip moves toward the open bite, however, it will divert the airstream to the contralateral side and result in a lateral distortion of sibilants.

The Role of Speech Therapy

Speech pathologists and dental professionals must work closely together to correct problems of speech related to the dentition in the child with a history of cleft lip and palate (Pinsky & Goldberg, 1977; Shprintzen et al., 1985). When there are speech distortions due to faulty dental structure, speech therapy will not be effective in correcting the speech (Shprintzen, 1991). Instead, correction of the structural problem of the dentition is required before there can be any improvement in speech. In fact, if the speech errors are all obligatory as a result of the faulty structure, then correcting the structure will correct the speech without the need for speech therapy. On the other hand, if there are compensatory errors as a result of the structural abnormality, then speech therapy will be required, preferably after correction of the dentition. Speech pathologists and dentists should coordinate their interventions to coincide with the stages of dental development, as outlined above (Shprintzen, McCall, & Skolnick, 1975). Coordination of treatment timing, sequencing, and follow-up is important to make efficient use of resources and to ensure the best overall outcome (Shprintzen, 1982).

Summary

Children with cleft lip and palate or other craniofacial anomalies are at risk for dental and oc-

clusal abnormalities that include missing teeth, supernumerary teeth, rotated teeth, crowding, anterior crossbite, Class III malocclusion, open bite, and protruding premaxilla. All of these abnormalities can affect speech by affecting the movement of the tongue tip or lips. Crowding of the oral cavity, particularly anterior crowding, can cause lisps and a palatal placement for tongue tip and sibilant sounds.

Because so many children with craniofacial anomalies have dental and speech problems, it is important for dental professionals and speech pathologists to work closely together. Interdisciplinary communication and coordination will help to determine the appropriate form of treatment needed to achieve a maximal outcome in aesthetics, mastication, and speech.

References

Berkowitz, S. (Ed.). (1996). *Cleft lip and palate, Perspectives in management* (Vols. 1 and 2). San Diego, CA: Singular Publishing Group.

Bloomer, H. (1971). Speech defects associated with dental malocclusions and related abnormalities. In L. Travis (Ed.), *Handbook of speech pathology and audiology* . New York: Appleton.

Cohen, M., Figueroa, A. A., & Aduss, H. (1989). The role of gingival mucoperiosteal flaps in the repair of alveolar clefts. *Plastic and Reconstructive Surgery, 83*(5), 812–819.

Cohen, M., Figueroa, A. A., Haviv, Y., Schafer, M. E., & Aduss, H. (1991). Iliac versus cranial bone for secondary grafting of residual alveolar clefts [see Comments]. *Plastic and Reconstructive Surgery, 87*(3), 423–427; Discussion 428.

Cohen, M., Polley, J. W., & Figueroa, A. A. (1993). Secondary (intermediate) alveolar bone grafting. *Clinics in Plastic Surgery, 20*(4), 691–705.

Cohen, S. R. (1999). Midface distraction. *Seminars in Orthodontics, 5*(1), 52–58.

Cooper, H. K., Long, R. E., Sr., Long, R. E., Jr., & Pepek, M. J. (1979). Orthodontics and oral orthopedics. In H. K. Cooper, R. L. Harding, W. M. Krogman, M. Mazaheri, & R. T. Millard (Eds.), *Cleft palate and cleft lip: A team approach to clinical management and rehabilitation of the patient* (pp. 359–430). Philadelphia: W.B. Saunders.

Cutting, C., Grayson, B., Brecht, L., Santiago, P., Wood, R., & Kwon, S. (1998). Presurgical columellar elongation and primary retrograde nasal reconstruction in one-stage bilateral cleft lip and nose repair [see Comments]. *Plastic and Reconstructive Surgery, 101*(3), 630–639.

Dado, D. V., Rosenstein, S. W., Alder, M. E., & Kernahan, D. A. (1997). Long-term assessment of early alveolar bone grafts using three-dimensional computer-assisted tomography: A pilot study. *Plastic and Reconstructive Surgery, 99*(7), 1840–1845.

Figueroa, A. A., & Polley, J. W. (1999). Management of severe cleft maxillary deficiency with distraction osteogenesis: Procedure and results. *American Journal of Orthodontic and Dentofacial Orthopedics, 115*(1), 1–12.

Figueroa, A. A., Polley, J. W., & Cohen, M. (1993). Orthodontic management of the cleft lip and palate patient. *Clinics in Plastic Surgery, 20*(4), 733–753.

Figueroa, A. A., Polley, J. W., & Ko, E. W. (1999). Maxillary distraction for the management of cleft maxillary hypoplasia with a rigid external distraction system. *Seminars in Orthodontics, 5*(1), 46–51.

Figueroa, A. A., Reisberg, D. J., Polley, J. W., & Cohen, M. (1996). Intraoral-appliance modification to retract the premaxilla in patients with bilateral cleft lip. *Cleft Palate Craniofacial Journal, 33*(6), 497–500.

Friede, H., Figueroa, A. A., Naegele, M. L., Gould, H. J., Kay, C. N., & Aduss, H. (1986). Craniofacial growth data for cleft lip patients infancy to 6 years of age: Potential applications. *American Journal of Orthodontic and Dentofacial Orthopedics, 90*(5), 388–409.

Gaggl, A., Schultes, G., & Karcher, H. (1999). Aesthetic and functional outcome of surgical and orthodontic correction of bilateral clefts of lip, palate, and alveolus. *Cleft Palate Craniofacial Journal, 36*(5), 407–412.

Gaggl, A., Schultes, G., Karcher, H., & Mossbock, R. (1999). Periodontal disease in patients with cleft palate and patients with unilateral and bilateral clefts of lip, palate, and alveolus. *Journal of Periodontology, 70*(2), 171–178.

Grayson, B. H., Bookstein, F. L., McCarthy, J. G., & Mueeddin, T. (1987). Mean tensor cephalometric analysis of a patient population with clefts of the palate and lip. *Cleft Palate Journal, 24*(4), 267–277.

Grayson, B. H., Cutting, C., & Wood, R. (1993). Preoperative columella lengthening in bilateral cleft lip and palate [Letter]. *Plastic and Reconstructive Surgery, 92*(7), 1422–1423.

Hathaway, R. R., Eppley, B. L., Hennon, D. K., Nelson, C. L., & Sadove, A. M. (1999). Primary alveolar cleft bone grafting in unilateral cleft lip and palate: Arch dimensions at age 8. *Journal of Craniofacial Surgery, 10*(1), 58–67.

Hathaway, R. R., Eppley, B. L., Nelson, C. L., & Sadove, A. M. (1999). Primary alveolar cleft bone grafting in unilateral cleft lip and palate: Craniofacial form at age 8. *Journal of Craniofacial Surgery, 10*(1), 68–72.

Ishii, K., & Vargervik, K. (1996). Nasal growth in complete bilateral cleft lip and palate. *Journal of Craniofacial Surgery, 7*(4), 290–296.

Jacobson, B. N., & Rosenstein, S. W. (1970). The cleft palate patient: Dental help needed. *ASDC Journal of Dentistry for Children, 37*(2), 105–115.

Jacobson, B. N., & Rosenstein, S. W. (1984). Early maxillary orthopedics for the newborn cleft lip and palate patient. An impression and an appliance. *Angle Orthodontist, 54*(3), 247–263.

Jacobson, B. N., & Rosenstein, S. W. (1986). Cleft lip and palate: The orthodontist's youngest patient. *American Journal of Orthodontic and Dentofacial Orthopedics, 90*(1), 63–66.

Katz, M. I. (1992). Angle classification revisited 2: A modified Angle classification [see Comments]. *American Journal of Orthodontic and Dentofacial Orthopedics, 102*(3), 277–284.

Kearns, G., Perrott, D. H., Sharma, A., Kaban, L. B., & Vargervik, K. (1997). Placement of endosseous implants in grafted alveolar clefts. *Cleft Palate Craniofacial Journal, 34*(6), 520–525.

Kindelan, J., & Roberts-Harry, D. (1999). A 5-year post-operative review of secondary alveolar bone grafting in the Yorkshire region. *British Journal of Orthodontics, 26*(3), 211–217.

King, B. F. D., Workman, C. H. D., & Latham, R. A. (1979). An anatomical study of the columella and the protruding premaxillae in a bilateral cleft lip and palate infant. *Cleft Palate Journal, 16*(3), 223–229.

Latham, R. A. (1980). Orthopedic advancement of the cleft maxillary segment: A preliminary report. *Cleft Palate Journal, 17*(3), 227–233.

Latham, R. A., Kusy, R. P., & Georgiade, N. G. (1976). An extraorally activated expansion appliance for cleft palate infants. *Cleft Palate Journal, 13,* 253–261.

Liao, Y. F., Huang, C. S., Liou, J. W., Lin, W. Y., & Ko, W. C. (1998). Premaxillary size and craniofacial growth in patients with cleft lip and palate. *Chang-Keng I Hsueh Tsa Chih (Tai-Pei), 21*(4), 391–396.

Mazaheri, M. (1979). Prosthodontic care. In H. K. Cooper, R. L. Harding, W. M. Krogman, M. Mazaheri, & R. T. Millard (Eds.), *Cleft palate and cleft lip: A team approach to clinical management and rehabilitation of the patient* (pp. 269–358). Philadelphia: W.B. Saunders.

McNamara, C. M., Foley, T. F., Garvey, M. T., & Kavanagh, P. T. (1999). Premature dental eruption: Report of case. *Journal of Dentistry for Children, 66*(1), 70–72.

Millard, D. R., Jr., & Latham, R. A. (1990). Improved primary surgical and dental treatment of clefts. *Plastic and Reconstructive Surgery, 86*(5), 856–871.

Millard, D. R., Latham, R., Huifen, X., Spiro, S., & Morovic, C. (1999). Cleft lip and palate treated by presurgical orthopedics, gingivoperiosteoplasty, and lip adhesion (POPLA) compared with previous lip adhesion method: A preliminary study of serial dental casts. *Plastic and Reconstructive Surgery, 103*(6), 1630–1644.

Monroe, C. W., Griffith, B. H., McKinney, P., Rosenstein, S. W., & Jacobson, B. N. (1970). Surgical recession of the premaxilla and its effect on maxillary growth in patients with bilateral clefts. *Cleft Palate Journal, 7,* 784–793.

Monroe, C. W., Griffith, B. H., Rosenstein, S. W., & Jacobson, B. N. (1983). The correction and preservation of arch form in complete clefts of the palate and alveolar ridge. *Annals of Plastic Surgery, 11*(5), 438–442.

Motohashi, N., & Kuroda, T. (1999). A 3D computer-aided design system applied to diagnosis and treatment planning in orthodontics and orthognathic surgery. *European Journal of Orthodontics, 21*(3), 263–274.

Mouradian, W. E., Omnell, M. L., & Williams, B. (1999). Ethics for orthodontists. *Angle Orthodontist, 69*(4), 295–299.

Ngan, P., Alkire, R. G., & Fields, H., Jr. (1999). Management of space problems in the primary and mixed dentitions. *Journal of the American Dental Association, 130*(9), 1330–1339.

Pinsky, T. M., & Goldberg, H. J. (1977). Potential for clinical cooperation between dentistry and speech pathology. *International Dental Journal, 27*(4), 363–369.

Polley, J. W., & Figueroa, A. A. (1997). Management of severe maxillary deficiency in childhood and adolescence through distraction osteogenesis with an external, adjustable, rigid distraction device. *Journal of Craniofacial Surgery, 8*(3), 181–185; Discussion 186.

Polley, J. W., & Figueroa, A. A. (1998). Rigid external distraction: Its application in cleft maxillary deformities. *Plastic and Reconstructive Surgery, 102*(5), 1360–1372; Discussion 1373–1374.

Poyry, M. (1996). Dental development in 0- to 3-year old children with cleft lip and palate. In S. Berkowitz (Ed.), *Cleft lip and palate: II. An introduction to craniofacial anomalies* (Vol. II, pp. 93–98). San Diego, CA: Singular Publishing Group.

Proffit, W. R., & Fields, H. W., Jr. (2000). *Contemporary orthodontics.* (3rd ed.). Chapel Hill, NC: Mosby-Year Book.

Proffit, W. R., & White, R. P., Jr. (1991). *Surgical-orthodontic treatment.* Chapel Hill, NC: Mosby-Year Book.

Reisberg, D. J., Figueroa, A. A., & Gold, H. O. (1988). An intraoral appliance for management of the protrusive premaxilla in bilateral cleft lip. *Cleft Palate Journal, 25*(1), 53–57.

Rosenstein, S., Dado, D. V., Kernahan, D., Griffith, B. H., & Grasseschi, M. (1991). The case for early bone grafting in cleft lip and palate: A second report. *Plastic and Reconstructive Surgery, 87*(4), 644–654; Discussion 655–656.

Rosenstein, S. W., Monroe, C. W., Kernahan, D. A., Jacobson, B. N., Griffith, B. H., & Bauer, B. S. (1982). The case of early bone grafting in cleft lip and cleft palate. *Plastic and Reconstructive Surgery, 70*(3), 297–309.

Ross, B., Hubert, E., & Chojnacka, A. (1977). Analysis of 160 cases of cleft lip, alveolar process and palate. *Czasopismo Stomatologiczne, 30*(5), 409–414.

Rygh, P., & Tindlund, R. (1982). Orthopedic expansion and protraction of the maxilla in cleft palate patients—A new treatment rationale. *Cleft Palate Journal, 19*(2), 104–112.

Santiago, P. E., Grayson, B. H., Cutting, C. B., Gianoutsos, M. P., Brecht, L. E., & Kwon, S. M. (1998). Reduced need for alveolar bone grafting by presurgical orthopedics and primary gingivoperiosteoplasty. *Cleft Palate Craniofacial Journal, 35*(1), 77–80.

Schultes, G., Gaggl, A., & Karcher, H. (1999). Comparison of periodontal disease in patients with clefts of palate and patients with unilateral clefts of lip, palate, and alveolus. *Cleft Palate Craniofacial Journal, 36*(4), 322–327.

Semb, G., & Ramstad, T. (1999). The influence of alveolar bone grafting on the orthodontic and prosthodontic treatment of patients with cleft lip and palate. *Dental Update, 26*(2), 60–64.

Semb, G., & Shaw, W. C. (1996). Facial growth in orofacial clefting disorders. In T. Turvey, K. Vig, & R. Fonseca (Eds.), *Facial clefts and craniosynostosis: Principles and management.* Chapel Hill, NC: W.B. Saunders.

Shashua, D., & Omnell, M. L. (2000). Radiographic determination of the position of the maxillary lateral incisor in the cleft alveolus and parameters for assessing its habilitation prospects. *Cleft Palate Craniofacial Journal, 37*(1), 21–25.

Shprintzen, R. J. (1982). Palatal and pharyngeal anomalies in craniofacial syndromes. *Birth Defects Original Article Series, 18*(1), 53–78.

Shprintzen, R. J. (1991). Fallibility of clinical research. *Cleft Palate Craniofacial Journal, 28*(2), 136–140.

Shprintzen, R. J., McCall, G. N., & Skolnick, M. L. (1975). A new therapeutic technique for the treatment of velopharyngeal incompetence. *Journal of Speech and Hearing Disorders, 40*(1), 69–83.

Shprintzen, R. J., Siegel-Sadewitz, V. L., Amato, J., & Goldberg, R. B. (1985). Anomalies associated with cleft lip, cleft palate, or both. *American Journal of Medical Genetics, 20*(4), 585–595.

Solis, A., Figueroa, A. A., Cohen, M., Polley, J. W., & Evans, C. A. (1998). Maxillary dental development in complete unilateral alveolar clefts. *Cleft Palate Craniofacial Journal, 35*(4), 320–328.

Strauss, R. P. (1998). Cleft palate and craniofacial teams in the United States and Canada: A national survey of team organization and standards of care. The American Cleft Palate-Craniofacial Association (ACPA) Team Standards Committee. *Cleft Palate Craniofacial Journal, 35*(6), 473–480.

Strauss, R. P. (1999). The organization and delivery of craniofacial health services: The state of the art. *Cleft Palate Craniofacial Journal, 36*(3), 189–195.

Teja, Z., Persson, R., & Omnell, M. L. (1992). Periodontal status of teeth adjacent to nongrafted unilateral alveolar clefts. *Cleft Palate Craniofacial Journal, 29*(4), 357–362.

Tindlund, R. S. (1989). Orthopaedic protraction of the midface in the deciduous dentition. Results covering 3 years out of treatment. *Journal of Cranio-Maxillo-Facial Surgery, 17*(Suppl. 1), 17–19.

Tindlund, R. S. (1994). Skeletal response to maxillary protraction in patients with cleft lip and palate before age 10 years. *Cleft Palate Craniofacial Journal, 31*(4), 295–308.

Tindlund, R. S., & Holmefjord, A. (1997). Functional results with the team care of cleft lip and palate patients in Bergen, Norway. The Bergen Cleft Palate-Craniofacial Team, Norway. *Folia Phoniatrica et Logopedica, 49*(3/4), 168–176.

Tindlund, R. S., Rygh, P., & Boe, O. E. (1993). Intercanine widening and sagittal effect of maxillary transverse expansion in patients with cleft lip and palate during the deciduous and mixed dentitions. *Cleft Palate Craniofacial Journal, 30*(2), 195–207.

Trost-Cardamone, J. E. (1997). Diagnosis of specific cleft palate speech error patterns for planning therapy of physical management needs. In K. R. Bzoch (Ed.), *Communicative disorders related to cleft lip and palate* (Vol. 4, pp. 313–330). Austin, TX: Pro-Ed.

Trotman, C. A., Papillon, F., Ross, R. B., McNamara, J. A., Jr., & Johnston, L. E., Jr. (1997). A retrospective comparison of frontal facial dimensions in alveolar-bone-grafted and nongrafted unilateral cleft lip and palate patients. *Angle Orthodontist, 67*(5), 389–394.

Trotman, C. A., & Ross, R. B. (1993). Craniofacial growth in bilateral cleft lip and palate: Ages six years to adulthood. *Cleft Palate Craniofacial Journal, 30*(3), 261–273.

Turvey, T. A., Vig, K. W. L., & Fonseca, R. J. (1996). *Facial clefts and craniosynostosis: Principles and management.* Chapel Hill, NC: W.B. Saunders.

Turvey, T. A., Vig, K., Moriarty, J., & Hoke, J. (1984). Delayed bone grafting in the cleft maxilla and palate: A retrospective multidisciplinary analysis. *American Journal of Orthodontics, 86*(3), 244–256.

Vadiakas, G., & Viazis, A. D. (1992). Anterior cross-bite correction in the early deciduous dentition. *American Journal of Orthodontic and Dentofacial Orthopedics, 102*(2), 160–162.

Vargervik, K. (1981). Orthodontic management of unilateral cleft lip and palate. *Cleft Palate Journal, 18*(4), 256–270.

Vargervik, K. (1983). Growth characteristics of the premaxilla and orthodontic treatment principles in bilateral cleft lip and palate. *Cleft Palate Journal, 20*(4), 289–302.

Vig, K. W. (1980). Treatment planning principles for orthodontic-surgical correction of dento-facial anomalies. *Australian Orthodontic Journal, 6*(4), 137–146.

Vig, K. W. (1999). Alveolar bone grafts: The surgical/orthodontic management of the cleft maxilla. *Annals of the Academy of Medicine, Singapore, 28*(5), 721–727.

Vig, K. W., & Turvey, T. A. (1985). Orthodontic-surgical interaction in the management of cleft lip and palate. *Clinics in Plastic Surgery, 12*(4), 735–748.

CHAPTER

10

Psychosocial Aspects of Cleft Lip/Palate and Craniofacial Anomalies

Janet R. Schultz, Ph.D., ABPP

CONTENTS

When a baby is born, the infant is not just born to his parents. A child is born into a family, a social network, and society. These layers of context into which we all are born are also forces that impact on the individual child's development. The child also brings into the world his or her genetic endowment and the characteristics developed during intrauterine life. Among these are temperament, certain instinctual behaviors, and physical appearance. For some children, one aspect is a cleft lip and/or palate. The child's contribution interacts with the complex context into which he or she is born so that the developing individual is both affected by and affecting that environment.

Family Issues

Initial Shock and Adjustment

The birth of a child is typically a happy event. Parents' first questions almost always include "Is the baby all right?" When a baby is born with either a unilateral or bilateral cleft lip and/or palate, there is typically immediate knowledge and distress. When an infant is born with a cleft of the velum or a submucous cleft, hours (or longer) may elapse before the parents are informed that there is a problem. When something is wrong with the baby, there is often a period of shock and sadness. For many families, there is also a period of mourning the anticipated child and adjustment to the situation in which they find themselves (van Staden & Gerhardt, 1995). Usually, resolution of these feelings comes after the beginning of the whirlwind demand of medical concerns that characterize early infancy for many children with a cleft lip or palate. Many parents of babies with clefts had never heard of clefts before their child's birth (Middleton, Lass, Starr, & Pannbacker, 1986). They have never seen a cleft before the repair and know little about the problem other

than what they are told at the time of the baby's birth. Adjustment of parents is affected by the extent of the deformity, elapsed time before seeing the baby, their coping style, and the social support they receive. Family support has been found to be a significant factor in overall adjustment (Bradbury & Hewison, 1994). Strong feelings of love, hurt, fear, disappointment, existential betrayal, resentment, protectiveness, and guilt are often present but negative feelings tend to subside fairly rapidly without impairing the parent-child relationship on a long-term basis (Clifford, 1969, 1971). One reason for this relatively rapid resolution is the "fixable" quality of clefts at this point in history. On the other hand, there are some mixed findings that mothers may be less responsive to and interactive with infants with clefts than they are with babies without anomalies. Children with any kind of physical anomalies appear to be more at risk of physical abuse than normal children.

For a few families, the birth of a child with a cleft is a serious disruption, but for most, it is a difficult but manageable time. Mothers of babies with clefts reported higher levels of stress and more concerns about their competence as parents than mothers of healthy babies (Speltz, Armsden, & Clarren, 1990). The same mothers also reported a higher degree of marital conflict. There is little evidence however, that the divorce rate is higher in these families. In several studies, about 10% of parents reported that their marriage was adversely affected, while a quarter to a third reported that the birth of a child with a cleft brought the parents closer together. Reproductive plans generally were unaltered by the birth of child with a cleft (Andrews-Casal et al., 1998).

Feeding problems, discussion of surgery and appliances, and the question of how to talk to other people about the baby's anomaly color the experience of the first few weeks of their baby's life. Parents may find themselves supporting grandparents or other relatives, rather than receiving support themselves. Sometimes families pull together, but other times there are questions or worse, accusations about the reason for the cleft, perhaps with finger pointing at the other side of the family. Parents of infants with visible differences are likely to experience the staring of other adults and some children when they take their babies out in public. These experiences may serve to confirm the fears of social rejection, which tend to rise rapidly in the minds of parents at their first contact with the baby. Parents may also have other children to attend to during this time. Parents often find it difficult to explain to siblings that the baby looks different and has something wrong, even when they reassure them that the doctors are going to fix it. Whenever there is a new baby, parents also have to balance the time required to take care of the baby with the needs of the other children. That can be a more daunting task if the baby requires longer to feed, has frequent ear infections, or requires surgery and other medical visits. Intervening with parents who are experiencing considerable stress may have a preventive effect, in that later on parents' stress correlates with adjustment problems in the child's life.

Health care professionals, generally nurses or pediatricians, can be important sources of support and information for parents in the early months. Focusing more on what is "right" with the baby than what is "wrong" is often helpful, as is consistent availability. But parents also want to talk, to show their feelings, and to check out their fears. In addition, many parents want contact with other parents of children with clefts (Strauss, Sharp, Lorch, & Kachalia, 1995). It is comforting to talk to people who have been through the same experiences. Parents seem less afraid to "look stupid" in the eyes of sympathetic veterans of the process and may voice more of their fears and questions with them. A number of hospitals have systems in place to help parents of newborns with clefts link with veteran parents of somewhat older children. Parents compare experiences and solutions to problems and daily care challenges. A common activity is sharing pictures, which the newer parents often use as a peek into the future of their own child.

Cleft Palate as a Chronic Medical Condition

Dealing with the medical system is a common event in the lives of parents with babies with clefts. Visits to physicians may be experienced as reminders of the baby's anomaly or as evaluation of their efficacy as parents. Charting the infant's growth is important but may be more threatening when feeding has been a major challenge. Contacts with health professionals also raise the possibility, regardless of actual probability, of hearing more bad news. It is very important to parents that health care professionals relate to their child as a person, not an assortment of physical problems.

The first surgery, (when relevant, usually closing the lip), is often a stressful and frightening time for family members. Having a helpless, little baby taken from their arms for surgery reawakens many of the sad, frightened, and protective feelings that may have quieted since the birth. Moreover, it places the parents and other family members in direct confrontation with their powerlessness to fix the baby's problems themselves. Parents and grandparents "make it all better" for their children for many of the normal challenges of growing up. This role is impossible when surgery is required. Parents have to trust the surgeon and all of the professionals involved and let go, often leaving them feeling out of control of the situation. There is always at least a bit of concern that something may go wrong and that the baby could die. The decision for parents as to whether surgery is worth the risk only becomes more complicated as the child grows older and the emphasis is more on appearance.

Additionally, children with a history of cleft have been found to show negative mood and behavior changes following surgery. In one of the rare longitudinal studies of children with a history of cleft who have had surgery, Koomen and Hoeksma (1993) found changes in behavior that primarily had to do with the increased desire of the infants to be in the presence of or in contact with their mothers. They interpreted their findings as suggesting that attachment to parents may be impaired by cleft repair and its attendant hospitalization. On the other hand, their findings were inconsistent and their significance outside the laboratory of some question.

Helping parents recognize that they hold a unique role with their children that no health professional can take over is often important, especially in the case of prolonged hospitalizations. Practical advice about staying with the infant during the entire hospitalization, preparing siblings for the event and the baby's changed appearance, and caring for the baby after surgery can increase a parent's sense of being able to contribute to the child's well-being. For the baby, having a parent or other familiar adult available during the entire time he or she is in the hospital for surgery is important for security and comfort.

Some aspects of dealing with the medical system will continue to be problematic for parents for years. Even when there are positive relationships between health care professionals and parents, the medical system is still often quite overwhelming. The demands of the system in terms of paperwork and insurance approval, the expense involved, the complexity of the layout of many hospitals, and the experience of seeing their child as others, especially plastic surgeons, see their child can lead to a variety of negative feelings. Frustration with the system can be directed at important professionals as anger and even lead to nonadherence to the medical regimen.

The intensity of the family members' negative feelings about the child's cleft and the associated stressors usually diminishes over time, with resurgent peaks at times of surgery, social rejection, or the child's own distress. Parents often experience some fatigue during the whole process and are eager for everything to be done. Conflict or disagreement between the mother and father or between parents and the older child about medical decisions is not unusual, especially during the teen years. Fears may be reawakened when the teenager or adult with a history of a cleft moves into a serious relationship where reproductive and, hence, genetic issues are important.

When a parent has a history of cleft, these issues have an added dimension. It usually, if not accurately, resolves the question of why the child had a cleft. Although the parent is in an unusually good position to be knowledgeably empathic with the child's situation, there is also the risk that unresolved negative experiences from the parent's past may color his or her responses to the challenges facing the child. Sometimes parents make decisions that reflect an attempt to "get it right this time." It is particularly important to help the parent see differences between his or her situation and that of the child's. An important factor here is the advancement of surgical techniques since the parent's own repair.

Although having a child with a cleft is stressful, there is no evidence that it leads to a higher frequency of psychiatric symptoms in parents. An older study (Goodstein, 1960) compared the personality profiles of parents of children with a history of cleft to those of parents of children with no known abnormalities. Using the *Minnesota Multiphasic Personality Inventory*, the researchers found no significant differences between the groups and no unique patterns emerged. Similarly, a large interview study found that parents of children with a history of cleft, as a group, reported the same kinds of social life, recreation, and entertainment as the group of parents of children without anomalies.

School Issues

Knowledge and Expectation of Teachers

Teachers have reported not knowing very much about cleft lip and palate (like most of the population). They often have little information, and some of it may be incorrect. Teachers as a group have also been found to underestimate the intelligence of children with a history of cleft, especially when either appearance or speech is quite impaired. They also may expect less from the children who look different than those who appear normal (Richman & Eliason, 1982). These underestimates shape their expectations for the children and may result in lower performance and less positive evaluation of the children's academic performance. Several studies have found that children with clefts do not achieve to the level that would be predicted by intelligence alone.

Learning Ability and School Performance

Intelligence, as measured by formal IQ tests, seems to be in the average range for children with a history of cleft but no other identified syndromes. By contrast, children with various syndromes that may include clefts tend to score lower on intelligence tests. Children with a history of cleft, however, generally score lower on test sections that require verbal skills, especially oral responses, than they do on more performance-based sections. In particular, children with cleft palate only show more speech and language disorders than both nonaffected peers and those with cleft lip and palate (Broen, Devers, Doyle, Prouty, & Moller, 1998; Estes & Morris, 1970; Goodstein, 1961; Lamb, Wilson, & Leeper, 1973; Ruess, 1965; Wirls, 1971). They are also more likely to have serious reading disabilities, often evident in the primary grades

(Richman & Millard, 1997). Some studies have found that over half of children with cleft palate only show significant reading problems in first- and second-grade years. A full third still show reading problems at age 13. However, many of the supporting studies are older and may not have differentiated children with syndromes, such as velocardiofacial syndrome, confounding the results. Other studies have found that children with a history of cleft and speech problems often lack self-confidence in reading aloud, which may influence the teacher's evaluation of their abilities.

Teenagers with a history of cleft do not show a greater dropout rate than their unaffected peers. As a group they attain the same educational levels as other young adults. In fact, one study in Europe found persons with a history of cleft had a lower rate of dropping out than their peers (Ramstad, Ottem, & Shaw 1995b).

Social Interaction

In the early years of a child's life, the social issues are mainly experienced by the parents. They are the ones who note the stares or answer the questions about the child's condition. By the preschool years, however, the child starts to be asked directly about what happened to his or her lip. Sometimes the question comes from well-meaning adults who believe the child's scar to be from a fall or a minor accident. Other times, it comes from curious peers who notice a difference in the child's appearance. While preschool children prefer attractive children as friends, they are rarely cruel or tease their peers. They notice differences in appearance, speech, and behavior, but unless the differences interfere, they are not generally important for play relationships. One of the advantages of enrolling children with a history of cleft in good preschool or day care programs is the opportunity to build social skills and confidence when parents are not present at a time when teasing and rudeness is rare.

By school age, a significant number of children with a history of cleft do not have as many friendships as other children their age. This situation appears to be a result of the interaction of several factors. First, children with a history of cleft, especially girls, seem to be more socially inhibited than their peers. They are sometimes reluctant to risk new friendships; other times, they have difficulty in initiating and maintaining new friendships. Second, the lack of friends may relate to the interaction challenges associated with hearing impairment and speech difficulties. Third, appearance may be a contributor as well. Joyce Tobiasen (1988, 1989) showed pictures of children to second through fourth graders. Some of the children in the pictures had no cleft, some had a unilateral cleft, and some had a bilateral cleft visible in the photographs. The viewers rated the pictured children on personal qualities. Children rated those with a bilateral cleft as having fewer positive attributes than those with a unilateral cleft, and both cleft groups fared worse than the children without a visible cleft. The younger viewers were harsher in their ratings than the somewhat older ones. The degree of facial impairment is strongly correlated with perceptions of attractiveness and social desirability. On the other hand, an individual child's social relationships cannot be accurately predicted on the basis of facial attractiveness alone. The child's temperament, family support, social skills, and coping strategies also make a difference in that regard. Interestingly, children with a history of cleft tend to describe having more friends than their peers acknowledge. This may reflect misjudgment of what constitutes friendship or perhaps lower expectations for what constitutes a friend.

In most studies, older children and teenagers reported significant concerns about interpersonal relationships. The trend toward overinhibition and shyness continues into adolescence. Although the frequency of dating relationships among young people with a history of cleft relative to their peers has not been studied, it appears that teens with a history of cleft show more self-doubts and have lower expectations for relationships than their peers. Adults with a history of cleft have been found to marry later than their peers and siblings. In studies in other countries, adults have been seen as generally showing good psychological adjustment, but fewer were in long-term relationships or married. Women, in particular, worried about their appearance.

Teasing

Teasing is one social problem that parents worry about from early times. Most children, regardless of cleft status, are teased at least occasionally by peers. On the other hand, longstanding, cruel teasing that results in ostracism is not a common childhood occurrence. Although the conclusion is not as solid as some, it appears that children with a history of cleft are teased more often than their peers without a cleft. It seems to be at least influenced by physical appearance and speech differences because children tend to report less teasing after surgeries that address those problems. Other factors that affect teasing appear to be the child's personality and social standing, response to teasing, and adult response to peer teasing. Children who laugh off teasing or respond in kind appear to be teased less than those who respond with distress or helpless anger. Use of humor seems to be particularly helpful. Similarly, attributing teasing to a flaw in the person who does the teasing rather than to him- or herself is protective of the child's self-esteem. Recognizing that cruel comments about a cleft reflect ignorance about a topic well understood by the child as well as a lack of either compassion or kindness puts the blame squarely on the person making the comments, rather than the person commented upon.

Adult response, especially at school, influences the likelihood of teasing. Helping the child to present information about the cleft and the various surgeries can reduce teasing, especially among children in lower grades. It reduces the uncertainty of peers, activates empathy in some of the children, and generally reduces the status of the cleft as a sensitive spot to hit when teasing. Children of any age reduce the frequency of teasing when school officials take an active role in demonstrating that respect for all students is expected. On the other hand, when teasing is viewed as an inevitable behavior of children ("Kids will be cruel, there's not much we can do about it."), teasing is more likely to continue or increase.

Teasing tends to diminish or take on a friendlier tone by high school for all adolescents, including those with a history of cleft. There is a greater understanding of clefts and a generally greater acceptance of differences. When unpleasant teasing does continue, however, it can take on a cruel edge and even a group acceptance that may result in social withdrawal. Some social scientists see this kind of teasing as having the same power and domination quality as more general "bullying." Most adults report that teasing and social intimidation are not part of their lives.

Self-Perception

All children develop a concept of themselves over time and part of that concept is the worth that they feel themselves to have. Because children have not developed a clear sense of self at early ages, most studies begin at school age. Children with a history of cleft have been consistently found to have more negative self-concepts compared to their unaffected peers (Broder & Strauss, 1989; Kapp-Simon, 1986). They see themselves as less acceptable to their peers and more often report that they are sad or angry. Broder and Strauss (1989) found that children with both cleft lip and palate scored lower than those with an "invisible" cleft palate

only, but children with a history of any type of cleft rated themselves less well than children without any cleft. Higher levels of acceptance of the cleft were associated with better self-concepts. In school-aged children with a history of cleft, greater physical attractiveness correlated with better overall adjustment (Pillemer & Cook, 1989). Similarly, satisfaction with their own appearance was related to the adjustment and older teens and young adults were more satisfied than their younger counterparts (Thomas, Turner, Rumsey, Dowell, & Sandy, 1997). There is some evidence that having appearance-altering surgeries before the teen years contributes to better self-esteem and less social isolation (Pertschuk & Whitaker, 1982).

Teenagers who view themselves "realistically," that is, in agreement with their peers and familiar adults tend to be better adjusted. Generally teenagers have been found to have more negative feelings about themselves than younger children. Brantley and Clifford (1979) asked teenagers to report what they thought their parents felt and experienced when they were born. Teens with a history of cleft said that their parents experienced predominantly negative emotions and did not care to nurture them. Relative to teens with asthma, obesity, or no physical problems, adolescents with a history of cleft reported their parents had higher levels of apprehension and felt less pride in them. Physical appearance concerns are consistently greater in persons with a history of cleft across the life span, but in later adolescence and adulthood, women report greater feelings of self-consciousness than their male counterparts. Clifford, Crocker, and Pope (1972) found that dissatisfaction with appearance centered on the face, especially the mouth. Adults with a history of cleft lip were less satisfied with facial appearance than those with a history of cleft palate only, while people with a history of cleft palate were more displeased with their speech than those with a history of cleft lip only. More dissatisfaction with their mouth, teeth, lips, voice, and speech was expressed by both cleft groups than the control group of adults with no a history of cleft.

Adults with a history of cleft continue to report some levels of psychological distress. Ramstad, Ottem, and Shaw (1995a) surveying Norwegian adults with a history of cleft found higher levels of anxiety and depression than in unaffected controls. Their symptoms were strongly associated with more concerns about appearance, dentition, speech, and the hope of more treatment. The same researchers (1995b) also reported that adults with a cleft were less likely to marry than adults without a history of cleft and when they did marry, it was often later in life. This was particularly true of the group with bilateral cleft lip and palate. Other studies, in other countries have found similar results. Although education and employment per se did not differ between those with a history of cleft and the controls, people with a history of cleft appeared to make less money.

It should be noted that the rates of diagnosed psychiatric disorders for children and teens with a history of cleft appears no different than that of the population of children as a whole. In one study of the 600 most disturbed children in a large urban school district, not one had a cleft. More typical studies, comparing children with a history of cleft to children with other physical problems or to children with no medical difficulties, have found little difference among the groups. Research to identify a "cleft palate personality" has consistently failed to yield evidence of a consistent or specific organization or style of personality in children, adolescents, or adults with a history of cleft. The biggest risk appears to be for social competence problems, including those relating to development of friendships and participating in organizations (Richman & Eliason, 1982).

Societal Issues

Physical Attractiveness

One of the forces at work for a child with a cleft is society's response to facial difference.

Physical attractiveness, especially facial beauty, is an area that has been well researched, with findings among the most reliable and robust in the psychological literature. Some characteristics that people see as attractive or unattractive are cross-cultural; for example, there is no group of people known to find highly blemished skin to be attractive. Other characteristics considered attractive vary considerably among cultures, but even then, attractiveness tends to focus on facial features and body shape. There is some evidence that mouth shape is especially important across cultures, even though the specific standard for beauty may differ. Dental differences certainly carry meaning for adults, although it is less clear in the case of children.

Within a culture, there is considerable consensus about general characteristics of attractiveness. This consensus develops early. By preschool age, children know the standards of beauty that the adults hold and share those values. In fact, until recently one of the items on a commonly used intelligence test for children required them to choose the picture of the "pretty" woman from two choices. This could serve as a developmental test only because the cultural concept of beauty normally is learned prior to age 4.

More important than the consensual nature of cultural standards of beauty are the meanings associated with being considered either attractive or unattractive. In a nutshell, beauty is equated with goodness. More attractive people are rated as smarter, more friendly, nicer, more likely to be a good friend, and kinder than those who are less attractive. Ethnologists have found that characteristics in babies, such as a round head, large eyes, and short and narrow features are rated as "cute" (witness how most people respond to pandas) and elicit caregiving behaviors from adults. Infants considered to be highly attractive tend to be rated as more likable, smarter, and less problematic. The significance of these meanings lies in their power to shape the behavior and attitudes of people, directly and indirectly. These, in turn, become part of the feedback loop that shapes how an individual behaves and views himself or herself.

Physical attractiveness is important across the life span. Cute babies are attributed characteristics that their less attractive peers are not. Preschoolers prefer attractive children as their friends and the social power of attractiveness continues to increase until early grade school years and then tends to hold steady until adolescence. Teachers also have more favorable expectations of attractive children than unattractive children (Clifford, 1975). Teachers may respond differentially to more physically attractive children and their grades are often higher than those of less attractive peers. Being seen with attractive people increases a person's social desirability. Attractive teens are more likely to be elected to school office than other youth and, no surprise to most people, date more frequently and have a higher number of partners. Unattractive people are more likely to be found guilty of crimes and get less help from strangers in time of need. Physical attractiveness affects the likelihood of being hired for a job, even when public contact is not a major factor. It may also influence job performance evaluations. The power of physical attractiveness appears to hold in middle and older age as well, but this is less well established. People sometimes hope that this influence only holds at first impression, but research suggests that this is not the case. Although physical attractiveness is only one of many variables contributing to social responses to a person, it is a powerful force indeed.

Speech Quality

The quality of a person's speech is a factor rather similar to physical attractiveness. First, the quality of a person's speech impacts on social judgments of others, which in turn help shape behaviors and attitudes. Second, good speech appears to be associated in the minds of listeners with the assumption that the speaker has positive characteristics. While children are less likely to initiate conversations with those with impaired speech, adults associate children's speech problems with undesirable personal characteristics. Many adults with dysarthric speech have commented that, no matter what it is they are saying, they feel their comments are discounted or they are assumed to be retarded or "stupid." This experience has also been noted by adults with acquired speech disorders. Although cultural differences exist in these stereotypes, listeners often believe that people with speech disorders are more likely to be emotionally disturbed (Bebout & Bradford, 1992).

Although the area has not been thoroughly researched, it appears that speech quality and facial appearance interact with each other socially. Facial attractiveness may not change ratings of speech quality, but impaired speech seems to lower ratings of physical attractiveness of the speaker. Hypernasality appears to be particularly unattractive to listeners, so that ratings of social desirability of a speaker decrease steadily as nasality increases. Clifford (1987), a well-known psychologist studying effects of cleft lip and palate, called the results of the combination "a lack of perceived competence."

Hearing Impairment

Although speech quality is, of course, not entirely independent of hearing impairment, being hard of hearing appears to have some unique addition to the social judgments people make. Many children with a history of cleft have some degree of hearing impairment, which may vary with the frequency of recurrent ear infections. Negative stereotypes exist of people who have hearing impairments, with or without visible hearing aids. More importantly however, hearing is central to many aspects of social interactions among members of the general population. Misunderstanding of overall meaning or nuance shapes the next phase of interaction. When a person is perceived as missing the intention of a communication, he or she is often viewed as annoying or

Case Study: The Social and Emotional Effect of Facial Anomalies and Speech Defects

Sandy was a 14-year-old Caucasian girl who was born with a bilateral cleft lip and palate. When she came to the Craniofacial Team meeting, she was minimally interactive and looked down rather than establishing eye contact. She was cooperative in answering questions and allowing professionals to examine her, however. She said that she wanted any surgery that would improve her appearance or speech.

Her mother reported that Sandy had always seemed shy and somewhat withdrawn. She had one long-time neighborhood girl friend, but no one else called or came over to play. When she was in first and second grade, she was teased a great deal, especially by two boys who seemed to enjoy making her cry. Their favorite epithet was "Flat Nose" but they had a variety of insults and imitated her speech. When she was teased on the playground, she moved nearer the playground supervisor but never told her what was happening. The school bus was the worst, and when Sandy was younger, her mother had arranged for her to sit near the driver to reduce the cruelty.

Sandy's grades were in the average range, but the teachers reported that she did not speak in class unless called upon by name. Even then, she tended not to respond.

At home, Sandy was generally well behaved. She interacted freely with family members, displaying a good sense of humor. She was loyal to her family members and had a specially close relationship with her 3-year-old niece. The family rarely talked about her cleft because it was "not a big deal" to them and they didn't want to upset Sandy. They realized she was having a hard time and tried to be supportive, telling her to ignore the people who teased her because they hadn't taken the time to get to know her as a person.

Because Sandy was reluctant to talk at the team meeting, an appointment was made to see her individually. Eye contact was poor at first, but by the end of the first session, Sandy was able to talk about how she always felt different from the other kids. She sobbed as she described how she hated looking and sounding "different" and felt that it was understandable that no one wanted to be her friend. Teasing hurt her deeply and she felt she could avoid it if she didn't say anything or look at people. She said she was not suicidal but that the thought had crossed her mind when she considered going to high school next year where there would be new people and demands. She had begun to think about the future, feeling she might never be able to get a good job or get married because of her cleft. She also feared that if she had children, they would have a cleft and would have to go through the same things she did.

Sandy frequently wondered why the cleft had happened to her. When she was younger, she secretly blamed her mother because in health class, they had learned that alcohol can cause clefts. Through her contacts with Genetics at the team meetings, she had realized that this was not the cause in her case, but she still felt like she was being punished somehow, for something. She had been taught that God had created her the way she was for a reason, but it felt as if it were an act of cruel humor.

This case illustrates the kind of experiences, reactions, and feelings that may be associated with clefts. Although these may vary in degree and frequency, they are common for people with craniofacial anomalies. While psychological interviews can help to identify the issues so intervention is possible, the interactions with any professional treating the child may be influenced by emotional and social factors. In turn, those interactions may influence the person's psychological experience and functioning.

frustrating. With repetition, interactions may be avoided. This is another example of the importance of the social feedback loop.

Stigma

The concept of stigma is a common thread unifying all three areas described above. Stigma is the discrediting and objectifying of individuals based on difference from cultural standards. In the case of persons with craniofacial anomalies, they are evaluated in a negative fashion because of their visible difference from the cultural standards of beauty, speech, hearing, and/or social interactions. Stigma diminishes a person's social acceptability, negatively impacting self-esteem. Another effect is the reduction or blocking of social and economic opportunities. The impact of stigmatization may be felt in the absence of negative intent, as when people stare out of curiosity, ignorance, or sympathy. Essentially, it is a problem of people being defined by their stigma and coming to anticipate stigmatization as well. They then may behave accordingly, as if stigmatized, regardless of the behavior or attitudes of the other people involved in interactions. People who are disfigured are particularly vulnerable to stigma. Some studies have suggested that mouth differences may be particularly open to negativity.

Summary

If a child is born with a cleft lip and/or palate, it does not mean that he or she is certain to develop psychopathology. However, having a facial difference complicates life and presents challenges on many levels, challenges that children without medical problems generally do not face. These challenges are not restricted to the child, but extend to the family of the child as well. In fact, early in the child's development, the majority of the psychological "fallout" of a child's cleft is its effect on the family, rather than on the child. Later, the challenges to the individual seem most often to be related to school achievement (especially reading) and peer relationships. People with a history of cleft appear to be particularly at risk of diminished social interaction and sense of social competence.

Because of the prevalence and intensity of the feelings and problems affecting people with a history of cleft and their families, it is strongly recommended that craniofacial or cleft palate teams have a psychologist or similar professional as a member. Additionally, the cognitive differences that may affect learning and social interactions can often best be addressed through the work of the team psychologist. If a psychologist cannot be included as a member of the team, the next best option is to have a skilled pediatric psychologist, trained in issues related to clefts, available on a referral basis. In any case, the psychologist needs to communicate with other team members to facilitate continuity of care and to address the behaviors and attitudes that can interfere with optimal outcome.

References

Andrews-Casal, M., Johnston, D., Fletcher, J., Mulliken, J. B. , Stal, S., & Hecht, J. T. (1998). Cleft lip with or without cleft palate: Effect of family history on reproductive planning, surgical timing, and parental stress. *Cleft Palate Craniofacial Journal, 35*(1), 52–57.

Bebout, L., & Bradford, A. (1992). Cross-cultural attitudes toward speech disorders. *Journal of Speech and Hearing Research 35*(1), 45–52.

Bradbury, E. T., & Hewison, J., (1994). Early parental adjustment to visible congenital disfigurement. *Child Care Health and Development, 20*(4), 251–266.

Brantley, H. T., & Clifford, E. (1979). Maternal and child locus of control and field dependence in cleft palate children. *Cleft Palate Journal, 16,* 183–187.

Broder, H., & Strauss, R. (1989). Self-concept of early primary school age children with visible or invisible defects. *Cleft Palate Journal, 26*(2), 114–117.

Broen, P. A., Devers, M. C., Doyle, S. S., Prouty, J. M., & Moller, K. T. (1998). Acquisition of linguistic and cognitive skills by children with cleft palate. *Journal of Speech, Language, and Hearing Research, 41*(3), 676–687.

Clifford, E. (1969). Paternal ratings of cleft palate infants. *Cleft Palate Journal, 6,* 235–243.

Clifford, E. (1971). Cleft palate and the person: Psychological studies of its impact. *Journal of Southern Medical Association, 12,* 1516–1520.

Clifford, E. (1987). *The cleft palate experience: New perspectives on management.* Springfield, IL: Charles C. Thomas.

Clifford, E., Crocker, E. C., & Pope, B. A. (1972). Psychological findings in the adulthood of 98 cleft palate children. *Journal of Plastic and Reconstructive Surgery, 50,* 234.

Clifford, M. M. (1975). Physical attractiveness and academic performance. *Child Study Journal, 5,* 201–209.

Estes, R. E., & Morris, H. L. (1970). Relationships among intelligence, speech proficiency, and hearing sensitivity in children with cleft palates. *Cleft Palate Journal, 7,* 763–773.

Goodstein, L. D. (1960). MMPI differences between parents of children with cleft palate and parents of physically normal children. *Journal of Speech and Hearing Research, 3,* 31–38.

Goodstein, L. D. (1961). Intellectual impairment in children with cleft palates. *Journal of Speech and Hearing Research, 4,* 287–294.

Kapp-Simon, K. (1986). Self-concept of primary school age children with cleft lip, cleft palate or both. *Cleft Palate Journal, 23*(1), 24–27.

Koomen, H., & Hoeksma, J. (1993). Early hospitalization and disturbances of infant behavior and the mother-infant relationship. *Journal of Child Psychology and Psychiatry, 34*(6), 917–934.

Lamb, M., Wilson, F., & Leeper, H. (1973). The intellectual function of cleft palate children compared on the basis of cleft type and sex. *Cleft Palate Journal, 10,* 367.

Middleton, G. N., Lass, N. J., Starr, P., & Pannbacker, M. (1986). Survey of public awareness and knowledge of cleft palate. *Cleft Palate Journal, 23,* 58–63.

Pertschuk, M. J., & Whitaker, L. A. (1982). Social and psychological effects of craniofacial deformity and surgical reconstruction. *Clinical Plastic Surgery, 9*(3), 297–306.

Pillemer, F. G., & Cook, K. V. (1989). The psychosocial adjustment of pediatric craniofacial patients after surgery. *Cleft Palate Journal, 26*(3), 201–207.

Ramstad, T. E., Ottem, E, & Shaw, W. C. (1995a). Psychosocial adjustment in Norwegian adults who had undergone standardised treatment of complete cleft lip and palate: II. Self-reported problems and concerns with appearance. *Scandinavian Journal of Plastic and Reconstructive Surgery and Hand Surgery, 29*(4), 329–336.

Ramstad, T. E., Ottem, E., & Shaw, W. C. (1995b). Psychosocial adjustment in Norwegian adults who had undergone standardised treatment of complete cleft lip and palate: I. Education, employment and marriage. *Scandinavian Journal of Plastic and Reconstructive Surgery and Hand Surgery, 29*(3), 251–257.

Richman, L. C., & Eliason, M. (1982). Psychological characteristics of children with cleft lip and palate: Intellectual, achievement, behavioral, and personality variables. *Cleft Palate Journal, 19,* 249.

Richman, L. C., & Millard, T. (1997). Brief report: Cleft lip and palate: Longitudinal behavior and relationships of cleft conditions to behavior and achievement. *Journal of Pediatric Psychology, 22*(4), 487–494.

Ruess, A. L. (1965). A comparative study of cleft palate children and their siblings. *Journal of Clinical Psychology, 21,* 354.

Speltz, M. G., Armsden, G. C., & Clarren, S. S. (1990). Effects of craniofacial birth defects on maternal functioning postinfancy. *Journal of Pediatric Psychology, 15*(2), 177–196.

Strauss, R. P., Sharp, M. C., Lorch, S. C., & Kachalia, B. (1995). Physicians communication of "bad news"—Parent experiences of being informed of their child's cleft lip/palate. *Pediatrics, 96*(1), 82–89.

Thomas, P. S., Turner, S. R., Rumsey, N., Dowell, T., & Sandy, J. R. (1997). Satisfaction with facial appearance among subjects affected by a cleft. *Cleft Palate Craniofacial Journal, 34*(3), 226–231.

Tobiasen, J. M. (1988). Psychosocial outcome of craniofacial surgery in children: Discussion. *Plastic and Reconstructive Surgery, 82*, 745–746.

Tobiasen, J. M. (1989). Scaling facial impairment. *Cleft Palate Journal, 26*(3), 249–254.

van Staden, F., & Gerhardt, C. (1995). Mothers of children with facial cleft deformities: Reactions and effects. *South American Journal of Psychology, 25*(1), 39–46.

Wirls, C. J. (1971). Psychosocial aspects of cleft lip and palate. In W. C. Grabb, S. W. Rosenstein, & K. Bzoch (Eds.), *Cleft lip and palate* (p. 119). Boston: Little, Brown.

PART III

Interdisciplinary Care

CHAPTER

11

The Team Approach to Assessment and Treatment

CONTENTS

Individuals with craniofacial anomalies, including cleft lip and palate, have a variety of medical, surgical, dental, psychological, and communication problems. It is not possible for one professional to deal with all of these areas of concern. Therefore, patients with craniofacial anomalies require evaluation and treatment from a variety of professionals, and this is needed over a long period of time (Paynter, Wilson, & Jordan, 1993). Even the most knowledgeable of families would have difficulty coordinating the multitude of appointments and procedures for their child if the care was provided without the benefits of an interdisciplinary team. Without interdisciplinary communication and coordination of treatment procedures, the ultimate outcome of treatment could also be negatively affected.

The main purpose this chapter is to impress upon the reader the importance of the team approach in the management of patients with cleft lip/palate or craniofacial anomalies. This chapter discusses the advantages and some of the problems with team management. The types and characteristics of teams are described. Finally, information is given on how to find a specialty team in order to refer a child for further assessment and intervention as appropriate.

Need for Team Management

There are many qualified professionals throughout the United States, and in fact the world, who can care for patients with craniofacial anomalies. However, as part of the habilitation process, it is common for the treatment of one professional to have an impact on the treatment of the other professionals. In addition, the sequence of treatment from each discipline must be considered. Therefore, services to this population of patients must be provided in a coordinated and integrated manner over a period of years for maximum benefit to the patient. To accomplish this, the team approach to management is required for these patients.

With the team approach, the patient is more likely to receive quality services, continuity of care, and long-term follow-up to achieve the best ultimate outcome. In addition, the team approach allows the care to focus on the whole child, and not just the cleft or one particular abnormality.

The importance of team management for patients with cleft lip and palate was first recognized by H. K. Cooper, who founded the Lancaster Cleft Palate Clinic in the early 1930s (Krogman, 1979). Many cleft palate or craniofacial teams were formed across the country in subsequent years. In 1987, the Surgeon General of the United States recognized the need for a team approach to the management of patients with special health care needs, and articulated this need in a report (Surgeon General's Report, 1987). This report emphasized that these children require comprehensive, coordinated care provided by health care systems that are accessible and responsive to the patients and their families.

In response to this report, the Maternal and Child Health Bureau provided funding to the American Cleft Palate-Craniofacial Association (ACPA) to develop recommended practices in the care of patients with craniofacial anomalies. To accomplish this, a large group of various professionals from around the country was convened for a consensus conference in 1991. This meeting resulted in a comprehensive document published by the ACPA containing parameters for evaluation and treatment of patients with clefts or craniofacial anomalies (American Cleft Palate-Craniofacial Association, 1993). One of the fundamental principles contained in this document is that the "management of patients with craniofacial anomalies is best provided by an interdisciplinary team of specialists" (p. 5).

There is general consensus among professionals regarding the importance of a team approach to the care of patients with cleft lip/palate or craniofacial anomalies. This approach has the advantages of multidisciplinary teamwork, centralization of services, team continuity, long-term treatment planning from birth to adulthood, comprehensive documentation from all professionals involved in the patient's care, interdisciplinary evaluations, follow-up studies, and interdisciplinary research and quality assurance (Tindlund & Holmefjord, 1997). The team approach makes the care of patients easier for the provider, yet more effective for the patient.

Characteristics of Teams

Types of Teams

A team of professionals can be multidisciplinary or interdisciplinary, depending on the working relationship of the members and the structure of the team. A *multidisciplinary team* is a group of professionals from various disciplines who work independently in evaluating and treating patients with complex medical needs. The members of this type of team have well-defined roles and cooperate with each other, but there is little communication and interaction among the team members (Bardach et al., 1984; Strauss, 1999). The biggest problem with a multidisciplinary team is that the patent receives a series of evaluations and recommendations, but there is no integration of the information or recommendations.

On the other hand, an *interdisciplinary team* is a group of professionals from various disciplines who work together to coordinate the care of a patient. In this model, there is collaboration, interaction, communication, and cooperation among the different specialists who are involved in the patient's care. There may or may not be a joint evaluation, but there definitely is a joint plan of care. This is developed when all members of the team come together to discuss the findings, impressions, and recommendations. The final plan of care is negotiated and based on the integration of all the recommendations (Strauss, 1999). With this

approach, the sequence of procedures and approximate timelines can be outlined for the patient and the family. Therefore, the interdisciplinary team model is felt to be the most effective one for management of patients with craniofacial anomalies.

A cleft palate or craniofacial team whose members work together for a period of time may even evolve into a *transdisciplinary team.* This type of team has members who truly understand the other disciplines and how they relate to the total care of the patient. Although team members cannot perform duties across disciplines, they can have an understanding of the various disciplines in order to see the "big picture." This is certainly a benefit for the ultimate care of the patient.

Cleft palate or craniofacial teams often serve as the primary *treating team* for their patients. In larger centers, the team may also serve as a *consulting team.* In the role as a consulting team, the team members as a group provide a second opinion regarding the total care of the patient. This is forwarded to the treating professionals for consideration. The treating professionals may be in the local community or may be far away. Regardless, there must be excellent communication between the team and the practitioners who will be following the patient for treatment and follow-up care.

Team Membership and Structure

Typically, cleft palate or craniofacial teams include medical, surgical, dental, speech, and psychosocial professionals in order to meet the complex needs of the patient and their families. Table 11–1 lists the various professionals who are often members of a cleft or craniofacial team, and it describes each professional's role in the management of these patients. In 1996, the membership of the ACPA established basic standards for what constitutes a cleft or a craniofacial team (American Cleft Palate-Craniofacial Association, 1993). Teams that meet these standards are listed in the ACPA Membership-Team Directory,

TABLE 11-1. Professional roles on a cleft palate or craniofacial anomaly team.

Audiologist: The audiologist is the person who is responsible for testing the child's hearing and middle ear function. Because individuals with craniofacial anomalies are at high risk for structural ear anomalies, middle-ear disease, and hearing loss, the audiologist works with the otolaryngologist in monitoring the hearing and middle-ear function of these individuals.

Pediatric Dentist: The role of the pediatric dentist (sometimes called pedodontist) is to be responsible for the general care of the child's teeth and the prevention and treatment of tooth decay. The pediatric dentist ensures that the child develops habits of good oral hygiene for the promotion of healthy teeth and gums. Even the primary teeth are important to protect and preserve since they act as placeholders for the permanent teeth. The pediatric dentist may be involved with managing misaligned cleft segments prior to the lip closure. When the child is in the primary or mixed dentition stages, the pediatric dentist is often the one to improve early malocclusion, which often includes moving the maxillary segments through palatal expansion.

Geneticist: A geneticist (dysmorphologist) is responsible for assessing patients with a history of cleft, velopharyngeal dysfunction, or craniofacial anomalies for a pattern to indicate a known syndrome. Once a syndrome is identified, the geneticist counsels the family regarding the diagnosis, the recurrence risk for additional offspring of the family and for offspring of the patient, and the prognosis.

Neurosurgeon: The neurosurgeon is important in the evaluation and treatment of patients with certain craniofacial syndromes, particularly those with craniosynostosis. The neurosurgeon monitors intracranial pressure and brain anomalies and surgically intervenes as necessary. The neurosurgeon and plastic surgeon often work together to perform cranial vault and orbital remodeling procedures.

Nurse: The nurse's role on the team is to assess the child's overall physical development. The nurse can determine if the child is growing normally and is in good general health. With the help of the speech pathologist, the nurse is often the professional who assists the family in feeding techniques. Finally, the nurse is usually the professional who counsels the family regarding surgical procedures and answers their specific questions.

Ophthalmologist: The ophthalmologist evaluates congenital eye anomalies, such as colobomas, epidermoid cysts and cranial nerve palsy, and other ophthalmologic conditions, such as strabismus. This professional evaluates and treats vision loss, including myopia, which is characteristic of Stickler's syndrome. In patients with craniosynostosis, the ophthalmologist monitors the effects of increased intracranial pressure on vision. Treatment of these conditions may include surgery to the globe or the eye musculature.

Oral Surgeon: The oral surgeon is the specialist who does bone grafts to the alveolar cleft areas when there is deficient bone in the line of the cleft. This professional also performs the orthognathic surgeries, including maxillary expansions and mandibular setbacks to normalize the occlusion between the maxillary and mandibular arches.

Orthodontist: The orthodontist treats dental and skeletal malocclusion and promotes normal jaw relationships. The orthodontist is responsible for aligning misplaced teeth and adjacent tissues to improve the dental and facial aesthetics and to improve the function of the dentition.

Otolaryngologist: The otolaryngologist, also known as the ear, nose, and throat (ENT) specialist, is responsible for monitoring middle-ear function and hearing and treating middle ear disease, which is common in children with a history of cleft or craniofacial anomalies. The otolaryngologist also assesses the structural aspects of the oral cavity, oropharynx, nasal cavity, and upper airway and treats anomalies, including adenotonsillar hypertrophy, pharyngeal masses, or vocal fold nodules. The otolaryngologist may be the surgeon involved in the nasal and oral reconstruction or surgery for velopharyngeal dysfunction. The otolaryngologist also manages upper airway obstruction, which is particularly common in infants with Pierre Robin sequence.

TABLE 11-1. *(continued)*

Pediatrician: The pediatrician is responsible for assessing the patient's overall medical health, growth, and development. The pediatrician determines if other aspects of medical care should be done prior to surgical intervention.

Plastic Surgeon: The plastic surgeon is responsible for the surgical repair of the lip, the palate, facial anomalies, and also for the surgery for correction of velopharyngeal dysfunction. This surgeon may do cranial surgery, bone grafts, and orthognathic surgery on the jaws. The plastic surgeon is responsible for not only the repair of the defects, but also for the improvement of the overall facial aesthetics, function, and speech through surgery.

Prosthodontist: Prosthodontics is a branch of dentistry that deals with the restoration of natural teeth or the replacement of missing teeth. The prosthodontist can develop prosthetic devices to replace or improve the appearance of not only the teeth, but also the surrounding oral and facial structures. The prosthodontist can also manufacture and fit devices to assist with feeding and with velopharyngeal closure.

Psychologist: The psychologist assesses the patient's psychosocial needs and assists the patient and family in dealing with the medical, social, and emotional challenges that occur due to the patient's anomalies. The psychologist often assists the physician in determining the preparedness of the patient for each surgical procedure.

Social Worker: The social worker helps families to deal with the many problems associated with the child's anomalies. The social worker may be the one to coordinate appointments and may also assist the families in dealing with insurance and other funding sources. The social worker may help the family to manage their stress and emotional reactions to the many problems and issues associated with the child's treatment.

Speech-Language Pathologist (SLP): The speech-language pathologist counsels the parents or guardians regarding what to expect with communication skills and how to stimulate normal development at home. The speech-language pathologist evaluates feeding and swallowing, general development, speech, language, resonance, and velopharyngeal function and makes recommendations for treatment when problems are identified. The speech-language pathologist provides therapy for communication problems and disorders of feeding or swallowing.

Team Coordinator: The team coordinator is typically the representative of the team to parents, other health care professionals and the community. This person is responsible for planning the meetings and scheduling patients for each meeting. The coordinator compiles the recommendations from each professional and puts this together in a comprehensive team report. The coordinator helps to counsel the family regarding the recommendations and ensures that there is follow-up on recommendations that are made by team members.

which is published annually (American Cleft Palate-Craniofacial Association, 1999).

One standard requirement is that each team must have a coordinator, usually a nurse or other health care professional. This person facilitates the scheduling of all team meetings and the documentation of impressions and recommendations for each patient. The coordinator ensures that the recommendations are

implemented and may also be the person who represents the team in communicating with the patient or family.

As part of the basic standards, the ACPA has determined which professionals must be members of the team in order to qualify as either a cleft palate team or a craniofacial team. Most teams have additional professional members and also take advantage of consultation with other specialists on an as-needed basis. (Figure 11–1 shows the members of the team from the Craniofacial Center, Cincinnati, Ohio.)

Cleft Palate Team: The ACPA has determined that a Cleft Palate Team (CPT) must have a surgeon, an orthodontist, a speech-language pathologist, and at least one additional specialist. Other members might include an audiologist, geneticist (dysmorphologist), nurse, oral surgeon (maxillofacial surgeon), otolaryngologist (ear, nose and throat specialist), orthodontist, pediatrician, prosthodontist, psychologist, or social worker.

Craniofacial Team (CFT): A Craniofacial Team, as defined by the ACPA, must consist of a craniofacial surgeon, an orthodontist, a mental health professional, and speech-language pathologist. Other members may include a neurosurgeon and an ophthalmologist, in addition to those professionals included in a cleft team.

Velopharyngeal Dysfunction (VPD) Team: The ACPA has made no specific recommenda-

tions for a team structure for children with the primary problem of velopharyngeal dysfunction (VPD), with or without a history of cleft palate. Patients with velopharyngeal dysfunction, regardless of etiology, are often managed effectively by a full cleft or craniofacial team. However, some of these patients can be effectively managed by a subset of these professionals through a velopharyngeal dysfunction team or VPI Clinic. This team should ideally include a speech pathologist, an otolaryngologist (or a plastic surgeon), and a geneticist. The geneticist is important because many children with velopharyngeal dysfunction of unknown origin have a previously unidentified syndrome, most commonly velocardiofacial syndrome.

In 1996, the American Cleft Palate-Craniofacial Association conducted a survey of all known cleft palate and craniofacial teams in the United States and Canada (Strauss, 1998). Of the 296 teams contacted, 247 (83.4%) responded by filling out a self-assessment sur-

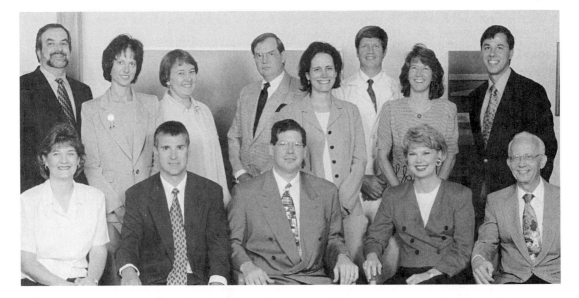

Figure 11–1. Members of the team of the Cincinnati Craniofacial Center, Cincinnati, Ohio, 2000.

vey. Based on the results of that survey, it was determined that 105 (42.5%) were functioning as cleft palate teams and 102 (41.3%) were functioning as craniofacial teams. The remaining 12 teams (4.9%) were either new teams, teams with low numbers due to their geographic location, or teams that merely consult, but do not provide treatment.

In addition to the professionals on the team, the parents or family are also key players in determining the treatment plan for the patient. It is important for the professionals on the team to gain the support and cooperation from the families. In fact, all decisions for treatment must be based on the patient's and family's wishes, in addition to the clinical indications (Sharp, 1995). If the family members are not active participants in the decision-making process, compliance with the team's recommendations can be affected (Nackashi & Dixon-Wood, 1989; Pannbacker & Scheuerle, 1993; Paynter, Jordan, & Finch, 1990; Paynter et al., 1993). On the other hand, appropriate family involvement can significantly improve compliance with the recommendations, which can ultimately improve the outcomes of treatment (Paynter et al., 1990; Paynter et al., 1993).

Team Leadership

The qualifications, personality, and skill of the team leader are highly important in determining the function and success of the team. There is little room for authoritarianism in clinical team leadership. Instead, the leader must be able to ensure that all team members are respected equally and that their opinions are heard and considered for the best patient outcome. A dominant team member can result in decisions that are made based on that person's opinion, rather than on team consensus. It is the responsibility of the team leader to be sure that that does not happen and that all members' opinions are heard and considered before decisions regarding the patient's care are

made (Strauss & Broder, 1985). The most effective teams function by consensus, even though each professional may view the needs of the patient differently (Noar, 1992; Strauss, 1999).

Team Responsibilities

To provide a truly integrated system of patient care, the ACPA has made a number of recommendations regarding the responsibilities of the team in its Parameters document (American Cleft Palate-Craniofacial Association, 1993). For example, the ACPA recommended that each team should have an office with a secretary or coordinator and a designated telephone number. The office should maintain all team documents and patient records. Patients should be evaluated at regular intervals, depending on the needs of the patient and the family. Although the patients may be examined individually by the professionals on the team, regularly scheduled team meetings must be held for discussion and negotiation of the plan of care. Communication of recommendations to the patient and family must be made verbally and in written form. There must be ongoing communication with the direct care providers in the patient's home community. The team should provide patients with information regarding resources for other services and financial assistance, as needed. Finally, the teams should provide educational programs for families, other care providers, and the general public.

Team Quality

The quality of the services provided by a team is difficult to measure or quantify. In many cases, quality is determined solely by the perception of the "customers." Although this is an important indicator of quality, there are other more measurable ways to assure quality of services. The guidelines listed in the Parameters document (American Cleft Palate-Craniofacial

Association, 1993) can help a team to achieve and maintain the basic requirements for an appropriate team, as determined by professional consensus from around the country.

Another way to ensure quality is for the team to develop and participate in a quality assurance program. In a recent survey of cleft and craniofacial teams in North America, 50% reported that they have a quality assurance program in place to measure treatment outcomes (Strauss, 1999). This type of a program provides a mechanism for teams to monitor, self-evaluate, and improve various aspects of patient care. Clinical pathways and algorithms of care have also been developed by some teams (Stal, Klebuc, Taylor, Spira, & Edwards, 1998).

The quality of the team is greatly determined by the quality of each individual member. It is important that all members of the team are licensed and certified in their individual areas of specialty. The education and experience required for specialization are determined by the various professional associations, specialty boards, and licensure boards. Each team must ensure that all members possess not only the appropriate and current credentials for practice, but also the requisite experience and skill in the evaluation and treatment of patients in the specialty area of craniofacial anomalies. If the professionals are not well-trained in this specialty area, their good intentions may not be enough to result in good decisions. In fact, these "experts" can actually do more harm than good due to the lack of specialty experience in this area (Sidman, 1995).

Another factor that affects the quality of a team is the number of patients seen per year and the number of team meetings per year. This has an impact on the experience base of the team and time commitment of the team members to craniofacial anomalies. In addition, teams with a large patient base usually have more members than those with few patients and they also have more disciplines represented on the team. Therefore, it is more likely that patients various treatment needs will be adequately and appropriately served by the team.

Of course, when the patient requires services by professionals not represented on the team, members must have the knowledge and resources to refer patient's to appropriate professionals outside of the immediate team.

The stability of the team and the longevity of team members can be a factor to consider. Because the patient's treatment typically begins at birth and may continue until adulthood, the consistency and longevity of team members becomes important for the consistency and continuity of care.

It is especially important that all members of the team stay current with recent developments in their respective disciplines, particularly as it relates to cleft and craniofacial care. Active membership in the American Cleft Palate-Craniofacial Association (ACPA) and attendance at annual meetings of the association is the best way to be informed. Members should also attend other continuing education programs and read the various journals with articles regarding the latest techniques in the evaluation and treatment of craniofacial anomalies. An interest in continuous learning is important in order to provide the best possible care for the patients.

Finally, the extent to which the team involves the parents or caregivers in the decision-making process affects the overall team quality. It has been found that when parents have a high opinion of the team and the services provided, compliance with recommendations is greatest. However, if the parents have a low opinion of the team, compliance is negatively affected (Paynter et al., 1990)

Team Process

The cleft or craniofacial team typically becomes involved in the management of the child's needs soon after birth. This begins with parent counseling and the management of feeding issues and airway problems. Team care should then continue until the physical growth of the individual has been completed, which is usually between the ages of 18 and 21. Care can continue through adulthood if there are remaining medical, surgical, dental, psychological, or communication problems that can be improved or resolved by the team members.

The method of scheduling and evaluating patients as a team differs in different settings. In most cases, each professional evaluates the patient through a separate consultation or screening, but this often occurs on the same day in a clinic setting. When the evaluations are done in a clinic, there is the opportunity for several professionals to work together in evaluating the patient (Figure 11–2). The interdisciplinary team members then meet to discuss impressions and recommendations and to negotiate a plan of treatment. The treatment priorities and appropriate sequence of treatment are determined. The coordinator, or another designated team member, is responsible for communicating the recommendations to the family and making sure that appropriate appointments are scheduled.

Although the team coordinator may be the primary contact person for the family, each person on the team in responsible for counseling the family on the concerns and the plan of treatment relative to that discipline. When the family members are involved and informed regarding the health care decisions for their children, it can reduce stress and improve treatment outcomes (Paynter, Edmonson, & Jordan, 1991; Walesky-Rainbow & Morris, 1978). The ultimate treatment plan is determined by the recommendations of the team members; the concerns, needs, and goals of the patient and the patient's family; and the limitations and restrictions of the third party payment sources.

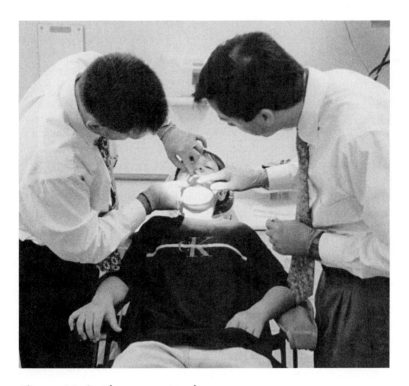

Figure 11–2. The team approach to assessment.

Advantages and Potential Problems of the Team Approach

Advantages of the Team Approach

The team approach to management offers many advantages to the patient and the patient's family (American Cleft Plate-Craniofacial Association, 1993; Borah, Hagberg, Jakubiak, & Temple, 1993; Chen, Chen, Wang, & Noordhoff, 1988; Colburn & Cherry, 1985; Kline, 1997; Lang, Neil-Dwyer, Evans, & Honeybul, 1998; Marsh, 1982; McWilliams, Morris, & Shelton, 1990; Pinsky & Goldberg, 1977; Sharp, 1995; Stal, Chebret, & McElroy, 1998; Strauss, 1998, 1999; Strohecker, 1993; Will, Aduss, Kuehn, & Parsons, 1989). First of all, the team offers an evaluation of the whole child and this is done through the individual evaluations of many professionals. The team evaluation is comprehensive, yet done with fewer visits and usually at a lower cost than individual evaluations. The plan of care is devised by professionals who work together and understand each other's disciplines. There is shared decision-making among the team members and decisions are based on more information than one professional would have independently (Sharp, 1995). There is usually better follow-up and monitoring of care, since this is the responsibility of the team coordinator. Teams usually consist of "experts" in the field who can provide state-of-the-art care. Teams promote better services through parent groups, special camps, and the provision of pamphlets and other educational materials. There is usually one main contact person on the team who can assist the family in communicating problems, questions, or concerns.

There are also many advantages of the team approach for the professionals. First, the team approach saves time by expediting the collaboration process. It also increases interprofessional communication. This helps to develop good working relationships among the team members and increases the knowledge of each professional. One of the most significant advantages of the team approach is that it makes it possible to keep good serial records (Brogan, 1988). The team can also be an effective vehicle for collaboration in research and publications. Some states have developed networks of teams for the purpose of collaboration in research endeavors and continuing education (Abdoney, Habal, Scheuerle, & Rans, 1988; Will & Aduss, 1987; Will & Parsons, 1991).

Potential Problems of the Team Approach

Although the advantages of the team approach far outweigh any disadvantage, there are some common inherent problems associated with interdisciplinary teams. One factor that can affect the function of the team is the perceived or ascribed status of various team members relative to other members. This can be based on characteristics such as age, gender, discipline, experience, or accomplishments (Cohn, 1991). If team members are not considered equals in status on the team, then the individuals with the ascribed higher status will tend to exert more influence on the decisions of the group than members of lower status (Cohn, 1991). This can have a negative impact on the quality of the group decision-making. For the team to be effective, there must be an atmosphere of equality and mutual respect among all of the team members.

Problems can also occur if the individual roles are not clearly defined within the team. If the roles are not clear, there may be interdisciplinary competition or "turf issues" at times. For example, there is often an overlap of skills between the plastic surgeon, the oral surgeon, and the otolaryngologist. As a team, it is helpful to define who does what, when it is done, and under what circumstances. This avoids conflicts over such things as who does the bone graft, who does the orthognathic surgery, or who does the flaps.

Case Report: The Value of the Team Approach

The value of a team approach to management is illustrated by the following case history. Barbara was a female who was born with a bilateral complete cleft lip and cleft palate. The lip and palate repairs were done at the appropriate time. She received speech therapy in grade school, but she was discharged from therapy with the notation that she was "doing as well as can be expected, given her velopharyngeal mechanism." Unfortunately, she was not followed by a craniofacial team at the time, and no referral was made for further assessment and treatment.

Barbara was finally seen at the age of 16 by the craniofacial team at Children's Hospital Medical Center in Cincinnati. Following the team evaluation, many treatment recommendations were made.

- The orthodontist reported that the patient had a Class III malocclusion with anterior open bite and linguaverted maxillary incisors. His recommendation was to align the maxillary arch with orthodontics.
- The speech pathologist reported that the speech was characterized by hypernasality and nasal air emission. Given those findings, the speech pathologist recommended a nasopharyngoscopy assessment and a pharyngeal flap for correction of velopharyngeal dysfunction. This was to be followed by postoperative speech therapy to correct articulation errors that were compensatory as a result of the malocclusion and velopharyngeal dysfunction.
- The oral surgeon reported that, with the discrepancy between the position of the maxillary and mandibular arches, a Le Fort I maxillary advancement was indicated to move the maxilla in appropriate position.
- The plastic surgeon noted that there was redundant vermilion in the line of the cleft and that the cupid's bow needed revision with an Abbe flap.
- The psychologist reported that, after talking with Barbara at length, she discovered that one of the things that really bothered her about herself was her flattened nose.

Given all of these concerns and recommendations, the plan of care had to be designed with the best overall results in mind. To achieve that, the appropriate sequencing of procedures had to be determined.

In this case, the first step was for the orthodontist to bring the teeth into alignment in preparation for the orthognathic (jaw) surgery. Bringing the teeth into proper alignment made the occlusion and profile actually worse, but this was an important first step for the best ultimate results. The next step was for the oral surgeon to perform a Le Fort I maxillary advancement. This normalized the occlusion and gave more support for the upper lip and base of the nose. Once the jaws were in alignment, the plastic surgeon did a pharyngeal flap to correct the velopharyngeal dysfunction, and then the lip and nose revision. About 6 weeks after the surgery, Barbara began speech therapy to correct the remaining compensatory articulation errors. She was discharged from therapy with normal speech after less than 2 months of therapy.

With this planned sequence, Barbara had the best overall outcome for both aesthetics and for speech. On the other hand, if the pharyngeal flap had been done prior to maxillary advancement, the position and effectiveness of the flap could have been compromised with the maxillary advancement. The maxillary advancement could also have had a detrimental effect on the lip and nose if those revisions had been done first. Therefore, the sequence and coordination of treatment is very important in patients who required the care from multiple specialists.

A different, but equally disruptive problem occurs when there are members on the team who are hypersensitive to feedback. This can be a problem, for example, when a surgical procedure was not as successful as was hoped, and needs to be revised. Team members must be able to speak honestly and express differences of opinion without hesitation.

Disagreements in the philosophy of care or in treatment protocols can have a major impact on the team's performance. Communication among members regarding procedures and protocols must take place so that there is consensus regarding the standards of care and continuum of care within the team. If necessary, an algorithm of care can be developed to help team members reach consensus on the management of various diagnoses and patient concerns.

All of the potential problems of the interdisciplinary team can and should be overcome for the team to be successful. This requires ongoing communication, honesty, and mutual respect. Ultimately, the focus of the team should be on the care and well-being of the patients, not on individual agendas and egos of the team members.

How to Be an Effective Team Member

Effective interdisciplinary team members are usually professionals who are very competent and knowledgeable in their particular discipline. When working on an interdisciplinary team that requires specialty knowledge, such as a craniofacial team, each member must have specialty expertise in that area. At the same time, an effective team member must show a strong interest in the knowledge of other disciplines, and have a desire to learn from other disciplines.

All team members should show respect for others and their opinions, especially when there is disagreement. Each team member must feel free to express his or her honest opinion, without the fear of offending someone. It is important to place quality patient care and appropriate patient management first and not be willing to compromise this due to a concern about personal feelings. When mistakes are made, as they will be, it is important that each team member feels comfortable enough to be able to admit mistakes, without worry about undue criticism. In addition, the team members must be comfortable enough with each other to be able to admit what they do not know to further learning and professional competence.

It is important for team members to be dependable and reliable, especially because all professionals are very busy. It is not well received when one person holds up the process or lets the other members down.

Finally, the use of humor can be very effective in developing camaraderie, and can also help to enhance respect and working relationships among the team members. This type of relationship among team members has an indirect, but very definite effect on the quality of services that are ultimately provided to the patients.

Resources for Services

How to Find a Craniofacial Team

Craniofacial teams are located all around the country, but particularly within teaching hospitals or pediatric hospitals. In most cases, it is not important that the team is located near the patient's home. In general, the team will need to see the patient for evaluation and consultation only once or twice a year during the active treatment process. Routine treatment, such as general dental care, orthodontics, speech therapy, and pediatric care, can usually be provided by professionals in the patient's own community, as long as there is regular communication and consultation with the team members. The closest cleft palate or craniofacial team can be determined by contacting the Cleft Palate Foundation (CPF), which is associated with the American Cleft Palate-Craniofacial Association. Information regarding this organization and others is listed in the Resources section in this book.

Funding Sources

Funding for the evaluation and treatment of the cleft lip, cleft palate, and other craniofacial anomalies can come from a variety of sources. Private insurance companies will usually cover most of the expenses associated with the medical care of the patient if the patient was born when the policy was in effect. Financial assistance can also be obtained through federal and state programs, such as Champus, Medicaid, the state's Children's Special Health Services (formerly Crippled Children's Services), Bureau of Vocational Rehabilitation, and through selected Shriners Hospitals across the country. Some private and nonprofit organizations provide funds or special services to meet the needs of children with clefts or craniofacial anomalies. Resources for financial aid can often be obtained through a social worker or team coordinator.

Identifying sources of funding and making sure that there is adequate funding is an important component in treatment planning. Recommending many expensive procedures that are not covered by insurance and are out of the family's financial reach is truly a disservice to the patient and the family.

Challenges to the Specialty Team Concept

With the changes in health care financing, there are some additional challenges to the team approach to the management of complex patients. Most people would agree that the fee-for-service system of health care funding was ineffective in either assuring quality or controling costs. However, the change to a managed care system has resulted in some additional concerns about the quality and costs of health care, particularly as it applies to specialty services.

Although the managed care system was designed to help to control the cost of health care, many critics would argue that this is hard to do when most of the managed care organizations exist as for-profit corporations. In fact, in many cases, the investors and the administrators of these organizations are reaping substantial profits. This may occur at the expense of the patients, who are not always receiving the services that they need. Critics of managed care would also argue that this system discourages the use of specialists in the care of complex disorders (Strauss, 1999). In fact, there are financial disincentives for primary care providers to seek specialty care for their patients. The managed care organizations seek to control costs by limiting the number and type of professionals that the patient can see and the number and type of procedures that the patient can have. This certainly has an impact on the specialty team approach.

An additional concern is that some third party payers limit access to physicians who are outside the network. If there are no specialists within the network to cover the particular medical needs, this may seriously affect the quality of care provided to the patient. It is an even greater problem when a whole team of professionals is required for quality care.

Some patients or parents are unable to move or change jobs due to a concern about changing insurance coverage. Managed care organizations often refuse to cover pre-existing conditions when the policy is new. As a result, the care of patients with cleft palate or craniofacial anomalies may not be covered. In addition, there is an incentive for managed care organizations to seek to enroll groups of patients who are at low financial risk due to few health problems. This may result in exclusion of the individuals who really need insurance coverage for medical services.

As the health care system continues to evolve in this country, it is difficult to predict the future and what it holds for specialty team care or even general medical care. With the efforts of professionals and various advocacy groups, it is hoped that the system will be refined so that the specific needs of the patient become a priority.

Summary

Over the last 50 years, the team approach to the management of individuals with craniofacial anomalies has evolved from a good idea to the accepted standard of care. Although there are some inherent difficulties that can occur when a group of professionals must work together, the advantages of this approach far outweigh the disadvantages. Without the interaction of various professionals through the team, the treatment of patients would become fragmented, and the outcomes would be negatively affected. Hopefully, as our health care system continues to change and develop, the team approach to cleft and craniofacial care will be supported and will thrive.

References

Abdoney, M., Habal, M. B., Scheuerle, J., & Rans, N. P. (1988). Cleft palate teams and the craniofacial centers in Florida: A state network. *Florida Dental Journal, 59*(2), 25–27, 53.

American Cleft Palate-Craniofacial Association. (1993). Parameters for evaluation and treatment of patients with cleft lip/palate or other craniofacial anomalies. *Cleft Palate Craniofacial Journal, 30*(Suppl.), 1–16.

American Cleft Palate-Craniofacial Association. (1999). *Membership-Team directory.* Chapel Hill, NC: American Cleft Palate-Craniofacial Association.

Bardach, J., Morris, H., Olin, W., McDermott-Murray, J., Mooney, M., & Bardach, E. (1984). Late results of multidisciplinary management of unilateral cleft lip and palate. *Annals of Plastic Surgery, 12*(3), 235–242.

Borah, G. L., Hagberg, N., Jakubiak, C., & Temple, J. (1993). Reorganization of craniofacial/cleft care delivery: The Massachusetts experience. *Cleft Palate Craniofacial Journal, 30*(3), 333–336.

Brogan, W. F. (1988). Team approach to the treatment of cleft lip and palate. *Annals of the Academy of Medicine, Singapore, 17*(3), 335–338.

Chen, Y. R., Chen, S. H., Wang, C. Y., & Noordhoff, M. S. (1988). Combined cleft and craniofacial team—Multidisciplinary approach to cleft management. *Annals of the Academy of Medicine, Singapore, 17*(3), 339–342.

Cohn, E. R. (1991). Commentary on team acceptance of recommendations by Dixon-Wood et al. *Cleft Palate Craniofacial Journal, 28*(3), 290–292.

Colburn, N., & Cherry, R. S. (1985). Community-based team approach to the management of children with cleft palate. *Child Health Care, 13*(3), 122–128.

Kline, R. M., Jr. (1997). Management of craniofacial anomalies. *Journal of the South Carolina Medical Association, 93*(9), 336–341.

Krogman, W. M. (1979). The cleft palate team in action. In H. K. Cooper, R. L. Harding, W. M. Krogman, M. Mazaheri, & R. T. Millard (Eds.), *Cleft palate and cleft lip: A team approach to clinical management and rehabilitation of the patient* (p. 145). Philadelphia: W.B. Saunders.

Lang, D. A., Neil-Dwyer, G., Evans, B. T., & Honeybul, S. (1998). Craniofacial access in children. *Acta Neurochirurgica, 140*(1), 33–40.

Marsh, J. L. (1982). Interdisciplinary care for craniofacial deformities. *Missouri Medicine, 79*(9), 623–628, 630.

McWilliams, B. J., Morris, H. L., & Shelton, R. L. (1990). *Cleft palate speech.* Toronto, Canada: B.C. Decker.

Nackashi, M., & Dixon-Wood, V. (1989). The craniofacial team: Medical supervision and coordination. In K. Bzoch (Ed.), *Communicative disorders related to cleft lip and palate* (pp. 63–73). Boston: College-Hill Press.

Noar, J. H. (1992). A questionnaire survey of attitudes and concerns of three professional groups involved in the cleft palate team. *Cleft Palate Craniofacial Journal, 29*(1), 92–95.

Pannbacker, M., & Scheuerle, J. (1993). Parents' attitudes toward family involvement in cleft palate treatment. *Cleft Palate Craniofacial Journal, 30*(1), 87–89.

Paynter, E. T., Edmonson, T. W., & Jordan, W. J. (1991). Accuracy of information reported by parents and children evaluated by a cleft palate team. *Cleft Palate Craniofacial Journal, 28*(4), 329–337.

Paynter, E. T., Jordan, W. J., & Finch, D. L. (1990). Patient compliance with cleft palate team regimens. *Journal of Speech and Hearing Disorders, 55*(4), 740–750.

Paynter, E. T., Wilson, B. M., & Jordan, W. J. (1993). Improved patient compliance with cleft palate team regimes. *Cleft Palate Craniofacial Journal, 30*(3), 292–301.

Pinsky, T. M., & Goldberg, H. J. (1977). Potential for clinical cooperation between dentistry and speech pathology. *International Dental Journal, 27*(4), 363–369.

Sharp, H. M. (1995). Ethical decision-making in interdisciplinary team care. *Cleft Palate Craniofacial Journal, 32*(6), 495–499.

Sidman, J. D. (1995). The team approach to cleft and craniofacial disorders—The down side [Editorial]. *Cleft Palate Craniofacial Journal, 32*(5), 362.

Stal, S., Chebret, L., & McElroy, C. (1998). The team approach in the management of congenital and acquired deformities. *Clinics in Plastic Surgery, 25*(4), 485–491, vii.

Stal, S., Klebuc, M., Taylor, T. D., Spira, M., & Edwards, M. (1998). Algorithms for the treatment of cleft lip and palate. *Clinics in Plastic Surgery, 25*(4), 493–507, vii.

Strauss, R. P. (1998). Cleft palate and craniofacial teams in the United States and Canada: A national survey of team organization and standards of care. The American Cleft Palate-Craniofacial Association (ACPA) Team Standards Committee. *Cleft Palate Craniofacial Journal, 35*(6), 473–480.

Strauss, R. P. (1999). The organization and delivery of craniofacial health services: The state of the art. *Cleft Palate Craniofacial Journal, 36*(3), 189–195.

Strauss, R. P., & Broder, H. (1985). Interdisciplinary team care of cleft lip and palate: Social and psychological aspects. *Clinics in Plastic Surgery, 12*(4), 543–551.

Strohecker, B. (1993). A team approach in the treatment of craniofacial deformities. *Plastic Surgery Nursing, 13*(1), 9–16.

Surgeon General's Report (1987, June). *Children with special needs.* Washington, DC: Office of Maternal and Child Health, U.S. Department of Health and Human Services, Public Health Service.

Tindlund, R. S., & Holmefjord, A. (1997). Functional results with the team care of cleft lip and palate patients in Bergen, Norway. The Bergen Cleft Palate-Craniofacial Team, Norway. *Folia Phoniatrica et Logopedica, 49*(3/4), 168–176.

Walesky-Rainbow, P. A., & Morris, H. L. (1978). An assessment of informative-counseling procedures for cleft palate children. *Cleft Palate Journal, 15*(1), 20–29.

Will, L. A., & Aduss, M. K. (1987). Illinois Association of Craniofacial Teams: A new state organization. *Cleft Palate Journal, 24*(4), 339–341.

Will, L., Aduss, M. K., Kuehn, D. P., & Parsons, R. W. (1989). The team approach to treating cleft lip/palate and other craniofacial anomalies in Illinois. *Illinois Dental Journal, 58*(2), 112–115.

Will, L. A., & Parsons, R. W. (1991). Characteristics of new patients at Illinois cleft palate teams. *Cleft Palate Craniofacial Journal, 28*(4), 378–383; Discussion 383–384.

PART IV

Assessment Procedures: Speech, Resonance, and Velopharyngeal Dysfunction

CHAPTER

12

Perceptual Assessment

CONTENTS

The evaluation of resonance and velopharyngeal function must begin with a speech pathology evaluation. In this evaluation, a perceptual assessment is done to determine whether resonance is normal or abnormal. Resonance can be said to be abnormal if the quality or the intelligibility of speech is affected by inappropriate transmission of acoustic energy in the vocal tract. A speech pathology evaluation is also necessary to determine if there are any other characteristics of velopharyngeal dysfunction, such as nasal air emission or compensatory articulation productions. The perceptual evaluation of speech and resonance should be done by a qualified and experienced speech pathologist.

Listener judgment is the most important test of velopharyngeal dysfunction as it relates to impaired communication. In fact, in a survey of speech pathologists in the United States and Canada, 90% of the those associated with a cleft palate team reported that they rely primarily on listener judgment, oral examination, and articulation testing in the diagnosis of velopharyngeal insufficiency (Schneider & Shprintzen, 1980). If there is no abnormality, as judged by a perceptual evaluation, then it does not matter what the instrumental procedures show. It is only when the perceptual evaluation shows an abnormality that treatment is initiated.

The goal of the perceptual evaluation is to determine if an abnormality exists, and if so, the type and severity of the disorder. Based on the results of the evaluation, further assessment may be recommended using instrumental procedures to determine the specific cause of the problem. The ultimate goal of the evaluation is to determine an appropriate treatment plan.

The purpose of this chapter is to review the perceptual evaluation process for individuals who have a history of cleft lip/palate or craniofacial anomalies. This information also applies to individuals who have a resonance disorder due to other causes. This chapter provides practical suggestions for a thorough assessment of resonance and the articulation correlates to velopharyngeal dysfunction. The word "child" is used throughout this section, but it should be

understood that the same procedures are also used when testing an adult.

Direct Versus Indirect Measures for Evaluation

Prior to discussing the perceptual assessment procedures, it may be helpful to describe the types of measures available for assessment of resonance and velopharyngeal function. There are two basic categories of procedures for evaluation of velopharyngeal function: those that give direct information and those that give indirect information.

Procedures that give direct information are those that allow the examiner to visualize aspects of velopharyngeal function. These *direct measures* include videofluoroscopy and nasopharyngoscopy procedures. Through these procedures, the examiner can view the anatomical and physiological defects that cause velopharyngeal dysfunction. Because there is a wide spectrum of anatomic and physiologic causes for velopharyngeal dysfunction, it is important to obtain this information so that the appropriate and most effective treatment can be determined. Although the structures and function of the velopharyngeal valve can be seen through these measures, the evaluation of what is seen is still subjective and open to interpretation. More information can be found in Chapter 16, Videofluoroscopy, and Chapter 17, Nasopharyngoscopy.

In contrast to direct measures, procedures that provide indirect information do not allow visualization of the structures. However, these *indirect measures* give objective data regarding the results of velopharyngeal function, such as airflow, air pressure or acoustic output. The Nasometer and pressure/flow equipment are examples of instrumentation that provide indirect, yet objective information. The advantage of objective data is that it can be compared to standardized norms for interpretation. In addition, these instruments can be used to collect objective data for pre- and post-treatment comparison. See Chapters 14 and 15 on Nasometry and Aerodynamics for more information.

Although instrumental assessment is important, the most important tool that we have for making decisions regarding velopharyngeal function and the need for management is the examiner's ear (Moller, 1991). From a thorough analysis of speech, a determination can be made regarding the status of velopharyngeal function and its potential for change. In the perceptual evaluation, the ear is used to analyze the acoustic product of velopharyngeal function in order to make inferences about the adequacy of the velopharyngeal mechanism. If the human ear can be considered an instrument in the broadest sense of the word, then listener judgment should be considered an indirect measure of velopharyngeal function (Dalston, 1997). Although a perceptual assessment is an indirect approach, it has face validity in that velopharyngeal dysfunction is usually not a problem unless it affects speech.

Timetable for Assessment

This section addresses the timetable for assessment of children with identified craniofacial anomalies at birth, including cleft lip and palate. Individuals who present with resonance disorders later in life can be evaluated as soon as the disorder becomes apparent.

Children with a history of cleft lip/cleft palate or craniofacial anomalies are at risk for communication disorders. If the child had a cleft of the primary palate, this risk is due to the possibility of dental abnormalities. If the cleft was of the secondary palate, the risk is related to the possibility of a fluctuating hearing loss that may accompany eustachian tube malfunction and velopharyngeal dysfunction. There may be other problems, such as mental retardation or neurological dysfunction, especially if the child has features of a craniofacial syndrome. These problems might further affect speech and language development and overall communication skills. Because of the structural and functional problems that are typical of cleft lip and palate or craniofacial syndromes, the child may be at risk for problems in the areas of articulation, language, phonation, and resonance. Feeding and swallowing abilities might also be affected.

First Year

During the first year, the primary speech pathology concerns are feeding and the development of the prerequisites for verbal communication. A professional from the cleft palate or craniofacial team is responsible for instructing the family on feeding methods and making sure that these methods are effective. If feeding continues to be a problem, despite the recommended feeding modifications, this should be evaluated immediately by the speech pathologist or another qualified professional and resolved quickly. In addition to feeding, the infant's development should be monitored throughout the first year. This can be done by parent report, through direct observation, or through the use of infant scales. If problems in development are noted, further assessment and intervention should be initiated.

The first year is usually a time of great joy for the parents. However, there is also significant anxiety over the uncertainty of what will happen in the future and the ultimate results of treatment. Because most people cope better with information rather than uncertainty, the parents should be counseled by various professionals, usually cleft palate team members, soon after the birth and again early in the first year. These professionals should explain the diagnosis, the effect of the anomalies on function, what might happen in the future, what will be done about it, and the ultimate prognosis. The speech pathologist should also discuss methods of speech and language stimulation. In particular, instructions for stimulating sound production after the palate repair are important to include in this discussion. However, it should be emphasized that during the first 3 years, language development needs to be the primary focus. In other words, the quantity of speech is more important than the quality of speech during those early years. The speech pathologist should reinforce this discussion with a handout that summarizes the information and provides additional suggestions.

At Cincinnati Children's Hospital Medical Center, these counseling sessions are done through the Infant/Toddler Meetings, where six to eight sets of parents attend each session. At these meetings, various team members give a brief lecture and then are available for questions and discussion. A particular benefit of these group meetings is that the parents are able to meet other families who are going through a similar experience and develop a support network. Many long-term relationships have developed through some of these meetings.

Annual Screenings and Periodic Evaluations

Children with a history of cleft lip/palate or craniofacial anomalies should receive at least a screening evaluation of speech and language skills on an annual basis until the age of 4 years (American Cleft Palate-Craniofacial Association, 1993). This is often done during the annual visit to the cleft palate or craniofacial team. If problems are suspected during these assessments, the child should be scheduled for a more in-depth evaluation.

Around the age of 3, the child should receive a comprehensive evaluation of speech and language. If the child is communicating with connected speech and is able to produce a variety of sounds, this is also the appropriate time to evaluate resonance and velopharyngeal function. On the other hand, if the child's speech development and expressive language development are delayed, the assessment of resonance and velopharyngeal function should be done at a later time in order to obtain accurate results. When hypernasality or nasal air emission are noted as a result of the perceptual evaluation, further assessment of velopharyngeal function

is usually done through instrumental measures prior to making recommendations for treatment.

A perceptual assessment, along with instrumental measures, should be done prior to any surgery that is designed to improve speech, such as a pharyngoplasty, or surgery that might affect speech, such as orthognathic surgery. It is very important to document baseline information regarding speech and resonance prior to the surgical procedure. A postoperative assessment should also be done to determine the effect of the surgery on speech and whether any further treatment is indicated.

The Diagnostic Interview

The perceptual evaluation is usually preceded by an interview with the child or a family member as appropriate. Many clinics send the family a pre-evaluation questionnaire prior to the appointment to determine the current concerns about speech, medical and developmental history, feeding, and the history of treatment. This information helps the examiner to prepare for the evaluation and can shorten the interview process.

Whether a comprehensive evaluation is being done or merely a screening evaluation in a cleft palate clinic, the examiner can obtain valuable information by interviewing the parents or child regarding their observations and concerns. This should be done even if background information was received through a referral or pre-evaluation questionnaire. Assuming the patient is a child, examples of interview questions can be found in Table 12–1.

Parents are usually very good observers of their own children, and can often effectively compare their child's communication skills with those of siblings or peers. A study by Glascoe (1991) showed that identification of the parent's concern and skillful observation of the child is sensitive to many speech and language problems. A simple rule of thumb is that if the parents are worried about their child's speech, there probably is a good reason.

Language Screening

Children with a history of cleft lip/palate or craniofacial anomalies are at risk for early language delay; therefore, it is important to be sure that these children receive regular and routine language screening. This should be done throughout the preschool years and can be done at the time of the yearly visits to the cleft palate team. If language problems are suspected from the screening evaluation or interview, or if the parents have concerns about language development, a comprehensive language evaluation is indicated. A comprehensive evaluation should also be done if the child has additional risk factors for language disorders, such as hearing loss, developmental delay, or neurological problems. This type of evaluation cannot be done adequately in a clinic setting; therefore, a separate appointment with the speech-language pathologist is usually needed. If a language disorder is identified, intervention should be initiated as soon as possible to ensure the best outcome.

The methods for language evaluation are beyond the scope of this text. Instead, the interested reader should consult one of the many books available on this subject. However, a discussion regarding screening methods may be helpful, particularly as it applies to a clinic setting.

Parent Questionnaire

One way to screen the language of infants and toddlers is to seek information from the parents through a questionnaire format. The questions must be understandable for the parents to answer with confidence and detailed enough to be of value to the examiner. Scherer and D'Antonio (1995) investigated the efficacy of a parent questionnaire as a component of early language screening, using the MacArthur Communicative Development Inventory (Fenson et al., 1989). They found that the parent questionnaire can be a valid means of screening language development when compared with a speech-language screening.

Informal Language Screening

Although formal screening tests provide structure and a set format, they are not necessary for the experienced examiner. It should be kept in mind that the purpose of a screening test is to determine whether more comprehensive testing is indicated. Most experienced examiners can make this determination through parent interview, observations of the child, and informal testing. The behaviors of the child, as noted through observation and report, can be compared to developmental norms to estimate the child's developmental level.

An informal screening assessment can be done "on the spot" and without the need for materials or special props. Speech and language can be screened informally by:

- Observing play behaviors, and the type and complexity of gestures (Scherer & D'Antonio, 1997).
- Asking the child to point to certain objects or follow certain commands.
- Having interesting toys available and observing spontaneous vocalizations and utterances.
- Listening to the child's spontaneous speech while he or she is talking to the parent.
- Eliciting communication by asking questions or asking for explanations. (See Table 12–2 for examples.)
- Having the child repeat words or sentences, such as those listed in the articulation-screening test. (See Table 12–3.) Even in repeating, the child will usually revert to his or her own form of syntax and morphology, which gives an indication of expressive language abilities.

Through some of these methods, the examiner should determine the primary mode of communication. This could be gestures, single

TABLE 12–1. Sample questions for use in a diagnostic interview.

Current Concern

- What concern's you about your child's speech?
- When did you first become concerned?
- Who referred your child for the evaluation and what was that person's concern?

Articulation

- What types of sounds does your child use during vocal play, vowels only or some consonants?
- If consonants, what are some of the consonants that you hear?
- Are they produced individually or over and over?
- Does the child jabber or use jargon?
- Does your child leave out sounds in words?
- Do you understand your child's speech all of the time, most of the time, some of the time, or hardly at all?
- How well do strangers understand his or her speech?
- Are there any particular sounds that are difficult for the child to produce?

Resonance

- Does your child sound "nasal" to you? If yes, does it sound like he or she is talking through the nose, or talking as if he or she has a cold?
- When did you first notice the problem with nasality?
- If the onset was sudden, what event preceded it?
- Does it vary with the weather, allergies, fatigue, or any other factor?
- Do you ever hear air coming through the nose during speech?

Language

- Does your child communicate with gestures, single words, short phrases, incomplete sentences, or complete sentences?
- When your child is talking, how many words does he or she put together at a time?
- Does your child leave out the little words (such as "of," "to," "the," "is") in the sentence?
- Is your child communicating as well as other children his or her age?
- Have you ever had a concern about how well your child understands the speech of others or follows directions?

Medical History

- Was your child born with any congenital problems? If so, what were they? How and when were they treated?
- Does your child have any medical problems, medical diagnoses, or conditions?
- What surgeries has your child undergone?
- Does your child take any medications on a regular basis? If so, what are they for?
- Does your child hear normally? When was the last hearing test?
- Has your child had many ear infections? If so, how were they treated?
- Does your child have any problems with vision?
- Where is your child on the growth chart?

Developmental History

- When your child was an infant, was he or she quiet, very vocal, or about average?
- Did you have any concerns about initial speech development?

270

TABLE 12–1. *(continued)*

Developmental History *(continued)*

- Did your child begin to use words before or after the first birthday?
- When your child was learning to sit up, stand, and walk, did it seem normal or behind other children?
- Did your child walk before or after the first birthday?
- Does your child have any difficulty learning in preschool or school?

Feeding and Oral-Motor Skills

- Does your child have any difficulty chewing, sucking, or swallowing?
- Is there a history of feeding problems?
- Does your child drool or keep the mouth open during the day?

Airway

- Does your child snore at night?
- Does your child ever gasp for breath at night or sleep restlessly?
- Does your child like to breathe through the mouth or through the nose?
- Is your child's breathing ever noisy during the day?
- Does your child have allergies, asthma or chronic congestion?

Treatment History

- Has your child ever had a speech evaluation or speech therapy?
- Is your child currently receiving speech therapy? If yes, what are the goals?
- Has your child's speech improved in the last 6 months? If so, in what way?

or multiple signs, single words, short utterances, short sentences, or compete sentences. The approximate mean length of utterance should be determined. If the child is communicating with sentences, the examiner should note if the sentences are complete or merely telegraphic. If there are syntax or morphology errors, this should also be noted by the clinician and compared to the expectations for the child's chronological age.

Formal Language Screening Tests

There are several formal screening tests that may be of value to the examiner. These tests allow the examiner to sample the child's communication abilities using a structured format. Some examples of screening tests include the *Receptive-Expressive Emergent Language Scale (REEL)* (Bzoch & League, 1991), the *Early Language Milestone (ELM) Scale* (Coplan, 1987), and the *Rossetti Infant-Toddler Language Scale* (Rossetti, 1990). These tests are used to screen children from birth to age 3 through observation and parent report. The *Fluharty Preschool Speech and Language Screening Test* (Fluharty, 1978) can be used to screen children from the ages of 2 to 6 in the areas of articulation, vocabulary, and receptive and expressive language.

Speech Samples

When assessing resonance and the articulation effects of velopharyngeal dysfunction, it is important to select an appropriate speech sample to obtain the information that is needed for a definitive diagnosis. When testing a child, the speech sample must be developmentally appropriate. It should contain appropriate speech

TABLE 12–2. Sample questions and requests to elicit speech.

What do you like best . . .

- puppy dogs or kitty cats?
- baby dolls or teddy bears?
- cookies or cupcakes?
- chocolate chip cookies or peanut butter cookies?
- singing or dancing?
- baseball or basketball?

What do you want to be when you grow up? Why?

What does a fireman do? What does a policeman do? What does a teacher do?

Tell me how you make a peanut butter and jelly sandwich.

Explain the game of baseball to me.

TABLE 12–3. Sample sentences for assessment of articulation and resonance.

Have the patient repeat the following sentences while noting articulation errors:

p	Popeye plays in the pool.
b	Buy baby a bib.
m	My mommy makes lemonade.
w	Wade in the water.
y	You have a yellow yo yo.
h	He has a big horse.
t	Take teddy to town.
d	Do it for Daddy.
n	Nancy is not here.
k	I like cookies and cream.
g	Go get the wagon.
ng	Put the ring on her finger.
f	I have five fingers.
v	Drive a van.
l	I like yellow lollipops.
s	Sissy sees the sun in the sky.
z	Zip up your zipper.
sh	She went shopping.
ch	I eat cherries and cheese.
j	John told a joke to Jim.
r	Randy has a red fire truck.
er	The teacher and the doctor are here.
th	Thank you for the toothbrush.
blends	splash, sprinkle, street

sounds, a reasonable length, and appropriate syntax for the child's developmental level.

Formal Articulation Tests

The speech evaluation often begins with the single word articulation test. In most cases, an articulation test with known articulatory targets should be used for a full assessment, rather than using only connected speech. The results of the articulation test can then be compared to what is heard in conversation. The advantage of a formal articulation test is that it can provide data for the clinician to develop a therapy program that is realistic and structured.

Several formal articulation tests have been developed specifically for the assessment of resonance and the characteristics of velopharyngeal dysfunction. The *Iowa Pressure Articulation Test*, a part of the *Templin-Darley Tests of Articulation* (Templin & Darley, 1960), is a test that is loaded with high-pressure consonants, making it very sensitive to nasal air emission. Another test that can be used for this purpose is the *Bzoch Error Pattern Diagnostic Articulation Tests* (Bzoch, 1979). This test was also designed to sample plosives, fricatives and affricates, which are most likely to be affected by velopharyngeal dysfunction.

Although these tests have some utility for evaluation of individuals with suspected velopharyngeal dysfunction, any articulation test can be used. An informal test of articulation can be just as useful, if not more so, in some cases. Regardless of the test that is used, the examiner should test all speech sounds that are age-appropriate.

Syllable Repetition

The examiner may want to test phonemes at the syllable level to isolate out the effects of other sounds. This is done by having the child produce consonant phonemes, particularly plosives, fricatives, and affricates, in a repetitive manner (such as "pa, pa, pa, pa"). Each of the pressure-sensitive phonemes can be tested with the low vowel and then again with a high vowel. This type of test allows the examiner to test both articulation and the presence of nasal air emission on each individual phoneme.

Sentence Repetition

The examiner should have a battery of sentences that test each consonant phoneme, as can be found in Table 12–3. It is best if these sentences contain phonemes that are similar in articulatory placement (such as "Take Teddy to town"). By asking the child to repeat these sentences, the examiner can quickly and easily test articulation, nasal air emission, and resonance in a connected speech environment.

When evaluating for nasal air emission and the other related characteristics (weak consonants or short utterance length), the sample should contain many pressure-sensitive consonants, particularly those that are voiceless (such as "Sissy sees the sun in the sky"). When testing for hypernasality, the sample should contain a high number of voiced, oral sounds. To separate out the effects of nasal air emission or compensatory errors, the examiner could use a sample with a large number of low-pressure consonants (such as "How are you? Where are you? Why are you here?"). Sample sentences with low-pressure sounds can be found in Table 12–4. To test for hyponasality, the examiner should use sentences with a high frequency of nasal phonemes (such as "My mama made lemonade for me"). Sample sentences loaded with nasal sounds can be found in Table 12–5.

Counting and Rote Speech

Spontaneous, connected speech is often difficult to obtain in the evaluation, especially with young children. However, connected speech can often be elicited by having the child count from 1 to 20 or say the alphabet. Reciting "Happy Birthday" can also provide a connect-

ed speech sample. Counting from 60 to 70, or repeating these numbers after the examiner, can be particularly informative because these numbers contain a combination of sibilants, velar plosives, and alveolar plosives. Another option is to have the patient simply repeat "60, 60, 60, 60." These sounds require a build-up and continuation of intraoral air pressure, which can particularly tax the velopharyngeal mechanism and may overwhelm a tenuous velopharyngeal valve. Counting from 70 to 79 can be

TABLE 12–4. Sample of low-pressure sentences for evaluation of resonance without the complication of nasal air emission.

How are you?

Who are you?

Where are you?

Why are you here?

You are here.

They are here.

Where are they?

They are where you are.

TABLE 12–5. Sentences for evaluation of hyponasality, denasality, or cul-de-sac resonance.

My mama made lemonade for me.

My name is Amy Minor.

My mama takes money to the market.

Many men are at the mine.

Ned made nine points in the game.

My nanny is not mean.

Nan needs a dime to call home.

My mom's home is many miles away.

Many men are needed to move the piano.

diagnostic as this series contains a nasal phoneme followed by an alveolar plosive. If there are timing difficulties, this may become apparent in this speech sample as assimilated hypernasality. If there are concerns regarding possible hyponasality, counting from 90 to 100 allows the examiner to assess the production of the nasal /n/ in connected speech.

Spontaneous Connected Speech

Although a single word test helps the examiner to isolate each phoneme and the individual's ability to produce that sound, it is also very important to assess articulation, and particularly resonance, in connected speech. Connected speech increases the demands on the velopharyngeal valving system to achieve and maintain closure. The examiner may note an increase in hypernasality and nasal air emission in connected speech when compared to single words. An increase in articulation errors is also common during the production of continuous utterances.

Some children are naturally loquacious and little or no effort is needed to elicit connected speech. Other children need some prodding. The examiner should begin by asking the child questions that require only a short response. Either/or questions (e.g., "What do you like best, baseball or basketball?") can be particularly helpful in getting the child to talk. Once the child is responding, questions that require a longer response can be asked (e.g., "How do you play the game of baseball?"). If this fails, it may be best to allow the parent to try to engage the child in conversation while the examiner appears to be not listening.

Analysis of Articulation and Nasal Air Emission

In conducting a perceptual evaluation, the examiner must listen for several aspects of speech at the same time. In addition to listening to resonance, the examiner must also assess articulation, nasal air emission, and phonation. If there are articulation errors, it is important to determine if the errors are obligatory errors, compensatory errors, placement errors, phonological errors, errors due to oral-motor dysfunction, or merely developmental errors. A description of compensatory errors is found in Chapter 7. Trost-Cardamone (1987) has an instructional videotape in which compensatory productions are nicely demonstrated.

The following sections describe the observations that should be made when assessing for articulation errors and nasal air emission. Correctly identifying the type of errors and the potential cause is important because this can impact the recommendations for treatment.

Compensatory Articulation Productions

Compensatory articulation errors are common in individuals with velopharyngeal dysfunction; therefore, it is important to specifically look for these errors in this population. When there is velopharyngeal dysfunction, the compensatory productions are produced by making use of the airstream in the pharynx before it is lost through the velopharyngeal port. One of the best ways to identify the placement of compensatory errors is to try to imitate the sound. By imitating the production, the examiner can usually determine the place of production and, therefore, identify the compensatory error.

Some compensatory productions can be coarticulated so that it appears that there is normal placement, even though the actual placement is posterior, usually in the pharynx or glottis. To determine the true placement of the sound, the examiner should listen carefully and watch the production of each phoneme. Some of the compensatory productions can even be felt. For example, the child may appear to be producing a normal /p/ phoneme with bilabial closure, while coarticulating the plosive portion with a glottal stop. This can be determined by looking for exaggerated laryngeal movements or by feeling for increased laryngeal activity on the child's neck during articulation.

Glottal stops can also be confused with a simple consonant omission. To make a distinction between a glottal stop and an omission, it should be remembered that glottal stops are produced with a quick sound and rapid voice onset time. If the phoneme is completely omitted, the voice onset is smooth with the initiation of the vowel. There is also an obvious difference between a consonant omission and glottal stop in the duration of the following vowel. If the phoneme is merely omitted, the vowel will be longer in duration than if the consonant is substituted by a glottal stop. A final clue to the production of glottal stops is the observation of increased laryngeal activity that can be seen in the throat area. Again, this can be felt if the examiner places a hand on the individual's throat as he or she is speaking.

A pharyngeal fricative can sound similar to a lateral lisp to an inexperienced listener. To make this distinction, the examiner should determine whether the airstream is in the oral or pharyngeal area. If the examiner cannot find the airstream at either side of the dental arch, then the sound is probably produced in the pharynx.

Obligatory Articulation Errors

As noted previously, an obligatory error is one that occurs as the result of a structural abnormality or dysfunction. When assessing articulation, placement and voicing are not affected directly by velopharyngeal dysfunction. However, the manner is often affected due to the lack of velopharyngeal closure. In particular, oral phonemes are often "nasalized" if the velopharyngeal valve is open. As a result, attempts to produce voiced plosives may result in the production of their nasal cognates (m/b, n/d, ng/g). Even voiceless plosives and other oral sounds can be nasalized due to the open velopharyngeal valve. Whenever there is a predominate use of nasal phonemes during con-

nected speech, the examiner should suspect a significant velopharyngeal opening due to these obligatory errors.

Nasal Air Emission

As part of the articulation assessment, the speech pathologist should assess for the presence of audible nasal air emission. If it is present, it is important to determine whether the nasal emission is the unobstructed type, which is usually the result of a larger velopharyngeal opening, or whether it is the "bubbly" nasal rustle (turbulence), which is usually the result of a small opening (Kummer, Curtis, Wiggs, Lee, & Strife, 1992). The examiner should also note the occurrence of a nasal snort, which is produced most often with /s/ blends. A nasal grimace commonly accompanies nasal air emission and this should be reported if it is observed.

The consistency of the nasal air emission should be noted during the articulation test. If nasal air emission occurs during the production of most pressure-sensitive phonemes, then it is considered consistent. If it occurs occasionally on most pressure-sensitive phonemes, then it is inconsistent. If it occurs consistently, but only on specific phonemes, then it may be phoneme-specific nasal air emission (PSNAE), which is related to faulty articulation rather than velopharyngeal dysfunction.

It is always important to assess for nasal air emission in connected speech. Many individuals are able to achieve velopharyngeal closure for short segments and therefore, nasal air emission may not be noted on even the sentence level during the examination. Because connected speech increases the demands on the velopharyngeal mechanism, nasal air emission is more likely to be noted at this level.

Weak Consonants

The adequacy of intraoral air pressure should be evaluated by listening to the force of production of the pressure-sensitive consonants.

Having the individual repeat sentences loaded with these consonants is a good way to test oral pressure. If these consonants seem to be weak in intensity and pressure, it might be assumed that intraoral air pressure is compromised due to velopharyngeal dysfunction. Weak consonants are usually associated with both nasal air emission and hypernasality; therefore, there is usually a significant velopharyngeal opening as the cause.

Short Utterance Length

If there is significant nasal air emission, it can also have an effect on utterance length. This can be determined by observing the phrasing of utterances in connected speech. If the individual seems to take breaths frequently during speech, this may be due to the loss of air pressure through the velopharyngeal valve and the need to replenish this air pressure more frequently. Utterance length can be tested by asking the individual to count to 20. Most normal speakers can count at least to 15 on one breath. If more than two breaths are needed, this may indicate a significant loss of air pressure during speech due to velopharyngeal dysfunction.

Oral-Motor Function

Symptoms of velopharyngeal dysfunction may be obscured by significant articulation errors secondary to a verbal apraxia (apraxia of speech). Individuals with verbal apraxia typically demonstrate multiple inconsistent articulation errors involving the placement, manner, and voicing of the phonemes. The errors are often noted to increase with an increase in phonetic length or phonemic complexity. This type of oral-motor dysfunction is not uncommon in individuals with craniofacial syndromes, and seems to be particularly prevalent in individuals with velocardiofacial syndrome.

There are several formal tests of verbal apraxia that go from a nonspeech oral level up to the sentence level of production (Hickman, 1997;

Kaufman, 1994), but this can also be tested informally. The individual can be asked to repeat individual oral movements (e.g., lateralizing the tongue) and to sequence movements (e.g., moving the tongue to the corner of the mouth and then to the upper lip). Diadochokinetic exercises can be used to assess the ability to sequence syllables. The individual can be asked to repeat two syllable combinations (e.g., "puh tuh, puh tuh") or three syllable combinations (e.g., "puh tuh kuh, puh tuh kuh, puh tuh kuh"). Young children will often refuse to imitate nonsense syllables, so the use of real words usually works better. The child can be asked to repeat certain words three to five times in a row (e.g., "patty cake," "puppy dog," "teddy bear," "kitty cat," "bubble gum"). For older children and adults, more complex words or phrases should be used (e.g., "basketball," "peanut butter and jelly," "Encyclopedia Britannica," or even a fun word such as "supercalifragilisticexpialidocious").

Stimulability

An assessment of stimulability is a critical component of the perceptual evaluation since some articulation errors actually cause nasal air emission and even hypernasality. In fact, it has been shown radiographically that, when producing glottal stops, there is less velopharyngeal movement than during the production of oral sounds (Henningsson & Isberg, 1991). Articulation errors that cause nasal air emission or hypernasality are often the result of faulty learning of oral-motor movements, rather than a primary velopharyngeal valving disorder. In this case, the child will usually be stimulable for a reduction or elimination of nasal air emission with a change in articulatory placement. This is often found in individuals who demonstrate phoneme-specific nasal air emission (PSNAE) due to the use of a posterior nasal fricative as a substitution for oral sounds.

Stimulability should be assessed by attempting to normalize the placement of the articulation on single phonemes. If the child is able to produce the sound without nasal air emission or hypernasality merely by changing placement, this suggests a good prognosis for correction with speech therapy.

Recording the Results of Testing

The scoring of an articulation test is traditionally done by using phonetic diacritics from the International Phonetic Alphabet (IPA) (Bronsted et al., 1994). However, this system does not include symbols for compensatory productions that are typical of individuals with velopharyngeal dysfunction. Therefore, a set of diacritic symbols for compensatory productions was proposed by Trost (1981) and Trost-Cardamone (1997). The examiner may choose to use fine diacritics, but it is also acceptable to describe the speech characteristics in words, such as, "This child demonstrates the use of pharyngeal fricatives as a substitution for sibilant sounds (s, z,

---

Case Report: Velocardiofacial Syndrome and Oral-Motor Dysfunction

Katie, age 2 years 3 months, had a diagnosis of Velocardiofacial syndrome. Medical history was consistent with this diagnosis and included a submucous cleft, a ventricular septal defect (VSD), and an interrupted aortic valve. Katie was small for her age and was under the 10th percentile for both weight and height. She had a history of airway problems as an infant. Early feeding problems were also reported and Katie continued to have difficulty with certain textures.

Although the development of gross motor milestones was essentially within normal limits, speech and language development were delayed and fine motor skills were abnormal. Although she could put words together and even sing nursery rhymes, Katie's speech was mostly unintelligible. Therefore, she communicated primarily by gestures, signs, and pointing to pictures. According to the parents, Katie's understanding of language seemed normal.

A speech assessment revealed a severe articulation disorder. Katie's phonemic repertoire was extremely limited and consists of nasal consonants (m, n), /h/, glottal stops, and vowels. Occasionally she is able to produce a /d/ approximation. Vowels were on target most, but not all, of the time. When attempting to imitate sounds or oral placement, there was evidence of significant oral-motor dysfunction. Although Katie was able to produce nasal sounds in isolation, she was unable to produce them in certain word positions or with certain vowels. She was also unable to combine them for words such as "money, naming," or "many." When attempting to imitate oral pressure sounds or blow, there was only nasal air emission. Voice quality was noted to be normal, but resonance was judged to be mildly hypernasal.

Although it was felt that Katie would probably need surgical intervention for correction of the velopharyngeal dysfunction, given her age and size, her history of airway obstruction, and the evidence of severe oral-motor dysfunction, it was decided to delay this decision. Instead, a period of intensive speech therapy was recommended to improve oral-motor skills and articulation. It was felt that after a period of therapy, a more informed decision could be made regarding whether the hypernasality was due to a structural or oral-motor cause.

sh, ch, j)." This may be a more appropriate form of description for the diagnostic report, which usually goes to physicians, family members, and other readers who are unfamiliar with the symbols.

For nasal air emission, the examiner should report the type of nasal air emission and the consistency. If it occurs only on certain phonemes, this is also important to note.

Evaluation of Resonance

Evaluation of resonance is best done by listening to connected speech. Connected speech increases the demand on the velopharyngeal valving system, and as a result, deficiencies may become apparent on this level, even though they were not noted during the production of single words or short utterances.

Types of Resonance

The examiner should first determine the type of resonance by listening to connected speech, or sentences loaded with oral sounds and then those loaded with nasal sounds. Resonance should be judged as normal, hypernasal, hyponasal, denasal, cul-de-sac, or mixed resonance. It should be noted that these types of resonance are distinct types and are not different points on a continuum. As a general rule, if nasal sounds are heard more frequently than normal or if they are substituted for oral-type sounds, the resonance is hypernasal. On the other hand, if oral-type sounds are heard as a substitution for nasal sounds, the resonance is hyponasal. Mouth breathing is also indicative of airway obstruction and hyponasality. Cul-de-sac resonance sounds as if the voice is very muffled and remains in the head. For comparison, a type of cul-de-sac resonance can be simulated by imitating hypernasal speech while closing the nose.

Rating Scales of Severity

Several authors have suggested the use of an equal-appearing interval scale, with up to seven levels, to rate the severity of deviant resonance (McWilliams, Morris, & Shelton, 1990; Morris, Shelton, & McWilliams, 1973; Subtelny, Van Hattum, & Myers, 1972). McWilliams et al. (1990) provided a table (p. 316) of several types of rating scales that can be used to assess severity. Although these rating scales have a high degree of face validity, the reliability of these scales is in question. In fact, the more levels on the scale, the less reliable the scale will be. Therefore, other authors and clinicians feel that the best way to assess resonance is to make a decision that the problem is either present or absent (Bzoch, 1979). As a compromise, the examiner may choose to use a simple 4-point scale that includes normal, and then mild, moderate, and severe as descriptors of severity.

Regardless of the type of rating scale used, it should be noted that there is poor correlation between the perceived degree of hypernasality and the size of the velopharyngeal opening (Andrews & Rutherford, 1972; Carney & Morris, 1971; Kummer et al., 1992). This is due to many factors, including the use of compensatory articulation productions and the compounding effect of nasal air emission. In addition, a small velopharyngeal gap can cause a nasal rustle or turbulence, which is a loud bubbly sound. This can cause the speech to be perceived as more severely abnormal than when there is nasal air emission due to a larger gap.

Although the perceptual assessment of resonance is critically important, it is understandably difficult for the untrained ear. The use of training tapes for judgments of speech characteristics or collaboration with more experienced professionals may help to establish intra- and interjudge agreement. McWilliams and Phillips (1979) developed an excellent series of audiotapes that can be used for training both students and professionals in the identification of various types of resonance and various aspects of velopharyngeal dysfunction. Despite training, rating perceptual qualities remains a very difficult task.

Evaluation of Phonation

Breathiness and hoarseness may develop in individuals with mild velopharyngeal dysfunction as a result of vocal nodules (McWilliams, 1969; McWilliams, Lavorato, & Bluestone, 1973). These individuals may employ laryngeal hyperfunction in an attempt to compensate for the acoustic effects of velopharyngeal dysfunction. The use of glottal stops may also contribute to the development of vocal fold nodules. Finally, individuals with craniofacial anomalies may have anomalies of the larynx and vocal tract. Therefore, phonation should always be assessed as part of a complete resonance evaluation.

Phonation can be assessed in connected speech or by having the child prolong a single vowel. The child should sustain the vowel as long as possible without taking another breath. The examiner should also have the child glide on a vowel from low to high pitch and then back down the scale to see if pitch changes affect the quality of phonation.

In evaluating phonation, the examiner should listen for characteristics of dysphonia, including hoarseness, breathiness, glottal fry, hard glottal attack, inappropriate pitch level, restricted pitch range, diplophonia, or inappropriate loudness (Kummer & Marsh, 1998). When present, these abnormalities can be rated on a severity scale from mild to severe (Stemple, Glaze, & Gerdeman, 1995; Wilson, 1987). The ability to sustain phonation should also be observed. Dysphonic characteristics may not be noted until the end of the prolonged vowel as the child begins to run out of air pressure. Finally, the quality of breath support and the type of breathing pattern should be noted.

Supplemental Tests

At this point in the evaluation, the clinician may have an impression of the normal and abnormal characteristics of speech. However, supplemental tests are often needed to more clearly identify the type of resonance and the presence of nasal air emission, including nasal rustle (turbulence). The following supplemental tests may be helpful since they are sensitive to velopharyngeal valving problems.

Auditory Detection

- *Cul-de-Sac Test*: The cul-de-sac test (Bzoch, 1979, 1997) can be used to assess for hypernasality, hyponasality, and nasal air emission. To evaluate for hypernasality, the test is done by having the child prolong a vowel or repeat a sentence that is devoid of nasal consonants. The same speech segment is then repeated with the nostrils occluded by pinching the nares with the fingers (Figure 12–1). In normal speech, there should be no perceptible difference in the quality of the production since the nasal cavity is already closed by the velopharyngeal mechanism. If there is a difference in quality with closure of the nares, this suggests that resonance is hypernasal, since there is sound resonating in the nasal cavity. If resonance is perceived as abnormal but closure of the nares results in no change in quality, this does not necessarily rule out velopharyngeal dysfunction. The problem could include hyponasality or cul-de-sac resonance, in which case there is already blockage; therefore, further closure of the nares has no additional effect on the resonance.

  To assess for nasal air emission, the cul-de-sac test is done during the production of pressure-sensitive consonants. If there is an increase in oral pressure with closure of the nose, this is suggestive of velopharyngeal dysfunction.

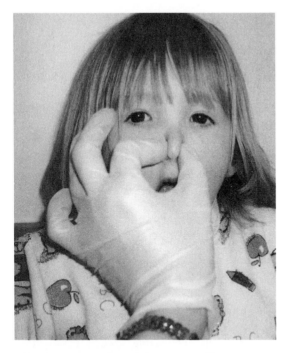

Figure 12–1. The cul-de-sac test. The examiner asks the patient to produce a speech segment and then repeat the segment with the nostrils occluded.

The cul-de-sac can also be used to a limited degree to assess hyponasality. In this case, the child is asked to produce a nasal sound repetitively (such as "ma, ma, ma") and then repeat this speech segment with the nose closed. If there is little or no difference in the quality, this suggests significant hyponasality.

- *Stethoscope:* If a stethoscope is available, it can be used to listen for nasal air emission or hypernasality. This is done by placing the stethoscope on one side of the nose and then on the other side and listening during the production of oral sounds and sentences. Hypernasality and nasal air emission, particularly a nasal rustle, can be heard with this instrument. The stethoscope can also be placed just under the nostrils to pick up nasal air emission.

- *Straw:* A straw can assist the examiner in the detection of nasal air emission. The straw is placed in the child's nostril as he or she produces pressure-sensitive sounds (Figure 12–2). If there is nasal air emission, this can be heard through the straw. If a lateral lisp is suspected (which often sounds like nasal air emission), the examiner can place a straw at different positions on the side of the dental arch during the production of a prolonged sibilant. If the air stream is lateralized, it will be heard through the straw at the side of the mouth.

- *Listening Tube:* A plastic tube can be a very helpful tool in evaluating nasal air emission and even hypernasality. One end of the tube is place in the child's nostril or even just at the entrance to the nostril, and the other end is place in the examiner's ear (Figure 12–3). As the child produces sounds or sentences, the examiner can hear occurrences of nasal air emission or hypernasality very clearly. This procedure is actually the most effective and most practical of all of these suggestions, and therefore, it is highly recommended.

Visual Detection

- *Dental Mirror:* A dental mirror can be held under the nares during speech in order to evaluate nasal air emission based on condensation (Figure 12–4). The examiner should place the mirror under the child's nose during the production of pressure-sensitive sounds. If the mirror clouds up, it indicates nasal air emission. Unfortunately, this is not a very practical technique because the mirror fogs as soon as the child breathes at the end of an utterance.

- *Air Paddle*: In addition to listening for nasal emission, the examiner can actually see nasal emission by using an "air paddle," as first described by Bzoch (1979). An air paddle can be cut from a piece of paper and placed underneath the nares during the production of repetitive syllables with pressure-sensitive consonants (i.e., "pa pa pa; ta ta ta; ka

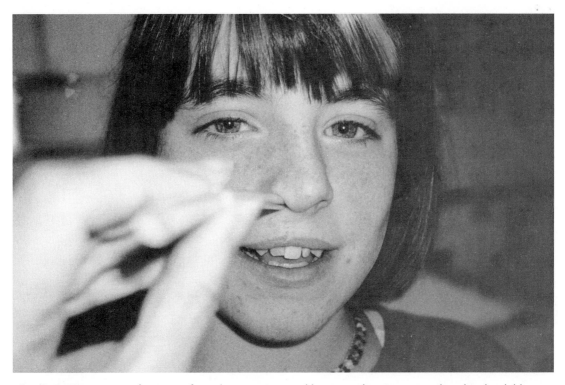

Figure 12–2. A straw for a test of nasal air emission and hypernasality. A straw is placed in the child's nostril as he or she produces pressure-sensitive sounds. If there is nasal air emission or hypernasality, this can be heard through the straw.

ka ka") (Figure 12–5). It is best to use voiceless consonants since these consist of more air pressure and are therefore most likely to show nasal air emission. If the paddle moves during the production of these sounds, this indicates that there is nasal air emission.

- *See Scape*: If a See Scape (Pro Ed, 1986, Austin, Texas) is available, the examiner can view the occurrence of nasal air emission with this instrument. A nasal olive is placed in the child's nostril. The nasal olive is attached to a flexible tube that is connected to a rigid vertical tube. As the child repeats pressure-sensitive phonemes, a styrofoam stopper rises in the vertical tube if there is nasal air emission (Figure 12–6). It is important to

keep in mind that, at the end of the utterance, the child will exhale slightly through the nose. Therefore, the stopper may rise slightly at this point, but this is normal.

Tactile Detection

- *Feel the Sides of the Nose:* Nasal air emission or hypernasality can sometimes be felt by placing the index fingers lightly on the individual's nose, in the area of the cartilage that is just below the bone (Figure 12–7). As the child repeats pressure-sensitive consonants or says "60, 60, 60," the examiner can feel for a vibration. If a vibration is felt during these repetitions, this suggests nasal air emission. Vibration can particularly be felt

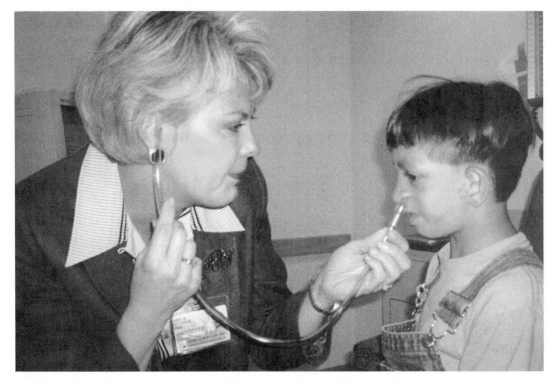

Figure 12–3. A "listening tube" for a test of nasal air emission and hypernasality. One end of a plastic tube is place in the child's nostril or at the entrance to the nostril, and the other end is place in the examiner's ear. As the child produces sounds or sentences, the examiner can hear occurrences of nasal air emission or hypernasality.

when a nasal rustle or turbulence occurs. The examiner can also feel the side of the nose as the child prolongs a vowel sound. If nasal vibration is felt during the production of the vowel, this suggests hypernasality.

These supplemental tests can provide additional information to help the examiner to make a determination regarding resonance and nasal air emission with confidence.

Differential Diagnosis

In every evaluation of resonance, the examiner must determine not only the perceptual features of the resonance disorder, but also the apparent source or cause of the problem. It certainly cannot be assumed that hypernasality and nasal air emission are always due to velopharyngeal dysfunction. The cause of the problem is important to determine because it will have a direct impact on the treatment recommendations.

Oronasal Fistula Versus Velopharyngeal Dysfunction

If there is an oronasal fistula, it is important to rule out the fistula as a cause of hypernasality or nasal air emission. The size of an oronasal fistula should always be noted, because this is one factor that can determine the effect on speech. If the fistula is large, approximately 5 mm or more in diameter, nasal air emission

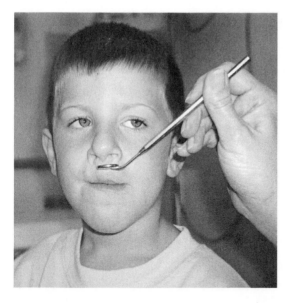

Figure 12–4. A dental mirror for testing nasal air emission. A dental mirror can be held under the nares during speech in order to evaluate nasal air emission during speech based on the appearance of condensation.

may be noted with the production of pressure-sensitive consonants. If the fistula is very large, there may be hypernasality as well.

The position of the fistula can also determine whether there is an effect on speech. If the fistula is in the area of the incisive foramen, which is very common, there may be nasal air emission during the production of lingual-alveolar sounds due to the fact that the tongue pushes air into the opening as it elevates for production. A mid-palatal fistula can result in the use of a palatal-dorsal placement for many sounds as a compensatory strategy to close the fistula with the tongue. A posterior fistula may be less symptomatic because there are fewer posterior sounds in speech to force the airstream upward.

A fistula usually does not have the same type of detrimental effect on speech as a velopharyngeal opening. When comparing a fistula to a velopharyngeal gap of the same size, the velopharyngeal opening will be far more sympto-

matic than the fistula. This difference has to do with position. With the velopharyngeal gap, there is air pressure traveling superiorly in the pharynx, perpendicular to the velopharyngeal opening. Therefore, even a small opening will be symptomatic. In contrast, an oronasal fistula is in the oral cavity where the airstream is flowing anteriorly, so that it is parallel to and under the fistula. Therefore, unless the fistula is large or the tongue pushes the airstream into it with articulation, it may not be symptomatic for speech.

There are a few techniques that can be used to determine if a fistula is symptomatic. First, if there is hypernasality, it is unlikely that it is coming from the fistula, unless the fistula is very large. If there is nasal air emission, the examiner can compare its occurrence on anterior sounds versus posterior sounds. If there is no difference, then the source of the nasal air emission is probably velopharyngeal dysfunction. However, if there is more nasal emission on anterior sounds than on the posterior sounds that are behind the fistula, this suggests the fistula as the cause.

Another way to evaluate the effect of a fistula is to temporarily close it with chewing gum or dental wax. A comparison of the speech with and without occlusion can be done perceptually, through nasometry, pressure-flow measures, or informal measures. If occlusion of the fistula results in a reduction in nasal air emission or hypernasality, then it is obvious that the fistula is at least partly to blame for the deviant speech and resonance. If hypernasality or nasal air emission are still noted with total occlusion of the fistula, then velopharyngeal dysfunction is implicated as the cause.

One complicating factor in evaluating the effect of a fistula versus velopharyngeal dysfunction is the combined effect of the two. When there is a leak in the system as a result of a fistula, this can also cause the velopharyngeal mechanism to function less efficiently (Moller, 1991). Therefore, unless the fistula is closed or obturated, it can be difficult to evaluate the ca-

A

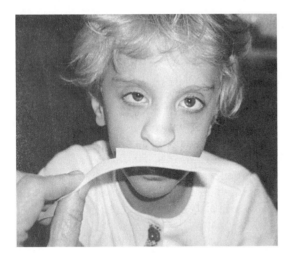

B

Figure 12–5. A. An "air paddle" to be used in testing for nasal air emission. The paddle can be cut (or even torn) from a piece of paper. **B.** The paddle is placed underneath the nares during the production of repetitive syllables with pressure-sensitive consonants. If the paddle moves during speech, this indicates nasal air emission.

pabilities of velopharyngeal mechanism. It often takes a multidisciplinary approach to determine the symptomatology that is directly due to the fistula and to formulate the appropriate treatment plan (Folk, D'Antonio, & Hardesty, 1997).

Mislearning Versus Velopharyngeal Dysfunction

When there are characteristics of velopharyngeal dysfunction, this reflects what the child is doing with the velopharyngeal mechanism,

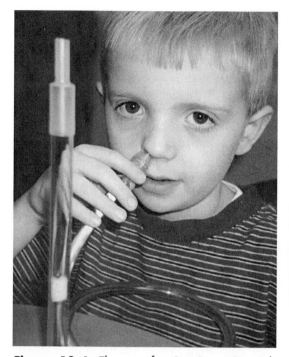

Figure 12–6. The use of a See Scape (Pro Ed, Austin, TX) for testing nasal air emission. The patient places the nasal olive at the entrance to the nostril. If there is nasal air emission during speech production, the sytrofoam stopper will rise in the tube.

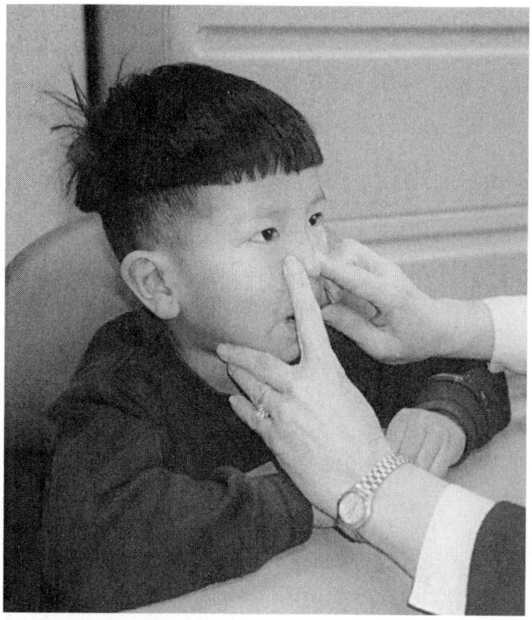

Figure 12–7. A tactile test of nasal air emission and hypernasality. Nasal air emission or hypernasality sometimes be felt by placing the index fingers lightly on the individual's nose, in the area of the cartilage that is just below the bone. As the child repeats pressure-sensitive consonants or says "60, 60, 60," the examiner can feel the vibration of nasal air emission or hypernasality.

but it does not necessarily reflect what the individual is capable of doing. If the characteristics of velopharyngeal dysfunction are due to mislearning or faulty articulation, this is very important to determine so that speech therapy, rather than a surgical procedure, is recommended for treatment.

Stimulability testing is the key to determining whether the characteristics are due to a structural or physiological defect or due to mislearning disorder. For example, if nasal air emission is noted only on certain sounds, but there is good oral pressure and no nasal air emission on other pressure-sensitive phonemes, this suggests the possibility of an articulation disorder rather than velopharyngeal dysfunction. In addition, if nasal air emission is eliminated by a change in articulation placement, this is a good indication that the disorder is functional, not structural. For specific suggestions on changing articulatory placement to eliminate nasal air emission, see Chapter 21.

Follow-Up

Recommendations

Once the speech pathology evaluation is completed, the examiner must make a decision as to whether to recommend speech therapy or to refer for further evaluation. If the child demonstrates hypernasality or nasal emission and does not respond to stimulability probing, speech therapy alone is usually not appropriate. Instead, a further evaluation of velopharyngeal function may be recommended with consideration of surgical management. Depending on the other observations during testing and the other test results, additional recommendations might also be made. These could include assessments by a developmental specialist, psychologist, neurologist, geneticist, otolaryngologist, plastic surgeon, oral surgeon, dentist, or orthodontist. The examiner might also recommend other diagnostic procedures, such as a sleep study, a videofluoroscopic swallow study, or an endoscopic evaluation of speech or swallowing. If the child was evaluated through a screening, further assessment of speech and language skills could be recommended. Treatment recommendations might include surgical management, prosthetic management, or speech therapy. A special preschool or educational setting may be part of the overall treatment plan or the examiner may refer the child and family to other community resources. Prior to making the referrals for additional evaluations or for other forms of treatment, the speech pathologist should discuss the recommendations with the primary care physician and the referring physician. This is not only common courtesy, but is consistent with the "medical model" where the primary care physician manages the child's overall plan of care.

Recommendations should always be based on the cause and severity of the speech or resonance disorder, its effect on the child's quality of life, the potential for improvement, the associated risks, and the desires of the child and the family. The examiner must be careful not to impose his or her own value system and personal preferences on the child and the family. They are the ones who have to live with the consequences of the decision.

Family Counseling

One important aspect of the speech and resonance evaluation is family education. Counseling the child and family members following the evaluation is not optional. Instead, it is one of the most important components of the evaluation. Unfortunately, it often does not receive the emphasis from healthcare professionals that it should. In order to include the child and family members as part of the team, which most professionals agree is appropriate, thorough counseling becomes a prerequisite. Considering the fact that the child and family hold the deciding vote on all treatment options, yet are the least informed regarding these options, education is critically important and the key to successful treatment of the child.

Counseling is usually done immediately following the evaluation. The family members and child (as appropriate) should be informed of the results of the evaluation, the implications of those results, the examiner's impressions, and finally, the recommendations for treatment. When treatment is recommended, the risks and benefits should be carefully explained. Because most family members want to be a part of the treating team, it is important to include instructions on how they can help, and what their role will be in the treatment process. For children under the age of 3, methods of speech and language stimulation should be explained to the parents and demonstrated if possible.

Many professionals make the mistake of using professional or medical terminology when talking to the family. Even speech pathologists, who are experts in communication, are often guilty of this error. Counseling will never be successful, however, if the family members do not understand the terminology. Although the appropriate terms should be used to describe the anatomy or diagnosis, these terms should be carefully explained and defined. It is important to phrase explanations using simple and direct language as much as possible. The use of

Case Report: Phoneme-Specific Nasal Air Emission

Jeff was a 36-year-old man with a history of "nasality" although he was not born with a cleft palate. His parents were told that he would need surgery to correct the problem, but they opted not to have that done. In his early 20s, Jeff sought another opinion and was again told that he would require surgery for correction. Due to his hesitancy to go through with the procedure, the surgery was never done. When he came to our clinic at the age of 36, Jeff reported that his speech had been a barrier in his work and social life, and therefore, he was finally ready for the surgery.

On examination, the velum appeared to be normal. An assessment of speech revealed the substitution of a posterior nasal fricative for sibilant sounds (s, z, sh, ch, j). This production was accompanied by nasal air emission. All other speech sounds were produced correctly with normal air pressure and no evidence of nasal air emission. An assessment of resonance revealed normal oral resonance and no evidence of hypernasality. Given these findings, it was surmised that this patient was demonstrating phoneme-specific nasal air emission rather than velopharyngeal dysfunction with either an anatomic or physiological etiology.

To test this assumption, stimulability testing was done. Jeff was asked to repeat various pressure-sensitive phonemes in sequence (pa pa pa, ta ta ta, etc.) with his hand in front of his mouth to note the oral air pressure. He was then instructed to produce an isolated /t/ sound repetitively and in a forceful manner, while still feeling the air pressure during production. In the next step, Jeff was told to produce the /t/ forcefully with the teeth closed while still maintaining velopharyngeal closure. He was able to perform all of these tasks easily with good oral pressure and no nasal air emission. Therefore, he was instructed to produce the /t/ with the teeth closed and then prolong the end, making it a /tsssss/. Again, he was able to do this easily, and the /s/ sound was produced orally with no nasal air emission. The final step was to eliminate the starter /t/. This was the hardest part for Jeff, but within a few minutes, he was able to produce the /s/ and all of the other sibilants in isolation with normal oral pressure and no nasal air emission. This was suggestive of a functional learning problem since, with instruction, he was able to achieve complete velopharyngeal closure on all speech sounds.

Rather than undergoing a surgical procedure, as was recommended in the past, Jeff was enrolled in speech therapy. Within a few months, he had eliminated the use of posterior nasal fricatives and was producing sibilants normally without nasal air emission. In essence, the "nasality" was "cured" without the need for surgery.

This case illustrates the importance of a differential diagnosis. In Jeff's case, it is fortunate that he did not follow through with the recommendation for surgery, because it would not have corrected the problem. On the other hand, it is unfortunate that he was misdiagnosed and that speech therapy was not done when he was a child.

handouts is a method to ensure that the family members understand and remember the information that was given to them in the counsel-ing session. Handouts with labeled drawings are particularly useful in helping the family to understand the anatomy and any surgical procedures that are being proposed. Many centers give out their own handouts and brochures that contain specific information regarding their program and facility, as can be seen in the example in Appendix 12–1. In addition, many informational brochures are available through the Cleft Palate Foundation (CPF) of the American Cleft Palate-Craniofacial Association. Information regarding the CPF is found in Appendix A of this book, and a selected bibliography for parents is found in Appendix B.

Evaluation Report

The perceptual evaluation is only as good as the information in the report, since that is what is primarily communicated to the family and other professionals. Therefore, the report must be accurate, succinct, clear, and concise. Many professionals fail to consider their "customers" when writing the report. Long reports are usually not read and are definitely not appreciated by busy professionals. The report should contain appropriate language and medical terminology, but should also be understandable to the readers. If the physicians, parents, and other professionals are unfamiliar with the terminology that is used, they will not be able to clearly understand what the examiner is trying to communicate. The report should focus on the evaluation results, the examiner's impressions, and the recommendations. Most of all, it is important to be correct and confident in the stated conclusions and recommendations, as this will often result in surgical management.

Some centers are beginning to generate computer-based reports. At Cincinnati Children's Hospital Medical Center, we worked with two software development companies to develop a comprehensive software program that computerizes all patient documentation, including diagnostic reports, through what is now called Chart Links Rehabilitation Software (Version 3.1, Chart Links, New Haven, CT). As part of this software, there are preset evaluation sections and formats with selected words to fill in the blanks. This makes report generation very easy and cost-effective. Computerized reports can help to guide the examiner through the evaluation and ensure that the evaluation, and thus the report, is done completely and with good consistency among all speech pathologists.

Evaluation reports are often sent to the treating speech pathologist in the child's community. Since evaluations as part of a cleft palate or craniofacial team meeting are often screening evaluations to determine the need for further testing or the type of intervention, these evaluations may not include in-depth speech or language testing. Therefore, the team speech pathologist may recommend further assessment of communication skills. The team speech pathologist should offer to assist the treating therapist by providing information, answering questions, and offering suggestions for a treatment approach as needed.

Summary

A perceptual assessment of resonance gives the examiner information regarding the presence of velopharyngeal dysfunction and the effect on speech production. However, this type of evaluation does not allow the examiner to determine the cause, size, or location of the velopharyngeal opening. Therefore, direct instrumental assessment may be helpful in determining the treatment plan. However, instrumental measures will never replace the perceptual evaluation. In the end, the ear remains the best judge of abnormal speech and resonance, and intervention for correction is only initiated based on judgments made by the ear.

References

American Cleft Palate-Craniofacial Association. (1993). Parameters for evaluation and treatment of patients with cleft lip/palate or other craniofacial anomalies. *Cleft Palate Craniofacial Journal, 30* (Suppl.), 1–16.

Andrews, J. R., & Rutherford, D. (1972). Contribution of nasally emitted sound to the perception of hypernasality of vowels. *Cleft Palate Journal, 9,* 147–156.

Bronsted, K., Grunwell, P., Henningsson, G., Jansonius, K. J. K., Meijer, M., Ording, U., Sell, K., Vermeij-Zieverink, E., & Wyatt, R. (1994). A phonetic framework for the cross-linguistic analysis of cleft palate speech. *Clinical Linguistics and Phonetics, 8,* 109–125.

Bzoch, K. R. (1979). Measurement and assessment of categorical aspects of cleft palate speech. In K. R. Bzoch (Ed.), *Communicative disorders related to cleft lip and palate* (Vol. 2, pp. 161–191). Boston: Little, Brown.

Bzoch, K. R. (1997). Clinical assessment, evaluation and management of 11 categorical aspects of cleft palate speech. In K. R. Bzoch (Ed.), *Communicative disorders related to cleft lip and palate* (Vol. 4, pp. 261–311). Austin, TX: Pro-Ed.

Bzoch, K. R., & League, R. (1991). *Receptive-Expressive Emergent Language Test: A method for assessing the language skills of infants* (2nd ed.). Austin, TX: Pro-Ed.

Carney, P. J., & Morris, H. L. (1971). Structural correlates of nasality. *Cleft Palate Journal, 8,* 307–321.

Chart Links Rehabilitation Software (Version 3.1) [Computer software]. New Haven, CT: Chart Links.

Coplan, J. (1987). *Early Language Milestone (ELM) Scale.* Austin, TX: Pro-Ed.

Dalston, R. M. (1997). The use of nasometry in the assessment and remediation of velopharyngeal inadequacy. In K. R. Bzoch (Ed.), *Communicative disorders related to cleft lip and palate* (Vol. 4, pp. 331–346). Austin, TX: Pro-Ed.

Fenson, L., Dale, P. S., Reznick, J. S., Thal, D., Bates, E., Hartung, P., Pethick, S., & Reilly, J. S. (1989). *The MacArthur Communicative Development Inventory.* San Diego, CA: Development Psychology Lab, San Diego State University.

Fluharty, N. B. (1978). *Fluharty Preschool Speech and Language Test.* Boston: Teaching Resources Corporation.

Folk, S. N., D'Antonio, L. L., & Hardesty, R. A. (1997). Secondary cleft deformities. *Clinics in Plastic Surgery, 24*(3), 599–611.

Glascoe, F. P. (1991). Can clinical judgment detect children with speech-language problems? *Pediatrics, 87*(3), 317–322.

Henningsson, G., & Isberg, A. (1991). A cineradiographic study of velopharyngeal movements for deviant versus nondeviant articulation. *Cleft Palate Craniofacial Journal, 28*(1), 115–117; (Discussion 117–118).

Hickman, L. A. (1997). *Apraxia profile: A descriptive assessment tool for children.* San Antonio, TX: Communication Skill Builders.

Kaufman, N. R. (1994). *Kaufman Speech Praxis Test for Children (KSPT).* Detroit, MI: Wayne State University Press.

Kummer, A. W., Curtis, C., Wiggs, M., Lee, L., & Strife, J. L. (1992). Comparison of velopharyngeal gap size in patients with hypernasality, hypernasality and nasal emission, or nasal turbulence (rustle) as the primary speech characteristic. *Cleft Palate Craniofacial Journal, 29*(2), 152–156.

Kummer, A. W., & Marsh, J. H. (1998). Pediatric voice and resonance disorders. In A. F. Johnson & B. H. Jacobson (Eds.), *Medical speech-language pathology: A practitioner's guide.* New York: Thieme.

McWilliams, B. J. (1969). The role of otolaryngological problems in speech disorders associated with cleft palate. *Transactions of the American Academy of Ophthalmology and Otolaryngology, 73*(4), 720–723.

McWilliams, B. J., Lavorato, A. S., & Bluestone, C. D. (1973). Vocal cord abnormalities in children with velopharyngeal valving problems. *Laryngoscope, 83*(11), 1745–1753.

McWilliams, B. J., Morris, H. L., & Shelton, R. L. (1990). Diagnosis of phonation and resonance. In B. J. Williams, H. L. Morris, & R. L. Shelton (Eds.), *Cleft palate speech* (pp. 311–319). Philadelphia: B.C. Decker.

McWilliams, B. J., & Phillips, B. J. (1979). Velopharyngeal incompetence. *Audio Seminars in Speech Pathology.* Philadelphia: W. B. Saunders.

Moller, K. T. (1991). An approach to the evaluation of velopharyngeal adequacy for speech. *Clinics in Communication Disorders, 1*(1), 61–65.

Morris, H. L., Shelton, R. L., & McWilliams, B. J. (1973). Assessment of speech. *Speech, language and psychosocial aspects of cleft lip and palate: State of the art. Asha Reports, 9.*

Rossetti, L. (1990). *The Rossetti infant-toddler language scale.* East Moline, IL: Lingui Systems.

Scherer, N. J., & D'Antonio, L. L. (1995). Parent questionnaire for screening early language development in children with cleft palate. *Cleft Palate Craniofacial Journal, 32*(1), 7–13.

Scherer, N. J. & D'Antonio, L. L. (1997). Language and play development in toddlers with cleft lip and/or palate. *American Journal of Speech-Language Pathology, 6*(4), 48–54.

Schneider, E., & Shprintzen, R. J. (1980). A survey of speech pathologists: Current trends in the diagnosis and management of velopharyngeal insufficiency. *Cleft Palate Journal, 17*(3), 249–253.

Stemple, J. C., Glaze, L. E., & Gerdeman, B. K. (1995). *Clinical voice pathology: Theory and management.* San Diego, CA: Singular Publishing Group.

Subtelny, J. D., Van Hattum, R. J., & Myers, B. B. (1972). Ratings and measures of cleft palate speech. *Cleft Palate Journal, 9*(1), 18–27.

Templin, M. C., & Darley, F. (1960). *Screening and diagnostic tests of articulation.* Iowa City, IA: Bureau of Educational Research and Service Extension Division, State University of Iowa.

Trost, J. E. (1981). Articulatory additions to the classical description of the speech of persons with cleft palate. *Cleft Palate Journal, 18*(3), 193–203.

Trost-Cardamone, J. E. (1987). *Cleft palate misarticulations; A teaching tape* [Videotape]. Northridge, CA: California State University, Northridge, Instructional Media Center.

Trost-Cardamone, J. E. (1997). Diagnosis of specific cleft palate speech error patterns for planning therapy of physical management needs. In K. R. Bzoch (Ed.), *Communicative disorders related to cleft lip and palate* (Vol. 4, pp. 313–330). Austin, TX: Pro-Ed.

Wilson, D. K. (1987). *Voice problems of children.* (Vol. 3). Baltimore, MD: Williams & Wilkins.

Appendix 12-1

The Effects of Cleft Lip/Palate on Communication Development: Information for Parents

A history of cleft lip or palate can affect the child's ability to develop verbal communication skills. The following aspects of verbal communication can be defective:

- **Articulation (Speech)**—the physical production of sounds to form spoken words.
- **Language**—the message conveyed back and forth in talking. This includes the ability to understand the speech of others and the ability to express thoughts through words and sentences.
- **Voice**—the sound that results from the vibration of the vocal folds (phonation).
- **Resonance**—the vibration of voiced sound in the oral cavity (mouth) and nasal cavity (nose).

There are three main causes of communication disorders in children with a history of cleft lip and palate. These are as follows:

1. Dental Abnormalities

If the cleft extended into the alveolus (gum ridge), dental development may be affected. This may result in dental abnormalities such as:

- missing teeth
- supernumerary (extra) teeth
- malocclusion (poor closure of the top and bottom jaws)

Dental abnormalities may cause speech errors as follows:

- a lisp type of distortion on sibilant sounds (s, z, sh, ch, j).
- difficulty producing lip sounds (p, b, m).
- difficulty producing teeth to lip sounds (f, v).
- difficulty producing tongue-tip sounds (t, d, n, l)

These distortions can usually be corrected with a combination of dental and orthodontic treatment, and speech therapy.

2. Hearing Loss

Children with a history of cleft palate often have chronic ear infections called otitis media. This is due to the loss of function of the tensor veli palatini muscle in the soft palate. This muscle is responsible for opening the eustachian tube between the ear and the back of the throat to allow air into the ear and fluids out. If this muscle does not function well, the eustachian tube does not open. Negative pressure builds up in the middle ear, causing a build-up of fluids, ear infections, and a conductive hearing loss.

A conductive hearing loss can affect a child's ability to develop receptive and expressive language skills. In addition, articulation development may be disrupted due to the difficulty in hearing the fine differences between individual speech sounds.

To avoid potential middle ear problems, pressure equalizing (PE) tubes are often inserted in the eardrum at an early age. This helps to prevent fluids from building up in the ear to cause infection and hearing loss.

3. Velopharyngeal Dysfunction (VPD), Also Known as Velopharyngeal Insufficiency (VPI)
In order to close off the nose from the mouth during speech, several structures come together to achieve "velopharyngeal closure." These include the following:

- velum (soft palate)
- lateral pharyngeal walls—side walls of the throat
- posterior pharyngeal wall—the back wall of the throat

Through sphincterlike closure, these structures close off the oral cavity (mouth) from the nasal cavity (nose) during speech. This allows the speaker to build up air pressure in the mouth to produce various consonant sounds with normal pressure and normal oral resonance. Velopharyngeal closure also occurs during other activities, such as swallowing, gagging, vomiting, sucking, blowing, and whistling.

After a cleft palate repair, the velum (soft palate) may still be too short or may not move well enough to reach the posterior pharyngeal wall (back wall of the throat). This results in velopharyngeal dysfunction (VPD) which causes problems with speech.

Effects of Velopharyngeal Dysfunction on Speech

Velopharyngeal dysfunction can cause the following speech characteristics:

- hypernasality or too much sound in the nose during speech,
- nasal air emission during consonant production,
- weak or omitted consonants due to inadequate air pressure in the mouth, and
- compensatory articulation productions.

Treatment of Velopharyngeal Dysfunction (VPD)

Treatment of VPD may include speech therapy or surgical intervention. Prosthetic devices can also be used on a temporary or permanent basis in some cases.

Summary

Communication disorders secondary to a history of cleft lip or palate can be successfully treated with early and appropriate intervention. If a communication or swallowing disorder is suspected at any age, an evaluation should be done. Prior to age 3, language development should be the primary focus. After age 3, speech and resonance should be evaluated. If therapy or further surgery is indicated, it is often done in the preschool years. In most cases, the speech disorder can be greatly improved and often corrected by the time the child begins school. The team approach to management is particularly important for the best overall outcome since coordination of multiple disciplines is required to meet a variety of needs.

CHAPTER

13

Orofacial Examination

CONTENTS

An intraoral examination should always be done as part of a speech or resonance evaluation. Knowledge of the oral structures and their potential effect on speech production and resonance is extremely important in order to make appropriate recommendations for treatment. If there are structural factors that cause or contribute to the deviant speech or resonance, these structural problems should be corrected, if possible, prior to starting speech therapy. In some cases, correcting the structure results in correction of the speech without the need for further intervention. In other cases, the compensatory productions need to be corrected with therapy after the structure is normalized.

In performing an intraoral assessment, the examiner should be aware, however, that a judgment regarding velopharyngeal function cannot be made based on this examination alone. Velopharyngeal closure occurs behind the velum, usually on the plane of the hard palate, and is therefore well above the level that is viewed through the oral cavity. In addition, the examiner cannot see the point of maximum lateral pharyngeal wall movement from an intraoral perspective. In fact, at the oral level, the lateral pharyngeal walls may actually appear to bow outward during phonation. Finally, velopharyngeal function cannot be judged during a sustained vowel, such as "ah." An intraoral examination does not provide an adequate view of the structures to truly evaluate function, and even if it did, the function of the velopharyngeal mechanism must be evaluated based on the movement and closure during connected speech

Despite these limitations, the examiner can evaluate all of the oral structures that can affect speech and resonance production, including the status of labial competence, dental occlusion, the hard palate, the oral surface of the velum, the uvula, the tonsils, and the tongue. Therefore, an intraoral assessment can result in valuable information that can impact the examiner's overall impressions and recommendations from the assessment.

This chapter discusses methodology for a comprehensive examination of relevant structures and function for the production of normal speech and resonance. In addition, it seems appropriate to include information here regarding procedures for infection control.

General Methodology

Tools for an Orofacial Examination

An intraoral examination can often be done effectively without instruments. However, some instruments are very helpful and should be available for oral examinations. The tools for an intraoral examination include:

- **gloves:** for protection of the patient and the examiner.
- **flashlight:** for illumination of the oral cavity.
- **tongue blades:** to assist in holding the tongue down to observe the velum and uvula and to put between the buccal sulcus to observe dentition. Flavored tongue blades are now available and seem to be better received by young patients.
- **dental mirror:** to use like a tongue blade in depressing the tongue; also to use to look up into the pharynx, or to inspect the palate for a fistula with the help of the reflection.
- **alcohol swabs:** to clean contaminated surfaces or equipment.

Visual Inspection of the Oral Cavity

If done correctly, a physical examination of morphology and function of the oral cavity can reveal important information. An adequate examination, therefore, involves more than a quick look in the mouth. It involves careful inspection of the structures that relate to speech production and viewing of these structures during function.

When conducting an intraoral examination, most health care professionals ask the patient to say "ah" in order to inspect the structure. This vowel works well for evaluation of the hard palate and the anterior oral structures, but is less appropriate for evaluating the structure of the velum and the uvula. Although the "ah" vowel is considered a low vowel, it is primarily the jaw and tip of the tongue that are in a low position. The back of the tongue can be high and retracted so that it obstructs the view of the posterior section of the oral cavity and pharynx. Furthermore, this vowel makes it impossible to bring the tongue forward and out of the way for an adequate view. Because of these problems, a tongue blade is usually required to depress the back of the tongue so that it is low enough for the examiner to visualize the tip of the uvula.

If the vowel "aah" is used for the examination instead, the patient can be instructed to stick the tongue out and down as far as it will go (Figure 13–1). A young child can be instructed to point his tongue to his shoes. Although this does not allow the examiner to see "typical" velar movement, it does provide the examiner with a better view of the velum, uvula, and pharynx as the base of the tongue moves down and forward. This can be especially important when evaluating for a submucous cleft, because the examiner can better evaluate for diastasis of the muscles of the velum and this allows the examiner to see down to the tip of the velum. In addition to providing a better view of the structures, this technique allows the examiner to see the structures without the use of a tongue blade in many cases. Many patients, including adults, have a strong aversion to the use of tongue blades for fear of gagging.

If a tongue blade is needed, however, the blade should be placed approximately three

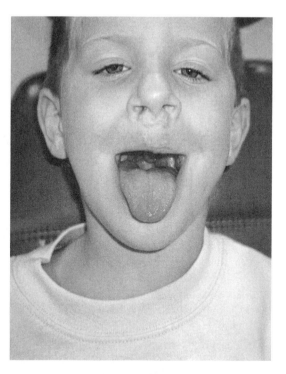

Figure 13–1. The vowel "aah" should be used for the examination of the velum and uvula. The patient should be instructed to stick the tongue out and down as far as it will go. A young child can be asked to point it to his shoes. Although this does not allow the examiner to see "typical" velar movement, it does provide the examiner with a better view of the velum, uvula, and pharynx as the base of the tongue moves down and forward.

quarters of the way back. If the blade is placed too far forward, which is a common mistake, it causes the posterior part of the tongue to mound up so as to obscure, rather than expose, the pharynx. If the tongue blade is placed behind the *circumvallate papilla*, a line of prominent taste buds that form an inverted "V" on the posterior tongue, it often elicits a gag reflex. The gag can give the examiner a good view, but it is a quick view and is not appreciated by the patient. The correct technique for using a tongue blade is to press the tongue downward firmly, while scooping it forward at the same time. The tongue is a strong, muscular organ, so firm pressure is often required to push against resistance.

As the individual phonates in producing a single vowel, there may be vigorous movement of the velum, or very little movement, even in normal speakers. To stimulate movement, the child can be asked to produce the vowel repetitively. If this does not seem to stimulate movement, then the examiner can ask the child to do a big yawn with the tongue protruded. This will help to elevate the velum to its fullest extent.

Positioning of the patient is another consideration when performing an intraoral examination. The patient's head should be tilted slightly backward so that the examiner can look directly to the back of the pharynx. The examiner should be slightly below the patient so that his or her eye level is at the level of the patient's oral cavity. If the patient is a very young child, it is sometimes helpful to have the parent or caregiver hold the child in a supine position with the head slightly lower than the rest of the body. This will usually promote an open-mouth posture, but the tongue may fall back into the pharynx. On rare occasions when an examination is needed and the patient refuses to open his or her mouth, the examiner should place the tongue blade between the upper and lower incisors and apply steady pressure. The muscles closing the mouth are powerful, but fatigue rapidly, so that constant, firm pressure will allow insertion of the tongue blade within a few seconds. When the blade reaches the posterior tongue, the gag reflex will cause the mouth to open fully.

Palatal Palpation

One purpose of palatal palpation is to determine if there is a notch in the border of the hard palate, which would suggest a submucous cleft (Mason & Grandstaff, 1971; Mason & Simon, 1977). Palpation might also be done to further

explore a fistula to determine whether it is patent. If the examiner is inexperienced or not well trained in this area, palatal palpation can be difficult for the examiner and even more difficult for the patient. The key to successful palpation is to be gentle and slow in feeling the palatal structures. Surprises in the area of the gag reflex are not well received by the patient! However, carefully feeling the roof of the mouth with a gloved finger does not cause pain or even discomfort. If there is an open cleft or a fistula, it should be remembered that this is a variation in the structure and not an open wound.

In preschool and school-aged children, it is best to use the fifth (or little) finger for palpation. This finger is long enough to reach the back of the palate of children in this age group. In addition, this finger is narrow enough to feel a small notch in the palatal bone. For teenagers and adults, the fifth finger is usually not long enough to reach to the back of the hard palate. Therefore, the index finger must be used.

To begin the examination, it is important to wash hands thoroughly and then to don gloves. For a young child, the examiner should begin by merely rubbing or stimulating the outside gums above the maxillary teeth. This helps the patient to become more comfortable and accepting of the examiner's finger in the mouth. The examiner should then stimulate the alveolar ridge behind the teeth by moving the finger from the front of the ridge to the back in the area of the molars. Once the patient is comfortable with that amount of stimulation, the examiner should glide the finger directly behind the last molar, and then slowly move the finger along the back edge of the hard palate until it reaches the midline. This is the point where the notch should be felt if it exists. To feel for the notch, the examiner should try to gently probe the midpoint of the posterior border of the hard palate. With the little finger, the examiner is more likely to feel a small or narrow defect than if the larger index finger is used.

Examination for a Fistula

If the patient has a history of cleft palate, the examiner should rule out the presence of an oronasal (palatal) fistula. This is done by having the patient put the head back as far as possible so that the entire hard palate can be visualized. A dental mirror can be especially helpful in visualizing the palate (Figure 13–2). Once the palate can be seen, the examiner should look carefully for evidence of a hole anywhere in the line of the cleft. At times, there may be a furrow or a small depression in the palate. This may appear to be a fistula, but it may actually be a blind pouch that does not go through to the nasal cavity.

The patency of an apparent oronasal fistula can often be determined partly by patient history. If the patient or parent report that the coloring of food is sometimes seen in the nostril area, this is an indication of a patent fistula. (Chocolate milk, chocolate pudding, and spaghetti seem to be primary offenders.) It should be noted that regurgitation of food does not usually occur with velopharyngeal dysfunc-

tion. The size of a fistula is often difficult to estimate. It may appear narrow on the oral surface but open considerably on the nasal surface. With gloved fingers, the examiner can sometimes feel the extent of a large palatal fistula.

In addition to inspecting the palate for a fistula, the examiner should also look for a fistula in the alveolar bone, just under the upper lip and in the line of the cleft. This type of fistula, called a nasolabial fistula or just labial fistula, is common before the alveolar bone grafting is done. It does not typically cause problems with speech because it is in an anterior position and the upper lip drapes over the opening. To inspect the alveolar ridge for a labial fistula, the examiner should use a tongue blade or dental mirror to gently raise the upper lip. The fistula can be seen or palpated by feeling the anterior gum ridge under the buccal sulcus with a gloved finger.

Important Observations

When conducting an orofacial or intraoral examination, it is important to keep in mind that there are normal variations in structure. Therefore, the examiner may observe characteristics that are unusual, but not necessarily abnormal. In addition, there may be abnormalities that have no relevance to speech or resonance. Although the examiner should focus on assessing for abnormalities that can contribute to a speech or resonance disorder, other abnormalities should also be noted. This is particularly important if they provide evidence for the diagnosis of a syndrome (i.e., hypertelorism) or if they require additional referral and follow-up (i.e., dental caries). Although the speech pathologist is not qualified to make a diagnosis of a syndrome based on observations of abnormalities, the speech pathologist can and should discuss the observations with the primary care physician and referring physician. A genetics evaluation may be suggested if it has not been done.

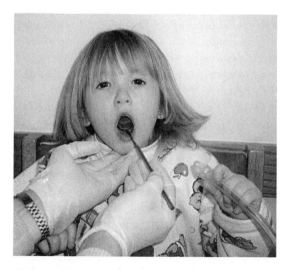

Figure 13–2. A dental mirror can be especially helpful in visualizing the palate in order to see a palatal fistula.

Case Report: Oronasal Fistula

Gerald presented as a new patient at the age of 11. He had a history of bilateral complete cleft lip and palate, which were repaired in another state. He had also had a pharyngeal flap for correction of velopharyngeal insufficiency at the age of 4. Gerald received speech therapy for several years in school. The mother reported that her primary concern was Gerald's nasality.

Upon examination, Gerald's speech was found to be minimally intelligible. His articulation pattern consisted of backing of anterior phonemes. Many compensatory productions were used. Resonance was hyponasal and mouth breathing was noted, suggesting upper airway obstruction. An obstructing pharyngeal flap was suspected.

The surprise came with the intraoral inspection, however. When examining the hard palate, a very large palatal fistula was observed. However, this was packed with food. Gerald was taken to the otolaryngologist, who spent some time cleaning out the fistula and the nasal cavity.

Once the fistula was cleaned out and opened, the speech was re-evaluated and found to be hypernasal with nasal air emission. The pattern of backing of phonemes was obviously developed as a means to compensate for the position of the open fistula. Nasopharyngoscopy showed both lateral ports to be stenosed, which was the cause of the hyponasality and upper airway obstruction when the fistula was impacted. With this information in mind, a fistula repair and lateral port revisions were recommended.

This case study illustrates the importance of an intraoral examination. At times, observations made in the intraoral examination relate directly to the cause of the speech or resonance disorder.

An examination of the oral mechanism begins with observation of the external anatomy, particularly the anatomy of the face. The facial structures should be observed initially at rest. The examiner should then watch the facial gestures, the tongue, and the teeth during articulation. In addition to observing the mouth, the examiner should inspect the eyes, ears, nose, and facial profile for evidence of abnormality or dysmorphology. Once this is completed, an intraoral examination should be done to assess the hard palate, velum, pharyngeal walls, tongue, and finally, dentition and occlusion.

Eyes

The spacing between the eyes can be abnormal in certain craniofacial syndromes. Normally, the eyes should be about one eye's width apart. An individual with a craniofacial syndrome may demonstrate excessive spacing between the eyes, called *hypertelorism*, or too little spacing between the eyes, which is called *hypotelorism*. The opening between the eyelids, called *palpebral fissures*, should also be observed. Narrow palpebral fissures are a phenotypic feature in congenital conditions, such as velocardiofacial syndrome. Finally, the presence of *epicanthal folds* might be noted. These are excess folds of tissue that extend from the upper eyelid to the lower part of the orbit at the inner *canthus* or corner of the eye. This is often seen in Down's syndrome and other syndromes, although epicanthal folds are normal in the Asian population.

Ears

The shape and location of the ears should be observed. Many craniofacial syndromes include malformed ears, such as a simplified helix, or *microtia*, which is hypoplasia or absence of the pinna or auricle of the ear. This is often accompanied by *aural atresia*, which is the congenital absence of the external auditory canal. Aural atresia usually results in a conductive hearing loss, and of course, this can have an impact on the quality of speech and possibly resonance when it is bilateral. Ears that are low set, or below the level of the eyes, may also be suggestive of a syndrome.

Nose and Airway

The *nasal bridge*, or *nasion*, should be observed, since a flat nasal bridge can affect the nasal airway, causing upper airway obstruction and hyponasality. A bulbous nasal tip is often associated with syndromes. On the other hand, a flattened nasal tip may be noted if the columella is short due to a history of cleft lip. The nares should be inspected for evidence of stenosis that could affect resonance and cause hyponasality.

An open-mouth posture secondary to upper airway obstruction is common in individuals with a history of cleft palate or craniofacial anomalies. When this occurs, the tongue will often be forced to an anterior position and the mandible may be positioned down and forward in order to open the airway further. The anterior tongue position can ultimately result in an anterior open bite. Additional characteristics of upper airway obstruction include suborbital coloring, which makes the patient appear to be tired, pinched nostrils, and a face that appears elongated and narrow due to the position of the mandible. These characteristics have been referred to as the "adenoid facies," because they are commonly seen in individuals with upper airway obstruction due to adenoid enlargement. Other signs of upper airway obstruction include strident breathing, snoring at night, and, of course, hyponasality.

To test the nasal airway, the examiner can ask the patient to close the lips and breathe nasally for several minutes. The examiner should observe whether there is any difficulty with nasal breathing. Prior to opening the mouth, the patient should then inspire deeply through the nose and then exhale through the nose. Again, the examiner should observe any difficulty. The patency of each nostril can be assessed by having the child close one nostril and then forcibly inspire through the other nostril. If there is obstruction, this will be difficult to do and will result in a high-pitched sound, with the highest sound in the most obstructed nostril. Another test is to ask the patient to prolong an /m/ with the lips closed to see if there is blockage. If there is significant blockage, the patient will be unable to do this easily.

Facial Bones and Profile

The bony structures of the face are important to assess, particularly as they relate to each other. Flattened zygomas, or cheekbones, are often seen in individuals with a history of cleft lip and palate or other craniofacial syndromes. The facial profile can give an indication of the dysmorphology of the other facial bones. This can be evaluated by having the patient turn so that the examiner is viewing the side of the person's face. For a normal profile, imaginary points on the forehead, bridge of the nose, base of the nose, and chin button should all line up in a vertical plane. If these points do not line up, the examiner should determine whether this is due to protrusion or retrusion of particular facial bones, particularly the maxilla or mandible. Discrepancy in the relationship between the maxilla and mandible can be particularly problematic for speech. Because the tongue always resides within the arch of the mandible, the position of the maxilla in relationship to the mandible can affect the amount of space available for the tongue tip to articulate.

Lips

The lips should be assessed for the ability to achieve bilabial closure at rest and during speech. If the upper lip is short relative to the length of the maxilla, bilabial closure may be difficult to accomplish and maintain. When there is a history of cleft lip, there may be excess scarring, the cupid's bow may be asymmetrical or flat, or the vermilion may extend into the philtral suture lines. The examiner should always look for lip pits, which are small depressions in the bottom lip. This finding is indicative of Van der Woude's syndrome, which also includes cleft palate. This syndrome has a 50% recurrence risk for future pregnancies; therefore, the finding of lip pits is significant.

If the lips are apart and the upper lip is not short, the problem may be related a skeletal discrepancy and resultant malocclusion. The open-mouth posture may also be due to poor facial tone or oral-motor dysfunction. There may be drooling associated with the lack of adequate tone or motor skills. A chronic open-mouth posture can actually increase the production of saliva, which further exacerbates the drooling.

There may be reduced mobility of the lips due to scarring. To assess labial movement, the patient can be asked to sustain exaggerated /i/ and /u/ sounds. The examiner should observe the symmetry and range of lip and facial movements. Observing the patient produce quick repetitions of the /p/ or /b/ sounds will allow the examiner to assess the ability to make rapid movements with the lips (Mason & Simon, 1977).

Additional External Anatomy

Additional external anomalies should be noted, because they may be relevant to a syndrome. Some anomalies may not be readily seen, but may be recorded in the medical history or reported by the parents. For example, when velocardiofacial syndrome is suspected, an examination of the fingers may reveal the characteristic long and slender digits. The child's size and stature may also be important to note, as short stature is another phenotypic feature of this syndrome.

Hard Palate

The palatal vault should be evaluated, especially in relationship to the size of the tongue. If the palatal vault is low and flat, this can reduce the space available for the lingual articulation. This can also be a problem if the maxillary arch is narrow relative to the tongue size. To compensate for intraoral crowding, the mandible will often lower and tongue may be forced down and forward.

A prominent longitudinal ridge in the middle of the hard palate may be observed in some individuals. Although this can appear very unusual and may look like an abnormality, it is actually a normal variation, called a *torus palatinus*. It is not a concern because it does not interfere with speech or any other function. If a palatal fistula is noted anywhere in the palate, its size and location are important to determine. Size and location are the primary determinants of whether the fistula will be symptomatic for nasal regurgitation or for speech.

The position of the alveolar ridge, as it relates to the position of the tongue tip, should be determined. If the alveolar ridge is not just above the tongue tip, as commonly occurs when there is significant maxillary retrusion or protrusion, difficulty with the production of lingual-alveolar and sibilant sounds might be expected.

Velum and Uvula

In an intraoral examination, the clinician should determine velar integrity. As noted previously, a normal velum may have a white line down the middle, called the median palatine raphe. This is the area where the levator veli palatini muscles interdigitate in the midline. If there was a cleft palate, it is important to rule out a fistula in the velum in addition to the hard palate. A fistula that is anterior to the velar dimple is likely to be symptomatic, as this location is near the area of maximum air pressure as it enters the oral cavity. On the other hand, a fistula that is posterior to the area of the velar dimple will not affect resonance, because it is below the area of velopharyngeal closure and in the area of velar redundancy as it contacts the posterior pharyngeal wall.

If there is no history of cleft palate, the examiner should always look for characteristics of a submucous cleft. At times, the submucous cleft will be readily apparent through a quick inspection. At other times, the findings may be very subtle and require more careful examination. Even when there is no apparent evidence of a submucous cleft through an intraoral examination, it cannot be ruled out. There may be an occult submucous cleft in the muscles or mucosa on the nasal side of the velum. This can only be detected though nasopharyngoscopy or during a surgical procedure.

The most common sign of a submucous cleft is an abnormal uvula. As noted previously, a bifid uvula is a relatively common finding in the general population (Bagatin, 1985; Meskin, Gorlin, & Isaacson, 1964; Saad, 1980; Shapiro, Meskin, Cervenka, & Pruzansky, 1971; Wharton & Mowrer, 1992). At times, the uvula will be intact, but is hypoplastic, appearing to be very short and stubby. More often, however, the submucous cleft will include a bifid uvula where there is a split in the uvula, resulting in two tags. In some cases, the uvula may appear to be intact due to the fact that the saliva helps to "glue" the tags of a bifid uvula together. If the examiner suspects that the uvula is bifid but is unsure, this can often be determined by taking a tongue blade gently behind the uvula and then flipping it forward (Mason & Simon, 1977). If there are two tags, they will separate with this maneuver. This must be done very carefully and only in a very cooperative individual.

Additional signs of a submucous cleft include a zona pellucida, which is a bluish appearing area in the middle of the velum. This appearance is due to the fact that the velum is thin and somewhat transparent as a result of the lack of muscle in this area. In palpating the posterior nasal spine, the examiner may feel a notch in the bony structure that would suggest a submucous cleft. During phonation, the velum may appear to "tent up" in an inverted V-shape if there is a submucous cleft that extends through the velum. This occurs because the levator veli palatini muscles have a forward attachment and are inserted on the edge of the posterior hard palate, rather than in the midline of the velum. If the submucous cleft extends into the hard palate, the examiner may note an inverted V-shape under the mucosa of the velum and extending into the bony hard palate. It is important to recall that many individuals with a bifid uvula or other characteristics of a submucous cleft will have normal speech. However, these individuals are at increased risk for hypernasality following an adenoidectomy.

After examining the basic morphology of the velum, both velar length and mobility should be observed during phonation. The "effective length" of the velum is the distance between the hard palate and the velar dimple during velopharyngeal closure (Mason & Grandstaff, 1971). It contains the portion of the velum that serves to obturate the nasopharyngeal port during speech. The *velar dimple* is the point on the oral side of the velum that corresponds to the place where it bends during phonation or velopharyngeal closure. Of note is the fact that, when two lateral dimples are observed, it suggests diastasis of the levator veli palatini muscles, which is consistent with a submucous cleft (Boorman & Sommerland, 1985). The section of the velum that is posterior to the velar dimple does not help to reach toward closure, but does help in maintaining firm closure across a vertical surface. During sustained phonation, the velar dimple should appear to be back approximately 80% of the length of the soft palate (Mason & Grandstaff, 1971; Mason & Simon, 1977) or just above the uvula. If the velar dimple is closer to the hard palate rather than to the uvula, it suggests that the place of bend is not back far enough for the velum to reach the posterior pharyngeal wall. The resulting short effective length can cause velopharyngeal insufficiency.

During phonation, the velum should raise symmetrically in a superior and posterior direction. When poor velar movement is noted during phonation, it suggests the possibility of velopharyngeal incompetence or it may be a nonsignificant finding. Even with a normal speaker, the velum may not appear to move well during phonation of a single vowel. The examiner should have the person produce the "ah" repetitively or phonate with a yawn to stimulate the full potential of velar movement. Even with this, only a general impression of velopharyngeal movement can be obtained from an intraoral examination during sustained phonation. Eliciting the gag reflex may show the maximum excursion of the velum and pharyngeal walls. However, this does not correlate well with movement potential for speech and a diminished gag reflex is not necessarily indicative of a problem with velopharyngeal function.

If the velum does not appear to move well, despite all attempts to elicit movement, and the patient has normal resonance, it may be because the patient has a sagittal form of closure. In this case, the lateral pharyngeal walls move medially to close in midline and there is little need for velar movement. Another possible cause for poor velar movement may be enlarged adenoids, which can interfere with the upward movement of the velum during speech. In individuals with a history of cleft palate, poor velar movement could be due to poor muscle function, despite a palatoplasty to repair the velum. Dysarthria, apraxia, or any form of oral-motor dysfunction can also result in poor velar mobility. Little or no velar movement may suggest a velar paralysis.

Asymmetrical velar movement of the velum may also suggest velopharyngeal incompetence. If there is unilateral paralysis or *paresis* (weakness), the velum will pull up on the unaffected side and droop on the affected side. With normal velar movement, the uvula should be noted to be in midline and hanging straight down. With asymmetrical velar movement, the uvula will point to the functional side. The examiner should particularly rule out unilateral paralysis or paresis of the velum in individuals with hemifacial microsomia. This finding is very important to note prior to planning surgical intervention because unilateral paralysis or paresis will cause a lateral, rather than central, velopharyngeal gap.

Regardless of the appearance of the velum or its mobility, the examiner should remember that one can only guess at the implication for velopharyngeal function. This is because the oral view is below the level of velopharyngeal closure, and it is impossible to know the curve of the posterior pharyngeal wall or the basic closure pattern from an intraoral perspective alone.

Epiglottis

Although it appears infrequently, at times the epiglottis can be viewed when a child protrudes the tongue to say "aah." The epiglottis is located just below the base of the tongue and is relatively high in the hypopharynx in young children. As the tongue goes forward, the epiglottis is pulled upward toward the oropharyngeal isthmus. Therefore, the epiglottis can often be viewed with an intraoral assessment of a child. The epiglottis is not usually seen in adults, because the larynx descends in the neck with age, minimizing its ability to be viewed during oral examinations.

Posterior and Lateral Pharyngeal Walls

The depth of the posterior pharyngeal wall can be judged relative to the possible length of the velum during phonation. In cases of severe velopharyngeal insufficiency, the examiner can almost look up into the nasopharynx due to the severe discrepancy between velar length and pharyngeal depth. However, in most cases, the examiner can only guess how the pharynx curves as it courses superiorly and then anteriorly to form the nasal cavity. The pharynx may appear to be very deep on the oral level, but may curve sufficiently during the incline so that velopharyngeal closure can be obtained. In addition, the velum may be closing against the adenoid pad rather than the posterior pharyngeal wall. The best way to assess the depth of the pharynx is through lateral videofluoroscopy.

Lateral and posterior pharyngeal wall movement can be observed during phonation. There may be very vigorous movement of the pharyngeal walls, which may indicate good pharyngeal movement higher up in the area of velopharyngeal closure. This can also substantiate that the nervous supply to the pharynx is intact. However, there is no way to know whether there is complete velopharyngeal closure as a result of the movement. On the other hand, poor movement of the pharyngeal walls is not necessarily an indication of a problem. In fact, at the oral level, the lateral pharyngeal walls may actually bow outward during phonation, while bowing inward at a higher plane to assist with closure.

At times, a Passavant's ridge can be observed to bulge forward from the posterior pharyngeal wall during phonation. This ridge appears with muscular contraction of the entire velopharyngeal sphincter. Finkelstein, Hauben, Talmi, Nachmani, and Zohar (1992) reported that an up-and-down movement of the posterior pharyngeal wall can often be observed when there is a Passavant's ridge. They termed this the "shutter sign" and noted that it occurs when the individual phonates or during the gag reflex. Unfortunately, if a Passavant's ridge can be observed from an intraoral view, it is not positioned high enough to assist with velopharyngeal closure. Therefore, in this case, it is no more than an interesting observation. The inferior border of the adenoid pad can occasionally, although infrequently, be observed on the posterior pharyngeal wall. It appears as lobulated tissue just behind and under the point of velar contact.

Tonsils

As noted previously, the tonsils are located between the anterior and posterior faucial pillars. They tend to be largest in preschool or school-aged children. They usually begin to gradually atrophy as the child gets older and may suddenly shrink around puberty. Tonsils are virtually nonexistent in most adults.

With the oral examination, the presence of tonsils should be noted. If they are present, their relative size can be judged on a 4-point scale. If the tonsils are absent, the rating would be 0. Tonsils that are small and fit within the confines of the faucial pillars are considered to be Grade 1 in size. If the tonsils extend to the edge of the pillars, they are rated as Grade 2. If they are beyond the pillars, they are rated as Grade 3, and if they are very large and meet in midline, they would be judged as a Grade 4 in size. The tonsils are generally not a problem for speech unless they extend beyond the faucial pillars or are so large that they interfere with the transmission of sound into the oral cavity.

The two tonsils are not always symmetrical in size. In fact, one may be significantly larger than the other. When this is the case, the size of each should be judged. In addition, if one tonsil is very large, the examiner should note whether it is affecting velar movement. A very large tonsil can pull the velum upward on that side or even intrude into the pharynx and interfere with velopharyngeal closure. When the velum is stretched upward by the tonsil, the uvula will point to the side of the large tonsil. Markedly asymmetric tonsils may be a sign of malignancy and, therefore, require further evaluation.

Dentition and Occlusion

Dental occlusion should always be assessed as part of an intraoral examination because occlusion can have a significant effect on articulation. Malocclusion is a common contributor to speech problems in patients with a history of cleft palate. Anterior and lateral crossbites, missing teeth, and supernumerary teeth, are often seen in this population.

To examine the dentition, the examiner should first assess the skeletal relationships between the maxillary and the mandibular arches during biting. The best way to examine the relationships of the two arches is to have the patient bite down on the "back teeth." The examiner should make sure that the bite is with the molars, and not with the incisors. Then, by inserting a tongue blade between the lateral teeth and the cheeks, the examiner can pull the cheeks away from the teeth to view the occlusal relationships (Figure 13–3).

The position of the molar teeth is important to observe because once they erupt, they be-

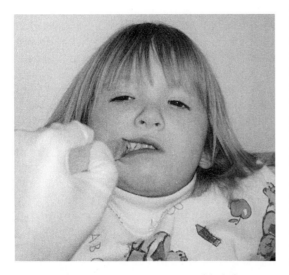

Figure 13–3. By inserting a tongue blade between the lateral teeth and the cheeks, the examiner can pull the cheeks away from the teeth to view the occlusal relationships.

come the key to alignment for the rest of the dentition (Mason & Simon, 1977). In normal occlusion, the mandibular molar should line up to be one half of a tooth in front of the maxillary molar. If one or more molars have not yet erupted or have been extracted, the examiner can look at the relationships between the canine teeth in the same way. A normal occlusal relationship is termed a Class I occlusion according to Angle's classification (Bloomer, 1971). If the mandible is behind where it should be in relationship to the maxillary arch, this is considered a Class II occlusal relationship. On the other hand, if the mandible is forward in relationship to the maxilla, this is considered a Class III malocclusion.

In addition to assessing the anterior-posterior skeletal relationships, the examiner should determine if there is any evidence of dental malocclusion. In the cleft population, *crossbite*, where the maxillary teeth are inside the mandibular teeth, is very common. There can be an *anterior crossbite*, involving the maxillary incisors, or a *lateral crossbite*, due to a narrow maxillary arch relative to the mandibular arch. The examiner should rule out a *deep bite*, where there is excessive vertical overlap, as this can cause crowding in the oral cavity and restrict tongue movement. The examiner should also note an *overjet* where the incisors are labioverted, or an *underjet* where the incisors are linguaverted. If the individual had a bilateral cleft of the lip and alveolus, the position of the premaxilla should be assessed. In many cases, the premaxilla is positioned in a way that affects speech. It may be in an anterior position so that it makes bilabial closure very difficult, if not impossible, or it may be retruded so that the teeth are linguaverted. In this case, labio-dental sounds could be affected. An *open bite*, where the maxillary teeth do not occlude or overlap the mandibular teeth, should be noted because this can affect the position of the tongue at rest and during speech. The effect of these dental conditions on tongue position and movement during speech is very important to determine as it will have an impact on the recommendations for speech therapy versus physical management.

The examiner should note the presence of supernumerary teeth, especially if the tooth is in a place where it might interfere with tongue movement, and whether there are any missing teeth in the line of the cleft, or elsewhere. The status of oral hygiene should also be determined. When the examiner observes poor oral hygiene or obvious caries, a referral for dental care must be included in the overall recommendations following the assessment.

Tongue

Both the structure and the function of the tongue should be assessed. The size of the tongue should be evaluated in relationship to the mandibular arch, the palatal arch, and the overall oral cavity space. It should be remembered that the infant's tongue is considerably larger relative to the oral cavity space than the tongue of an older child or adult. In addition, the tongue reaches maturation at around the age of 8, while the mandible continues to grow for several more years (Mason & Simon, 1977). Therefore, at various points during development, the tongue may appear to be relatively large. However, if the tongue is significantly larger than the oral cavity space so that it does not fit with attempts to close the teeth, this might indicate a macroglossia. A large tongue relative to the mandibular space can affect the dentition, so this should also be evaluated.

The tongue should be further evaluated for multiple lobes if there is a history of a syndrome. If the patient has had a tongue flap for closure of an oronasal fistula, the scarring and effect on function should be noted. The lingual frenulum under the tongue should be inspected for the location of the attachment. If there is evidence of ankyloglossia, where the frenulum has an anterior attachment or is very short, this will also be noted with lingual protrusion. As the tongue is protruded, the tip will course inward so that the tongue is in the shape of the top of a heart. When ankyloglossia is noted, the examiner should determine if this affects tongue tip elevation for production of an /l/ or tongue tip protrusion for production of a /th/. However, an effect on speech is actually unlikely. There is a common misconception that ankyloglossia often affects speech production and is a common cause of speech problems. The truth is that it rarely affects speech. Instead, it is more likely that it will affect feeding by restricting the ability to move a bolus around in the mouth or remove a bolus from the *buccal sulcus*, which is the area between the cheeks and teeth.

Oral-Motor Function

In examining the function of the tongue, the examiner can ask the child to protrude, elevate, depress, and lateralize the tongue tip. The examiner can also evaluate the function of the lips by having the patient purse or smack the lips. However, what is most important is to evaluate the individual's ability to sequence motor movements for speech. This can be done through the use of diadochokinetic exercises, which require the person to produce a sequence of syllables rapidly. The syllables "puh," "tuh," and "kuh" have been used for years to assess motor movements for speech. The examiner can use one syllable and have the patient produce it over and over (e.g., puh, puh, puh, puh, etc.) or the syllables can be combined (i.e., puh-tuhkuh, puhtuhkuh, puhtuhkuh, etc.). Using meaningless syllables can be difficult for young children. Therefore, having the child repeat common multisyllabic words over and over (i.e., patty cake, kitty cat, puppy dog, teddy bear, basketball, or baseball bat) may be more effective.

In diadochokinetic testing, it is more important to look at the accuracy of production than the number of repetitions. If consonants are omitted, substituted, or reversed with an increase in utterance length or phonemic complexity, the possibility of verbal apraxia should be considered.

During the examination, the examiner should also look for more subtle signs of oral-motor dysfunction, such as those that might indicate a dysarthria. Some of the signs include a chronic open-mouth posture in the absence of upper airway obstruction. Usually when there is an open-mouth posture, the tongue is also in an anterior position in the mouth. With the open mouth and anterior tongue position, drooling is a common observation. This can be subtle, with just a little moisture on the chin, or it can be copious so that the child wears a bib or carries a cloth. If the child has feeding difficulties, by history or by observation, this could also be an indication of oral-motor dysfunction.

If the individual demonstrates an open-mouth posture and anterior tongue position, the possibility of a tongue thrust should be ruled out, especially if there is also an anterior open bite. This can be determined by gently stimulating the tip of the tongue with a tongue blade, and then having the child take a drink of water. The examiner then asks the child to report whether the tongue tip went up (against the alveolar ridge), forward (against or between the incisors), or down (against the mandibular incisors). If the child consistently reports that the tongue goes forward or down with the swallow, a tongue thrust should be suspected (Neiva & Wertzner, 1996). If the child is unable to report the direction of the tongue movement, it can be observed by asking the child to swallow with the lips open. This is particularly easy to observe if there is also an anterior open bite.

Putting It All Together

Once the oral and peripheral examination is complete, the examiner must put the information together for a diagnostic profile. In particular, it is important to determine if there are physical factors that could potentially be interfering with articulation and resonance.

If multiple anomalies are noted, in addition to a speech or resonance disorder, the examiner should consider the possibility of a syndrome if one has not already been diagnosed. Because speech, resonance, and learning problems are some of the primary characteristics of velocardiofacial syndrome, it is very common for the speech pathologist to be the first to identify individuals with this syndrome (Carneol, Marks, & Weik, 1999).

Infection Control During the Examination

A discussion of the intraoral examination would not be complete without a section on infection control. Four communicable diseases make up the biggest concern in the health care environment, and can also cause concern in other settings, including the schools. These include the human immunodeficiency virus (HIV), hepatitis B virus (HBV), cytomegalovirus I (CMV), and tuberculosis (TB). Professionals must also be concerned about the transmission of minor diseases, such as a cold or influenza. Pediatric settings are a particular concern because children generally have poor personal hygiene habits, and yet are very susceptible to infection (Krewedl, 1991).

In 1988, the Centers for Disease Control and Prevention (CDC) in Atlanta (1987, 1988) developed guidelines for infection control, called the universal blood and body fluid precautions (UBBFP). These guidelines contain recommended precautions that are designed to protect the patient, the professional, and all others in a health care environment from the spread of infection. Since that time, the American Speech-Language-Hearing Association (ASHA) (1990) has adopted these guidelines and recommended them to its membership.

Handwashing

The role of the human hands in the transmission of infection was recognized even before the establishment of microbiology as a science (Kerr, 1998). For many years, handwashing has been considered the single most important means of preventing the spread of infection in a health care setting (Gallagher, 1999; Ginsberg & Clarke, 1972; Horton, 1995). Handwashing reduces the number of potential pathogens on the hands and interrupts the opportunity of transferring organisms to patients. If all health care providers used the proper technique for handwashing and this became a habit, infection rates in health care facilities would drop dramatically (Brown & Persivale, 1995). The Centers for Disease Control (1986) have issued guidelines on appropriate handwashing in a hospital environment. Unfortunately, health care workers are not always compliant in washing their hands as often as they should. This is one reason why *nosocomial infections* (infections that are acquired while in the hospital) continue to be a principal cause of morbidity and even mortality in health care settings.

Hands should be washed before and after every patient contact and especially before and after an intraoral examination. In addition, hands should be washed after contact with potentially contaminated surfaces, after accidental contact with body fluids, and any time the hands are soiled. The use of examination gloves does not eliminate the need for handwashing (Bowman & Nicholas, 1990; Hopkins, 1989; Ripper, 1988; Shogren, 1988). It is important to wash hands before putting on gloves because there can be a perforation in the glove that is not readily visible. It is also necessary to wash hands after glove removal, because the warm, moist environment in the glove is conducive to rapid bacterial multiplication (Mayone-Ziomek, 1998).

Routine handwashing is accomplished by wetting hands with water and applying an antibacterial soap. If soap and water are not immediately available, there are products on the market that can be used for hand disinfection. Antimicrobial handwashing products (e.g., 2% chlorhexidine gluconate, triclosan) should be used before contacts with newborns, immunocompromised patients, patients on high-risk

units, and prior to an invasive procedure, including an intraoral examination. The hands should be washed using friction for a minimum of 10–15 seconds, and then rinsed thoroughly with water to remove any residual soap. The hands should be dried thoroughly with fresh paper towels. The towels should be used to turn off manual faucets in order to avoid recontamination.

Gloves

With the universal precautions approach to infection control, the examiner should assume that all human secretions, including saliva, could potentially be infectious or contain bloodborne pathogens. Therefore, the examiner must wear personal protective equipment (PPE) when performing any task that has the risk of contact with the patient's secretions. Protection must be worn when the professional is engaged in any type of evaluation or treatment that requires physical contact with the mouth or nose of patient.

The best form of protection for the examiner is a pair of gloves. Until recently, latex gloves were used in most health care settings. However, latex allergies are not uncommon. To minimize the sensitization of health care workers and exposure to latex-sensitive patients, most institutions have now eliminated the use of latex gloves. Gloves should always be worn during an intraoral examination and also while performing a nasopharyngoscopy exam. They should be changed as needed during patient care and immediately if holes, rips, or tears are visible. Because all gloves are designed for single patient use, they are discarded in the waste can after each patient. When removing gloves, they should be pulled off so that they are inside out, and then immediately discarded. This prevents physical contact with the contaminated surface of the gloves.

Patient Equipment and Supplies

Tongue blades, dental mirrors, and other tools for an intraoral assessment should not be placed directly on a desk or table after use. Instead, these tools should be placed on a clean paper towel or tissue until they can be cleaned or discarded. Patient equipment and supplies should be stored in a clean and safe manner that protects the items from exposure or contamination to body fluids, known soiled items, dust, particulate matter, and even moisture. Supplies should always be stored a minimum of 4–6" off the floor to enable floor cleaning and protection from accidental damage due to rolling carts, being stepped on, and contamination with floor cleaning solutions.

Disposable items, such as tongue blades, should be used for intraoral examinations or manipulation whenever possible. It is easier to dispose of an item and use a new one for the next person than to wash and disinfect the item between uses. Items that are manufactured to be disposable cannot usually be adequately washed or disinfected. Therefore, all disposable items are for single-patient use and should be discarded immediately after use. It is important to discard these items appropriately and not leave contaminated items sitting on a desk or table.

Nondisposable items, such as a dental mirror, should be thoroughly cleaned after use. Items that are placed in the mouth can be cleaned in a standard dishwasher. If washed by hand, disinfection can be done by using chlorine and water (1 part chlorine with 9 parts water) or by wiping the dental mirror with alcohol. Both ethyl alcohol and isopropyl alcohol have broad spectra of antimicrobial activity that includes vegetative bacteria, fungi, and viruses (including HIV) (Widmer & Frei, 1999). Alcohol has many qualities that make it suitable for low level and intermediate-level disinfection, including the fact that it is fast acting (15 to 30 seconds), and it readily evaporates. Sterilization, as opposed to disinfection, is required to destroy bacterial spores, but because intact mucous membranes are resistant to bacterial spores, this is not necessary for a dental mirror.

Summary

The structure and function of the oral articulators and the oral cavity have a direct impact on the quality and intelligibility of speech. In addition, the function of the velopharyngeal valve is critical for normal speech and resonance. Therefore, when speech or resonance problems are noted, a thorough intraoral examination must be done. The examiner must rule out structural abnormalities that may require surgical or orthodontic treatment prior to the initiation of speech therapy. In addition, a keen eye and a thorough examination can help to detect previously undiagnosed conditions with the help of the physician.

References

American Speech-Language-Hearing Association, (1990). AIDS/HIV: Implications for speech-language pathologists and audiologists. *Asha*, 46–48.

Bagatin, M. (1985). Submucous cleft palate. *Journal of Maxillofacial Surgery*, 13(1), 37–38.

Bloomer, H. (1971). Speech defects associated with dental malocclusions and related abnormalities. In L. Travis (Ed.), *Handbook of speech pathology and audiology* (pp. 608–652). New York: Appleton.

Boorman, J. G., & Sommerland, B. C. (1985). Levator veli palati and palatal dimples: Their anatomy, relationship and clinical significance. *British Journal of Plastic Surgery*, 38, 326–332.

Bowman, A. M., & Nicholas, T. J. (1990). Improving compliance with universal blood and body fluid precautions in a rural medical center. *Journal of Nursing Quality Assurance*, 5(1), 73–81.

Brown, J. W., & Persivale, E. J. (1995). Managing the front line of infection control: Handwashing. *Director*, 3(1), 36–37.

Carneol, S. O., Marks, S. M., & Weik, L. (1999). The speech-language pathologist: Key role in the diagnosis for velocardiofacial syndrome. *American Journal of Speech-Language Pathology*, 8(1), 23–32.

Centers for Disease Control. (1986). Guidelines for handwashing and hospital environmental control. *Infection Control*, 7(4), 231–235.

Centers for Disease Control. (1987). Recommendations for prevention of HIV transmission in health-care settings. *Morbidity and Mortality Weekly Review, 36*(Suppl. 25).

Centers for Disease Control.(1988). Perspectives in disease prevention and health promotion. *Morbidity and Mortality Weekly Review, 37*, 377–388.

Finkelstein, Y., Hauben, D. J., Talmi, Y. P., Nachmani, A., & Zohar, Y. (1992). Occult and overt submucous cleft palate: From peroral examination to nasendoscopy and back again. *International Journal of Pediatric Otorhinolaryngology, 23*(1), 25–34.

Gallagher, T. (1999). This is the way we wash our hands. *Nursing Times, 95*(10), 62–65.

Ginsberg, F., & Clarke, B. (1972). Handwashing is simple, effective infection control, so why won't people wash their hands? *Modern Hospital, 119*(4), 132.

Gravens, D. L. (1978). Handwashing and infection control. *Professional Sanitation Management, 9*(5), 2p.

Hopkins, C. C. (1989). AIDS. Implementation of universal blood and body fluid precautions. *Infectious Disease Clinics of North America, 3*(4), 747–762.

Horton, R. (1995). Handwashing: The fundamental infection control principle. *British Journal of Nursing, 4*(16), 926, 928, 930–933.

Kerr, J. (1998). Handwashing. *Nursing Standards, 12*(51), 35–39; Quiz 41–42.

Krewedl, A. (1991, August 23). Infection control in pediatric settings. *Advance*, pp. 26–27.

Mason, R. M., & Grandstaff, H. L. (1971). Evaluating the velopharyngeal mechanism in hypernasal speakers. *Language, Speech, and Hearing Services in the Schools, 2*(4), 53–61.

Mason, R. M., & Simon, C. (1977). An orofacial examination checklist. *Language, Speech, and Hearing Services in the Schools, 8*(3), 155–163.

Mayone-Ziomek, J. M. (1998). Handwashing in health care. *Dermatological Nursing, 10*(3), 183–188.

Meskin, L., Gorlin, R., & Isaacson, R. (1964). Abnormal morphology of the soft palate: The prevalence of a cleft uvula. *Cleft Palate Journal, 3*, 342–346.

Neiva, F. C., & Wertzner, H. F. (1996). A protocol for oral myofunctional assessment: For application with children. *International Journal of Orofacial Myology, 22*, 8–19.

Ripper, M. (1988). Universal blood and body fluid precautions. *Journal of Advances in Medical Surgical Nursing, 1*(1), 21–25.

Saad, E. F. (1980). The underdeveloped palate in ear, nose and throat practice. *Laryngoscope, 90*(8, Pt. 1), 1371–1377.

Shapiro, B. L., Meskin, L. H., Cervenka, J., & Pruzansky, S. (1971). Cleft uvula: A microform of facial clefts and its genetic basis. *Birth Defects Original Article Series, 7*(7), 80–82.

Shogren, E. (1988). An ounce of prevention is worth a pound of cure: Using universal blood and body fluid precautions in your work setting. *MNA Accent, 60*(2), 35–36.

Wharton, P., & Mowrer, D. E. (1992). Prevalence of cleft uvula among school children in kindergarten through grade five. *Cleft Palate Craniofacial Journal, 129*(1), 10–12; Discussion 13–14.

Widmer, A. F., & Frei, R. (1999). Decontamination, disinfection, and sterilization. In P. R. Murray, E. J. Baron, & R. H. Yolken (Eds.), *Manual of clinical microbiology* (pp. 138–146). Washington, DC: ASM Press.

CHAPTER

14

Nasometry

CONTENTS

The Nasometer (Kay Elemetrics Corp., Lincoln Park, NJ) is a computer-based instrument that provides data regarding the acoustic results of velopharyngeal function. Because it does not allow visualization of the velopharyngeal structures, it is considered an *indirect measure*. The advantage of the Nasometer is that it provides objective data that can be compared to standardized norms for interpretation. In addition, it can be used to collect data for pre- and post-treatment comparisons. The Nasometer is useful in an evaluation of resonance because it supplements what is heard through the perceptual evaluation and what is seen through direct instrumental measures.

The purpose of this chapter is to describe the Nasometer and nasometric procedures in the evaluation of individuals with resonance disorders.

Nasometric Procedures

Purpose

The first instrument to measure nasal and oral acoustic energy was developed by Samuel Fletcher in 1970. This instrument was called TONAR, which is an acronym for The Oral-Nasal Acoustic Ratio (Fletcher, 1970). The TONAR was later updated, revised, and then renamed the TONAR II (Fletcher, 1976a, 1976b). Although the TONAR and later the TONAR II were the first instruments to provide objective data regarding the acoustic product of speech, this instrumentation had some limitations. The data were reportedly affected by the orientation of the sound separator and the individual's face, making the measurements somewhat unreliable (Dalston, 1997). Therefore, based on his early work, Samuel Fletcher, Larry Adams, and Martin McCutcheon at the University of Alabama, Birmingham developed the next generation of instrumentation to measure the acoustic output of speech. This new instru-

ment, called the Nasometer, was introduced by Kay Elemetrics Corp. in 1987.

The *Nasometer* is a computer-based instrument that measures the relative amount of nasal acoustic energy in an individual's speech. By measuring the acoustic energy in both the nasal cavity and the oral cavity during speech, a ratio of nasal over total (nasal plus oral) acoustic energy is obtained. This is converted to a percentage value (by multiplying the decimal by 100) and is called the *nasalance score*. Since its introduction, the Nasometer has been a useful tool in the evaluation of velopharyngeal dysfunction (Dalston, Warren, & Dalston 1991b, 1991c; Dalston, 1997; Hardin, Van Demark, Morris & Payne, 1992; Karnell, 1995). It has also been used as a method of assessing upper airway obstruction and hyponasality through their acoustic correlates during speech (Dalston, Warren, & Dalston, 1991a, 1991b; Hardin, Van Demark, Morris, & Payne, 1992; Hong, Kwon, & Jung, 1997; Parker, Clarke, Dawes, & Maw, 1990). Nasometry has been suggested as a means of selecting at-risk individuals for adenoidectomy (Gonzalez-Landa, Santos Terron, Miro Viar, & Sanchez-Ruiz, 1990; Kummer, Myer, Smith, & Shott, 1993; Parker, Maw, & Szallasi, 1989; Williams, Eccles, & Hutchings, 1990), and as a tool for measuring surgical results (Heppt, Westrich, Strate, & Mohring, 1991; Williams et al., 1990).

Equipment

The basic Nasometer equipment is illustrated in Figure 14–1. The Nasometer requires the use of either an IBM-compatible or Apple computer. The equipment consists of a Nasometer box, which is connected by a cable to an interface printed circuit board in the computer. The Nasometer software is then installed on the computer's hard drive.

The Nasometer also has a headset that is designed to be worn by the individual during data collection (Figure 14–2). This headset is

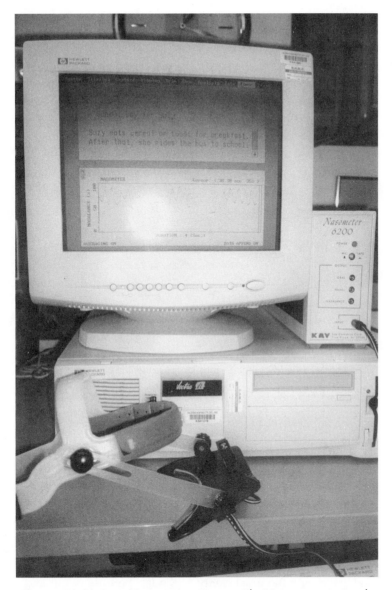

Figure 14–1. Basic Nasometer equipment. The Nasometer requires the use of either an IBM-compatible or Apple computer, a Nasometer box, which is connected by a cable to an interface printed circuit board in the computer, and a headset that is worn by the individual during data collection. Nasometer software is installed on the computer's hard drive.

plugged into the Nasometer box. The top part of the headset consists of a harness that encircles the forehead and a Velcro strip that attaches the headset in the back. There is an adjustable band that fits across the top of the head to hold the headset in place.

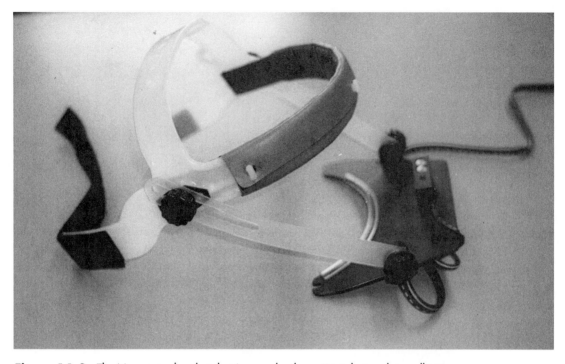

Figure 14–2. The Nasometer headset that is worn by the patient during data collection.

The bottom part of the headset has two directional microphones, one for the mouth and the other for the nose. These microphones are mounted on either side of a sound separator plate or baffle. This plate rests in a horizontal position between the upper lip and the nose. The part that comes in contact with the individual has a plastic guard that helps to soften the force against the face. During speech production, the microphones pick up acoustic energy from the oral cavity and the nasal cavity simultaneously. The sound separator plate provides about a 25-dB separation between the oral and the nasal signals (Kay Elemetrics Corporation, 1994).

Calibration

Prior to its first use, the Nasometer should be calibrated according to the manufacturer's instructions (Kay Elemetrics Corporation, 1994). This is necessary to be sure that the data collection and analyses are accurate. The Nasometer comes with a calibration stand that holds the headset during the calibration process. The headset is placed so that both microphones are equidistant from the box and about 12 inches in front of the calibration speaker on the Nasometer box (Figure 14–3). When a tone from the Nasometer box is presented to the microphones, both the nasal and oral microphones should register the tone equally, and therefore, the bar graph on the screen should indicate 50% for an exact balance. If the two microphones are not balanced so that the tone registers above or below the 50% mark, calibration adjustments are made at the side panel of the Nasometer box. Calibration is not required often, but it should be done periodically to insure a proper balance for accurate data collection.

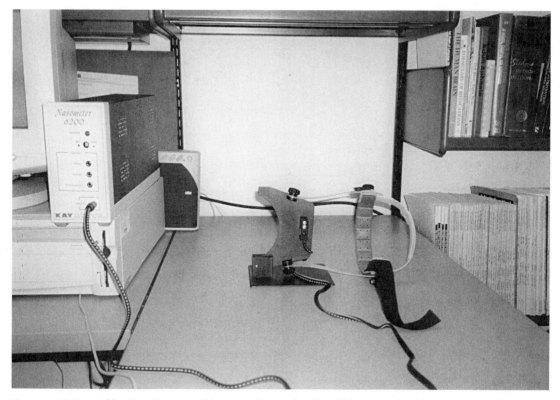

Figure 14–3. Calibration. During calibration, the headset should be placed so that both microphones are equidistant from the Nasometer box and about 12 inches in front of the calibration speaker.

Examination Procedure

Prior to placing the headset on the individual's head, the examiner should wipe the sound separator plate and plastic guard with an alcohol towelette or a germicidal wipe. This helps to prevent the spread of infection. The headset is then put on the individual's head and secured using the top adjustment band and the Velcro strip in the back. Once the top part of the headset is in place, the sound separator plate is secured by tightening the upper adjustment knobs. The plate is placed so that it is perpendicular to the face or in a horizontal position. The microphones should be directly in front of the mouth and the nose. Once this position is achieved, the plate is further stabilized by

tightening the lower adjustment knobs that are just above the plate. The proper placement of the headset is seen in Figure 14–4.

Positioning the headset on small children can be a challenge. In this case, it can be helpful to talk about this test as if it were a computer game. With this "game," it is necessary to talk in order to see blue mountains and valleys on the computer screen. The child should be told that to "talk" to the computer, it is necessary to talk into the computer's "ears," which of course are the microphones. It helps to have the child feel the plate and the plastic tubing that will come in contact with the face. The examiner can explain that this part of the headset will "hug" around the face so that it will stay on by itself. Having the headset "hug" the child's leg

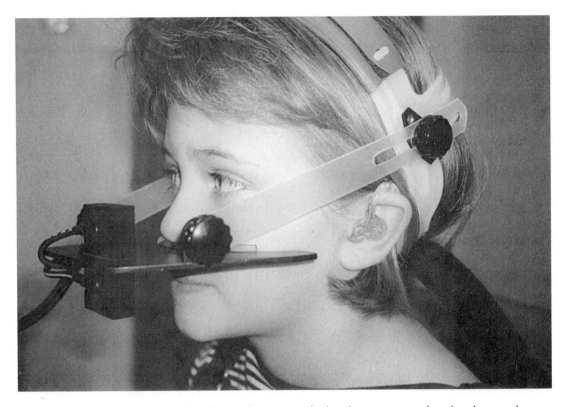

Figure 14–4. Placement of the headset on the patient. The headset is positioned so that the sound separator plate is perpendicular to the face or in a horizontal position. The microphones should be directly in front of the mouth and the nose.

or arm first can help to allay fears of the feel of it on the face. Once the headset is on, the examiner should praise the child and comment on how he or she looks. The child can be told that he or she looks like a pilot, like an astronaut, or even like Darth Vader with the headset in place. In pediatric facilities, it's often helpful to modify the headset so that it fits inside a baseball hat, a fireman's helmet, or anything else that would be appealing to young children. At times, the child will refuse to put the headset on. When this occurs, the parent can hold the sound separator plate at the appropriate position on the child's face while the child repeats a few syllables or short utterances. Even

a brief speech sample can result in the collection of data that can be useful.

Standardized Passages

Once the headset is in place, the individual is asked to read or repeat certain speech passages for data collection (Figure 14–5). Although any speech segment can be used informally, a standardized speech segment must be used to be able to compare the child's performance with normative data. There are several standardized passages that can be selected as noted below. These can be displayed on the screen along with pictures for children (Figure 14–6).

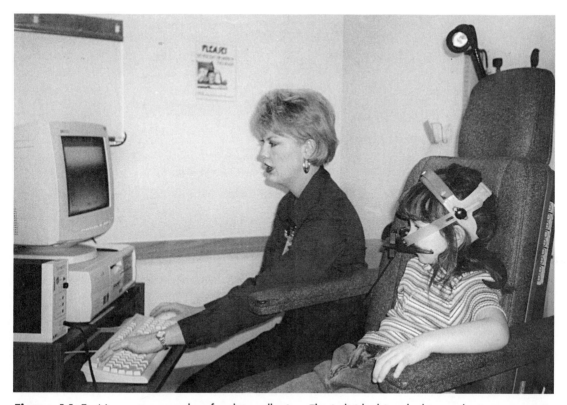

Figure 14–5. Nasometer procedure for data collection. The individual is asked to read or repeat certain speech passages for data collection.

Nasometric norms were first established for three passages; the Zoo Passage (Fletcher, 1972), the Rainbow Passage (Fairbanks, 1960) and Nasal Sentences (Fletcher, 1978). These passages and their norms can be found in Appendix 14-1. For these passages, the Nasometer manual includes the mean scores and standard deviations that were obtained from a population of normal speaking children and adults (Adams, Fletcher, & McCutcheon, 1989).

The Zoo Passage consists of sentences that are devoid of nasal phonemes. This passage allows the examiner to determine if velopharyngeal closure can be achieved and maintained throughout connected speech. Of course, without nasal consonants, this passage does not test

the effects of the timing of closure with the transitions between nasal and oral phonemes. If there are problems with velopharyngeal timing or movement, this is more likely to be demonstrated with the Rainbow Passage. In this passage, 11.5% of the consonants are nasal consonants, which is representative of the percentage of nasal consonants in Standard American English. If hyponasality is suspected, the Nasal Sentences passage is used because it is heavily loaded with nasal consonants. In fact, 35% of the phonemes in this passage are nasal consonants, which is more than three times as many nasal sounds as would normally occur in standard American English. This passage allows the examiner to test the individual's abil-

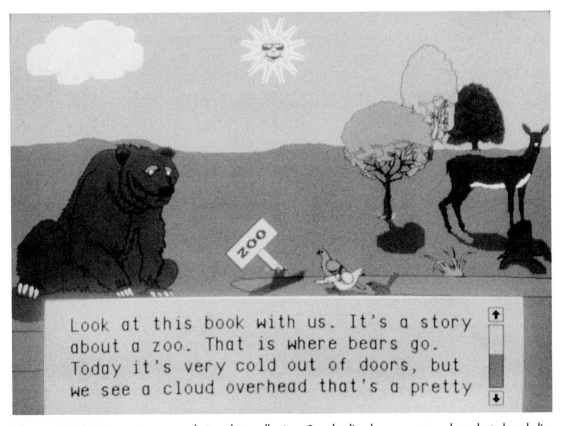

Figure 14–6. Nasometer screen during data collection. Standardized passages can be selected and displayed on the screen along with pictures for children.

ity to open the velopharyngeal port for normal nasal resonance. In addition to giving information regarding resonance, this score also has implications for the presence of nasal obstruction.

Although the original passages are still commonly used and work well in many cases, they have certain disadvantages. The Zoo and Rainbow Passages are long and awkward. Some of the sentences are semantically and syntactically complex, and some of the words are difficult to pronounce. This makes the passages hard to read or even repeat accurately, increasing the possibility of production errors. A pause with the use of "uhm" is particularly problematic. These original passages are especially hard to use with young children who cannot read, have a limited attention span, or may be noncompliant.

The phonetic heterogeneity of these passages limits their use in many ways. The passages are difficult for most preschool children to produce, because this age typically have incomplete phonological acquisition. When the passage is produced with articulation substitutions or deletions, the nasalance score associated with it loses some validity. In addition, long passages with a mixture of phonemes make it impossible to isolate the effects of phoneme-specific nasal emission, because the nasalance score is computed based on the average score for a variety of phonemes. Finally, with a mixture of phonemes, there is no way to determine the effects of a fistula on the nasalance score.

In an effort to determine the best and most efficient way to collect nasometric data while avoiding the pitfalls of the original passages, some investigators have found that reliable measures of nasalance can be obtained using much shorter stimuli (MacKay & Kummer, 1994; Watterson, Lewis, & Foley-Homan, 1999; Wozny, Kuehn, Oishi, & Arthur, 1994). In addition, it has been suggested that the Rainbow Passage does not provide clinically relevant information that cannot be obtained using the other speech samples (Dalston & Seaver, 1992).

Given the limitations of the first three standardized passages, the *Simplified Nasometric Assessment Procedures* (SNAP Test; MacKay & Kummer, 1994) was developed in a pediatric setting for the purpose of providing more appropriate standardized passages for children. This test can be found in Appendix 14-2. It was also designed to enhance the diagnostic value of nasometry by allowing the examiner to test nasalance using specific phonemes and thus avoid the problem of phonetic heterogeneity. The SNAP test is currently incorporated in the Nasometer Model 6200-3 software and is also included in the instruction manual.

The SNAP test consists of a battery of passages divided into three subtests: the Syllables Subtest, the Picture-Cued Passages Subtest, and the Paragraphs Subtest. Any or all of these subtests can be used by the examiner, but are usually selected based on the age of the child, the anticipated level of cooperation, the child's level of literacy, and the specific characteristics or etiologies that need to be evaluated.

The *Syllables Subtest* consists of simple consonant-vowel (CV) syllables, which contain either a pressure-sensitive phoneme (plosive, fricative, or affricate) or a nasal phoneme (m or n) combined with a vowel. The syllables are produced repetitively by the individual until the screen is full. The Syllables Subtest is particularly appropriate for individuals who have a limited attention span, limited cooperation, or a limited phonemic repertoire. The Syllables Subtest allows the examiner to isolate out the effects of misarticulation by evaluating nasalance on specific phonemes or phoneme groups. By comparing the relative nasalance on sibilant phonemes, particularly /s/, versus plosives sounds, the examiner can make a judgment as to whether nasal emission is phoneme-specific or is more generalized due to velopharyngeal dysfunction. If the individual has an anterior fistula and its effects on speech and resonance are unknown, the examiner can compare the nasalance score on anterior sounds (ta, ta, ta or sa, sa, sa) with those obtained on the posterior sounds (ka, ka, ka). Higher nasalance scores on phonemes anterior to the fistula suggest that the fistula is symptomatic for speech.

The examiner can also use the Syllables Subtest to determine if there are subtle abnormalities of velopharyngeal elevation and control by comparing nasalance scores on syllables with high vowels versus low vowels. Because low vowels require a lower point of velopharyngeal closure than high vowels, it is easier to achieve closure on low vowels, and therefore achieve normal nasalance scores. Although, high vowels normally have a higher degree of nasalance than low vowels, difficulties with velopharyngeal closure can be more apparent when syllables with high vowels are used. Therefore, if the examiner finds a significantly higher nasalance score, as compared to the norm, on high vowels than on low vowels, it may suggest difficulty with velopharyngeal function that increases with certain phonemic contexts. Finally, the nasal phonemes can be used effectively to evaluate individuals who have evidence of hyponasality due to upper airway obstruction. These syllable strings can be particularly useful in testing individuals following placement of a flap, which has the potential to cause these problems. Low scores on the nasal syllables can be an indication of both hyponasality and upper airway obstruction that should be medically evaluated and treated.

The *Picture-Cued Passages Subtest* consists of five sets of repeated carrier phrases to be used with simple pictures. Each set has a single carrier phrase and three different pictures to be named at the end of the carrier phrase. Each picture is listed twice so that the carrier phrase with a picture is produced six times in the set. The nasalance score is calculated after the individual completes the six sentences. This subtest allows the examiner to elicit a form of connected speech, yet it is very simple to use, even with young children. Because the pictures are easy to identify and the same carrier phrase is used for each set, this reduces the chance for production errors and increases validity. In addition, each set is phonologically homogeneous to aid the examiner in the diagnostic process by limiting or controlling the phonetic heterogeneity.

The *Paragraphs Subtest* consists of two short, simple passages that can be either read or repeated after the examiner. The first passage contains primarily plosive phonemes while the second passage contains a high incidence of sibilant (fricative and affricate) phonemes. The examiner can select either or both passages, depending on the articulation ability of the individual and the diagnostic goals of the examiner.

Nasometric Results

Display of the Speech Signal

As the individual is speaking, the speech signal enters the Nasometer microphones and the program computes the ratio of nasal acoustic energy to total (nasal plus oral) acoustic energy. The software then converts this ratio to a percentage by multiplying by 100. This percentage point is displayed on the computer screen in re-

al time as the individual is speaking (Figure 14–7). For normal speech and the production of only oral sounds, the data points are usually between the 10 to 20 percentage points above the baseline. For speech that contains primarily nasal consonants, the data points are between 55 and 65 points above the baseline.

The reason that normal oral speech results in a nasalance value of around 15% rather than 0% is that there is always some spillover between the microphones during the production of vowels and even with voiced consonants (Kay Elemetrics Corporation, 1994). The sound separator plate cannot totally block reception of the signal from one side to the other side of the plate. Because there is always some spillover between microphones, the scores of 0% or 100% will never be obtained unless one of the microphones is not working. Another reason that nasalance is noted with oral speech is that there is slight nasal resonance during the production of vowels.

Calculating Statistics

Once the passage has been read or repeated, the examiner can select "Analysis" from the menu and then view the calculation of statistics (Figure 14–8). The statistic that is listed as the "mean" is actually the mean of all of the percentage points for the entire passage. As noted previously, this mean is referred to as the nasalance score and it represents the relative amount of nasal acoustic energy in the person's speech. The nasalance score can be compared to normative data for analysis. This can help the examiner to determine if there is a problem and its approximate degree of severity. The calculations also include the minimum percent and the maximum percent of nasalance during the passage so that the examiner can view the range of nasalance in order to judge the variability of resonance.

Prior versions of the Nasometer included the standard deviation of the passage in the statistics. In a study to evaluate the value of the standard deviation scores, it was found that the standard deviation score could not distinguish speakers beyond a gross normal and abnormal resonance diagnostic category (Vallino-Napoli & Montgomery, 1997). Although the standard deviation score might give some indication of the amount of variability of resonance during production of the passage, it was concluded that the standard deviation value serves little overall clinical utility. Instead, the mean nasalance score continues to be the best measure of resonance.

Normative Studies

Many studies of normal speaking adults and children have shown that nasalance scores vary with dialect (Leeper, Rochet, & MacKay, 1992; Seaver, Dalston, Leeper, & Adams, 1991), with racial group or culture (Mayo, Floyd, Warren, Dalston, & Mayo, 1996), with age and gender (Hutchinson, Robinson, & Nerbonne, 1978), and with language (Anderson, 1996; Leeper et al., 1992; Nichols, 1999; Santos-Terron, Gonzalez-Landa, & Sanchez-Ruiz, 1990; van Doorn & Purcell, 1998). For example,

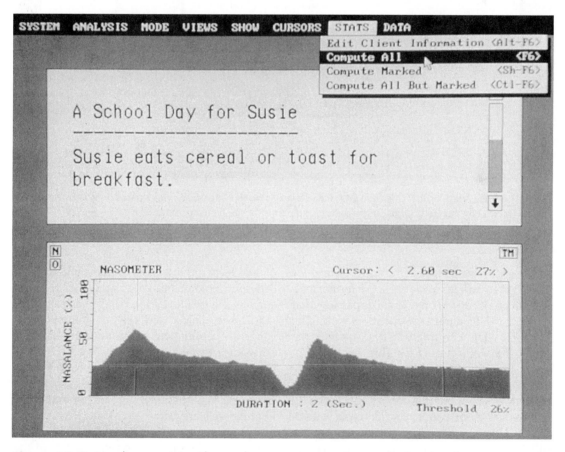

Figure 14–7. Nasalance statistics. The nasalance percentage points are displayed on the computer screen in real time as the individual is speaking. For normal speech and the production of only oral sounds, the data points are usually between the 10 to 20 percentage points above the baseline.

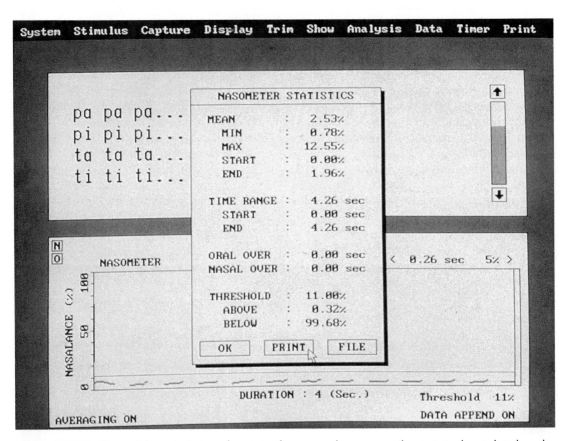

Figure 14–8. View of the calculation of statistics for a speech passage. The statistic that is listed as the "mean" is actually the mean of all of the percentage points for the entire passage.

in the study by Santos-Terron and colleagues (1990), the average nasalance score for normally speaking children on a Spanish passage that was devoid of nasal consonants was 22. The norm for American English speaking children on the Zoo Passage is 15.53. This represents an interesting difference.

It should be recalled that a portion of the nasalance score on oral passages is due to spillover of oral sound to the nasal microphone. However, this does not account for the differences in the scores. The differences in nasalance scores among various dialects and languages represent a difference in the amount of inherent nasal quality among speakers of different regions and languages. Because consonants are produced essentially the same, regardless of dialect, and even a slight velopharyngeal opening will cause audible nasal air emission during consonant production, these differences are necessarily in the production of the vowels. Some feel that nasalized vowels are the cause of a "nasal twang" in some dialects. High vowels are perceived as more nasal than low vowels due to the fact that the high tongue position results in increased impedance of the sound as it passes through the oral passage. As a result, there may also be increased bombardment of sound against the velum and some of the sound may go through the valve or even through the soft tissues (S. G. Fletcher, personal Communication, August 1999). At the same time, less oral resonance is achieved due to the high position of the tongue and the resulting reduction in the relative size of the oral cavity. In contrast, when the tongue is low in the oral cavity for the production of low vowels, there is considerably less impedance of the sound and the size of the oral cavity is larger so that oral resonance is more pronounced. Therefore, it might be assumed that dialects, accents or languages that use more high vowels or a higher tongue position might be expected to have higher nasalance scores as compared to those with a greater incidence of low vowels or a lower tongue position. There may also be a difference in dialects between the timing of closure when transitions are made between nasal consonants and vowels (Mayo et al., 1996).

Interpretation of Nasometric Data

Interpretation of the Nasalance Score

When one of the standardized passages is used, the nasalance score of the individual can be compared to normative data for that passage. However, there is no score that serves as the threshold between normal and abnormal resonance. If a child obtains a nasalance score of 25% on the Zoo Passage, it would represent two standard deviations above the mean. Yet the child may have very acceptable speech at that level. Vallino-Napoli and Montgomery (1997) suggested that a mean nasalance score in the high 20s could be used to differentiate speakers with borderline velopharyngeal function from those who are normal speakers. Dalston, Warren, and Dalston (1991c) used the score of 32 as the threshold of normal, but later, Dalston, Neiman, and Gonzalez-Landa (1993) used the

score of 28 as the threshold between normal and abnormal. Because nasalance and resonance are on a continuum, there is a "gray area" between normal and abnormal and therefore, there is no absolute or definitive "cutoff" point for normal. In fact, the score can be slightly high in the presence of perceptually normal speech, as noted before. On the other hand, the nasalance score can be in the normal range in the presence of audible nasal air emission, as long as the resonance is normal. Therefore, nasometry should always serve as a supplement to clinical judgment, not as a substitute for it. In fact, the results of nasometric testing must be interpreted by the speech pathologist in the context of the perceptual assessment of resonance, nasal air emission, phonation, and even articulation. Therefore, before nasometry testing is done, the examiner should complete a thorough perceptual evaluation.

An awareness of the individual's characteristics of resonance, articulation, and phonation will allow the examiner to interpret nasometric scores appropriately. If there is evidence of culde-sac resonance due to blockage in the pharynx, the nasalance scores may be essentially normal, since both oral and nasal resonance may be blocked and the nasalance score is a ratio of the two. A combination of hypernasality and hyponasality can also result in normal or near normal nasalance scores as both characteristics are combined for the average nasalance score. A combination of hyponasality and nasal emission can affect the nasalance score to a significant degree as well (Dalston et al., 1991a). When there is nasal turbulence (or a "nasal rustle"), it may result in a high nasalance score due to the degree of nasal distortion, even though it may be due to a small velopharyngeal opening. On the other hand, a large velopharyngeal opening may give a moderate nasalance score due to the lack of intensity of both oral and nasal acoustic energy. A breathy vocal quality or low volume can also influence the nasalance score to some degree.

Articulation errors can also affect the nasalance score. If velar fricatives are substituted for sibilant phonemes, the nasal emission associated with this articulation production will produce an elevated nasalance score. It should be kept in mind that this particular type of air emission may be due to faulty articulatory placement rather than true velopharyngeal dysfunction. In fact, phoneme-specific nasal air emission is not uncommon, and is merely an articulation disorder. However, this cannot be distinguished from velopharyngeal dysfunction on the nasometer. Because so many factors can affect the nasalance score, the examiner should always interpret the score based on a thorough knowledge of the individual's resonance and articulation characteristics.

Sensitivity and Specificity of the Nasalance Score

Several studies have evaluated the sensitivity and specificity of the nasalance score as it is correlated to another measure that serves as the guide. The *sensitivity* refers to the extent to which the score correctly identifies individuals with abnormal resonance. The *specificity* refers to the extent to which the score correctly excludes individuals with normal speech from being included in the abnormal group.

Dalston and colleagues (Dalston et al., 1991c) conducted a study to determine the extent to which nasometric results corresponded with aerodynamic estimates of velopharyngeal orifice area. Using an oral speech passage and a cutoff nasalance score of 32, the sensitivity of the Nasometer scores in correctly identifying the presence or absence of velopharyngeal areas in excess of 0.10 cm^2 was 0.78 and the specificity was 0.79. As a second part of the study, the nasalance results were compared to clinical judgments of hypernasality. Again, using the score of 32 as the threshold of abnormality, the sensitivity and specificity of nasometry in correctly identifying subjects with more than mild hypernasality in their speech was 0.89 while

the specificity was 0.95. Hardin and others (Hardin et al., 1992) conducted a similar study, but used a cutoff score of 26. In this study a sensitivity coefficient of 0.87 and a specificity coefficient of 0.93 were obtained. Ninety-one percent of the nasometry-based classifications accurately reflected listener judgments of hypernasality. Watterson, McFarlane, and Wright (1993) also found a significant correlation between nasalance and judgments of hypernasality on an oral speech passage. These results suggest that the Nasometer is an instrument that can be of value in assessing individuals suspected of having velopharyngeal impairment.

Dalston and associates (Dalston et al., 1991b) conducted a complementary study to determine the extent to which nasometric scores corresponded with clinical judgments of hyponasality and aerodynamic measurements of nasal cross-sectional area. Among the 38 adult subjects with moderate to severe nasal airway impairment as identified by aerodynamic studies, the sensitivity of the nasalance scores in correctly identifying these individuals was 0.38, whereas the specificity was 0.92. Among a group of 76 individuals, the sensitivity and specificity of nasometry in correctly identifying the presence or absence of hyponasality, as determined by perceptual assessment, were 0.48 and 0.79, respectively. However, when individuals with audible nasal emission were eliminated from analysis, the sensitivity rose to 1.0 and the specificity rose to 0.85. This study suggests that the sensitivity of nasometry in the identification of hyponasality with nasal air emission is not as strong as the sensitivity for identification of hypernasality.

Karnell (1995) suggested that one reason for a lack of agreement between perceptual measures and the nasalance results is that nasometry does not permit discrimination between nasal acoustic energy due to hypernasality and nasal acoustic energy due to turbulent nasal airflow. Hypernasal resonance occurs on vowels and nasal air emission occurs during the production of consonants. However, the presence of either can give the impression of "hypernasality," as judged by the listener. To test resonance, without the effect of nasal air emission, he used a "low pressure" speech sample that contained only consonants that do not require intraoral air pressure. The nasalance results from this sample were compared to the results of the "high pressure" sentences from the Zoo Passage. He found that the scores for some individuals were significantly different in the two passages. From this study, he suggested that individuals with hypernasal resonance will obtain elevated nasalance scores on the low-pressure and high-pressure speech samples, because the resonance occurs primarily on the vowels. In contrast, individuals with normal resonance but nasal air emission, especially the turbulent nasal rustle, will have low scores or normal scores on the low-pressure sample, but will have higher nasalance scores on the speech sample with high-pressure consonants. This observation seems true in our clinical experience and is another reason to consider the nasalance score based on what is heard perceptually.

Interpretation of the Nasogram

The *nasogram* is a contour display on the computer screen that represents the nasalance results of the spoken passage. It shows the individual data points in sequence as they were collected during the production of a passage. The configuration of the nasogram can be useful when the results of the passage are displayed on the screen. Some general guidelines in interpretation are as follows:

- Normal oral resonance, in a passage without nasal phonemes, is typically between 10–20% nasalance.
- The higher the contour is on the screen, the higher the degree of nasal resonance will be. On the other hand, the lower the contour is on the screen, the greater the nasal resist-

ance will be. A very low contour suggests a great degree of nasal resistance (probably due to nasal obstruction) and very little nasal resonance or even hyponasality.

- During production of an oral passage: If the contour is high and the data points are toward the top of the screen, this represents hypernasality.
- During the production of a nasal passage: If the data points are low and remain toward the bottom of the screen, it indicates hyponasality and can also suggest upper airway obstruction.
- During production of an oral passage: If most of the data points appear to be normal at around the 15% mark, but there are occasional high peaks, this suggests normal resonance but inconsistent nasal air emission.
- A gradual rise in the curve throughout the passage suggests muscle fatigue, which could indicate neuromotor problems.
- Significant variations in the height and valleys of the configuration in a passage that contains oral and nasal phonemes may suggest difficulty with the timing of closure.
- Having the individual prolong an /s/ or /sh/ sound can be enlightening, since with normal velopharyngeal closure, there should be no data points during this production. However, if there is a break in velopharyngeal closure, this will be seen on the screen.

The nasogram can be particularly helpful in counseling individuals and their families. With the visual display, it is easier for the examiner to explain what is happening during speech and the relative severity of the problem.

Use in Therapy

Although the Nasometer is a very useful diagnostic tool, its use in therapy must also be mentioned. It can provide the individual with valuable real-time visual feedback and tangible goals during the treatment process. It can be particularly helpful in eliminating a nasal rustle (turbulence), especially if this is due to a small, inconsistent velopharyngeal opening. This form of biofeedback can be used to modify resonance in certain cases of velopharyngeal incompetence (Heppt et al., 1991). However, it should be noted that biofeedback is only effective if the individual's velopharyngeal mechanism is anatomically and physiologically capable of achieving normal velopharyngeal closure. For more information regarding the use of nasometry in treatment, please refer to Chapter 21.

Summary

Nasometric testing is an easy, noninvasive procedure to obtain objective data regarding the results of velopharyngeal function. The nasalance score can be compared to normative data to gauge the type and degree of abnormality. Nasometry is an excellent means of substantiating the subjective findings of the speech pathologist. In addition, the Nasometer provides a visual display that is helpful in counseling individuals and families. Finally, nasometry is an excellent means for providing visual biofeedback regarding the results of velopharyngeal function during speech. Therefore, it can be very useful during treatment.

Although nasometry can be a very valuable part of an evaluation of resonance and velopharyngeal function, it should not be viewed as an independent diagnostic measure. Because the nasalance score can be affected by articulation errors, production errors, mixed nasality, and other factors, the objective measurements provided by nasometry should be interpreted based on an accompanying perceptual evaluation by a qualified speech pathologist. In addition, just like with aerodynamic instrumentation, nasometry can give objective scores, but cannot show the cause of velopharyngeal dysfunction, or the location and size of the defect, as the direct measures can do. It would be inappropriate to conclude that hypernasality or nasal airway obstruction exist solely on the basis of the nasalance score. Instead, the results of the nasometry testing must be integrated into a test battery for a complete evaluation of velopharyngeal function.

References

Adams, L., Fletcher, S. G., & McCutcheon, S. (1989). Cleft palate speech assessment through oral-nasal acoustic measures. In K. R. Bzoch (Ed.), *Communicative disorders related to cleft lip and palate* (pp. 24–257). Boston: College-Hill Press.

Anderson, R. T. (1996). Nasometric values for normal Spanish-speaking females: A preliminary report. *Cleft Palate Craniofacial Journal, 33*(4), 333–336.

Dalston, R. M. (1997). The use of nasometry in the assessment and remediation of velopharyngeal inadequacy. In K. R. Bzoch (Ed.), *Communicative disorders related to cleft lip and palate* (Vol. 4, pp. 331–346). Austin, TX: Pro-Ed.

Dalston, R. M., Neiman, G. S., & Gonzalez-Landa, G. (1993). Nasometric sensitivity and specificity: A cross-dialect and cross-culture study. *Cleft Palate Craniofacial Journal, 30*(3), 285–291.

Dalston, R. M., & Seaver, E. J. (1992). Relative values of various standardized passages in the nasometric assessment of patients with velopharyngeal impairment. *Cleft Palate Craniofacial Journal, 29*(1), 17–21.

Dalston, R. M., Warren, D. W., & Dalston, E. T. (1991a). The identification of nasal obstruction through clinical judgments of hyponasality and nasometric assessment of speech acoustics. *American Journal Orthodontics and Dentofacial Orthopedics, 100*(1), 59–65.

Dalston, R. M., Warren, D. W., & Dalston, E. T. (1991b). A preliminary investigation concerning the use of nasometry in identifying patients with hyponasality and/or nasal airway impairment. *Journal of Speech and Hearing Research, 34*(1), 11–18.

Dalston, R. M., Warren, D. W., & Dalston, E. T. (1991c). Use of nasometry as a diagnostic tool for identifying patients with velopharyngeal impairment [published Erratum appears in *Cleft Palate Craniofacial Journal*, 1991, 28(4), 446]. *Cleft Palate Craniofacial Journal*, 28(2), 184–188; Discussion 188–189.

Fairbanks, D. (1960). *Voice and articulation drill book* (p. 127). New York: Harper and Row.

Fletcher, S. G. (1970). Theory and instrumentation for quantitative measurement of nasality. *Cleft Palate Journal*, 7, 601–609.

Fletcher, S. G. (1972). Contingencies for bioelectronic modification of nasality. *Journal of Speech and Hearing Disorders*, 37, 329–346.

Fletcher, S. G. (1976a). "Nasalance" vs. listener judgments of nasality. *Cleft Palate Journal*, 13, 31–44.

Fletcher, S. G. (1976b). Theory and use of Tonar II: A status report. *Biocommunications Research Reports*, 1, 1–38.

Fletcher, S. G. (1978). *Diagnosing speech disorders from cleft palate*. New York: Grune & Statton.

Gonzalez-Landa, G., Santos Terron, M. J., Miro Viar, J. L., & Sanchez-Ruiz, I. (1990). [Post-adenoidectomy velopharyngeal insufficiency in children with velopalatine clefts]. *Acta Otorrinolaringology Español*, 41(3), 159–161.

Hardin, M. A., Van Demark, D. R., Morris, H. L., & Payne, M. M. (1992). Correspondence between nasalance scores and listener judgments of hypernasality and hyponasality. *Cleft Palate Craniofacial Journal*, 29(4), 346–351.

Heppt, W., Westrich, M., Strate, B., & Mohring, L. (1991). [Nasalance: A new concept for objective analysis of nasality]. *Laryngorhinootologie*, 70(4), 208–213.

Hong, K. H., Kwon, S. H., & Jung, S. S. (1997). The assessment of nasality with a nasometer and sound spectrography in patients with nasal polyposis. *Otolaryngology—Head and Neck Surgery*, 117(4), 343–348.

Hutchinson, J. M., Robinson, K. L., & Nerbonne, M. A. (1978). Patterns of nasalance in a sample of normal gerontologic subjects. *Journal of Communication Disorders*, 11(6), 469–481.

Karnell, M. P. (1995). Nasometric discrimination of hypernasality and turbulent nasal airflow. *Cleft Palate Craniofacial Journal*, 32(2), 145–148.

Kay Elemetrics Corporation. (1994). *Instruction manual: Nasometer Model 6200-3*. Lincoln Park, NJ.

Kummer, A. W., Myer, C. M. I., Smith, M. E., & Shott, S. R. (1993). Changes in nasal resonance secondary to adenotonsillectomy. *American Journal of Otolaryngology*, 14(4), 285–290.

Leeper, H. A., Rochet, A. P., & MacKay, I. R. A. (1992). Characteristics of nasalance in Canadian speakers of English and French. *Proceedings of the International Conference on Spoken and Language Processes*, 5, 49–52.

MacKay, I. R. A., & Kummer, A. W. (1994). Simplified nasometric assessment procedures. In Kay Elemetrics Corp. (Ed.), *Instruction manual: Nasometer Model 6200-3* (pp. 123–142). Lincoln Park, NJ: Kay Elemetrics Corp.

Mayo, R., Floyd, L. A., Warren, D. W., Dalston, R. M., & Mayo, C. M. (1996). Nasalance and nasal area values: Cross-racial study. *Cleft Palate Craniofacial Journal*, 33(2), 143–149.

Nichols, A. C. (1999). Nasalance statistics for two Mexican populations. *Cleft Palate Craniofacial Journal*, 36(1), 57–63.

Parker, A. J., Clarke, P. M., Dawes, P. J., & Maw, A. R. (1990). A comparison of active anterior rhinomanometry and nasometry in the objective assessment of nasal obstruction. *Rhinology*, 28(1), 47–53.

Parker, A. J., Maw, A. R., & Szallasi, F. (1989). An objective method of assessing nasality: A possible aid in the selection of patients for adenoidectomy. *Clinical Otolaryngology*, 14(2), 161–166.

Santos-Terron, M. J., Gonzalez-Landa, G., & Sanchez-Ruiz, I. (1990). Nasometric patterns in the speech of normal child speakers of Castilian Spanish. *Revista Espanola de Foniatrica*, 4, 71–75.

Seaver, E. J., Dalston, R. M., Leeper, H. A., & Adams, L. E. (1991). A study of nasometric values for normal nasal resonance. *Journal of Speech and Hearing Research*, 34(4), 715–721.

Vallino-Napoli, L. D., & Montgomery, A. A. (1997). Examination of the standard deviation of mean nasalance scores in subjects with cleft palate: Implications for clinical use. *Cleft Palate Craniofacial Journal*, 34(6), 512–519.

van Doorn, J., & Purcell, A. (1998). Nasalance levels in the speech of normal Australian children. *Cleft Palate Craniofacial Journal*, 35(4), 287–292.

Watterson, T., Lewis, K. E., & Foley-Homan, N. (1999). Effect of stimulus length on nasalance scores. *Cleft Palate Craniofacial Journal, 36*(3), 243–247.

Watterson, T., McFarlane, S. C., & Wright, D. S. (1993). The relationship between nasalance and nasality in children with cleft palate. *Journal of Communication Disorders, 26*(1), 13–28.

Williams, R. G., Eccles, R., & Hutchings, H. (1990). The relationship between nasalance and nasal resistance to airflow. *Acta Otolaryngology (Stockholm), 110*(5/6), 443–449.

Wozny, C. G., Kuehn, D. P., Oishi, J. T., & Arthur, J. L. (1994, November). *Effect of passage length on nasalance values in normal adults.* Paper presented at the American Speech-Language-Hearing Association, New Orleans, LA.

Appendix 14-1.

Standard Nasometric Passages Supplied by Kay Elemetrics
Zoo Passage[1]

Look at the book with us. It's a story about a zoo. That is where bears go. Today it's very cold out of doors, but we see a cloud overhead that's a pretty, white, fluffy shape. We hear that straw covers the floor of cages to keep the chill away; yet a deer walks through the trees with her head high. They feed seeds to birds so they're able to fly.

(Mean Nasalance = 15.53   S.D. of Mean = 4.86)

Rainbow Passage[2]

When the sunlight strikes raindrops in the air, they act like a prism and form a rainbow. The rainbow is a division of white light into many beautiful colors. These take the shape of a long round arch, with its path high above, and its two ends apparently beyond the horizon. There is, according to legend, a boiling pot of gold at one end. People look, but no one ever finds it. When a man looks for something beyond his reach, his friends say he is looking for the pot of gold at the end of the rainbow.

(Mean Nasalance = 35.69   S.D. of Mean = 5.20)

Nasal Sentences[3]

Mama made some lemon jam.

Ten men came in when Jane rang.

Dan's gang changed my mind.

Ben can't plan on a lengthy rain.

Amanda came from Bounding, Maine.

(Mean Nasalance = 61.06   S.D. of Mean = 6.94)

---

[1]The Zoo Passage excludes nasal consonants.

[2]In the Rainbow passage, 11.5% of the consonants are nasal consonants.

[3]The Nasal Sentences Passage is loaded with nasal phonemes so that 35% of the total phonemes in these sentences are nasal consonants. This is more than three times as many as would be expected in standard American English sentences.

Appendix 14-2.

Score Sheet for SNAP Test.

This illustrates the types of passages and normal scores.

Simplified Nasometric Assessment Procedures
The MacKay-Kummer SNAP Test
by Ian MacKay, Ph.D., and Ann Kummer, Ph.D.

Table 6.4 - Score Sheet

Name _____ Date _____

Birthdate _____ Age _____ Sex _____

Pertinent History _____

_____

Examiner _____

Syllable-Repetition Subtest		Child Norms		Measured Nasalance								Comments
					Difference from Norm (SD's)							
					hyponasal			norm	hypernasal			
Passage		Mean	SD	Patient's Score	-3	-2	-1	Mean	+1	+2	+3	
A	pa, pa, pa...	7.2	2.3		0	2.6	4.9	7.2	9.5	11.8	14.1	_____
B	pi, pi, pi...	17.6	6.2		0	5.2	11.4	17.6	23.8	30.0	36.2	_____
C	ta, ta, ta...	8.3	2.8		0	2.7	5.5	8.3	11.1	13.9	16.7	_____
D	ti, ti, ti...	19.0	6.1		0	6.8	12.9	19.0	25.1	31.2	37.3	_____
E	ka, ka, ka...	8.6	3.0		0	2.6	5.6	8.6	11.6	14.6	17.6	_____
F	ki, ki, ki...	19.4	6.5		0	6.4	12.9	19.4	25.9	32.4	38.9	_____
G	sa, sa, sa...	7.1	2.4		0	2.3	4.7	7.1	9.5	11.9	14.3	_____
H	si, si, si...	17.1	5.9		0	5.3	11.2	17.1	23.0	28.9	34.8	_____
I	fa, fa, fa...	7.5	2.7		0	2.1	4.8	7.5	10.2	12.9	15.6	_____
J	fi, fi, fi...	16.1	5.9		0	4.3	10.2	16.1	22.0	27.9	33.8	_____
K	ma, ma, ma...	58.4	7.8		35.0	42.8	50.6	58.4	66.2	74.0	81.8	_____
L	mi, mi, mi...	78.7	7.4		56.5	63.9	71.3	78.7	86.1	93.5	00	_____
M	na, na, na...	59.3	8.6		33.5	42.1	50.7	59.3	67.9	76.5	85.1	_____
N	ni, ni, ni...	79.1	6.9		58.4	65.3	72.2	79.1	86.0	92.9	00	_____

Simplified Nasometric Assessment Procedures
The MacKay-Kummer SNAP Test
by Ian MacKay, Ph.D., and Ann Kummer, Ph.D.

Name Date _____

Picture-Cued Subtest	Child Norms		Measured Nasalance							Comments
			Patient's Score	Difference from Norm (SD's)						
				hyponasal			norm	hypernasal			
Passage	Mean	SD		-3	-2	-1	Mean	+1	+2	+3	
A Pick up...	11.0	3.5		0	4.0	7.5	111.0	14.5	18.0	21.5	_____
B Take a turtle...	11.3	3.7		0	3.9	7.6	11.3	15.0 1	18.7	22.4	_____
C Go get a cookie...	12.4	4.0		0	4.4	8.4	12.4	16.4	20.4	24.4	_____
D Suzy sees the scissors...	12.9	4.4		0	4.1	8.5	12.9	17.3	21.7	26.1	_____
E Mama made some mittens...	56.9	7.4		34.7	42.1	49.5	56.9	64.3	71.7	79.1	_____

Reading Subtest	Child Norms		Measured Nasalance							Comments
			Patient's Score	Difference from Norm (SD's)						
				hyponasal			norm	hypernasal			
Passage	Mean	SD		-3	-2	-1	Mean	+1	+2	+3	
A Bobby and Billy Play Ball	15.4	2.8		7.0	9.8	12.6	15.4	18.2	21.0	23.8	
B A School Day for Suzy	10.8	3.1		1.5	4.6	7.7	10.8	13.9	17.0	20.1	

Comments: _____

_____

_____

_____

_____

_____

CHAPTER

15

Speech Aerodynamics of Cleft Palate

David J. Zajac, Ph.D.

CONTENTS

Why Aerodynamic Assessment?

Aerodynamics is the branch of physics that deals with the mechanical properties of air and other gases in motion. Because speech production requires a buildup and release of air pressure at the various valving points in the vocal tract, aerodynamic principles can be used to study the speech process. Indeed, aerodynamic processes are responsible for all acoustic aspects of speech production. Beginning with inspiration, air enters the lungs due to the expansion of the thoracic cavity and the generation of negative air pressure relative to the atmosphere. During expiration, positive subglottal pressure (P_S) is generated due to passive relaxation of the thorax and, if needed, active contraction of the muscles of respiration. Positive P_s is responsible for the rapid displacement of the vocal folds that results in the quasi periodic release of air for all voiced speech sounds. The articulators of the upper vocal tract further modify airflow for sound production. During production of the stop-plosive /p/, for example, the lips momentarily impede airflow resulting in a buildup and release of pressure. The acoustic bursts resulting from the release of the articulators provide important intensity and frequency cues to the place of articulation of stop consonants. In addition, the articulators create relatively prolonged noise by constricting the size of the upper vocal tract. During production of the fricative /s/, for example, the tongue approximates the alveolar ridge, resulting in a reduction of cross-sectional area and the generation of turbulent airflow.

Adequate production of speech requires an effective velopharyngeal (VP) mechanism. During production of oral pressure consonants, the VP mechanism must separate the oral and nasal cavities. Conversely, during production of nasal consonants, the VP mechanism must allow some degree of oral-nasal coupling. As indicated by Sussman (1992) and others, the following perceptual speech symptoms commonly occur in individuals with cleft palate due to VP dysfunction: (1) weak pressure consonants, (2) nasal air emission, (3) hypernasality, (4) hyponasality, and (5) compensatory articulation (pp. 211–212). Although the first two symptoms have clear aerodynamic foundations, their perceptual characteristics are not well defined. Both occur during oral consonant production due to the physical coupling of the oral and nasal cavities. Sussman (1992) described weak pressure consonants as sounds that "appear muffled and lack clarity." As indicated by McWilliams, Morris and Shelton (1990), nasal air emission may or may not be audible depending on the status of the nasal passages. Even when audible, nasal air emission may be masked by or attributed to acoustic deviations resulting from faulty oral articulation, especially those related to sibilant production. Clearly, aerodynamics should be considered an essential assessment method to determine the extent of "weak pressure consonants" and "nasal air emission." Although hypernasality and hyponasality are complex acoustic-perceptual phenomena associated with vowels and nasal consonants, respectively, they too may have identifiable aerodynamic substrates.

Because of the above factors, we believe that aerodynamic techniques should form an important part of the diagnostic procedures for individuals with cleft palate when VP inadequacy is suspected. As described below, when aerodynamic techniques are appropriately employed, they provide objective documentation of intraoral air pressure levels, rates of nasal air emission, and estimates of VP orifice size during consonant production. In addition, aerodynamic methods can be used to provide information on (a) the timing aspects of VP function during certain phonetic contexts and (b) the patency of the nasal airways during breathing. Such information can provide a firm basis for diagnostic decisions and/or postmanagement evaluation of individuals with cleft palate.

The following sections describe (a) basic principles of the pressure-flow technique, (b) instrumentation and calibration of equipment,

(c) aerodynamic assessment of nasal respiration, and (d) aerodynamic assessment and characteristics of speech production in cleft palate. The first two sections lay the groundwork and theory of aerodynamic assessment techniques. The third section is included because, as indicated above, the nasal airway is an important component relative to the perceptual aspects of speech production. The final section provides a detailed examination of aerodynamic characteristics of normal and cleft palate speech.

Basic Principles of the Pressure-Flow Technique

Warren and DuBois (1964) were the first to describe the use of aerodynamic principles to study the dynamics of the velopharyngeal (VP) mechanism during speech. Their procedure has often been referred to as the *pressure-flow technique*. By placing small-bore catheters in the oral cavity and in the nostril, respectively, along with the insertion of a flow tube into the remaining nostril, estimation can be made of the cross-sectional area of the VP port. The technique, therefore, provides an indirect method of determining the presence and extent of VP inadequacy.

Derivation of the "Orifice Equation"

As described by Warren and DuBois (1964), the cross-sectional area of a constriction or an orifice can be calculated if the differential pressure across the orifice and rate of airflow are measured simultaneously. In an ideal situation as illustrated in Figure 15–1, the static pressures (i.e., pressures associated with the moving airstream) are determined before the orifice (Point A) and at the point of constriction (Point B). The difference between these pressures is the dynamic pressure loss. Assuming that airflow is steady or nonturbulent, the area of the orifice can be calculated using the dynamic pressure loss and a modification of Bernoulli's equation as follows:

$$A = \dot{V}/[2(p_1-p_2)/D]^{1/2}$$

where A is orifice area in cm^2, $\dot{V}$ is airflow in ml/s, p_1 is static pressure in dynes/cm^2 before the orifice, p_2 is static pressure in dynes/cm^2 at the orifice, and D is the density of air (.001 gm/cm^3). As indicated by Warren and DuBois (1964), however, ideal or "theoretical" conditions do not exist in the human anatomy. In addition, because of practical limitations in-

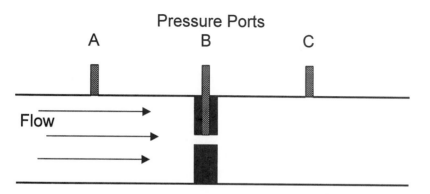

Figure 15–1. The area of a constriction can be calculated if the rate of airflow and the pressure loss across the constriction are measured. Either the dynamic pressure loss (from A to B) or the stagnation pressure loss (from A to C) are measured.

volving the placement of pressure probes, the static pressure at the constriction cannot be measured. The pressure-flow technique, therefore, uses a stagnation pressure (i.e., pressure associated with a low velocity or nonmoving air stream) detected at Point C in Figure 15–1 to determine the pressure loss. As noted by Yates, McWilliams and Vallino (1990), "the pressure loss created by the orifice is nearly equal to the dynamic pressure at the orifice" if the flow velocities before and after the orifice are small. Because these conditions are assumed in the human anatomy—and indirectly confirmed by Zajac and Yates (1991)—the substitution of a stagnation pressure for a static pressure is used in the pressure-flow technique.

As further noted by Warren and DuBois (1964), the substitution of a pressure measured downstream of the orifice is valid "if the kinetic energy of the gas passing through the orifice is lost due to turbulence on the nasal side of the orifice." Because the "theoretical" equation does not take turbulence into account, the calculated area will differ from the actual area. To overcome this problem, Warren and DuBois (1964) introduced a "correction factor k." This was a dimensionless coefficient, 0.65, derived from model tests of the upper vocal tract. Using short tubes that varied in area from 2.4 to 120.4 mm^2, they determined that an average value of 0.65 would suffice for the range of areas typically encountered in speakers with inadequate VP structures.[1] Based on their model tests, Warren and DuBois (1964) modified the "theoretical" equation as follows:

$$A = \dot{V}/k[2(p_1-p_2)/D]^{1/2}$$

where k is 0.65. Although Warren and DuBois (1964) referred to this as a "working equation," it has subsequently become known as the "orifice equation."

Application of the Pressure-Flow Technique

Air pressures during consonant production can be associated with a moving air stream (e.g., the fricative /s/) or a nonmoving air volume (e.g., the stop-plosive /p/). To detect these air pressures, small-bore catheters must be positioned behind the articulators of interest. To detect static pressures associated with fricative sounds, care must be taken to ensure that the opening of the catheter is positioned perpendicular to the direction of airflow. To detect stagnation pressures associated with stop consonants, the orientation of the catheter within the vocal tract is inconsequential—as long as it is behind the articulator of interest—due to equal pressure being exerted in all directions (Baken, 1987). Practical placement of the catheters, therefore, is an important issue that will be addressed below.

Warren and DuBois (1964) originally used a balloon-tipped catheter placed in the posterior oropharynx as illustrated in Figure 15–2. The catheter was passed through a nostril and secured at a level just below the resting velum by a cork. The catheter was then connected to a calibrated differential air pressure transducer referenced to atmosphere. A larger plastic tube was fitted to the speaker's other nostril and connected to a calibrated flowmeter. Because the catheter was positioned behind the tongue, stagnation pressures associated with the place of articulation of all stop sounds (i.e., bilabial, alveolar, and velar) could easily be detected. These pressures reflected the driving pressure before the VP orifice, corresponding to Point A in Figure 15–1. Warren and DuBois (1964) noted that the use of a thin-walled balloon reduced pressure measurements by approximately 3% as compared to an open-tip catheter. The balloon

[1]Although Yates et al. (1990) inferred that Warren and DuBois (1964) used "rectangular, thin plate orifices," Warren has clarified that the original model actually used short tubes to derive the k coefficient (personal communication, March 27, 2000)

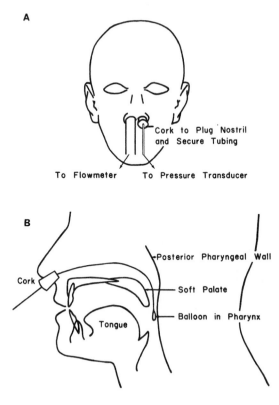

Figure 15–2. The pressure-flow method as originally described by Warren and DuBois (1964). **A.** Front view. **B.** Side view. A balloon-tipped catheter was placed in the oropharynx.

was used, however, to eliminate the possibility of saliva occluding the catheter. An additional advantage of using a transnasal placement of a catheter is that it does not interfere with tongue movements during articulation.

A disadvantage of the pressure-flow technique as illustrated in Figure 15–2 is that the differential pressure recorded during speech also includes a nasal pressure component when the VP portal is open. To overcome this problem, Warren and DuBois (1964) first instructed the speaker to breathe lightly through the nose

with the lips closed. The differential pressure and nasal airflow values obtained during breathing were then plotted as x and y coordinates. As noted by Warren and DuBois (1964), although the differential pressure in theory also contains a VP orifice component during breathing, at low rates of nasal airflow typical of speech, this component is too small to be recorded. During speech, the measured flow rate for a specific segment is used to determine the nasal pressure component from the breathing plot. This pressure is then subtracted from the differential pressure obtained during speech.

In a subsequent report by Warren (1964), the pressure-flow technique was modified to permit direct estimation of the differential pressure across the VP orifice during speech production. As illustrated in Figure 15–3, a catheter was placed in the oral cavity to detect oral-pharyngeal pressure below the VP orifice and another catheter was placed in one of the nostrils. The latter catheter was held by a cork stopper that also served to occlude the nostril and create a stagnation pressure downstream (i.e., above) of the VP orifice. The oral and nasal catheters were connected to a calibrated differential pressure transducer. The remaining nostril was used to detect nasal airflow as described above.

A final modification of the pressure-flow technique was described by Warren, Dalston, Trier and Holder (1985). Instead of recording differential oral-nasal pressure by means of a single transducer, they recorded oral and nasal pressures separately by using two pressure transducers—each referenced to atmosphere. The differential pressure needed for the orifice equation was then calculated from the oral and nasal pressure values. An advantage of this modification was that true oral air pressure was obtained which could be compared to normative data. An estimate of subglottal pressure, therefore, could also be inferred from the oral pressure value during production of voiceless stop consonants.

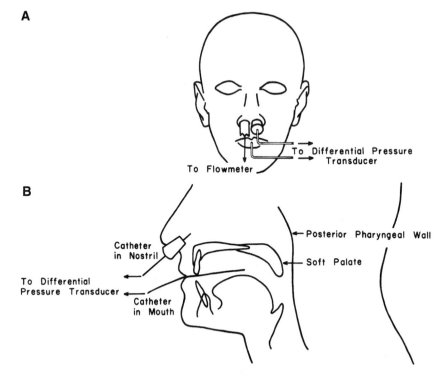

Figure 15–3. Front and side views of the pressure-flow method as modified by Warren (1964). Open-end catheters were placed in the nostril and the oropharynx.

Instrumentation and Calibration

Equipment

Contemporary measurement of air pressure and flow during speech production requires the use of appropriate transducers. *Transducers* convert the detected air pressure or flow into electrical signals for further processing. Transducers vary in construction, design, and performance characteristics. Figure 15–4 illustrates two types of differential air pressure transducers useful for speech work. A variable capacitance transducer (Figure 15–4A) consists of a diaphragm and an insulated electrode that forms a variable capacitor. As pressure is applied to the high (center) port relative to the low (or atmospheric) port, capacitance increases in proportion. Two of the transducers shown in Figure 15–4A have a pressure range of 0–15 inches of water (approximately 0–38 cm H_2O), useful for recording most pressures associated with speech activities. The upper limit of these transducers, for example, is approximately twice as high as pressures associated with even loud speech. The other two transducers shown have a pressure range of 0–0.5 inches of water, useful for recording the typically low airflow rates associated with speech. Solid state transducers are illustrated in Figure 15–4B. Again, two of the transducers have relatively high ranges required for speech pressures while two have lower ranges appropriate for recording speech airflow. Both types of transducers have good response

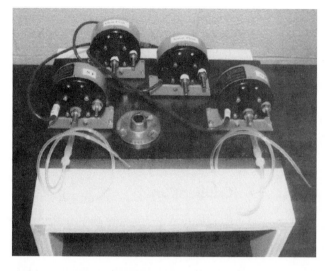

Figure 15–4. A. Four variable-capacitance differential pressure transducers. The two in the foreground are used to measure air pressures. The two in the background are used to measure airflows. **B.** Four solid-state differential pressure transducers. Two are used to measured air pressures and two are used to measure airflows.

A

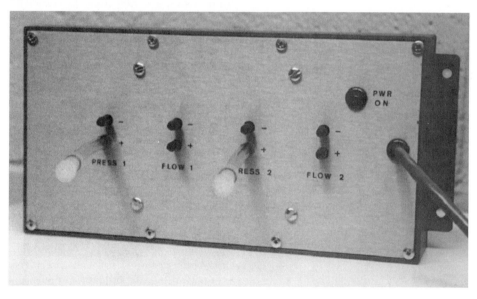

B

times (especially the solid state) and exhibit little drift (especially the variable capacitance).

The recording of speech airflow also requires the use of a heated *pneumotachograph*. This instrument, illustrated in Figure 15–5, provides a resistance by channeling airflow through a bundle of small diameter tubes housed within a larger conduit. The two pressure taps are connected to the ports of a differential pressure transducer. As indicated above, because the pressure drops associated with rates of airflow during speech are relatively low, a pressure

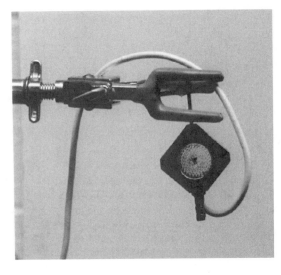

A

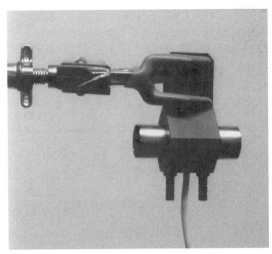

B

Figure 15–5. A. Front view of a bidirectional pneumotachograph showing resistive channels. **B.** Side view of pneumotachograph showing static pressure ports.

Higher rates of airflow will produce a proportionally higher pressure drop for the given resistance. Pneumotachographs are available in different sizes for different applications. As indicated by Baken (1987), the Fleisch #1 pneumotachograph (Figure 15–5) is appropriate for many speech applications. It has a maximum useful flow rate of 1.0 L/s, a resistance of 1.5 cm H_2O/L/s, and a dead space of 15 ml.

Calibration

Calibration of pressure-flow instrumentation is required to ensure that the output of the transducers is consistent with a known input. Calibration of pressure transducers is typically done using a *U-tube water manometer*. This device consists of a U-shaped glass tube partially filled with water. A scale—usually in centimeters of water (cm H_2O)—is positioned so that zero aligns with the meniscus of the water column. When a pressure is applied to one leg of the manometer, it depresses the column of water in that leg while simultaneously elevating the column of water in the other leg. The amount of applied pressure is determined by summing the magnitude of displacement in both legs of the manometer. If the first column was depressed by 3 cm, for example, and the second column was elevated by 3 cm, then a total pressure of 6 cm H_2O was applied. A *well-type manometer* (Figure 15–6) is similar to a U-tube but provides for the direct reading of applied pressures. This type of manometer has a calibrated reservoir (the left leg in Figure 15–6) filled with water or oil. Zero on a centimeter scale is aligned with the meniscus of the reservoir. When pressure is applied to the reservoir, it causes the fluid to rise in a connected column. The height of the column of fluid indicates the applied pressure.

Calibration of the pneumotachograph is typically accomplished by using a compressed air supply and *rotameter* to provide a known rate

transducer with a range of 0–0.5 or 0–1.0 inches of water is appropriate. The rate of airflow through the pneumotachograph is determined by measuring the differential pressure drop.

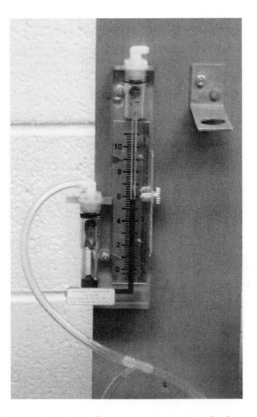

Figure 15–6. Well-type manometer. Applied pressure to the reservoir (left side) displaces the column of fluid on the right.

Calibration of computer-based aerodynamic systems also involves the use of software programs that will determine and store calibration (or scale) factors for the various pressure transducers. The numerical scale factors indicate the relationship between the electrical voltage output of the transducer and the known input (i.e., the applied air pressure or flow). Currently, there are several manufacturers of speech aerodynamic equipment. They typically provide the basic components, including calibration devices and software programs, for complete assessment of patients. If clinicians are not familiar with calibration procedures, it is suggested that they seek assistance from someone with the requisite background (e.g., electrical technician, mechanical engineer) to setup and calibrate instrumentation.

Assessment of the Nasal Airway

Nasal Airway Obstruction

Aerodynamic instrumentation can be used to evaluate nasal respiration and to quantify upper airway obstruction. Because nasal respiration involves resistance to airflow by both the nasal cavity and the velopharynx, obstruction may occur at either or both of these sites. Nasal airway obstruction is common in individuals with a history of cleft lip/palate or other craniofacial anomalies. This can be caused by maxillary retrusion, cranial base anomalies, a narrow hypopharynx, or enlarged adenoids, all of which restrict the nasopharyngeal airway. Other conditions, such as a septal deviation, choanal atresia, or a stenotic naris, restrict the size and patency of the nasal cavity. Even acute conditions, such as congestion or mucosal hypertrophy, can reduce nasal airway size. Any condition that obstructs and therefore attenuates the airflow through the nasopharynx or nasal cavity is a cause of nasal airway obstruction.

Individuals with cleft lip/palate are also susceptible to nasal airway obstruction as a conse-

of airflow as illustrated in Figure 15–7. A float or ball in the *rotameter* rises in proportion to the applied rate of airflow. A Gilmont rotameter is shown in Figure 15–7. This rotameter is calibrated in arbitrary units from 0 to 100. The units must be converted to ml/s (or L/s) by means of a calibration curve provided by the manufacturer. Other types of rotameters are available that are calibrated in units such as ml/s. A large volume syringe (e.g., 1–3 liters) may also be used to apply a known quantity of air across the pneumotachograph for calibration purposes. The advantage of this approach is that it eliminates the need for a compressed air supply that may not be available in all test settings.

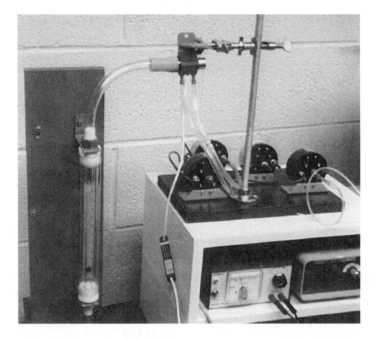

Figure 15–7. Calibration of pneumotachograph. A compressed air supply (not shown) delivers a known flow rate to a rotameter (left side in figure) that is coupled to a pneumotachograph and differential pressure transducer.

quence of the surgical procedures used to repair their defects. Indeed, work by Warren and colleagues indicated that children with a repaired unilateral cleft lip and palate have significantly reduced nasal airway size as compared to noncleft children (Warren, Hairfield, Dalston, Sidman, & Pillsbury, 1988). Individuals with a cleft of the soft palate who undergo secondary surgical procedures for residual velopharyngeal (VP) inadequacy are also at risk for posterior nasal airway obstruction. Such obstruction may not only result in hyponasal resonance, it may also interfere with health and daily living activities if severe enough to cause obstructive sleep apnea. Therefore, the evaluation of nasal resistance during respiration is of significance to both the speech-language pathologist and otolaryngologist.

Nasal Resistance and Rhinomanometry

Traditionally, measurements of nasal airway resistance have been obtained by using the techniques of anterior and posterior *rhinomanometry*. These techniques involve "the measurement of the pressure encountered by air passing through the nasal cavity" (Clement, 1984). During posterior rhinomanometry (Figure 15–8), the differential pressure between the oropharynx and the external nostrils along with the simultaneous rate of nasal airflow are determined. The resulting nasal airway resistance measure, therefore, includes components of both the velopharynx and the nasal cavities. As previously indicated, however, the relaxed velum typically produces a negligible pressure

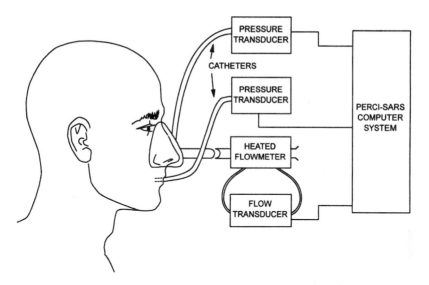

Figure 15–8. Posterior rhinomanometry. Both nostrils are evaluated simultaneously.

drop during quiet breathing. During anterior rhinomanometry (Figure 15–9), the differential pressure is obtained between the nasopharynx and the external nostrils. This is achieved by occluding one of the nostrils with a cork/catheter assembly. As previously described, this condition creates a stagnation pressure downstream of the velopharynx. This pressure serves as the upstream (or driving) pressure to atmosphere. Because of the need to occlude a nostril, anterior rhinomanometry measures the resistance of only the unoccluded nostril. To obtain resistance of the other nostril, the cork/catheter assembly and the nasal flow tube are reversed and the measurement is repeated. During either anterior or posterior rhinomanometry, it is important that the individual maintains lip closure while breathing in order to obtain valid results.

Once differential air pressure and nasal airflow measures are obtained by either anterior or posterior rhinomanometry, nasal resistance (R_n) may be calculated as:

$$R_n = P/\dot{V}_n,$$

where P is differential pressure in cm H_2O and $\dot{V}n$ is nasal airflow in L/s. Nasal resistance, therefore, is expressed in units of cm $H_2O/L/s$. As noted by Clement (1984), although this formula is universally accepted for the calculation of nasal resistance, it is valid only when turbulent flow conditions are not present during nasal respiration. Depending on the degree of respiratory effort (i.e., the driving pressure provided by the lungs), airflow through the nasal cavity may be laminar or turbulent. *Laminar flow* is steady and smooth due to the lack of significant resistance. With the convolutions and irregularities in the passages of the nasal cavities, this causes *turbulent flow*. When airflow is laminar in nature, the relationship between pressure and flow is linear and the above equation for nasal resistance is valid. When airflow becomes turbulent, however, the pressure-flow relationship is quadratic and the resistance equation must be modified accordingly. To overcome this problem, many clinicians will measure nasal resistance at relatively low rates of airflow to avoid turbulent conditions and to ensure that comparisons among individuals

A

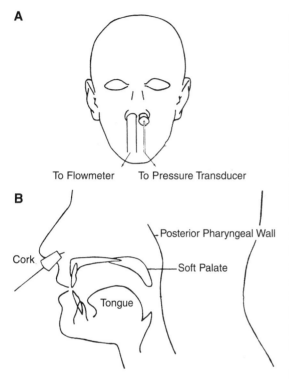

To Flowmeter   To Pressure Transducer

B

Posterior Pharyngeal Wall

Cork

Soft Palate

Tongue

Figure 15–9. A. Front view of anterior rhinomanometry. Each nostril is evaluated separately. **B.** Side view.

are valid (e.g., Allison & Leeper, 1990; Berkinshaw, Spalding, & Vig, et al., 1987; Warren Duany, & Fischer, 1969). Berkinshaw et al. (1987), for example, suggested that a flow rate of 0.250 L/s be used because it is laminar in nature and can easily be achieved by individuals even with nasal obstruction.

Estimation of Nasal Cross-Sectional Area

Warren (1984) demonstrated that the "orifice equation" could also be applied to pressure-flow measurements obtained during rhinomanometry to estimate nasal cross-sectional area. The use of an area measure effectively circumvents the problem of calculating nasal re-

sistance when airflow is turbulent. This approach, therefore, permits the calculation of nasal area at any point and at any flow rate in the breathing cycle. The approach assumes that the calculated area reflects the smallest cross-sectional area of the nasal cavity. The anatomical location of this area—called the "nasal valve"—is approximately 1 cm posterior to the entrance of the nose (Bridger, 1970). The boundaries of the nasal valve are the septal wall medially, the alar cartilage laterally, and the anterior portion of the inferior turbinate. Collectively, these structures form the smallest constriction of the normal nasal passage. Warren and colleagues reported a nonlinear relationship between nasal cross-sectional area and nasal airflow in adults with varying degrees of nasal obstruction (Warren, Hairfield, Seaton, & Hinton, 1987). Specifically, they showed that the rate of nasal airflow was controlled by nasal cross-sectional area when the nasal airway size was less than 0.40 cm^2.

Subsequent studies by Warren and colleagues have indicated that the size of the nasal airway is age dependent (Warren et al., 1988; Warren, Hairfield & Dalston, 1990). As with facial growth, nasal airway size appears to continue to increase up until about the age of 16–18. Warren et al. (1990), for example, used the pressure-flow technique to evaluate children between the ages of 6 and 15 years. They found that nasal airway size increased approximately 0.032 cm^2 each year and mean nasal cross-sectional area increased from 0.21 cm^2 at age 6 to 0.46 cm^2 at age 14. The percentage of nasal breathing also increased with age in these children. Age, therefore, should always be considered when assessing the status of the nasal airway in children and adolescents.

Clinical Procedures— Posterior Rhinomanometry

The specific procedures of posterior rhinomanometry using the pressure-flow technique are summarized as follows:

1. Nasal resistance and area are measured for both nostrils during inhalation and exhalation of quiet respiration.

2. A heated pneumotachograph is connected to a nasal mask, which is fitted snuggly over the patient's nose. The rate of nasal airflow is measured in L/s and recorded by a computer.

3. A catheter connected to a pressure transducer is placed in the patient's mouth. This catheter detects oropharyngeal air pressure. Pressure is measured in cm H_2O and recorded by the computer.

4. A second catheter connected to a pressure transducer is inserted through the wall of the nasal mask. This catheter detects mask pressure—or the pressure external to the nostrils.

5. During the examination, the patient breathes quietly through the nose while maintaining lip closure. Simultaneous recordings are made of the rate of nasal airflow, oropharyngeal pressure, and mask pressure.

The pressure-flow breathing records from an adult without nasal obstruction are illustrated in Figure 15–10. The figure shows oropharyngeal pressure, nasal (i.e., mask) pressure, nasal airflow, and calculated differential pressure from top to bottom, respectively. The three cursors labeled "I" indicate peak flow points during inspiration where measurements of nasal resistance and area were calculated. The three cursors labeled "E" show corresponding measurements made during expiration. All mea-0surements and means are printed at the bottom of the figure. In addition, the rectangular boxes labeled "E Means" and "I Means" on the left of the figure provide a summary of the mean measurements for each parameter except nasal resistance. The mean nasal areas of the individual were 62.2 and 67.5 mm² during expiration and inspiration, respectively. As indicated by Warren (1984), a mean nasal area of approximately 60 mm² is typical of adults without nasal impairment.

Clinical Procedures— Anterior Rhinomanometry

The specific procedures of anterior rhinomanometry using the pressure-flow technique are summarized as follows:

1. Nasal resistance and area are measured for *each* nostril separately during both inhalation and exhalation of quiet respiration.

2. A nasal flow tube connected to a heated pneumotachograph is placed snuggly in one nostril of the patient. The rate of nasal airflow is measured in L/s and recorded by a computer.

3. A cork/catheter assembly connected to a pressure transducer is placed in the patient's other nostril. This catheter detects nasopharyngeal air pressure. Pressure is measured in cm H_2O and recorded by the computer.

4. During the examination, the patient breathes quietly through the nose while maintaining lip closure. Simultaneous recordings are made of the rate of nasal airflow and nasopharyngeal pressures. The nasal flow tube and cork/catheter assembly are then reversed and the procedures repeated. As noted by Riski (1988), care must be taken when using anterior rhinomanometry to ensure that an airtight seal is obtained with the nasal flow tube and that the cork/catheter assembly does not deform the nasal valve area of the unoccluded nostril.

Using the above procedures, left and right nasal areas during inspiration for the individual illustrated in Figure 15–10 were 43.8 and 17.9 mm², respectively. Because the individual did not have posterior nasal airway obstruction, the summation of the left and right nasal areas (61.7 mm²) approximates the total nasal area (67.5 mm²) obtained by posterior rhinomanometry. It must be noted, however, that if an individual has significant posterior nasal obstruction, then the two techniques will not correspond. The use of both anterior and pos-

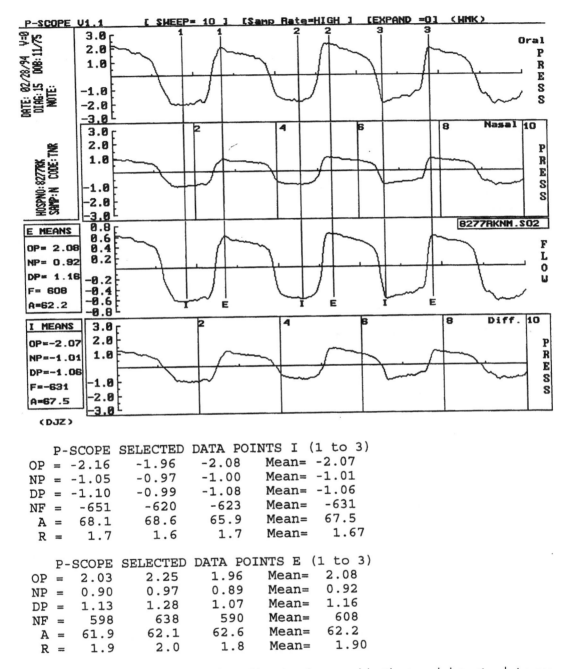

Figure 15–10. Pressure-flow recordings of breathing from an adult without nasal obstruction during posterior rhinomanometry. Calculated nasal area (A) is expressed in mm², calculated nasal resistance (R) is expressed in cm H₂O/L/s.

terior rhinomanometry, therefore, has the potential to identify the site of nasal obstruction in patients with clefts of either the primary and/or secondary palates. Although it is beyond the intended scope of this chapter, some clinicians have discussed the use of rhinomanometric techniques to partition the VP and nasal components of measured nasal resistance. The interested reader is referred to Smith, Fiala, and Guyette (1989).

Speech Aerodynamics and Velopharyngeal Function

The pressure-flow technique is ideally suited to document the magnitude of intraoral air pressure levels and the rates of nasal air emission during consonant production. It is important to realize, however, that intraoral air pressures vary with the type of consonant and phonetic context. Voiceless sounds are known to have greater intraoral pressure than voiced sounds due to the open glottis. In addition, intraoral air pressures tend to remain relatively constant at approximately 3.0 cm H_2O or higher, even in individuals with gross velopharyngeal (VP) dysfunction (Dalston, Warren, Morr, & Smith, 1988). This can be partly explained by the effects of increased nasal airway resistance, which is common in patients with a history of clefting as indicated above. Individuals with inadequate VP closure may also compensate for their oral pressure loss by increasing respiratory effort (Warren, Dalston, Morr, & Hairfield, 1989). Intraoral air pressures, therefore, may be affected by both increased nasal resistance and respiratory effort. Similarly, the rate of nasal airflow may be affected by increased nasal resistance. Measures of oral air pressure and/or nasal airflow, therefore, should be used

with caution as indicators of VP function. The pressure-flow technique, however, circumvents these limitations by providing estimates of the size of the VP orifice that are, in theory, unaffected by changes in either respiratory effort and/or nasal resistance.

Clinical Procedures

The pressure-flow technique is noninvasive and involves minimal risk to the patient.[2] It requires, however, a certain level of cooperation in that the patient must place a flow tube in the nose and pressure catheters in the mouth and nostril. Figure 15–11 illustrates placement of the flow tube and catheters along with a diagram of the equipment configuration. The specific pressure-flow procedures for estimating VP orifice size are as follows:

1. A plastic tube is inserted into the patient's more patent nostril. If anterior rhinomanometry has previously been performed, then the nostril with the larger area is selected. Otherwise, indirect estimation of the more patent nostril can be made using a mirror or detail reflector during quiet breathing with the mouth closed. The flow tube is connected to a heated pneumotachograph. The rate of nasal airflow is measured in L/s and recorded by a computer.
2. A cork/catheter assembly connected to a pressure transducer is placed in the patient's other nostril. This catheter detects a stagnation pressure downstream of the VP orifice. Pressure is measured in cm H_2O and recorded by the computer.
3. A catheter connected to a pressure transducer is placed in the patient's mouth. This catheter detects oral air pressure. Pressure is measured in cm H_2O and recorded by the computer.

[2]There is always the inherent risk that patients, especially children, may accidentally harm themselves around pressure-flow (or any laboratory) equipment. Standard safety precautions, therefore, should be followed. Care should also be taken to ensure that flow tubing and/or corks do not have sharp edges that may irritate or cut the nasal skin and/or mucosa.

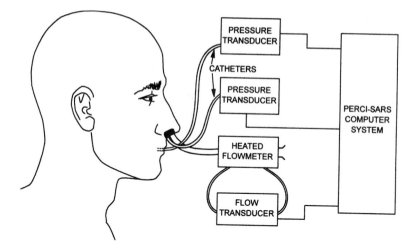

Figure 15-11. The pressure-flow technique to estimate velopharyngeal orifice areas during speech production.

As previously indicated, placement of the pressure catheter must be behind the articulator of interest in order to record a valid pressure. In addition, if the sound is associated with a moving airstream (e.g., /s/), then the open end of the catheter must be positioned perpendicular to the direction of airflow. Because of these requirements, clinicians most often evaluate VP function during production of the bilabial stop consonants. To evaluate the alveolar /s/ sound, the oral catheter should be occluded at the distal end, side holes placed in the catheter wall, and the catheter inserted to an area behind the alveolar ridge. Inserting the catheter from the side of the mouth during /s/ production will often reduce interference with articulation. To detect stagnation pressures associated with velar stops, a buccal-gingival catheter placement may be used. This approach, described below, permits valid detection of pressures associated with all oral consonants.

During the examination, simultaneous recordings are made of oral air pressure, nasal air pressure, and the rate of nasal airflow as the patient produces a series of speech samples designed to evaluate the VP mechanism. The speech samples typically employed by this author include the syllables /pi/, /pa/, /mi/, and /si/, the word "hamper," and the sentence "Peep into the hamper." The oral syllables are used because the VP mechanism must sustain closure during their repetition. The word "hamper" is tested because it contains the /mp/ sequence, which requires the speaker to rapidly adjust the VP mechanism from an open to closed configuration. Dynamic aspects of VP function, therefore, are assessed. The sentence is included to embed the word "hamper" in an utterance and thus approximate the conditions associated with continuous speech. The fricative /s/ is tested because this sound is most often associated with isolated nasal air emission seen in speakers with marginal VP function. In addition, the /s/ is also most often associated with phoneme-specific nasal air emission (PSNAE). This latter phenomenon is described below.

The following sections present actual pressure-flow recordings of speakers with adequate VP function and with varying degrees of

VP inadequacy. The pressure-flow data were collected using the PERCI P-SCOPE system (MicroTronics, Inc., Chapel Hill, NC). In the recordings, oral pressure, nasal pressure, and nasal airflow are illustrated from top to bottom, respectively. In some recordings, calculated differential oral-nasal pressure is displayed. The pressures are shown in units of cm H_2O; airflow is expressed in L/s. Estimated VP areas are expressed in mm². Measurements were made at peak oral pressures for all oral consonants and at peak nasal flow for all nasal consonants. The locations of measurements are indicated by numbered cursors in the recordings. As indicated by Warren (1997), estimated VP areas are most accurate when the measurements are taken at the point of peak flow, where the rate of flow change is zero. Peak pressures were used for oral consonants because (a) there is typically no nasal airflow for speakers with adequate

VP function, and (b) peak nasal airflow typically coincides with peak pressure for speakers with inadequate VP function. If the latter situation does not occur, however, then measurements should be made at the flow peak.

Speech Aerodynamics of Adequate Velopharyngeal Function

Figures 15–12 to 15–14 illustrate the pressure-flow recordings from an adult male speaker with adequate VP function saying the syllable /pi/, the word "hamper," and the sentence "Put the baby in the buggy," respectively. In Figure 15–12, the syllable is repeated eight times on a single breath. Except for the first intraoral air pressure pulse, the magnitude and shape of the pulses are strikingly consistent across the repeated productions. Typically, the first pulse in an utterance may have greater

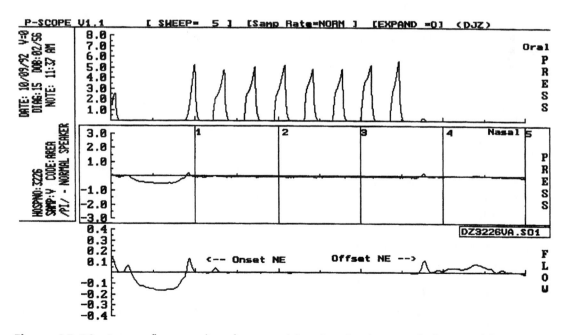

Figure 15–12. Pressure-flow recordings from an adult male with adequate velopharyngeal function. The syllable /pi/ was repeated eight times. Onset and offset nasal emission (NE) are evident at the beginning and end of the utterance.

magnitude than the following pulses due to higher relaxation pressure available at the beginning of a breath group. The rise in slope of the first pressure pulse may also be steeper due to the lack of voicing from a preceding vowel. As indicated above, voicing tends to reduce the magnitude of air pressure available to the oral cavity.

Figure 15–12 also illustrates that nasal air pressure and nasal airflow are present and in synchrony during respiration before and after the utterance. This confirms the patency of both nostrils required for valid estimation of VP orifice areas. Normal onset and offset nasal air emissions (NE) are evident at the beginning and end of the utterance. Onset NE reflects the transition of the VP mechanism from an open configuration during breathing to a closed configuration during speech. Offset NE reflects the converse transition from speech to breathing. Close examination of the nasal airflow signal reveals that the speaker exhibited approximately 40–50 ml/s of airflow during the beginning of the second pressure pulse. This type of inconsistent nasal airflow may have occurred due to several reasons. First, even in the presence of airtight VP closure, muscular contractions of the velum may displace the nasal volume of air (Lubker & Moll, 1965). As noted by Thompson and Hixon (1979) and Hoit, Watson, Hixon, McMahon, and Johnson (1994), however, this phenomenon is typically characterized by both positive and negative flows with rates less than ±10 ml/s. Second, the nasal airflow may have occurred due to inadvertent movement of the flow tube. Artifact airflow resulting from compression of the flow tube, however, would also be bidirectional and relatively small in magnitude. Third, the VP mechanism of the speaker may have actually opened momentarily. As reported by Bell-Berti and Krakow (1990), velar height is reduced for vowels as compared to pressure consonants. Indeed, as noted by Moll (1962), VP closure may not be complete for all vowels, especially low vowels.

Although the speaker produced the high vowel /i/, VP closure may still have been incomplete, giving rise to nasal emission when oral pressure increased to a level that was sufficient to overcome the resistance of the nasal cavity. This last explanation may be most likely because the nasal airflow occurred following the initial vowel and did not reoccur during any of the subsequent syllables. One may speculate, therefore, that the speaker was able to implement an online adjustment that was facilitated by auditory feedback, aerodynamic feedback, or some combination of both.

It should also be noted that there may be a gender bias for inconsistent nasal emission. McKerns and Bzoch (1970) reported that males achieved VP closure with relatively less velar contact against the posterior pharyngeal wall than females. Zajac and Mayo (1996), however, reported that males exhibited higher oral air pressures than females during production of "hamper." These findings suggest that subtle gender differences may exist relative to both respiratory and VP function. Such differences may cause males to be more prone to inconsistent nasal airflow than females. Although McWilliams et al. (1990) also acknowledged the various reports on gender differences and VP function, they further questioned the clinical significance of the differences.

Figure 15–13A illustrates the same speaker saying the word "hamper" five times. Nasal air pressure and airflow are evident throughout the nasalized segments of each word. P-SCOPE software was used to measure oral air pressure, nasal air pressure, nasal airflow, and to calculate VP orifice areas of the /m/ and /p/ segments. The three vertical cursors labeled "M" indicate peak nasal flow where measurements were made for the /m/ segments. The three vertical cursors labeled "P" indicate peak oral pressure where measurements were made for the /p/ segments. As expected, peak nasal airflow associated with /m/ occurred before peak oral pressure for /p/. In addition, anticipatory

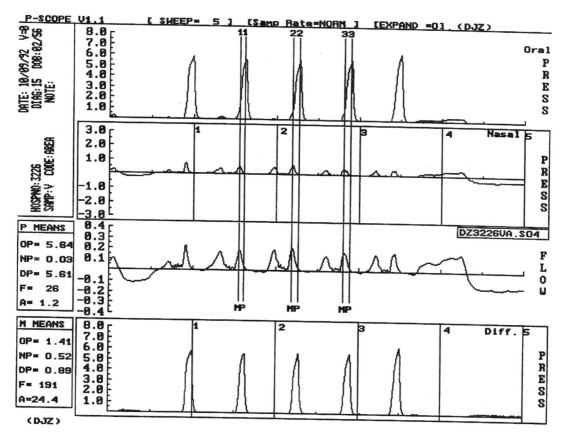

A

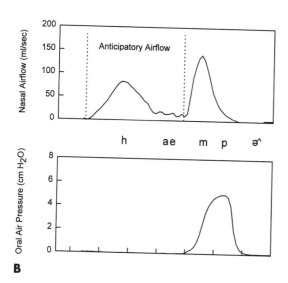

Anticipatory Airflow

h   ae   m   p   ɚ

B

Figure 15–13. A. Pressure-flow recordings from an adult male with adequate velopharyngeal function. The word "hamper" was repeated five times. **B.** Pressure-flow recordings of a single production of "hamper" with phonetic notation.

nasal airflow occurred during the phonetic segments preceding peak nasal flow for /m/. Figure 15–13B illustrates a single production of "hamper" with accompanying notation to indicate the phonetic segments. As illustrated, nasal airflow was higher during the voiceless /h/ than during the vowel immediately preceding the nasal consonant. This was expected due to increased resistance provided by the vocal folds during voicing. Nasal airflow reached its peak during the /m/ segment when lip closure occurred. Although not shown in the illustration, the simultaneous acquisition of the speech audio signal facilitated the identification of phonetic segments. This capability is available in a newer version of the software (PERCI-SARS, MicroTronics, Inc., Chapel Hill, NC).

As indicated in the measurements of Figure 15–13A, mean oral pressure of the speaker during /p/ averaged approximately 5–6 cm H_2O. This value is typical of noncleft adult speakers saying "hamper" (Zajac & Mayo, 1996). Children typically average higher oral pressures (7–8 cm H_2O) than adults, depending on their specific age (Zajac, in press). The reason for higher pressures is most likely due to the smaller surface area of children's vocal tracts. As explained by Müller and Brown (1981), a smaller surface area means that higher pressures must be generated to overcome the increased mechanical impedance to airflow. Nasal airflow of the speaker during the /p/ segments averaged 26 ml/s and estimated VP area was 1.2 mm^2. Although these values are typical of both children and adults (Zajac, in press), children tend to exhibit even lower rates of nasal airflow and smaller VP areas. This may be due to the fact that children typically possess greater amounts of adenoid tissue than adults. Nasal airflow of the speaker during the /m/ segments averaged 191 ml/s and the estimated VP area was 24.4 mm^2. Again, these are typical values for adult speakers. During /m/ production, children tend to show relatively reduced rates of nasal airflow and smaller VP areas.

eas. This is not surprising given that children tend to have larger adenoid tissue mass and smaller nasal cross-sectional areas than adults.

Finally, Figure 15–14 shows an example of continuous speech. The sentence "Put the baby in the buggy" was produced by the previous speaker. To record the oral pressures associated with the various consonants, a polyethylene catheter was heated and then molded so that its distal end approximated a 90° angle. The catheter was placed along the buccal-gingival sulcus with its angled end around the last mandibular molar, approximating the midline of the posterior oropharynx behind the tongue. This placement and orientation of the catheter permitted the valid recording of both static and stagnation pressures associated with all of the consonants regardless of place of articulation. As illustrated in Figure 15–14, the voiceless consonants were associated with higher oral pressures than voiced consonants. This effect was most evident during production of /p/ and /b/, sounds that differ only in voicing. Consistent with adequate VP function, Figure 15–14 also revealed the absence of nasal air pressure and flow during the utterance except for the nasal segment.

Speech Aerodynamics of Inadequate Velopharyngeal Function

Figure 15–15 illustrates the pressure-flow recordings from a 12-year-old boy with a repaired bilateral cleft lip and palate while repeating the syllable /pi/. Perceptually, the boy's speech was characterized by consistent but mild hypernasality, suggesting marginal VP function. Oral air pressures were somewhat reduced and variable during the utterance, ranging from approximately 2.5 to 5.5 cm H_2O. Consistent nasal emission of air occurred during the /p/ and vowel segments, averaging approximately 75 and 40 ml/s, respectively. In Figure 15–15, nasal emission during /p/ segments is reflected by the flow peaks and numbered vertical cursors. Nasal emission during

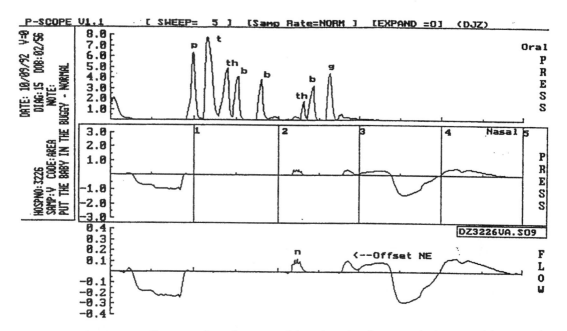

Figure 15–14. Pressure-flow recordings from an adult male with adequate velopharyngeal function. The sentence, "Put the baby in the buggy," was produced.

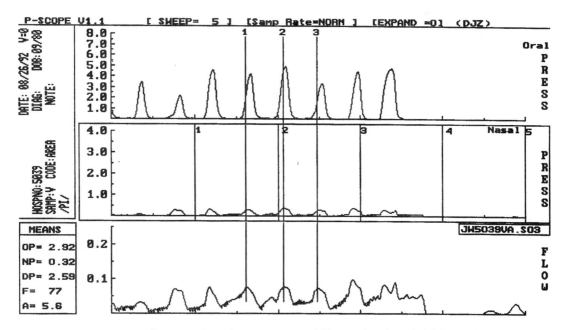

Figure 15–15. Pressure-flow recordings from a 12-year-old boy with repaired cleft lip and palate. The syllable /pi/ was repeated eight times. Estimates of velopharyngeal area were calculated at peak nasal airflow associated with the /p/ segments.

vowels is reflected by the variable flow occurring between the flow peaks. It must be noted that nasal airflow during vowel segments may not be readily detected by the pressure-flow method. This occurs because oral resistance to airflow is generally less than nasal resistance. Most of the airflow, therefore, will be shunted through the oral cavity even in the presence of a VP gap. The appearance of consistent nasal airflow during vowels in the speaker suggests the use of increased respiratory effort and/or altered lingual articulation as compensatory behaviors. Because of the consistent nasal air loss during /p/ production, however, the oral pressure measures may not be good indicators of overall respiratory effort.

The estimated size of this boy's VP gap was approximately 6 mm^2 during production of the /p/ segments. Based on this VP area, the boy's VP function would be categorized as "borderline adequate" according to criteria proposed by Warren et al. (1989). They suggested that VP areas under 5.0 mm^2 reflected adequate VP function, 5.0–9.9 mm^2 was borderline adequate, 10.0–19.9 mm^2 was borderline inadequate, and greater than 20 mm^2 was inadequate. It must be emphasized that these categories refer to the "respiratory requirements" of speech production, not perceptual aspects. The boy illustrated in Figure 15–15, for example, while clearly sounding "hypernasal," was nevertheless capable of generating borderline adequate oral air pressures demanded of speech production. This is an important distinction that clinicians must bear in mind when interpreting the VP area categories suggested by Warren et al. (1989). Overall, the pressure-flow records of the boy clearly indicate the marginal nature of his VP function. Borrowing a diagnostic term from Morris (1984), the boy illustrated in Figure 15–15 may be considered to exhibit VP function that is "almost but not quite" adequate.

Figure 15–16 illustrates another example of a speaker with marginal VP function. The pressure-flow records are from a 7-year-old girl with a repaired bilateral cleft lip and palate while repeating the syllable /pi/. Perceptually, she exhibited inconsistent hypernasality and moderate hoarseness. The girl repeated the syllable eight times. Because the P-SCOPE software was set to trigger automatically on a positive oral air pressure value, only partial pressure-flow data were recorded for the first syllable. The seven numbered cursors in the figure, therefore, indicate pressure-flow measurements that were made for the last seven syllables. These measurements are listed at the bottom of the figure. Initially, the girl exhibited relatively low rates of nasal airflow during both consonant and vowel segments of the syllables. Estimated VP orifice areas during /p/ production were also well under 5 mm^2 for the second (cursor #1) and third (cursor #2) syllables. During production of the fifth syllable (cursor #4), however, VP orifice size increased dramatically to almost 40 mm^2, causing a drop in oral pressure to 1.42 cm H_2O. Beginning with the next syllable (cursor #5), the girl appeared to use a compensatory strategy as evidenced by a rise in oral pressure with concomitant decreases in both nasal airflow and estimated orifice size. By production of the seventh syllable (cursor #6), she had achieved essentially airtight VP closure. It should be noted that the duration of her oral air pressure pulses increased during this process. Warren et al. (1989) have suggested that increased respiratory effort is a compensatory strategy employed by speakers with inadequate VP function. The increased duration of the oral air pressure pulses suggests that some type of respiratory strategy occurred. Such a strategy, however, may also result in laryngeal hyperfunction and perceived dysphonia. Indeed, as previously noted, the girl exhibited vocal hoarseness. Again, using the diagnostic terms of Morris (1984), the VP function of this speaker may be categorized as "sometimes but not always" adequate.

The pressure-flow characteristics of a speaker with gross VP inadequacy are presented in

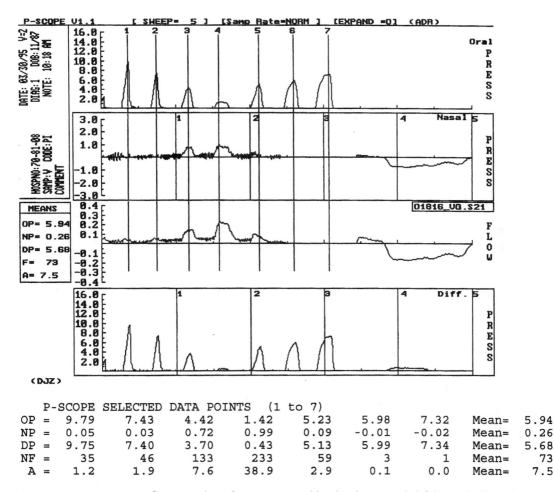

P-SCOPE SELECTED DATA POINTS (1 to 7)

OP =	9.79	7.43	4.42	1.42	5.23	5.98	7.32	Mean=	5.94
NP =	0.05	0.03	0.72	0.99	0.09	-0.01	-0.02	Mean=	0.26
DP =	9.75	7.40	3.70	0.43	5.13	5.99	7.34	Mean=	5.68
NF =	35	46	133	233	59	3	1	Mean=	73
A =	1.2	1.9	7.6	38.9	2.9	0.1	0.0	Mean=	7.5

Figure 15–16. Pressure-flow recordings from a 7-year-old girl with repaired cleft lip and palate. The syllable /pi/ was repeated eight times.

Figures 15–17 and 15–18. The speaker was an almost 5-year-old girl with an unrepaired submucous cleft palate and hypernasal speech. Videofluoroscopy confirmed VP inadequacy. In Figure 15–17, she repeated the syllable /pa/ four times. Because of the extent of her VP inadequacy, nasal air pressures (2.86 cm H_2O) were slightly but consistently higher on average than oral air pressures (2.84 cm H_2O). This finding—relatively rare except in cases of severe inadequacy—invalidates the estimated VP orifice area shown in the figure. Nasal air-

flow during /p/ production was 181 ml/s on average. It should also be noted, however, that relatively little nasal airflow was evident during vowel productions, as seen by the essentially baseline levels between the flow peaks.

In Figure 15–18, the same speaker repeated the word "hamper" five times. Because P-SCOPE software was set to an automatic trigger mode, pressure-flow data associated with the initial syllable in the first "hamper" were not recorded. The most striking feature of Figure 15–18 is the complete overlap of oral

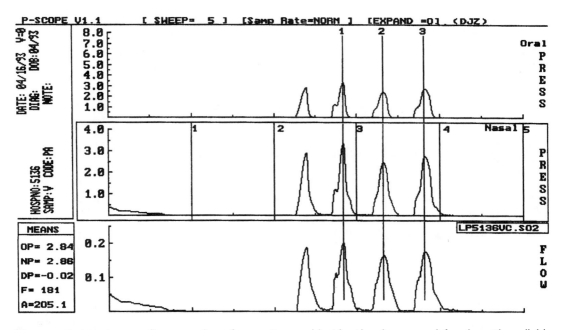

Figure 15-17. Pressure-flow recordings from a 5-year-old girl with submucous cleft palate. The syllable /pa/ was repeated four times.

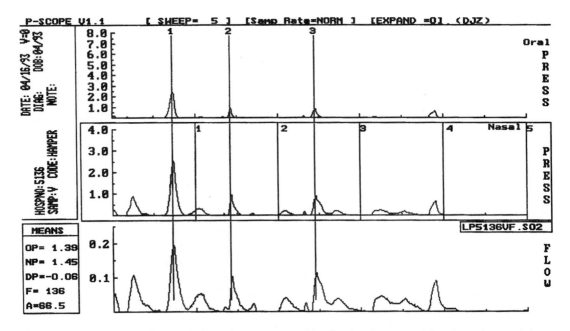

Figure 15-18. Pressure-flow recordings from a 5-year-old girl with submucous cleft palate. The word "hamper" was repeated five times.

pressure, nasal pressure, and nasal airflow during the /mp/ segments as indicated by the numbered vertical cursors. In essence, oral-nasal coupling was so complete that the speaker was unable to aerodynamically distinguish the /m/ from the /p/ segments in the words. Warren et al. (1989) showed that this overlap of pressure and airflow is a distinctive feature of inadequate VP function when orifice areas exceed 20 mm^2. Zajac and Mayo (1996) provided normative pressure-flow and timing data for the /mp/ segment in adult speakers. They reported a mean temporal separation of the nasal airflow and oral pressure pulse of approximately 70–75 ms. Finally, also demonstrated in Figure 15–18 is the speaker's inability to generate adequate oral air pressures. This is especially apparent after the initial productions of "hamper" when oral pressures dropped from approximately 2.5 cm H$_2$O (cursor #1) to 1.0 cm H$_2$O (cursor #2).

The pressure-flow recordings of "hamper" from a 10-year-old girl with a repaired cleft palate and a superior-based pharyngeal flap are illustrated in Figure 15–19. Perceptually, the girl's speech was characterized by hyponasality, suggesting an obstructive pharyngeal flap. The aerodynamic correlate is clearly seen as a severe reduction in nasal airflow associated with the /m/ segments. In addition, expected anticipatory nasal airflow was entirely absent. Because rhinomanometric testing indicated normal nasal airway size prior to the secondary palatal surgery, these findings confirmed the suggestion of an obstructive pharyngeal flap.

Finally, Figure 15–20 illustrates the pressure-flow recordings of a 6-year-old boy without a history of cleft palate who exhibited a pattern of phoneme-specific nasal air emission (PSNE). Although the boy exhibited adequate VP function, his findings are presented because they

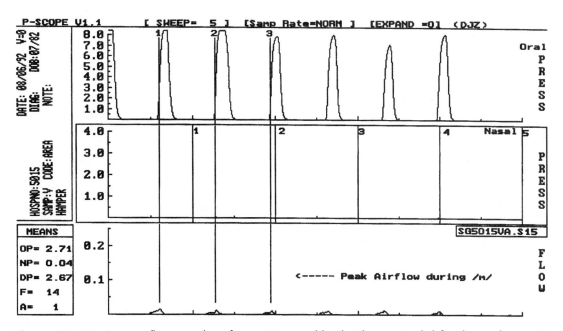

Figure 15–19. Pressure-flow recordings from a 10-year-old girl with a repaired cleft palate and a superior-based pharyngeal flap. The word "hamper" was repeated seven times.

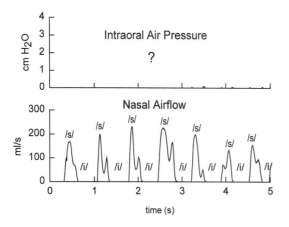

Figure 15–20. Pressure-flow recordings from a 6-year-old boy who exhibited a pattern of phoneme-specific nasal air emission. The syllable /si/ was repeated seven times. Oral air pressures were not detected due to deviant articulation.

have differential diagnostic value. The boy's speech was characterized by audible nasal air emission associated with all sibilant speech sounds. Trost (1981) has described this type of articulation as a "posterior nasal fricative." All stop-plosive sounds and the /f/ and /v/ fricative sounds, however, were produced orally, indicating a learned articulatory pattern for the posterior nasal fricatives. The pressure-flow recordings in Figure 15–20 illustrate production of the target syllable /si/. Nasal airflow was evident during all expected /s/ segments (nasal pressure is not shown in the figure). More interesting, however, was the virtual lack of oral air pressures. As previously noted, oral air pressure is typically maintained at some minimal level even in the presence of severe VP inadequacy. The boy, however, had learned a pattern of PSNAE that included the simultaneous articulation of a mid-dorsum palatal stop during the posterior nasal fricative. This pattern of oral stopping was confirmed by subsequent perceptual and acoustic analyses of the separate oral and nasal audio signals obtained from the microphones of a Nasometer.

In essence, the oral air pressure recordings were nearly atmospheric because the oral catheter was positioned at the alveolar ridge in anticipation of /s/. This anterior placement of the catheter did not detect the pressure buildup at the palatal location of stop articulation.

Precautions and Limitations of the Pressure-Flow Technique

There are several factors of which the clinician must be aware during the acquisition and interpretation of pressure-flow measures. First, as previously indicated, to obtain accurate measures, the equipment must be properly calibrated. During the examination of patients, all tubing, masks, corks, and catheters must be intact, snuggly fitted to the patient, and securely connected to other instrumental components. As Warren (1997) noted, tubing must be free of kinks and nasal masks must not be so tight that they distort the nasal valve. To estimate VP orifice size, both nostrils of the patient must be patent. Another concern is that the accuracy of VP orifice size estimations decreases significantly with openings that are 0.8 cm² or above (Warren, 1997). This occurs due to the limits of the pressure transducers in detecting small pressure changes. As indicated above, however, most perceptual characteristics of VP inadequacy are clearly evident when orifice size exceeds 20 mm² (0.2 cm²).

There is also debate in the literature about the appropriate value of the correction factor *k* to be used in the orifice equation. As noted by Müller and Brown (1981) and Yates et al. (1990), 0.65 may not be the most appropriate value for the geometry of the human VP orifice. Because of this uncertainty, it should be emphasized that VP area estimates are only *relative* measures. That is, as long as speakers exhibit similar VP orifice geometries, a relative comparison among individuals is possible using any value of *k*. Indeed, some researchers have omitted the *k* value entirely (e.g., Hixon, 1966).

Last, it must be reemphasized that, although aerodynamic procedures have the advantage of providing objective pressure-flow data, they do not provide direct information about perceptual aspects of speech production. As indicated throughout the previous examples, evaluation of voice quality, resonance, and articulation must be done using perceptual and/or other appropriate instrumental techniques.

Summary

Since the original report by Warren and DuBois (1964), aerodynamic measures have been used by many researchers and clinicians to study the function of the velopharyngeal mechanism. The pressure-flow technique can give the examiner objective information regarding velopharyngeal function and respiratory parameters. Because of this, it should be considered an invaluable tool in the assessment of patients with cleft palate and/or suspected velopharyngeal dysfunction.

References

Allison, D. L., & Leeper, H. A. (1990). A comparison of noninvasive procedures to assess nasal airway resistance. *Cleft Palate Journal, 27*, 40–44.

Baken, R. J. (1987). *Clinical measurement of speech and voice.* Boston, MA: College-Hill Press.

Bell-Berti, F., & Krakow, R. A. (1990). Anticipatory velar lowering: A coproduction account. *Haskins Laboratories Status Report on Speech Research, SR-103/104*, 21–38.

Berkinshaw, E. R., Spalding, P. M., & Vig, P. S. (1987). The effect of methodology on the determination of nasal resistance. *American Journal of Orthodontic Dentofacial Orthopedics, 92*, 196–198.

Bridger, G. P. (1970). Physiology of the nasal valve. *Archives of Otolaryngology—Head and Neck Surgery, 92*, 543–553.

Clement, P. A. R. (1984). Committee report on standardization of rhinomanometry. *Rhinology, 22*, 151–155.

Dalston, R. M., Warren, D. W., Morr, K. E., & Smith, L. R. (1988). Intraoral pressure and its relationship to velopharyngeal inadequacy. *Cleft Palate Journal, 25*, 210–219.

Hixon, T. J. (1966). Turbulent noise sources for speech. *Folia Phoniatrica, 18*, 168–182.

Hoit, J. D., Watson, P. J., Hixon, K. E., McMahon, P., & Johnson, C. L. (1994). Age and velopharyngeal function. *Journal of Speech and Hearing Research, 37*, 295–302.

Lubker, J., & Moll, K. (1965). Simultaneous oral-nasal airflow measurements and cinefluorographic observations during speech production. *Cleft Palate Journal, 2*, 257–272.

McKerns, D., & Bzoch, K. R. (1970). Variations in velopharyngeal valving: The factor of sex. *Cleft Palate Journal, 7*, 652–662.

McWilliams, B. J., Morris, H. L., & Shelton, R. L. (1990). *Cleft palate speech* (2nd ed.). Philadelphia, PA: B.C. Decker.

Moll, K. L. (1962). Velopharyngeal closure on vowels. *Journal of Speech and Hearing Research, 17*, 30–77.

Morris, H. L. (1984). Marginal velopharyngeal incompetence. In H. Winitz (ed.), *Treating articulation disorders: For clinicians by clinicians.* Baltimore, MD: University Park Press.

Müller, E. M., & Brown, W. S. (1981). Variations in the supraglottal air pressure waveform and their articulatory interpretation. In N. Lass (Ed.), *Speech and language: Advances in basic research and practice.* (Vol. 4, pp. 317–389). New York: Academic Press.

Riski, J. E. (1988). Nasal airway interference: Consideration for evaluation. *International Journal of Orofacial Myology, 14*, 11–21.

Smith, B. E., Fiala, K. J., & Guyette, T. W. (1989). Partitioning model nasal airway resistance into its nasal cavity and velopharyngeal orifice areas during steady flow conditions and during aerodynamic simulation of voiceless stop consonants. *Cleft Palate Journal, 21*, 18–21.

Sussman, J. E. (1992). Perceptual evaluation of speech production. In L. Brodsky, L. Holt, & D. H. Ritter-Schmidt (Eds.), *Craniofacial anomalies: An interdisciplinary approach.* St. Louis, Mo: Mosby Yearbook.

Thompson, A. E., & Hixon, T. J. (1979). Nasal air flow during normal speech production. *Cleft Palate Journal, 16*, 412–420.

Trost, J. E. (1981). Articulatory additions to the classical description of the speech of persons with cleft palate. *Cleft Palate Journal, 18,* 193–203.

Warren, D. W. (1979). Perci: A method for rating palatal efficiency. *Cleft Palate Journal, 16,* 279–285.

Warren, D. W. (1984). A quantitative technique for assessing nasal airway impairment. *American Journal of Orthodontics, 86,* 306–314.

Warren, D. W. (1997). Aerodynamic assessments and procedures to determine extent of velopharyngeal inadequacy. In K. R. Bzoch (Ed.), *Communicative disorders related to cleft lip and palate.* (4th ed.). Austin TX: Pro-Ed.

Warren, D. W., Dalston, R. M., Morr, K., & Hairfield, W. (1989). The speech regulating system: Temporal and aerodynamic responses to velopharyngeal inadequacy. *Journal of Speech and Hearing Research, 32,* 566–575.

Warren D. W., Dalston, R. M., Trier, W. C., & Holder, M. B. (1985). A pressure-flow technique for quantifying temporal patterns of palatopharyngeal closure. *Cleft Palate Journal, 22,* 11–19.

Warren, D. W., Duany, L. F., & Fischer, N. D. (1969). Nasal pathway resistance in normal and cleft lip and palate subjects. *Cleft Palate Journal, 6,* 134–140.

Warren, D. W., & DuBois, A. (1964). A pressure-flow technique for measuring velopharyngeal orifice area during continuous speech. *Cleft Palate Journal, 1,* 52–71.

Warren, D. W., Hairfield, W. M., & Dalston, E. T. (1990). Effect of age on nasal cross-sectional area and respiratory mode in children. *Laryngoscope, 100,* 89–93.

Warren, D. W., Hairfield, W. M., Dalston, E. T., Sidman, J. D., & Pillsbury, H. C. (1988). Effects of cleft lip and palate on the nasal airway in children. *Archives of Otolaryngology—Head and Neck Surgery, 114,* 987–992.

Warren, D. W., Hairfield, W. M., Seaton, D. L., & Hinton, V. A. (1987). The relationship between nasal airway cross-sectional area and nasal resistance. *American Journal of Orthodontic Dentofacial Orthopedics, 92,* 390–395.

Yates, C. C., McWilliams, B. J., & Vallino, L. D. (1990). The pressure-flow method: Some fundamental concepts. *Cleft Palate Journal, 27,* 193–198.

Zajac, D. J. (in press). Pressure-flow characteristics of /m/ and /p/ production in speakers without cleft palate: Developmental findings. *The Cleft Palate Craniofacial Journal.*

Zajac, D. J., & Mayo, R. (1996). Aerodynamic and temporal aspects of velopharyngeal function in normal speakers. *Journal of Speech and Hearing Research, 39,* 1199–1207.

Zajac, D. J., & Yates, C. C. (1991). Accuracy of the pressure-flow method in estimating induced velopharyngeal orifice area: Effects of the flow coefficient. *Journal of Speech and Hearing Research, 34,* 1073–1078.

CHAPTER

16

Videofluoroscopy

CONTENTS

Velopharyngeal dysfunction can be accurately diagnosed with a perceptual speech examination. However, a wide spectrum of anatomical and physiological abnormalities can cause velopharyngeal dysfunction. Before one can determine the appropriate form of intervention, it is important to specifically define the cause of the problem and the size and location of the defect (Van Demark et al., 1985).

Videofluoroscopy is a radiographic procedure that can be used to diagnose the cause of velopharyngeal dysfunction. This technique allows visualization of all aspects of the velopharyngeal portal during speech, through the use of several views (Skolnick, 1970; Skolnick & Cohn, 1989; Skolnick & McCall, 1971). Because there is visualization of velopharyngeal function during speech through this procedure, it is considered a *direct measure*. Videofluoroscopy can help the examiner to assess both the anatomical and physiological abnormalities that are causing velopharyngeal dysfunction so that the optimal surgical or prosthetic treatment for the patient can be determined.

The purpose of the chapter is to explain how radiographic images have been used in the past and how they are used currently in the evaluation of velopharyngeal function. The specific procedures for a videofluoroscopic speech study are reviewed. Most importantly, the interpretation of the images are discussed as they relate to the diagnosis and treatment of velopharyngeal dysfunction.

Radiography

Radiography refers to the use of the roentgen ray (X ray) to image internal body parts. As the ray goes through the body, it exposes the film or fluoroscopic screen on the other side. The film then shows structures as light images and air space as a dark image. Due to the fact that the beam goes entirely through a structure, it will project the summation of all of the parts of that structure through which the beam passes. In other words, it will show matter whether the matter is consistent throughout or only occurs in a small portion of the line of the beam.

Most radiographic images are planar, or two-dimensional in nature. To image a volume structure adequately, it must be examined in three mutually perpendicular planes to fully appreciate that structure (Skolnick & Cohn, 1989). Of course, the velopharyngeal port is a structure of both dimension and volume.

Lateral Cephalometric Radiographs

Lateral cephalometric X rays are still images taken in the sagittal plane. The *sagittal plane* is the median, longitudinal plane of the body. Dental professionals, including orthodontists and oral surgeons, use lateral cephalometric radiographs to study and measure the craniofacial bones and parameters of growth. This has been done through a process called *laminography*, which involves careful tracing of the structures and measurement of the distances and angles between particular landmarks. This process is now computerized, so that the meticulous tracing and measurements are no longer done by hand.

In the 1950s, cephalometric radiographs were used extensively in cleft palate research (Yules & Chase, 1968). In fact, the role of adenoid tissue in velopharyngeal closure was better understood with the use of this procedure (Subtelny & Koepp-Baker, 1956). However, cephalometric radiographs are no longer used for assessment of velopharyngeal function for several reasons. First of all, lateral cephalometric radiographs are still images and, therefore, closure can only be viewed during the production of a single continuant, such as /s/. In addition, the movement of the velopharyngeal structures during speech cannot be evaluated with this procedure.

Another disadvantage with this type of X ray is that it shows only the midsagittal section of the velopharyngeal portal. Views to visualize the lateral pharyngeal walls are not possible using cephalometric radiographs because the structures cannot be seen with this type of radiograph. Since the velopharyngeal mechanism is a three-dimensional dynamic structure, it is therefore impossible to adequately evaluate it through the use of a lateral cephalometric X ray alone. In fact, it has been estimated that, when judgments are based on a lateral X ray alone, the examiner is likely to misdiagnose the presence or absence of velopharyngeal insufficiency on the order of 30% of the time, when compared to the use of a multiview technique (Williams & Eisenbach, 1981).

Cineradiography

The use of *cineradiography* as a method for evaluating velopharyngeal function was first introduced in the early 1950s. Often referred to as a *cine study*, this technique involved taking a series of 16 to 24 frames of radiographs per second, which were recorded on motion picture film (Shprintzen, 1995). Multiple views were taken so that several dimensions could be evaluated. This technique had the advantage of being able to show movement and show all the velopharyngeal structures through several views. Therefore, it was used extensively for clinical evaluations and was also a useful method for continuous research regarding velopharyngeal function (Bzoch, 1968; Dellon & Hoopes, 1970; Litzow & Darley, 1966; Lubker & Morris, 1968; Massengill & Bryson, 1967; Massengill, Quinn, Pickrell, & Levinson, 1968; McClumpha, 1969; McWilliams, Musgrave, & Crozier, 1968; Yules & Chase, 1968; Yules, Northway, & Chase, 1968). However, there was no way to simultaneous record sound, and thus the speech with this procedure, so correlating movement patterns with speech phonemes was not possible.

Videofluoroscopy

A significant methodological advancement was made when multiview *videofluoroscopy* was first introduced (Skolnick, 1969, 1970; Skolnick & McCall, 1971). The videofluoroscopic technique allows the radiographic images to be recorded on videotape. The advantages of this procedure over cineradiography include the addition of a simultaneous audio recording with the videotape. Because a videotape recorder is used for this procedure, the video and audio signals can be recorded simultaneously on the same tape. Another advantage is that, unlike cineradiography, film development is not required. Therefore, the radiologist can check the adequacy of the study before the patient leaves and the tape is available for review and analysis immediately. The best improvement with videofluoroscopy, however, is the significant reduction in radiation exposure with this technique as compared to cineradiography. This is due to the fact that a video recording system is very sensitive to light; therefore, it can record at lower light intensities and at lower radiation levels. As a result of these significant advantages over previous techniques, multiview videofluoroscopy became the standard for radiographic visualization of the velopharyngeal port. For an excellent resource on the use of videofluoroscopy in the evaluation of velopharyngeal function, please refer to the book by Skolnick and Cohn (1989).

Clinical Uses for Videofluoroscopy

Videofluoroscopy is a good technique for the evaluation of the structure and function of the velopharyngeal mechanism. Using multiview videofluoroscopy, the examiner can confirm the presence of a velopharyngeal opening and determine the size and relative shape of that opening. The cause of velopharyngeal dysfunction can also be differentiated between a short velum, poor velar movement, or poor lateral pharyngeal wall motion. Videofluoroscopy is particularly helpful in assessing the extent and symmetry of lateral pharyngeal wall motion. In comparison with nasopharyngoscopy, videofluoroscopy is superior in showing the upward movement of the velum during speech. It also provides a view of the entire length of the pharyngeal wall during closure.

Given what can be viewed with videofluoroscopy, it is a technique that can help to determine surgical and prosthetic options for the treatment of velopharyngeal dysfunction. It can be helpful in assessing the placement of a prosthetic device, particularly a palatal lift. It can also be used to evaluate the effects of surgical procedures, such as adenoidectomy, maxillary advancement, retropharyngeal implant, or pharyngeal flap.

Preparation of the Patient

Because most patients who require an evaluation of velopharyngeal function are children, special consideration must be taken in preparing the patient for the study and making the child comfortable during the procedure. Many centers help to orient the patient to the videofluoroscopy procedure by sending information in the mail at the time that the appointment is scheduled. Information in the form of a story book or coloring book is particularly well received by children. The speech pathologist can also help to prepare the patient by describing the procedure to the child so that he or she will know what to expect on the day of the appointment. Having the child repeat sentences while simulating the various positions for the views can also give the child an idea of what to expect.

During the examination, it is important that the technicians speak calmly to the child and reassure the child about the procedure. Telling the child what will happen before it happens is

always a good idea. Having the parents in the room during the procedure is often a help, but it can also be a hindrance. This has to be determined on an individual basis. The parents can always help by offering a reasonable reward for cooperation during the study.

Videofluoroscopy Procedure

The velopharyngeal port is a three-dimensional structure that operates as a sphincter, with movement from all sides of the port. Therefore, it is important to view all aspects of this sphincter in order to determine the point of deficiency (Skolnick, 1973, 1975; Shprintzen, Rakof, Skolnick, & Lavorato, 1977). With fluoroscopic imaging however, only two-dimensional views can be obtained. The only way to view all aspects of the velopharyngeal sphincter with fluoroscopy is to obtain multiple views. The use of three mutually perpendicular planes is usually recommended to fully evaluate the port (Skolnick & Cohn, 1989; Skolnick & McCall, 1971). These include the lateral view, the frontal view (also known as the anterior-posterior or AP view), and the base view. In addition to the standard views, there are some supplemental views that can also be used. These views are used if the information that is needed from the study is not adequately obtained with the standard views. Since multiple views are used, the examiner can evaluate the motion of the velum and posterior pharyngeal wall, and then assess the movement of the lateral pharyngeal walls during speech. Other supplemental views can be used for certain diagnostic circumstances.

Lateral View

The *lateral view* shows the velum and posterior pharyngeal wall in a midsagittal plane. The orientation of the lateral view is as if one were able to look through the side of the individual's head to view these structures.

For this view, the patient is ideally placed in an upright position. The fluoroscopic table is vertically positioned and the patient stands or sits between the table and the fluoroscopic screen (Figure 16–1). The head remains in a neutral position with the patient looking straight ahead. For a young child who has difficulty holding still, the child can lie on the table on his or her side (Figure 16–2). A special pillow is used to support and stabilize the head. The disadvantage of this position is the potential effect of gravity on velar movement, although this effect may be negligible. The examiner should always be sure that the rami of both sides of the mandible are superimposed on the view to be sure that the head is not rotated or tilted during the study. This is very important because, if a true lateral view is not obtained, it may appear that there is closure when there is not, due to the position of the head.

Frontal View

The *frontal view*, also called the *anterior-posterior* or simply the *AP view*, allows the examiner to visualize the lateral pharyngeal walls at rest and during speech. The orientation of this view is as if one is looking straight through the nose. The X-ray beam is directed so that it is tangential to the plane of the velar eminence, which is usually appreciated as an arc between the lateral pharyngeal walls.

If we think of the patient facing to the side of the X-ray beam for the lateral view, the patient is then turned 90° to face forward for the frontal view. The patient can be upright, or

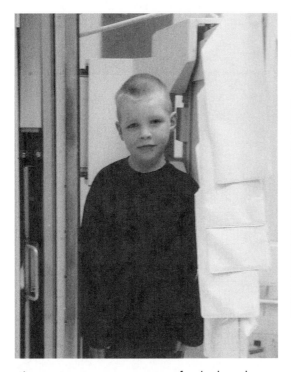

Figure 16–1. Patient position for the lateral view. The fluoroscopic table is vertically positioned and the patient stands or sits between the table and the fluoroscopic screen. The head remains in a neutral position with the patient looking straight ahead.

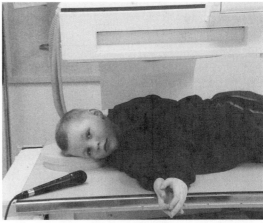

Figure 16–2. Alternate patient position for the lateral view. This is used if the patient needs more head support. For a young child who has difficulty holding still, the child can lie on the table on his or her side. A special pillow is used to support and stabilize the head. The disadvantage of this position is the potential effect of gravity on velar movement, although this effect may be negligible.

placed in a supine position (Figure 16–3). It is very important that the head is centered for the frontal projection and is not rotated. This can be determined by observing the nasal septum and making sure that it appears to be in midline. The septum should be equidistant from the lateral margins of the maxillary antra, and the incisor teeth should appear to be on either side of the nasal septum, allowing for deviations in structures. During nasal breathing, the lateral pharyngeal walls can be seen to bow outward on either side of the nasal septum. With speech, the lateral pharyngeal walls can be observed to move inward where they appear to meet the area of the nasal septum.

Base View

The *base view*, also called an *enface view*, allows the examiner to see the entire velopharyngeal sphincter as if looking up through the port. With this orientation, the relative contributions of the velum, the lateral pharyngeal walls and posterior pharyngeal wall to closure can be determined.

For the base view, the patient is placed on the X-ray table in a prone position. The patient is then asked to assume a "sphinx position" by pulling the head up and placing the upper body weight on the arms and elbows (Figure 16–4). The head and the back are then hyperextended so that the X-ray beam can be directed vertically through the base of the chin and then up through the velopharyngeal port. The correct positioning of the base view is actually very difficult, because the beam must be directly at right angles to the plane of closure. Otherwise, the port will not be visualized or the dimensions of the port will be severely distorted. The presence of large adenoids can also affect the interpretation of this view.

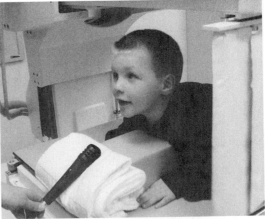

Figure 16–4. Patient position for the base view. The patient is placed on the X-ray table in a prone position and then asked to assume a "sphinx position" by pulling the head up and placing the upper body weight on the arms and elbows. The head and the back are then hyperextended so that the X-ray beam can be directed vertically through the base of the chin and then up through the velopharyngeal port. The correct positioning is important since the beam must be directly at right angles to the plane of closure.

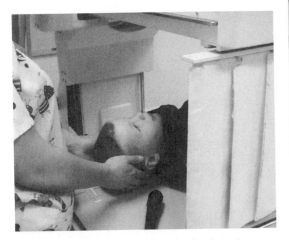

Figure 16–3. Patient position for the frontal or A-P view. The patient is placed in a supine position and the head is centered. This can be determined by observing the nasal septum through the fluoroscope and making sure that it appears to be in midline.

Towne's View

The *Towne's view* has been described as an alternative to the base view because it also provides an *en face* orientation (Stringer & Witzel, 1986, 1989). However, instead of looking up into the port, as is done with the base view, this view allows the examiner to look down into the port from above. The Towne's view is similar in orientation to the view that is seen through a nasopharyngoscope.

For the Towne's view, the patient is seated upright with the head hyperflexed and the chin tucked down. The beam goes through the top of the head and intersects the plane of the portal in a perpendicular manner. When the adenoids are large, the Towne's view may provide a better view of the velopharyngeal portal than the base view (La Rossa, Brown, Cohen, & Spackman, 1980; Stringer & Witzel, 1986, 1989).

Oblique View

The *oblique view* might be done if a satisfactory base view cannot be obtained due to large adenoids or the inability to hyperextend the neck (Skolnick & Cohn, 1989). As with the base view, this view also helps the examiner to relate the movements of structures seen on the lateral view to those on the frontal view. It can also be helpful in visualizing asymmetrical movement of the lateral pharyngeal walls, which is actually quite common. It has been estimated that about 15% of patients with velopharyngeal dysfunction have asymmetrical lateral wall movement (Argamaso, Levandowski, Golding-Kushner, & Shprintzen, 1994; D'Antonio, Muntz, Marsh, Marty-Grames, & Backensto-Marsh, 1988).

The oblique view is performed by having the patient sit facing forward. With the fluoroscopy on, the patient slowly rotates the head and body as a single unit so that it moves 45% to one side, back to the midline, and then 45 % to the other side. Because it is important to compare the movements on both sides with each other, a repetitive speech sample (i.e., pa pa pa pa pa) must be used. With this technique, the examiner can view the anterior half of the velopharyngeal valve as it closes during speech.

Use of Contrast Material

Radiopaque contrast material is not necessary for the lateral view, as the velum and posterior pharyngeal wall can be easily visualized without contrast. This is due to the fact that there is a column of air in the space between these structures. Because air is less absorbent of X-ray photons than the soft tissues of the velum and posterior pharyngeal wall, the air appears black, which provides contrast against the white structures. The frontal and base views, however, require the use of contrast to view the structures adequately.

The most commonly used radiopaque substance to view the nasopharyngeal structures is a suspension of colloidal barium sulfate. This can be purchased as a powder that is mixed with water or as a premixed liquid. Skolnick and Cohn (1989) recommend using a consistency of heavy cream. Flavoring is often added to the mixture as well.

Prior to instilling the barium into the nasopharynx, the patient is asked to blow his or her nose to discharge any secretions that could interfere with the exam. One way to instill the barium into the nasal passages is through a soft rubber catheter that is inserted in a nostril and then pushed through the nose to the nasopharynx. A spray of Pontocaine in the nose a few minutes prior to inserting the catheter can help to numb the nasal cavity for more comfortable insertion. In addition, a small amount of viscous lidocaine (Xylocaine) can be applied to the tip of the catheter to help ease it through the nasal meatus. These steps are not required, however, as there is very little discomfort with the catheter insertion. A large syringe is then used to squeeze the barium through the catheter (Figure 16–5). The advantage of this technique is that it places the barium directly in the position that is needed.

Another method is to simply drip the barium through the nares using a large nose dropper or pipette. The head is hyperextended or the patient is placed in a supine position so that gravity helps to push the barium back to the nasopharynx. The patient is asked to sniff the barium and the head of the patient is rotated to be sure that the soft palate and pharyngeal walls become adequately coated with the contrast material. This is important because, without an adequate and even coating of barium over all the structures, the view may be useless to the examiner. The drip method is usually less frightening to young children, but it can delay the procedure and may not result in adequate coverage of the tissues. Regardless of the method used, approximately 1 to 3 ml of barium is needed in each nostril for adequate coverage.

When barium is introduced in the nasopharynx through the nose, it causes the eyes to water and gives the sensation that is felt when wa-

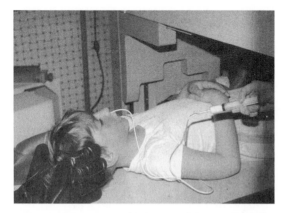

Figure 16–5. A method to instill barium into the nasopharynx is through the use of a large syringe and catheter. The barium is squeezed through the catheter to the nasopharynx.

ter goes into the nose. A burning sensation in the nasopharynx can last for an hour or more following its introduction. Although the barium can cause some discomfort and minor irritation, most children tolerate the procedure fairly well, especially if they are prepared with what to expect. However, if the child cries during this procedure, the secretions can wash the barium down. When that occurs, more barium needs to be squirted into the nasopharynx for the study.

Although contrast is essential in order to see the structures on the frontal and base views, it can also be helpful with the lateral view in some cases. The lateral view should always be done without contrast first, because the structures can actually be seen best with air as a contrast in this view. In addition, barium can mix with mucus and cause the velum to appear longer than it actually is. When the barium is added, however, it is sometimes helpful to repeat the lateral view. With the barium, a Passavant's ridge may become more obvious and the barium coating can also provide more information about posterior pharyngeal wall movement and palatal asymmetry (Cohn, Rood, McWilliams, Skolnick, & Abdelmalek, 1984).

Barium is particularly helpful in illustrating the patency of an oronasal fistula on the lateral view. This is done by first having the patient swallow some barium to see if there is any regurgitation through the fistula. Then the barium is instilled in the nasopharynx. If the fistula is patent, the barium can usually be seen as it drips from the nasal cavity through the fistula to the oral cavity (Skolnick, Glaser, & McWilliams, 1980). Barium can sometimes outline a defect in the nasal surface of the velum as a result of a submucous cleft.

Barium can also be helpful in the identification of small gaps. A disadvantage of videofluoroscopy is that it shows the sum of all of the parts that the beam goes through. Therefore, if the patient has a small, midline velopharyngeal gap, the lateral parts of the velum would close against the posterior pharyngeal wall. On lateral fluoroscopy, it would appear as if there is total closure. Fortunately, a small velopharyngeal gap usually results in a lot of air pressure being forced through the opening, which causes bubbling of the barium. Although a small gap may not be visualized directly with videofluoroscopy, its effect can usually be seen with this bubbling. In fact, whenever there is reflux of barium in the nasopharynx, it is always associated with a velopharyngeal gap. However, the absence of reflux is not similarly diagnostic. When there is a larger velopharyngeal gap, there is less concentrated air pressure going through the opening and therefore, bubbling is less likely to occur.

Since barium can produce artifacts or occasionally obscure structures, it is recommend that lateral videofluoroscopy always be performed without barium first and again with barium only if specific information is needed.

Speech Sample

During the projection for each view, the patient should first be asked to swallow. With the act of swallowing, the velopharyngeal structures come together forcefully and are easy to identify. This helps the technician to be sure that the orientation is correct, and it can also be useful when the study is interpreted because it orients the evaluators to the location of the structures. The X-ray technician then asks the patient to repeat syllables or standard sentences. A microphone is placed near the patient's head so that it can record the speech simultaneously with the visual images (Figure 16–6).

The speech pathologist does not need to be present during the examination in most cases. However, it is very important that the speech sample is selected by a speech pathologist. The speech sample should include a variety of pressure-sensitive phonemes in connected speech at the sentence level. Because the /s/ sound is most often affected by velopharyngeal dys-

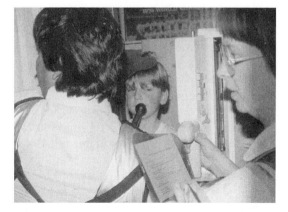

Figure 16–6. The X-ray technician asks the patient to repeat syllables and standard sentences. A microphone is placed near the patient's head so that it can record the speech simultaneously with the visual images.

function, the sample should include at least one sentence with a frequent occurrence of this sound. A sentence such as "Sissy sees the sun in the sky" can be particularly useful because it not only contains many /s/ sounds, but it also contains an /s/ blend, which further challenges velopharyngeal closure. In addition, it has some nasal sounds in the middle of the sentence, so the velum has to go up, come down, and then go up again to reach its target. It is also helpful to have the patient repeat syllables with pressure-sensitive phonemes (i.e., pa pa pa; ta ta ta; ka ka ka; sa sa sa; etc.). Repeating "60, 60, 60" or counting from 60 to 70 can be especially taxing on the velopharyngeal mechanism as it requires the production of fricatives and plosives, with a blend and high vowel. Therefore, it is an excellent speech segment to include in the sample.

The composition of the speech sample is very important because, if it does not adequately tax the velopharyngeal mechanism, the study may not identify mild or inconsistent velopharyngeal dysfunction. It is tempting, therefore, to test all speech phonemes for a comprehensive speech examination. However, it is more important to keep the sample as short as possible to minimize the amount of radiation exposure to the patient (Isberg, Julin, Kraepelien, & Henrikson, 1989). If the sentences that are chosen contain many pressure-sensitive phonemes, no more than 20 seconds of speech is needed to obtain an adequate speech sample.

There is sometimes a need to augment the standard sentences that are determined for use with each patient during a videofluoroscopic examination. For example, a longer connected speech sample might be needed when there is inconsistent velopharyngeal function or velopharyngeal dysfunction with fatigue. In this case, rote speech, such as counting or the alphabet, can be used. The speech sample can also be designed to test the patient's specific speech errors based on the observations from the speech assessment.

Interpretation

Who Performs and Interprets the Study?

A videofluoroscopic speech study can be performed perfectly by the technician with good angles and good barium contrast. However, the study is only as good as the interpretation. Experience, skill, and careful analysis are required for interpretation of the study.

Although the radiologist or X-ray technician actually performs the study, both the radiologist and the speech pathologist need to work together to interpret the study. The radiologist has a thorough understanding of the anatomy, physiology, and imaging of the velopharyngeal structures. The speech pathologist also understands the anatomy and physiology, but particularly understands the physiology of normal and abnormal speech. The speech pathologist has a unique perspective regarding the correlation between velopharyngeal function and the acoustic product. With both perspectives, the

interpretation of the study is more complete and accurate.

Interpretation of the Lateral View

On the lateral view, the examiner should observe the length, thickness, and contour of the velum, both at rest and during phonation. During phonation, the velum should elevate to the approximate level of the hard palate. There should be a bend in the velum at a point which is about two thirds of the distance from the hard palate to the tip of the uvula. This bend, or "knee action," is at the point of insertion of the levator veli palatini muscles and occurs as the levator sling contracts to pull the velum upward. When the velum makes contact with the posterior pharyngeal wall, the extent of contact between the velar eminence (the high point on the top of the "knee") down through the vertical part of the velum should be noted. The extent of the contact area gives an indication of the firmness of closure. If the contact area is small, it might be assumed that the closure is tenuous.

On the posterior pharyngeal wall, the presence and approximate size of an adenoid pad should be noted. The adenoid pad usually appears as a smooth, convex structure that is either on the same plane as the hard palate or slightly higher. If there is no adenoid mass, the depth and contour of the pharyngeal wall should be assessed. The examiner should note the relative depth of the pharynx during nasal breathing and then observe the anterior motion of the posterior pharyngeal wall, if this occurs, with speech. When a Passavant's ridge is present, it can be viewed as a shelflike projection on the posterior pharyngeal wall during speech. Tonsillar tissue can be seen somewhat on this view. It appears as an oval mass that is superimposed over the area of the posterior tongue.

Tongue movement during articulation should always be assessed from this view. In some cases, the posterior portion of the tongue can be observed to assist in elevating the velum during speech. If this is occurring, then the apparent movement of the velum and the resultant closure is actually very deceiving. In addition, the movement of the tongue tip, dorsum, the posterior tongue, and even the larynx should be observed to determine if there are compensatory productions, such as glottal stops, pharyngeal plosives, pharyngeal fricatives, or mid-dorsum palatal stops. Abnormal tongue movement, including backing of articulation or the use of the dorsum for articulation, should also be noted.

Evidence of abnormality may include a short velum relative to the posterior pharyngeal wall, a thin velum, or poor knee action of the velum during speech. Figure 16–7 shows a lateral view of a patient with a short velum relative to the posterior pharyngeal wall, resulting in velopharyngeal insufficiency. Figure 16–8 shows a velum with poor movement and little knee action, resulting in velopharyngeal in-

competence. The extent of the velopharyngeal opening as a result of these abnormalities should be noted.

On the lateral view, the examiner may also note evidence of a patent oro-nasal fistula if barium is used. Other abnormalities may include a localized indentation on the posterior pharyngeal wall following the removal of the adenoids. The appearance of hypertrophic tonsils or adenoids that intrude into the airway would also indicate a problem.

Interpretation of the Frontal View

On the frontal view, the examiner should assess the extent of lateral pharyngeal wall motion, the symmetry of movement between the two sides, and the approximate level of maximum motion. In most normal speakers, the point of maximum lateral pharyngeal wall motion is just below the plane of the velar eminence (Skolnick & Cohn, 1989). Poor lateral wall movement or the lack of lateral wall movement can suggest a problem with velo-

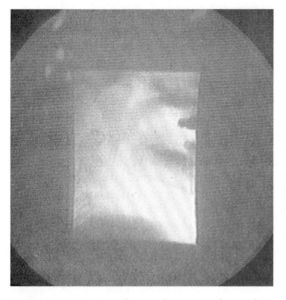

Figure 16–7. Lateral view showing a short velum relative to the posterior pharyngeal wall, resulting in velopharyngeal insufficiency.

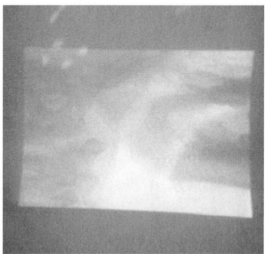

Figure 16–8. Lateral view showing a velum of normal length, but poor movement during speech, resulting in velopharyngeal incompetence.

pharyngeal closure. On the other hand, the patient may merely have a coronal pattern of closure, which requires only minimal lateral wall movement during closure. Figure 16–9 shows the frontal view of a patient. The barium-coated lateral pharyngeal walls are on either side of the septum. When there is a small velopharyngeal opening, bubbling of barium is often noted on this view. The examiner should note if the point of bubbling is in the midline or skewed to one side.

In some cases, the lateral pharyngeal walls will appear asymmetrical in their position at rest and may also be asymmetrical in the amount of medial movement noted during speech. Before making this judgment, however, it is important to be sure that the orientation of the view is appropriate and that the head was not turned slightly to give a false impression. Asymmetry in lateral wall movement can cause a lack of complete velopharyngeal closure on the side with the least medial movement. Another abnormality may be found when there is asymmetry in the vertical dimension. In this case, the level of maximum lateral wall movement is higher on one side than on the other. All of these observations are important to document because they have definite implications for appropriate surgical management. The examiner should remember that, because this view goes from the front to the back, the lateral wall on the right side of the screen is on the patient's left side and vice versa. The side of deficiency should be reported based on the patient's right or left, rather than the examiner's orientation.

Interpretation of the Base View

If the head is positioned properly so that the beam goes directly through the velopharyngeal port, the margins of the port can be viewed as an oval or round structure during nasal breathing. The lateral and posterior pharyngeal walls can be seen easily with this view if there is an adequate coating of the barium. On the top of the screen, the velum can also be seen, but it often appears light and is therefore harder to visualize than the pharyngeal walls. During speech, the structures can be observed to narrow and then close the lumen as a sphincter. Depending on the basic pattern of closure, a black horizontal line (with a coronal pattern), a vertical line (with a sagittal pattern), or a circle (with a circular pattern) will remain in the middle of the closure area. Figure 16-10 shows the nasopharyngeal port through the base view. Figure 16–10A shows the port entirely open. The port begins to close in Figure 16–10B and is entirely closed in Figure 16–10C, leaving a

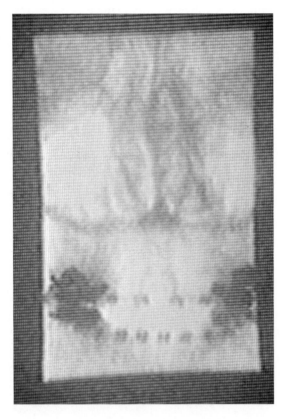

Figure 16–9. Frontal view showing the nasal septum in midline. The lateral pharyngeal walls are well coated with barium and bow outward during nasal breathing as noted in the frame.

small circle. The examiner should be careful not to confuse movement of the tongue and vocal folds with velopharyngeal movement on this view. In addition, the large foramen magnum can be seen on this view and this should not be mistaken for the velopharyngeal port.

When there is velopharyngeal dysfunction, the pharyngeal lumen does not appear to totally close. In fact, an opening during speech is a clear indication of velopharyngeal dysfunction. The examiner should also observe the symmetry of both sides of the port and note asymmetrical movement during speech. As

with the frontal view, the left lateral wall will be on the right side of the screen and vice versa. With a small velopharyngeal gap, bubbling of barium can often be seen on this view.

Interpretation of the Towne's View

Because the Towne's view is similar to the base view, only looking from above, the same observations and cautions apply. Again, the examiner should note that the lateral walls are on the opposite side of the screen as they are on the patient.

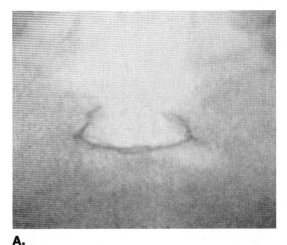

A.

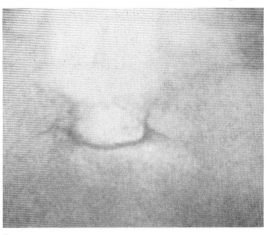

B.

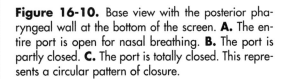

Figure 16-10. Base view with the posterior pharyngeal wall at the bottom of the screen. **A.** The entire port is open for nasal breathing. **B.** The port is partly closed. **C.** The port is totally closed. This represents a circular pattern of closure.

C.

Interpretation of the Oblique View

The oblique view can be difficult to interpret due to the superimposition of multiple structures over the area of interest. A coating of barium can make interpretation easier, however, and a swallow prior to the speech sample can help to orient the examiner to the structures of concern. As in the frontal view, the patient's right side will be seen on the left side of the screen and vice versa.

On the oblique view, the examiner should observe each lateral wall individually. The lateral wall should be viewed at rest and then during speech to determine if it closes against the velum. A notation should be made if there is an apparent gap between the lateral wall on that side and velum during speech. Of course, bubbling of the barium should be noted, because it indicates a small velopharyngeal opening.

Overall Results

Based on the information obtained from all views, the examiner must assimilate the information and make a determination of the extent of closure, the gap size, the gap location, and the basic closure pattern. This information is used to determine the appropriate type of treatment. If surgical intervention is planned, this information is especially important because it allows the surgeon to design the correction based on the abnormality.

Interpretation of the various views typically involves subjective analyses only. Direct measurement is difficult to do since the image on the screen is not life size and depends on a variety of factors. However, measurements are sometimes needed for research purposes. This can be done by putting a ruler or something of a known dimension in each view. For the view that is of interest, the examiner can then take a stop-frame at rest and again at the patient's best attempt at closure. The structures can then be traced off of the monitor onto a sheet of acetate paper. From this hard copy, quantifiable measurements can be made, using the object with a known dimension as the reference (Williams, Henningsson, & Pegoraro-Krook, 1997).

Reporting the Results

Some centers report the results of videofluoroscopy with a narrative report, using a few short paragraphs. Other centers use a scale to rate various parameters of structure and function as noted on each view. The first published rating scale was developed by McWilliams-Neely and Bradley (1964). Since that time, others have made additions and modifications to this basic scale. In 1990, a group of clinicians was assembled by the American Cleft Palate-Craniofacial Association to develop a standardized method for interpreting and reporting the results from videofluoroscopy and nasopharyngoscopy (Golding-Kushner et al., 1990). A procedure was developed which attempts to quantify the movement of the velopharyngeal structures relative to each structure's resting position and the resting position of the opposing structure. This is done as a ratio rather than as an absolute measurement. For example, the resting position of the velum is at the 0.0 point and the point of closure against the pharyngeal wall is 1.0. If the velum raises and closes 50% of the opening, then velar displacement is at a rating of 0.5 along the trajectory toward the posterior pharyngeal wall. This estimation is done for each lateral wall and for the posterior pharyngeal wall as well. Although this system may be used by some, it is somewhat complicated and the reliability of these fine judgments, especially for less experienced clinicians, comes into question. Therefore, it is not used by all centers.

Whether a specific rating scale is used or a narrative report is done, it is important to be consistent in the observations that are made and in the way that they are reported. This is particularly important if preoperative and postoperative studies are done for comparison.

Advantages and Limitations of Videofluoroscopy

Videofluoroscopy has the particular advantage of providing a view of the relationship between the velum and posterior pharyngeal wall through the lateral view. With this view, it is easy to determine if there is velopharyngeal insufficiency due to a short velum or velopharyngeal incompetence due to poor velar movement. In comparison with nasopharyngoscopy, videofluoroscopy is superior in showing the upward movement of the velum during speech. It also provides a view of the entire length of the posterior pharyngeal wall during closure.

Videofluoroscopy is also particularly helpful in assessing the extent and symmetry of lateral pharyngeal wall motion. Using both videofluoroscopic and nasopharyngoscopy, Henningsson and Isberg (1991) compared the observations of velopharyngeal movements during speech for 80 subjects with hypernasality. They found that videofluoroscopy was a better means for evaluating the movements of the lateral pharyngeal walls than nasopharyngoscopy. This was due, at least in part, to the angle of view through the nasopharyngoscope and the presence of adenoid tissue.

A primary disadvantage of videofluoroscopy is the radiation exposure. As with any X-ray procedure, there is always the concern about the amount of radiation exposure associated with the test. However, as noted previously, videofluoroscopy results in significantly less radiation exposure to the patient than the old procedure using cineradiography. In fact, videofluoroscopy requires about one tenth the radiation dosage as the same amount of cineradiography (Skolnick & Cohn, 1989). It has been estimated that for 1 minute of videofluoroscopy in the lateral view the radiation exposure is between 0.025 rad and 0.5 rad. For the frontal and base views, which require a higher radiation level for adequate resolution, the ex-posure can range from 0.125 rad to 1.00 rad (Skolnick & Cohn, 1989).

In most studies, the likely radiation exposure is about 0.1 rad per minute for the lateral view and about 0.45 rad per minute for the frontal and base views. Assuming a study of 1 minute per view for a total of 3 minutes (which is probably 3 times longer than what is actually needed), the patient would be exposed to approximately 1 rad of radiation. By way of comparison, a single lateral cephalometric X ray is about 0.25 rad and a single CT slice is between 1 and 4 rads. Therefore, although X-ray procedures are not innocuous and can potentially result in somatic and genetic damage, the dosage for videofluoroscopy is extremely low in comparison to many other types of X-ray procedures. In addition, the benefits gained from this procedure, despite the radiation exposure, must be weighed against the consequences of deciding on a course of treatment without adequate information.

Another disadvantage of videofluoroscopy is that the overall resolution of a radiographic procedure is not as good as a direct view. In fact, the ability to visualize structures, such as the velum and posterior pharyngeal wall, depends on these structures being surrounded by air (Skolnick & Cohn, 1989). However, as the velopharyngeal port narrows for closure, the amount of air between the velum and pharyngeal wall is markedly reduced and finally disappears during contact. Therefore, the ability to distinguish the margins of each structure becomes more difficult, if not impossible. As a result, small velopharyngeal gaps are not easily seen, and in fact, it may appear as if there is closure when there is not. In addition, the X-ray beam goes through all of the structures in the plane, as noted previously. As a result, the image represents a sum of all the parts. Therefore, if the velum touches the posterior pharyngeal wall at any point in the coronal plane, it will look as if there is complete closure, even if the velum does not contact the pharyngeal wall at all points. This is also the reason that the adenoid pad appears as a smooth shape, even though it is actually very convoluted in shape.

Videofluoroscopy is not a good procedure to evaluate the placement and the function of a pharyngeal flap either. It is very difficult to see a flap with this procedure unless there is a very good coating of barium. In fact, the presence of a pharyngeal flap could actually be missed altogether.

Although videofluoroscopy shows all of the velopharyngeal structures and their function through the use of multiple views, the examiner has to essentially extrapolate information from each view in order to imagine the three-dimensional structure and its function. Videofluoroscopy does not provide a clear view of all the structures as they function in the multidimensional pharynx. Because of the limitations of videofluoroscopy and the relative advantages of nasopharyngoscopy, this X-ray procedure seems to be used less frequently as a primary means of evaluating velopharyngeal function.

Summary

Videofluoroscopy provides a method to directly evaluate the structures and function of the velopharyngeal valve. It allows the examiner to identify the anatomical and physiological abnormalities that cause velopharyngeal dysfunction. It also gives the examiner information regarding the size and location of the velopharyngeal opening. This information is required before an appropriate plan of intervention can be determined for each patient.

References

Argamaso, R. V., Levandowski, G. J., Golding-Kushner, K. J., & Shprintzen, R. J. (1994). Treatment of asymmetric velopharyngeal insufficiency with skewed pharyngeal flap. *Cleft Palate Craniofacial Journal, 31*(4), 287–294.

Bzoch, K. R. (1968). Variations in velopharyngeal valving: The factor of vowel changes. *Cleft Palate Journal, 5*, 211–218.

Cohn, E. R., Rood, S. R., McWilliams, B. J., Skolnick, M. L., & Abdelmalek, L. R. (1984). Barium sulphate coating of the nasopharynx in lateral view videofluoroscopy. *Cleft Palate Journal, 21*(1), 7–17.

D'Antonio, L. L., Muntz, H. R., Marsh, J. L., Marty-Grames, L., & Backensto-Marsh, R. (1988). Practical application of flexible fiberoptic nasopharyngoscopy for evaluating velopharyngeal function. *Plastic and Reconstructive Surgergy, 82*(4), 611–618.

Dellon, A. L., & Hoopes, J. E. (1970). The palate analogue: An approach to understanding velopharyngeal function. *British Journal of Plastic and Surgery, 23*(3), 256–261.

Golding-Kushner, K. J., Argamaso, R. V., Cotton, R. T., Grames, L. M., Henningsson, G., Jones, D. L., Karnell, M. P., Klaiman, P. G., Lewin, M. L., Marsh, J. L., & et al. (1990). Standardization for the reporting of nasopharyngoscopy and multiview videofluoroscopy: A report from an International Working Group. *Cleft Palate Journal, 27*(4), 337–347; Discussion 347–348.

Henningsson, G., & Isberg, A. (1991). Comparison between multiview videofluoroscopy and nasendoscopy of velopharyngeal movements. *Cleft Palate Craniofacial Journal, 28*(4), 413–417; Discussion 417–418.

Isberg, A., Julin, P., Kraepelien, T., & Henrikson, C. O. (1989). Absorbed doses and energy imparted from radiographic examination of velopharyngeal function during speech. *Cleft Palate Journal, 26*(2), 105–109.

La Rossa, D., Brown, A., Cohen, M., & Spackman, T. (1980). Video-radiography of the velopharyngeal portal using the Towne's view. *Journal of Maxillofacial Surgery, 8*(3), 203–205.

Litzow, T. J., & Darley, F. L. (1966). Evaluation of velopharyngeal competence after primary repair of the palate. *Mayo Clinic Proceedings, 41*(8), 524–535.

Lubker, J. F., & Morris, H. L. (1968). Predicting cinefluorographic measures of velopharyngeal opening from lateral still X-ray films. *Journal of Speech and Hearing Research, 11*(4), 747–753.

Massengill, R., Jr., & Bryson, M. (1967). A study of velopharyngeal function as related to perceived nasality of vowels, utilizing a cine-fluorographic television monitor. *Folia Phoniatrica, 19*(1), 45–52.

Massengill, R., Jr., Quinn, G. W., Pickrell, K. L., & Levinson, C. (1968). Therapeutic exercise and velopharyngeal gap. *Cleft Palate Journal, 5*, 44–47.

McClumpha, S. L. (1969). Cinefluorographic investigation of velopharyngeal function in selected deaf speakers. *Folia Phoniatrica, 21*(5), 368–374.

McWilliams, B. J., Musgrave, R. H., & Crozier, P. A. (1968). The influence of head position upon velopharyngeal closure. *Cleft Palate Journal, 5*, 117–124.

McWilliams-Neely, B. J., & Bradley, D. P. (1964). A rating scale for evaluation of videotape recorded X-ray studies. *Cleft Palate Journal, 1*, 88–94.

Shprintzen, R. J. (1995). Instrumental assessment of velopharyngeal valving. In R. J. Shprintzen & J. Bardach (Eds.), *Cleft palate speech management: A multidisciplinary approach* (Vol. 4, pp. 221–256). St. Louis, MO: Mosby.

Shprintzen, R. J., Rakof, S. J., Skolnick, M. L., & Lavorato, A. S. (1977). Incongruous movements of the velum and lateral pharyngeal walls. *Cleft Palate Journal, 14*(2), 148–157.

Skolnick, M. L. (1969). Video velopharyngography in patients with nasal speech, with emphasis on lateral pharyngeal motion in velopharyngeal closure. *Radiology, 93*(4), 747–755.

Skolnick, M. L. (1970). Videofluoroscopic examination of the velopharyngeal portal during phonation in lateral and base projections—A new technique for studying the mechanics of closure. *Cleft Palate Journal, 7*, 803–816.

Skolnick, M. L. (1975). Velopharyngeal function in cleft palate. *Clinics in Plastic Surgery, 2*(2), 285–297.

Skolnick, M. L., & Cohn, E. R. (1989). *Videofluoroscopic studies of speech in patients with cleft palate.* New York: Springer-Verlag.

Skolnick, M. L., Glaser, E. R., & McWilliams, B. J. (1980). The use and limitations of the barium pharyngogram in the detection of velopharyngeal insufficiency. *Radiology, 135*(2), 301–304.

Skolnick, M. L., & McCall, G. N. (1971). Radiological evaluation of velopharyngeal closure. *Journal of the American Medical Association, 218*(1), 96.

Skolnick, M. L., McCall, G. N., & Barnes, M. (1973). The sphincteric machanism of velopharyngeal closure. *Cleft Palate Journal, 10*, 286–305.

Stringer, D. A., & Witzel, M. A. (1986). Velopharyngeal insufficiency on videofluoroscopy: Comparison of projections. *American Journal of Roentgenology, 146*(1), 15–19.

Stringer, D. A., & Witzel, M. A. (1989). Comparison of multi-view videofluoroscopy and nasopharyngoscopy in the assessment of velopharyngeal insufficiency. *Cleft Palate Journal, 26*(2), 88–92.

Subtelny, J. D. & Koepp-Baker H. (1956). The significance of adenoid tissue in velopharyngeal function. *Plastic and Reconstructive Surgery, 17*, 235.

Van Demark, D., Bzoch, K., Daly, D., Fletcher, S., McWilliams, B. J., Pannbacker, M., & Weinberg, B. (1985). Methods of assessing speech in relation to velopharyngeal function. *Cleft Palate Journal, 22*(4), 281–285.

Williams, W. N., & Eisenbach, C. R. D. (1981). Assessing VP function: The lateral still technique vs. cinefluorography. *Cleft Palate Journal, 18*(1), 45–50.

Williams, W. N., Henningsson, G., & Pegoraro-Krook, M. I. (1997). Radiographic assessment of velopharyngeal function for speech. In K. R. Bzoch (Ed.), *Communicative disorders related to cleft lip and palate* (Vol. 4). Austin, TX: Pro-Ed.

Yules, R. B., & Chase, R. A. (1968). Quantitative cine evaluation of palate and pharyngeal wall mobility in normal palates, in cleft palates, and in velopharyngeal incompetency. *Plastic and Reconstructive Surgery, 41*(2), 124–134.

Yules, R. B., Northway, W. H., Jr., & Chase, R. A. (1968). Quantitative cine radiographic evaluation of velopharyngeal incompetence. *Plastic and Reconstructive Surgery, 42*(1), 58–64.

CHAPTER

17

Nasopharyngoscopy

CONTENTS

Once hypernasality or nasal air emission are identified through a perceptual speech evaluation, further assessment of velopharyngeal function is indicated. Although velopharyngeal dysfunction can be identified from the speech evaluation based on the characteristics of the speech, it is important to determine the cause, the specific size, and the location of the velopharyngeal opening. This information is needed so that the appropriate form of intervention can be determined.

Nasopharyngoscopy is a minimally invasive endoscopic procedure that allows visual observation and analysis of the velopharyngeal mechanism during speech (D'Antonio, Achauer, & Vander Kam, 1993; D'Antonio, Chait, Lotz, & Netsell, 1986; D'Antonio, Muntz, Marsh, Marty-Grames, & Backensto-Marsh, 1988; David, White, Sprod, & Bagnall, 1982; McWilliams et al., 1981). Because the structures of velopharyngeal function can be viewed through nasopharyngoscopy, this procedure is considered a *direct measure*. Nasopharyngoscopy can help the examiner to assess both the anatomic and physiologic abnormalities that are causing velopharyngeal dysfunction so that the appropriate form of treatment for the individual can be identified. As such, nasopharyngoscopy can be a very powerful tool in the evaluation of velopharyngeal function and determining the cause of velopharyngeal dysfunction when it occurs. The same endoscopic technique can also be used to evaluate swallowing and the structure and function of the larynx and vocal folds.

The purpose of the chapter is to explain how nasopharyngoscopy is used in the evaluation of velopharyngeal function. The specific procedures for assessment are reviewed, including the procedure for preparing the individual and then inserting the endoscope. The interpretation of the observations is discussed as they relate to the diagnosis of velopharyngeal dysfunction and the recommendations for treatment.

Endoscopy

By definition, *endoscopy* is a procedure that allows the visualization of the interior of a canal or hollow organ by means of a special instrument called an *endoscope*. Physicians have used endoscopy for years to view anatomic structures and physiological function to make medical or surgical decisions regarding treatment. Speech pathologists are now using a form of endoscopy to assess the structures and function of the vocal tract. This particular procedure is called *nasopharyngoscopy* or *nasendoscopy*. With this procedure, the examiner is able to observe both the anatomical and physiological correlates of articulation, phonation, resonance, and swallowing to make a determination about the cause of abnormalities. The cause of deviant speech or resonance characteristics must be known before the speech pathologist can recommend or initiate any form of treatment.

Early Endoscopic Procedures

In 1966, Taub (1966) described the use of a *panendoscope* for the assessment of velopharyngeal function. The panendoscope consisted of an optical tube that could be placed in the mouth and then turned upward for visualization of the velopharyngeal sphincter. Of course, placement of the tube in the mouth interfered with the normal production of speech, and therefore, it had an effect on velopharyngeal function as well. Unfortunately, the optical tube was too big for nasal insertion. Another problem with this procedure was that the light bulb generated a dangerous amount of heat and there was also an electrical hazard for the individual. Therefore, this procedure did not gain wide acceptance.

In 1969, Pigott, Bensen, and White (1969) described the use of a rigid *endoscope* that was slender enough to be inserted through the nose, but large enough to allow observation of velopharyngeal portal at rest and during speech. This endoscope provided a view of the port from above at a fixed angle. One advantage of the rigid endoscope was that it provided a wide-angle view of 70°, which can include most of the port in one view (Pigott & Makepeace, 1982). However, despite the large cone of view, only one view of the port is possible with this scope. The rigid scope cannot be maneuvered for additional assessment of the lateral edges of the port or to see farther down into the pharynx or vocal tract. In addition, because the scope is very straight and the diameter of the nasal cavity is not, the rigid scope can be very difficult to insert.

This can be a particular problem if the individual has a septal deviation or stenosis of the naris. The pressure of the scope on the nasal septum and turbinates can also cause significant pain for the individual. Therefore, nasopharyngoscopy with a rigid scope is not an easy procedure to administer as an examiner, and it is not well tolerated by the individual.

Flexible Fiberoptic Nasopharyngoscopy

In the mid 1970s and the 1980s, the use of a flexible fiberoptic nasopharyngoscope (FFN) began to appear in the literature. The flexible scope is smaller than the rigid scope and, as a result, has a more restricted cone of view. However, its smaller circumference makes it much easier to insert and therefore, it is easier for individuals to tolerate. This is particularly advantageous when evaluating young children.

In 1975, a side-viewing flexible endoscope was described by Miyazaki, Matsuya, and Yamaoka (1975). With this design, the scope remained in a horizontal position and the opening at the side of the scope gave the examiner the same view as with the rigid scope. However, due to the side opening, the scope could not be manipulated easily to provide a view of both the horizontal and vertical aspects of the port.

In the late 1970s and the 1980s, the end-viewing flexible endoscope was described by several authors (Croft, Shprintzen, Daniller, & Lewin, 1978; Croft, Shprintzen, & Rakoff, 1981; Shprintzen, 1979; Shprintzen et al., 1979). The tip of this scope is flexible and with the use of a lever, the examiner can turn the tip down like a periscope to view the velopharyngeal port from various angles. It can even be moved farther down the pharynx for a view of the larynx and the vocal folds. This type of endoscope is used today.

Over the past 20 years, flexible nasopharyngoscopy has become a standard of care for the evaluation of velopharyngeal dysfunction in many craniofacial centers. In 1993, D'Antonio and colleagues (D'Antonio, Achauer, & Vander Kam, 1993) conducted a national survey of craniofacial teams concerning the use of nasopharyngoscopy in the evaluation of velopharyngeal dysfunction. At that time, 90% of the responding teams indicated that nasendoscopy was available and that it was indicated for difficult diagnostic problems at the very least. Forty-one percent of teams responded that endoscopic studies were appropriate for all individuals who require secondary palatal management. Since that survey, it is probable that more and more teams are using nasopharyngoscopy routinely as an adjunct to the perceptual evaluation of speech.

Equipment

Current nasopharyngoscopy equipment includes a flexible fiberoptic endoscope that consists of an eyepiece at one end of a long tube (or scope) (Figure 17–1). The diameter of the scope can vary from between just less than 2 mm to about 4 mm. The 3-mm scope is most commonly used since this size is easily tolerated by most individuals, including children, and it provides

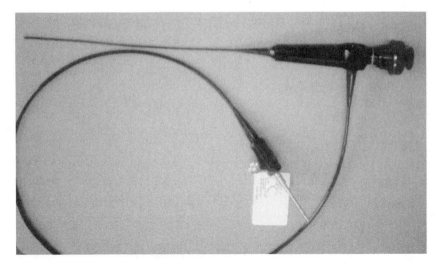

Figure 17–1. A flexible fiberoptic nasopharyngoscope. This instrument includes the long tubular endoscope. The body of the instrument, which is held in the examiner's hand, consists of an eyepiece and a control apparatus with a lever or wheel. The control apparatus allows the examiner to move the tip of the scope up and down like a periscope.

a wide scope of vision. However, for very young children and infants (when the procedure is done to evaluate swallowing), a smaller scope may be easier to use and better tolerated. Ideally, a variety of endoscopes should be available in a pediatric practice to ensure the ability to accommodate all children appropriately.

Looking at the end of the fiberoptic scope, one can see the small lens in the middle for gathering the image and a light source that encircles the lens. The scope is covered by a black vinyl covering. The end of the scope is very flexible and can be bent or turned easily without distorting the image. The body of the instrument, which is held in the examiner's hand, consists of an eyepiece and a control apparatus with a lever or wheel. The control apparatus allows the examiner to move the tip of the scope up and down like a periscope. The scope is plugged into a high-intensity cold-light source. This is necessary so that the light can travel through the scope without burning the individual as it reaches the pharyngeal area.

The nasopharyngoscope and cold-light source are the bare necessities for this examination. However, many authors, including this one, strongly recommend that a video camera, videotape player, and color monitor be added to the basic equipment. Figure 17–2 shows a complete system with monitor, video recording equipment, a cold-light source, and stroboscopy. With the complete equipment, the examiner can view the velopharyngeal structures on the video monitor rather than through a small, single ocular eyepiece. Other professionals can view the study during the procedure, or even later, including the surgeon, who may not be present during the examination. The parents and even the patient can view the examination, which can help when counseling the family regarding the problem and proposed treatment. An additional advantage is that the procedure can always be viewed again for further analysis.

Two types of cameras are currently available to record nasopharyngoscopy studies. The first kind is a standard camcorder. This type of recorder

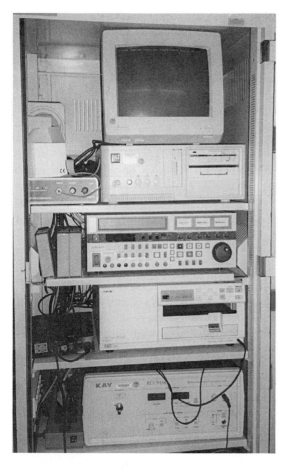

Figure 17-2. A complete system for nasopharyngoscopy, including (from top to bottom) monitor, computer and speakers, video recording equipment, a videoprinter, a cold light source and stroboscope, and finally, a keyboard.

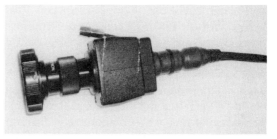

Figure 17-3. A very small, lightweight chip camera that can be attached directly to the eyepiece of a nasopharyngoscope.

For later assessment of the videotape, the audio of the speech must be as clear as the video of the velopharyngeal valve. Therefore, a microphone is attached to the individual or to the camera so that the speech recording is of good quality.

Clinical Uses for Nasopharyngoscopy

Flexible fiberoptic nasopharyngoscopy is now commonly used in clinical settings for the evaluation of velopharyngeal dysfunction. Nasopharyngoscopy provides a view of all of the structures of the velopharyngeal valve and their function during speech. Nasopharyngoscopy results are complementary to radiographic studies but in most cases, they are superior to those obtained through videofluoroscopy. This is due to the excellent clarity of the nasopharyngoscopy view and the maneuverability of the scope. Unlike videofluoroscopy, nasopharyngoscopy allows the examiner to see the configuration of the adenoid tissue and observe any fissures in the adenoid pad that affect the firmness of closure. Defects in the nasal surface of the velum or the presence of an oro-nasal fistula can be identified. The examiner can look directly into the port and can observe the movement of the velopharyngeal structures. Even very small gaps are easily visualized with this technique.

The observations made through nasopharyngoscopy provide a clear rationale for the design

is large and heavy and must be mounted on a tripod during the procedure. This camera can be used effectively with nasopharyngoscopic studies, and it is preferred by some clinicians (Shprintzen, 1995). Others prefer to use the chip cameras (Figure 17–3), which are very small, lightweight, and can be attached directly to the eyepiece. Once the camera is attached, it is hardly noticed by the examiner, yet it results in excellent optic quality.

and placement of pharyngoplasty surgery (Osberg & Witzel, 1981). In fact, by determining the location of the opening, the size of the opening, and the extent of lateral pharyngeal wall motion preoperatively, pharyngeal flaps can be "tailor-made" to fit the gap (Shprintzen et al., 1979). When the pharyngeal flap is prescribed according to observations seen through nasopharyngoscopy, it is more likely to be successful in correcting the defect. Nasopharyngoscopy is also an excellent technique for evaluating the effects of a pharyngeal flap, sphincteroplasty, or retropharyngeal implant, because the structures and results of surgery can easily be seen.

In addition to viewing the velopharyngeal structures, flexible endoscopy allows the examiner to view the larynx and vocal folds (Karnell, 1994; Karnell & Langmore, 1998). Because laryngeal abnormalities are often found in individuals with craniofacial anomalies and there is a high incidence of vocal nodules in individuals with velopharyngeal dysfunction, this should be done routinely with each exam. Because of the view of the pharynx and the larynx provided by this technique, this endoscopy procedure is often used in the evaluation of swallowing disorders. This is sometimes referred to as the *fiberoptic endoscopic evaluation of swallowing (FEES) procedure* (Aviv et al., 1998; Bastian, 1991, 1993, 1998; Kidder, Langmore, & Martin, 1994; Langmore, Schatz, & Olsen, 1988).

Nasopharyngoscopy procedures are used not only for diagnosis, but also during the treatment process. For example, nasopharyngoscopy can be used to help to design an obturator prosthesis (D'Antonio et al., 1988; Karnell, Rosenstein, & Fine, 1987). It can also be useful in therapy by providing biofeedback for the individual. This can help the individual to determine what is necessary to achieve velopharyngeal closure (Shelton, Beaumont, Trier, & Furr, 1978; Witzel, Tobe, & Salyer, 1988; Ysunza, Pamplona, Femat, Mayer, & Garcia-Velasco, 1997). These uses will be discussed in the Chapter 19 on Prosthetic Management and Chapter 21 on Speech Therapy.

Nasopharyngoscopy Preparation

Perceptual Evaluation

Prior to the endoscopy evaluation, the speech pathologist should complete a perceptual evaluation. This evaluation is important so that information regarding the speech characteristics can be obtained without the discomfort of the scope in place. If there is no evidence of abnormal resonance or airway obstruction as judged through the perceptual evaluation, then the nasopharyngoscopy procedure is not done. The information derived from the perceptual evaluation helps the examiner to focus on certain aspects during the endoscopy examination. For example, if the individual demonstrates nasal air emission on sibilants only, the examiner would want to test these sounds in particular and determine if, through instruction and biofeedback, closure can be obtained by altering the manner of production. On the other hand, if an element of hyponasality or cul-de-sac resonance is noted during the perceptual evaluation, then the examiner would want to actively look for a source of obstruction.

When working with a child, every effort should be made to help the child to feel relaxed, comfortable, and reassured throughout the evaluation. The perceptual evaluation gives the child an opportunity to do something that is painless, nonthreatening, and even fun. Therefore, it is an excellent time for the speech pathologist to develop a rapport with the individual and to help the child to become comfortable in the surroundings (D'Antonio et al., 1986; Lotz, D'Antonio, Chait, & Netsell, 1993).

Infection Control

Before even administering the topical anesthetic, the examiner should follow all of the Universal Blood and Body Fluid Precautions (UBBFP) for the prevention of the spread of disease (American Speech-Language-Hearing

Association, 1990; Centers for Disease Control, 1987, 1988; *Federal Register*, 1991). This is not only for the protection of the individual, but it is also for the protection of the examiner. Considering these guidelines, thorough hand washing should be done as the first step. The examiner should then wear gloves and keep the gloves on for the entire examination.

Once the endoscope has been used, care should be taken so that the scope is not placed on a surface that will be touched by others. Instead, the scope should be taken for immediate cleaning and disinfection. Guidelines for disinfection of the scope have been developed by the Association of Professionals in Infection Control and Epidemiology and also by the Association for the Advancement of Medical Instrumentation (American National Standard Institute, 1996; Rutala, 1996).

Nasal Anesthesia

Prior to the nasopharyngoscopy procedure, the nose is usually anesthetized with a form of topical anesthetic. These medications can be administered by the nurse or physician, or even by the speech pathologist. However, because they require a physician's prescription, the speech pathologist must work in close collaboration with the physician prior to administering these anesthetics. In addition, the speech pathologist should refer to the Code of Ethics of the American Speech-Language-Hearing Association (ASHA, 1992a) and the ASHA guidelines on the administration of topical anesthetics (ASHA, 1992b) prior to beginning this practice.

Before administering the topical anesthetic, the individual should be asked to blow his or her nose to discharge excess secretions that could interfere with the topical anesthetic or obscure the view through the nasopharyngoscope. Once the secretions have been eliminated as much as possible, the topical anesthetic is introduced into the nose. Most clinicians use some form of numbing solution prior to a nasopharyngoscopy procedure. However, it can

be done without topical anesthesia, especially with adults (Frosh, Jayaraj, Porter, & Almeyda, 1998). It is also helpful to open up the nasal passages as much as possible prior to the examination and this can be done with a topical decongestant.

Several methods for numbing the nasal cavity have been reported in the literature. Shprintzen and Golding-Kushner (1989) described a procedure where cotton packing is soaked in tetracaine (Pontocaine) and then inserted in the nose and left for approximately 5 minutes. Although this method is effective in numbing the nose, we have found that the process of packing the nose is often more traumatic for children than passing the scope. Other centers use a lidocaine (Xylocaine) gel, which is passed into the middle meatus with a long cotton swab. This can also be met with resistance from young children.

At Cincinnati Children's Hospital Medical Center, we recommend using a spray bottle to administer both the topical anesthesia and a decongestant at the same time (Figure 17–4). Children tolerate the introduction of numbing medicine best if a spray bottle is used. This is usually administered by the examiner, but it can also be administered by the parent or even by the child. It is helpful to have the child close the opposite nostril when one is sprayed and then sniff hard with the sprayed nostril to insure that the solution is distributed to the back of the nose. Three sprays are administered on each side so that there is adequate coating of the turbinates and the nasal septum. A wait of only 5 to 10 minutes is needed before the anesthetic takes effect. Because the spray coats the structures well and goes all the way to the back of the nose, anesthetic packing is usually not needed (Lotz et al., 1993).

The composition of the numbing spray and decongestant may vary. Our center uses a one-to-one mixture of oxymetazoline (Afrin) and 2% tetracaine (Pontocaine). Although several topical anesthetics can be used, tetracaine is

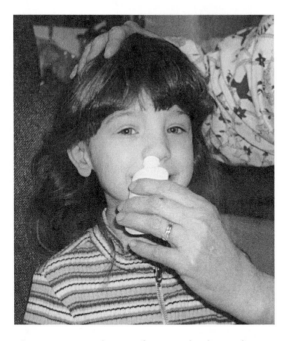

Figure 17–4. The use of a spray bottle to administer both the topical anesthesia and a decongestant prior to the nasopharyngoscopy procedure.

preferable because it acts quickly, has infrequent side effects, and does not have a noxious odor. This mixture is very effective in achieving the desired numbing effects, while opening up the nasal passages for the scope. By request, a pharmacy can dispense a mixture of oxymetazoline and 2% tetracaine in individual spray bottles that are disposed after use. Although limited dosing information is available, 0.3 mg/kg tetracaine has not produced any complications in our population. Just prior to inserting the scope in the nose, the end of the scope can be coated with viscous lidocaine. This not only helps in the numbing process, but it also smoothes the way for the scope to slide easily through the nose.

Using this technique, the examiner can ensure that the child has received adequate topical anesthesia to complete the procedure in comfort. Fortunately, the introduction of this mixture in the nasopharynx affects the sensation, but it does not affect velopharyngeal movement so it has no negative effect on the study.

Preparing a Child for the Procedure

The success of the nasopharyngoscopy procedure depends primarily on the individual's cooperation. Cooperation tends to improve with age so that obtaining a good examination with adults is usually not a problem. However, even adults can be very nervous and apprehensive before and during the test. Therefore, they may also need some comforting and reassurance.

In a pediatric setting, it is well known that preparing the child for what to expect can make the difference between a successful examination and one that is a waste of time, money, and everyone's patience. Many centers send a storybook or coloring book about the procedure to the child a few weeks before the examination. This can help the child and the parents understand what to expect.

Prior to starting the nasopharyngoscopy procedure, the examiner should carefully explain what will be done and what to expect so that there are no surprises. It is important to talk on the child's level and to keep the atmosphere as light as possible. For example, the child can be asked if he ever picks his nose in private and if so, if it hurts. The size of his or her nose-picking finger can then be compared to the size of the scope, which of course is much smaller. The child should be allowed to feel the end of the scope and even feel the sensation of the scope going up his or her sleeve.

Clear instructions on what will happen and what is expected of the child should be given prior to starting the procedure. It is important to be honest with the child, without alarming the child. For example, the explanation might be as follows: "You will feel the tube in your nose, but because we put the medicine in there, it shouldn't hurt. Instead, you will feel a little touch or some pressure. If it does hurt at any time, tell me so I can move it away from the part that hurts. When the tube is almost where it needs to be, there is a tight spot (the choana) and as the tube goes through it, it might make you want to sneeze. (In fact, many children do sneeze at this point, so it's helpful to stand clear!) It is very important to hold still, though, because if you move your head too much, it might make the tube bang around inside of your nose and that might hurt a little. Once the tube is in place, you will need to repeat some silly sentences and we will watch what happens on the monitor. When you finish saying all the sentences, we can take the tube out of your nose and you are done." Promising a reward, such as stickers, at the end of the procedure can also provide some motivation for cooperation.

With an adult, a nasopharyngoscopy examination can be done in a matter of a few minutes. When working with young children, however, nasopharyngoscopy takes a little more time and a lot more patience. If the examiner commits to spending whatever time is necessary, an adequate nasopharyngoscopy study can usually be obtained with most preschool and older children.

Nasopharyngoscopy Procedure

Passing the Scope

For best results in inserting the scope, the individual should be seated upright in a chair. For young children, it is best to have the child sit on the parent's lap and have the parent "hug" the child around his or her arms. This prevents the child from grabbing the scope during the procedure. At times, it is also helpful to have another person gently hold the child's head to be sure that it does not move erratically during the exam. The individual should be positioned in front of the monitor so that he or she can see it to watch the procedure (Figure 17–5).

The scope should always be passed through the most patent side of the nose. To determine

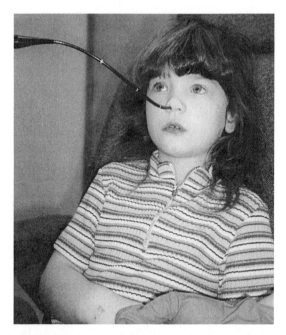

Figure 17–5. The position of the scope during the nasopharyngoscopy procedure.

which side has a larger opening, the examiner should put the scope at the entrance of each nostril to view the passageway. This can also be determined by having the individual close one nostril and then inspire deeply through the other. This should be done on both sides. The nostril with the higher pitch during inspiration is probably the one with the smallest passageway; therefore, the other nostril would be chosen for passage of the scope (Shprintzen, 1996). For individuals with a history of cleft lip, this is usually the noncleft side.

Once the largest side is determined and the end of the scope is coated with lidocaine gel, the end of the scope is held between the examiner's thumb and fingers and is gently passed into the nostril. The examiner should grasp the scope close to the individual's nose and can even rest his or her hand against the nose and face for maximum control. At this point, it is best to direct the child's attention to the television monitor, which can serve as a distraction to some extent. As the scope is passed through the nasal cavity, it is helpful to talk to the child about what he or she is seeing and perhaps liken the appearance of the nose to the inside of a cave.

The scope is usually guided into the middle nasal meatus and then back to the nasopharynx (Figure 17–6). If it goes through the inferior nasal meatus, which is on the floor of the nose, it will be on top of the velum when it reaches the port. In this position, the scope will usually bounce up and down with velar movement during speech, thus obscuring the examiner's vision of velopharyngeal function. The superior nasal meatus is too narrow for comfortable passage of the scope. Therefore, the middle nasal meatus is the passage of choice. The middle meatus is large enough to allow the scope to fit through it easily, and due to its position, it allows an unobstructed view of the port from above.

During insertion of the scope into the nasopharynx, the examiner should avoid contact with the septum as much as possible. This can be done by carefully observing the passage of the scope through the meatus and adjusting the

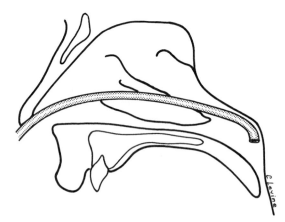

Figure 17–6. The pathway of the scope as it is guided through the middle nasal meatus and then back to the nasopharynx.

position of the scope accordingly. If contact occurs, it will be felt by the examiner as resistance against the scope, and it will be felt by the individual as pressure or mild pain. It is especially important to avoid hitting a bone spur or the base of the nasal septum in the area of the choana because these are particularly sensitive, even with good anesthetic coverage. It is always a good idea to tell the individual to let you know if it hurts or is especially uncomfortable so that appropriate adjustments can be made in the position of the scope. At times, the field of view will appear to be totally white during insertion into the meatus. This is due to the light bouncing off of a close object. If there is only white light in the field of view or if contact occurs, the examiner should withdraw the scope slightly and then reposition it before advancing the scope through the meatus.

Once the scope passes through the middle meatus, it finally reaches the choana at the back of the nasal cavity. This is the narrowest part of the canal and, therefore, can cause the most discomfort as the scope passes through. It can cause the individual's eyes to water and will often elicit a sneeze. Once the scope passes through the choana, the area opens up and there is less discomfort for the individual. At this point, the velopharyngeal port can be visualized. If the eyepiece only is being used to view the port, the velum will be seen at the bottom of the screen and the posterior pharyngeal wall will be seen at the top of the screen, because the view is from front to back. With this orientation, the left side of the screen will show the individual's right lateral pharyngeal wall and vice versa. If a chip camera is attached to the eyepiece, however, the entire view may be turned sideways or even upside down due to the position of the camera. When this occurs, the camera needs to be turned until the velum is seen at the bottom of the screen.

When the scope is first passed through the choana, it may be oriented in a horizontal position so that the view is of the nasopharyngeal wall rather than of the velopharyngeal port. To look down on the velopharyngeal port, the end of the scope needs to be turned down. This is done with control apparatus (lever or wheel) on the scope near the eyepiece. It is important that the end of the scope is perpendicular to the port so that the examiner can look down into the port rather than across the port. If the scope is not perpendicular to the port, it can cause significant error in interpretation because the examiner is not viewing the appropriate area (Henningsson & Isberg, 1991). Even if the scope is in good vertical position, the entire port may not be seen at one time. To examine the entire area, the instrument is rotated slightly from one side to the other so that each lateral border can be seen completely. Therefore, by moving the lever of the scope up and down, or by turning the entire scope from side to side, the examiner can view all areas of the velopharyngeal port from just one nostril.

During the examination, the examiner should remember that the velopharyngeal mechanism is a three-dimensional valve. Therefore, it is important to not only assess the depth and the width of the area, but also to assess the entire length of the valve. What is observed at the superior end of the valve may not accurately reflect what is occurring farther down in the valve. In addition, the examiner may make the mistake of having the scope too far down so that it is below the area of closure. This would give the false impression of velopharyngeal dysfunction, when the true closure is occurring above the level of view. Because of these concerns, the scope should be moved down and up in the area to be sure that the entire valve is adequately evaluated. At some point, the scope should be pulled up as high as possible. When the scope is pulled higher up, creating more distance between the end of the scope and the valve, more of the valve will be shown in the view.

Once the velopharyngeal valve has been adequately assessed, the scope is then passed down to the hypopharynx to observe the vocal folds. The individual is asked to prolong an "eeee" as long as possible so that vocal fold movement can be observed. If stroboscopy is also available, this allows the examiner to view the waveform of the vocal folds. Some children have difficulty with the concept of prolonging the sound. When this occurs and the child is not prolonging the sound, the speech pathologist can help by producing the sound simultaneously with the child in a contest to see who can hold it the longest.

During some examinations, the end of the scope will become very foggy and obscured by secretions. When this occurs, the first course of action is to ask the individual to sniff hard and then swallow to try to get rid of the secretions. If that does not work, then the scope is advanced into the oropharynx and the individual is asked to swallow. This is often sufficient to clear the scope. If this still does not clear the view, then the most effective course of action is to suction the individual's nose, if suction equipment is available. Suctioning can be done with the scope in place by putting the suction catheter in the same or opposite naris. If that still does not help, despite frequent swallows and suctioning, then it is necessary to remove the scope, wipe the end with alcohol or dip it in hot water, and then try again.

It is important to try to keep the child from crying during the examination so that an adequate assessment can be obtained. If the child is crying, the child will not cooperate adequately in order to repeat the speech sample. In addition, crying reduces the action of the velopharyngeal mechanism and can give a false impression of the status of velopharyngeal function. When the child begins crying, all the adults in the room have the tendency to try to talk to the child at once, and everyone ends up yelling over each other to the child. This can have the opposite effect of the one intended. It is best for one person, preferably the speech pathologist or person who will be eliciting the speech sample, to primarily communicate with the child. It is important to talk softly and calmly to the child to help the child to calm down. Asking the child to open his or her eyes to look at you often helps to break the fear. Turning down the lights can also promote a calmer atmosphere. Even distraction techniques can be useful. This might include a stuffed animal, puppet, or a bottle of bubbles. If the child will agree to blow some bubbles while the scope is in place, the act of blowing will necessarily stop the crying.

A successful examination is one in which there has been painless insertion of the scope and good patient cooperation. There must be good light saturation and good optical quality. There must be appropriate positioning of the scope so that there is good visualization of the airway and the velopharyngeal port. Finally, because the scope of view is limited to a portion of the velopharyngeal area, there must be good manipulation of the scope so that the entire sphincter has been adequately viewed (Shprintzen, 1995). For more information on the endoscopic procedure, please refer to the excellent book by Karnell entitled *Videoendoscopy: From Velopharynx to Larynx* (Karnell, 1994).

Speech Sample

Once the scope is in place, the velopharyngeal port should first be visualized at rest so that all the structures can be observed and the patency of the airway can be noted. Once this is done, the individual is asked to repeat sentences so that velopharyngeal function can be directly observed. As with videofluoroscopy, the speech pathologist should determine the speech sample based on the observations in the perceptual evaluation. However, unlike videofluoroscopy, there is no inherent danger to the individual with this procedure; therefore, there is no need to restrict the length of the speech sample, unless the individual's cooperation is limited. A combination of sentences loaded with pressure-sensitive phonemes, rote speech such as counting and the alphabet, and repetition of syllables can be used. It is particularly helpful to have the individual count from 60 to 70 to evaluate velopharyngeal function, because that

combination of sibilants and plosives in blends is particularly taxing on the velopharyngeal mechanism. Having the individual prolong an /s/ can be informative as, in some cases, the velopharyngeal closure that is initially achieved may break down with this task. If oral-motor dysfunction is suspected, having the individual repeat multisyllabic words with a combination of placement points can be helpful (i.e., baseball bat, kitty cat, puppy dog, teddy bear, patty cake, basket ball, ice cream cone, etc.). To test the effect of the fistula on the velopharyngeal valve, the speech sample can be done with the fistula open first and then it can be repeated with the fistula occluded so that a comparison can be made. Finkelstein and colleagues (Finkelstein, Talmi, Kravitz, Bar-Ziv, Nachmani, Hauben, & Zohar, 1991) recommend using the "forced sucking test (FST)" as an additional and complementary part of the endoscopic examination of the velopharyngeal valve. When the individual is asked to forcibly suck, it increases the appearance of some of the abnormal velopharyngeal characteristics, which can help in the analysis of velopharyngeal morphology.

If hyponasality or upper airway obstruction is a concern, the examiner should assess the patency of the velopharyngeal port during nasal breathing and during the production of nasal sounds. This can be done by having the individual repeat sentences with nasal phonemes, count from 90 to 100, repeat nasal syllables (e.g., ma, ma, ma) and then prolong an /m/ as long as possible. The examiner should also have the individual close the mouth and breathe as normally as possible through the nose for at least 30 seconds. Keeping the lips closed, the individual should then be asked to inspire deeply through the nose. During all of these activities, the relative opening of the pharyngeal port should be assessed. If a pharyngeal flap is in place, the patency of each lateral port should be examined.

Interpretation

Who Performs and Interprets the Procedure?

The nasopharyngoscopy procedure can be done by either a physician, such as a plastic surgeon or otolaryngologist, or by a speech pathologist who has been trained in the procedure. The speech pathologist should consult the ASHA training guidelines for endoscopic evaluations (ASHA, 1997). Adequate training and experience are important so that the procedure can be performed with good results and without causing discomfort for the individual.

Although some speech pathologists are performing this procedure around the country, the numbers probably remain few. In 1993, Pannbacker and colleagues (Pannbacker, Lass, Hansen, Mussa, & Robison, 1993) conducted a survey regarding nasopharyngoscopy. The survey was sent to speech-language pathologists who were randomly selected from the *Directory of the American Cleft Palate-Craniofacial Association* (ACPA, 104 South Estes Drive, Suite 204, Chapel Hill, NC 27514). Although the majority of respondents rated nasopharyngoscopy as important in the assessment of velopharyngeal function and said they also believed that it should be performed by speech-language pathologists, the majority did not perform nasopharyngoscopy examinations. Moreover, 40% had no academic preparation in the procedure and 20% had no clinical experience in nasopharyngoscopy. It is probable that, even today, those who are currently performing nasopharyngoscopy evaluations were trained by a mentor or another professional on the job. On-the-job training is not necessarily inappropriate in this case. It is impractical to train all graduate students in speech pathology in the procedure, because only a few will ever have the need or opportunity to perform nasopharyngoscopy. In addition, training is usually more effective if it is done in a clinical setting by someone who has clinical experience in both performing and interpreting nasopharyngoscopy.

For speech pathologists who are performing endoscopy evaluations, whether it's to evaluate velopharyngeal function, feeding, or the anatomic and physiological correlates of voice, it is important that they are skilled in basic competencies. The needed competencies to perform endoscopy evaluations are listed in the Training Guidelines for Laryngeal Videoendoscopy/ Stroboscopy, which has been developed by a committee of the American Speech- Language-Hearing Association (1998). This report also outlines educational modalities that can be used to prepare interested professionals to perform these studies. These activities include didactic or classroom learning, mentoring or a one-on-one relationship with another speech pathologist or otolaryngologist, supervised clinical experience, continuing education courses, videotape reviews of previous evaluations, and direct experience that ultimately leads to expertise.

Once the individual has been trained in nasopharyngoscopy, it is not difficult to pass the scope through the nose. The biggest challenge is the analysis and interpretation of the findings, and the formulation of appropriate recommendations. For this part of the evaluation, a team approach is definitely preferable. The team approach is advocated by most craniofacial professionals for the evaluation and treatment of craniofacial anomalies. The team approach is equally important for the evaluation and management of velopharyngeal dysfunction (D'Antonio et al., 1986). The most appropriate team for nasopharyngoscopy evaluations is the speech pathologist and a pediatric otolaryngologist. A plastic surgeon can also be an important member of the team.

Speech pathologists are trained to evaluate the velopharyngeal structures and function as they relate to the acoustic characteristics of speech, voice, and resonance. The gold standard for determining the need for intervention remains the perceptual quality of the speech. The speech pathologist can also determine if the individual is stimulable, which may suggest correction with speech therapy, or if the problem is functional, which definitely suggests correction with speech therapy. The speech pathologist is essential during the examination to determine the appropriate stimuli to emphasize the velopharyngeal closure defects. Finally, the speech pathologist can assist in determination of the appropriate recommendations for treatment.

The physician can assess the structural aspects of the oral cavity, pharynx, and nasal cavity with respect to the velopharyngeal valve and airway. Physicians are trained to assess the anatomy and physiology with a focus on disease and abnormality. They can determine the appropriate medical or surgical approaches to treatment for any abnormalities that are found. The physician can also identify associated problems, such as middle-ear effusion, vocal nodules, and adenotonsillar hypertrophy.

Because each professional views the structures and function with a different perspective, the nasopharyngoscopy assessment is most valuable when it is done by both professionals working together as a team. It makes no difference who passes the scope, as long as both professionals take a part in the interpretation of the results and formulation of the recommendations. Because speech, resonance, and phonation are highly dependent on the structures of the vocal tract, and because many of the problems are related to the ear, nose, or throat, it is especially helpful to have an otolaryngologist as part of the team. This way, a separate referral and evaluation are often avoided, and recommendations for treatment can be made on the spot after a thorough and comprehensive team evaluation.

Clinical Observations

With the endoscope in place in the nasopharynx, the examiner can view the velopharyngeal structures with the velum at the bottom of the

screen and the posterior pharyngeal wall at the top of the screen. The opening to the eustachian tube can often be seen in the view (Figure 17–7). As noted previously, the view through the scope is from the front of the individual to the back. Therefore, the left side of the screen is the individual's right side and vice versa. This is particularly important to keep in mind when reporting the location of an opening or growth, or reporting asymmetrical movement.

Nasopharyngoscopy shows the nasal surface of the velum, which can be scrutinized for signs of a submucous cleft palate or occult submucous cleft (Figure 7–8). This might include a hypoplastic musculus uvula, which appears as a flattening or concavity in the area where there should be a convex shape. There may also be a depression or a notch near the posterior border of the velum. A velopharyngeal opening during speech often corresponds to this area of deficiency in the midline (Gosain, Conley, Marks, & Larson, 1996; Lewin, Croft, & Shprintzen, 1980; Peterson-Falzone, 1985; Shprintzen, 1995;

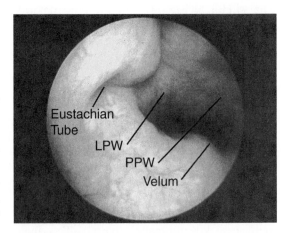

Figure 17–7. A nasopharyngoscopy view of normal velopharyngeal structures. The nasal surface of the velum is at the bottom of the screen and the posterior pharyngeal wall is at the top of the screen. The opening to the eustachian tube can be seen on the left side of the view.

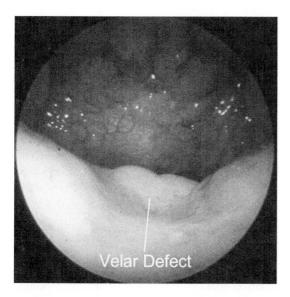

Figure 17–8. Nasopharyngoscopy view of a submucous cleft. Note the depression in the velum in the area where there should be a bulge from the musculus uvulae muscles.

Shprintzen, 1996; Shprintzen & Golding-Kushner, 1989).

The posterior pharyngeal wall can be examined from this perspective. The adenoid pad is evaluated for its size, surface, and location. The adenoid tissue may be large and blocking the nasopharynx, the opening of the choana, or the opening to one or both eustachian tubes. It may also have an irregular surface or fissures in the surface that prohibit the velum from achieving a tight velo-adenoidal seal. This is a particular concern in children who often achieve velar contact against the adenoids (Finkelstein, Berger, Nachmani, & Ophir, 1996; Gereau & Shprintzen, 1988; Mason, 1973; Morris, 1975; Siegel-Sadewitz & Shprintzen, 1986; Williams, Preece, Rhys, & Eccles, 1992).

If there is a Passavant's ridge during speech, this can often be observed, especially if there is a velopharyngeal opening. If there is complete or nearly complete closure, the Passavant's ridge usually cannot be seen through na-

sopharyngoscopy because it appears only with velopharyngeal closure and is usually located below the area of closure (Finkelstein et al., 1991; Finkelstein, Lerner, et al., 1993; Witzel & Posnick, 1989).

The posterior pharyngeal wall should always be observed at rest, particularly in individuals who have velopharyngeal insufficiency due to a submucous cleft of unknown origin. It is well documented that individuals with velocardiofacial syndrome often have medially displaced carotid arteries. In this case, one or both of the arteries can be seen pulsating on the posterior pharyngeal wall (D'Antonio & Marsh, 1987; Finkelstein, Zohar, et al., 1993; MacKenzie-Stepner, Witzel, Stringer, Lindsay, et al., 1987; Ross, Witzel, Armstrong, & Thomson, 1996; Witt, Miller, Marsh, Muntz, & Grames, 1998).

If the tonsils are very large and intrude into the oropharynx or nasopharynx, this can be seen through nasopharyngoscopy. At times, the tonsils are noted to be so large that they extend up to the area of velopharyngeal closure where they may interfere with closure by their placement between the velum and posterior pharyngeal wall. They can also interfere with lateral pharyngeal wall movement (Finkelstein, Nachmani, & Ophir, 1994; Henningsson & Isberg, 1988; Kummer, Billmire, & Myer, 1993; MacKenzie-Stepner, Witzel, Stringer, & Laskin, 1987). This mechanical interference with velopharyngeal closure can be corrected with a tonsillectomy.

The degree of velar, lateral pharyngeal wall, and posterior pharyngeal wall movement should be observed and the symmetry of lateral wall movement should noted. The relative contribution of all of these structures to closure should be assessed to determine the basic closure pattern (coronal, circular, or sagittal) (Croft et al., 1981; Finkelstein, Lerner, et al., 1993; Igawa, Nishizawa, Sugihara, & Inuyama, 1998; Shprintzen, Rakof, Skolnick, & Lavorato, 1977; Siegel-Sadewitz & Shprintzen, 1982; Skolnick, Shprintzen, McCall, & Rakoff, 1975; Witzel & Posnick, 1989). The basic closure pattern may determine the type of surgical management that is ultimately chosen.

The adequacy of closure of the velopharyngeal sphincter should be directly assessed during connected speech. If there is a velopharyngeal opening, the size and location of the opening are easy to visualize and important to report. These observations can determine the type of surgical management and the placement of the correction. For example, if the opening is small and skewed to the left, a relatively narrow pharyngeal flap can be placed to the left of center to make the flap fit the gap (Shprintzen et al., 1979).

A very small opening may not be seen immediately through nasopharyngoscopy. With connected speech, however, there will be bubbling of the secretions. Whenever bubbling is noted, the examiner can be sure that it is due to a velopharyngeal opening, which is usually small in size. This bubbling is due to air pressure being forced through a small velopharyngeal opening. If the opening were larger, there would be less friction and less bubbling. This bubbling, and the friction that goes with it, correspond to the perception of a nasal rustle, also called nasal turbulence (Kummer, Curtis, Wiggs, Lee, & Strife, 1992). Often, the opening will be to the left or right of midline. This is important to document because it has implications for surgical management.

If there is inconsistent closure, the examiner should analyze whether the opening occurs only on certain phonemes. If it is phoneme- specific (i.e., occurs only on certain sounds), this is usually due to faulty articulation (Peterson-Falzone & Graham, 1990). Therefore, the examiner should attempt to elicit closure on those phonemes using the video monitor for biofeedback. Inconsistent closure may also be due to fatigue with connected speech or prolonged speaking. In this case, the individual may be able to achieve closure, but is not able to maintain it over time. The examiner can assess this by having the patient count or produce a form of rote speech. Closure should be maintained throughout the utterance unless there is a nasal phoneme within the utterance. The examiner should observe whether the closure occurs at the beginning of an utterance and then begins to break down toward the end. Inconsistent closure can also be due to abnormal timing of closure in relation to the production of oral phonemes. The examiner should watch for this with the production of connected speech or the repetition of multisyllabic words. Longer or more complex utterances will test the timing and coordination of all of the articulators, including those for velopharyngeal closure.

Nasopharyngoscopy is a good procedure for evaluation of velopharyngeal function if the patient has undergone a surgical procedure, such as an adenoidectomy, pharyngeal flap, sphincteroplasty, or pharyngeal augmentation (see Chapter 18). Because nasopharyngoscopy allows direct visualization of the pharynx, the structural and functional results of the surgery can be accurately assessed through this procedure.

In all cases, the examiner should keep in mind that the closure that is seen through nasopharyngoscopy represents what the individual does with speech, not what the individual is capable of doing. The speech pathologist should try to determine potential before making assumptions that an opening is due to a structural problem. This is particularly true with individuals who have had surgical correction of velopharyngeal insufficiency. The examiner should keep in mind that changing structure does not change function. Therefore, surgical correction of velopharyngeal insufficiency may give the individual the structure to achieve closure, but he or she may require speech therapy to learn how to use the structure to achieve closure during speech.

Because of the high incidence of vocal nodules or voice disorders in individuals with velopharyngeal dysfunction (D'Antonio et al., 1988; Hirschberg et al., 1995; Lewis, Andreassen, Leeper, Macrae, & Thomas, 1993; Zajac & Linville, 1989), an evaluation of the larynx and vocal folds should also be performed as a matter of completeness. By viewing the vocal folds, the examiner can determine the presence of vocal nodules, or whether there is thickening or edema of the folds. The movement of the folds can be observed and the use of ventricular folds during phonation should be noted if it occurs. Any other anomalies of the vocal folds or their movement should also be noted.

Reporting the Results

As with videofluoroscopic speech studies, some centers report nasopharyngoscopy results with a narrative report. Several authors have suggested using either a numeric scale or a particular form to rate various parameters of structure and function (D'Antonio, Marsh, Province, Muntz, & Phillips, 1989; D'Antonio et al., 1988; Karnell, Ibuki, Morris, & Van Demark, 1983; Sinclair, Davies, & Bracka, 1982; Zwitman, Sonderman, & Ward, 1974). What is most important is that there is consistency in the observations that are made in each study and in the way that the studies are reported.

As noted previously, a multidisciplinary group of clinicians was assembled in 1990 by the American Cleft Palate-Craniofacial Association to address the question of standardizing reporting techniques for multiview videofluoroscopy and nasopharyngoscopy. Their report was an attempt to develop standards in the methodology for reporting results (Golding-Kushner et al., 1990). The proposed system was to rate the movement of the velum, the posterior pharyngeal wall and each lateral wall in relation to the structure that it is moving toward. The resting position of the structure is rated as 0.0 and the resting position of the opposing structure is 1.0. Using a ratio, the movement of the structure is scored according to the degree of its movement toward the resting position of the opposing structure. It is un-

clear how many centers are currently using this system, but its use may be somewhat limited due to its complexity.

The reliability of judgments from nasopharyngoscopy, regardless of the procedure used to report the results, seems to be greatly dependent on the experience of the evaluator (D'Antonio et al., 1989). Therefore, working with another experienced examiner initially is important to help the novice evaluator to develop the necessary skills. After that, practice is important to hone the skills required for observation and analysis.

Although results are reported to other professionals, they also need to be reported to the family. It is very important that the person who counsels the family uses clear, easy to understand language. All medical terms should be clearly defined. When discussing the function of the velopharyngeal mechanism, pictures and diagrams must be used. After the initial explanation, it may also be helpful to play the videotape of the procedure and point out the structures and their function.

Advantages and Limitations of Nasopharyngoscopy

Although videofluoroscopy is still used at various centers across the country, many centers, including the one at Cincinnati Children's Hospital Medical Center, are primarily using nasopharyngoscopy for assessments. With any radiographic procedure, there is some guesswork and the need to mentally extrapolate information from the X ray. In addition, several two-dimensional views must be considered individually to try to understand the three-dimensional structure. With nasopharyngoscopy, the structures and defects can be clearly seen in "living color." In contrast to videofluoroscopy, nasopharyngoscopy is done without radiation; therefore, there is no risk of harmful physical effects to the individual. Because there is no radiation involved, the examiner can take as much time as needed to determine the problem and the appropriate intervention. The procedure can also be repeated as often as needed for pre- and post-treatment assessments. Therefore, unless the examiner needs to see the entire length of the pharyngeal wall during speech, in our opinion, nasopharyngoscopy is usually a superior technique.

Because the patient can also see the monitor during the procedure, nasopharyngoscopy can be used as a biofeedback tool. The speech pathologist can give the individual instructions on placement and the patient can watch the velopharyngeal results on the monitor as he or she tries to follow the instructions. This is a particularly powerful procedure for the treatment of certain learned causes of velopharyngeal dysfunction (Brunner et al., 1994; D'Antonio et al., 1988; Kunzel, 1982; Rich, Farber, & Shprintzen, 1988; Shelton et al., 1978; Siegel-Sadewitz & Shprintzen, 1982; Witzel et al., 1988; Witzel, Tobe, & Salyer, 1989; Yamaoka, Matsuya, Miyazaki, Nishio, & Ibuki, 1983; Ysunza et al., 1997). For more information on the use of nasopharyngoscopy in therapy, please see Chapter 21.

The risks or limitations associated with nasopharyngoscopy are minimal. The transmission of infectious disease is always possible, but highly preventable if the Universal Blood and Body Fluid Precautions are followed and if the equipment is disinfected appropriately as noted above. It is possible for an individual to have an allergic reaction to the nasal anesthetic. Obtaining a history of drug allergies will minimize this risk. Other possible, but highly unlikely risks include a nosebleed or a vasovagal response, causing fainting. Nosebleeds could occur if the examiner is not careful in the passage of the scope and forcibly pushes it against the mucosa. Even when this occurs, the bleeding usually is slight and resolves quickly. Fainting is usually the result of individual anxiety and can be avoided by watching the individual carefully and giving the individual a great deal of reassurance if needed. If the patient appears ashen, the procedure should be terminated immediately. Although the risk of medical complication is very slight, this procedure should be performed in a setting where medical support is available.

Nasopharyngosopy requires a moderate degree of cooperation from the individual to successfully complete the study. Getting the scope through to the right place is not difficult. However, getting a child to talk and repeat sentences with the scope in place and without crying is the biggest challenge. Although nasopharyngoscopy should not be a painful procedure, it can cause some discomfort, especially if the scope hits a nasal spur or the base of the nasal septum. It can also be a very scary procedure for young children. However, with a good coating of topical anesthesia and with previous preparation as to what to expect, the nasopharyngoscopy procedure is usually well tolerated by children, even as young as 3 years of age.

Summary

Instrumental assessment is not required for identification of velopharyngeal dysfunction in most cases because it can be determined through a perceptual assessment of resonance. However, nasopharyngoscopy is a very effective procedure for the determination of the cause of velopharyngeal dysfunction, and the size and location of the opening. Nasopharyngoscopy can be used to determine the presence of obstruction in the vocal tract, which can also affect resonance. Therefore, in many centers across the country, nasopharyngoscopy has become a standard evaluation procedure for individuals who exhibit resonance disorders or characteristics of velopharyngeal dysfunction.

References

American National Standard Institute. (1996). Safe use and handling of flutaraldehyde-based products in health care facilities. *ANSI/AAMI, ST58*. New York: Author.

American Speech-Language-Hearing Association. (1990, December). Report update. AIDS/HIV: Implications for speech-language pathologists and audiologists. *Asha, 32*(Suppl. 9), 46–48.

American Speech-Language-Hearing Association. (1992a). Code of ethics of the American Speech-Language-Hearing Association. *Asha, 34*(Suppl. 9), 1–2.

American Speech-Language-Hearing Association. (1992b). Sedation and topical anesthetics in audiology and speech-language pathology. *Asha, 34*(Suppl. 7), 41-42.

American Speech-Language-Hearing Association. (1997). Training guidelines for laryngeal videoendoscopy/stroboscopy. *ASHA desk reference.* Rockville, MD: Author.

American Speech-Language-Hearing Association. (1998). Training guidelines for laryngeal videoendoscopy / stroboscopy. *Asha, 40*(Suppl. 18), III–154—154g.

Aviv, J. E., Kim, T., Thomson, J. E., Sunshine, S., Kaplan, S., & Close, L. G. (1998). Fiberoptic endoscopic evaluation of swallowing with sensory testing (FEESST) in healthy controls [see Comments]. *Dysphagia, 13*(2), 87–92.

Bastian, R. W. (1991). Videoendoscopic evaluation of patients with dysphagia: An adjunct to the modified barium swallow. *Otolaryngology—Head and Neck Surgery, 104*(3), 339–350.

Bastian, R. W. (1993). The videoendoscopic swallowing study: An alternative and partner to the videofluoroscopic swallowing study. *Dysphagia, 8*(4), 359–367.

Bastian, R. W. (1998). Contemporary diagnosis of the dysphagic patient. *Otolaryngology Clinics of North America, 31*(3), 489–506.

Brunner, M., Stellzig, A., Decker, W., Strate, B., Komposch, G., Wirth, G., & Verres, R. (1994). [Video-feedback therapy with the flexible nasopharyngoscope. The potentials for modifying velopharyngeal closure and phonation deficiencies in cleft patients]. *Fortschritte de Kieferorthopadei, 55*(4), 197–201.

Centers for Disease Control. (1987). Recommendations for prevention of HIV transmission in health-care settings. *Morbidity and Mortality Weekly Review, 36*(Suppl. #25).

Centers for Disease Control. (1988). Perspectives in disease prevention and health promotion. *Morbidity and Mortality Weekly Review, 37*, 377–388.

Croft, C. B., Shprintzen, R. J., Daniller, A. I., & Lewin, M. L. (1978). The occult submucous cleft palate and the musculus uvulae. *Cleft Palate Journal, 15*, 150–154.

Croft, C. B., Shprintzen, R. J., & Rakoff, S. J. (1981). Patterns of velopharyngeal valving in normal and cleft palate subjects: A multi-view videofluoroscopic and nasendoscopic study. *Laryngoscope, 91*(2), 265–271.

D'Antonio, L., Chait, D., Lotz, W., & Netsell, R. (1986). Pediatric videonasoendoscopy for speech and voice evaluation. *Otolaryngology—Head and Neck Surgery, 94*(5), 578–583.

D'Antonio, L. D., & Marsh, J. L. (1987). Abnormal carotid arteries in the velocardiofacial syndrome [Letter]. *Plastic and Reconstructive Surgery, 80*(3), 471–472.

D'Antonio, L. L., Achauer, B. M., & Vander Kam, V. M. (1993). Results of a survey of cleft palate teams concerning the use of nasendoscopy. *Cleft Palate Craniofacial Journal, 30*(1), 35–39.

D'Antonio, L. L., Marsh, J. L., Province, M. A., Muntz, H. R., & Phillips, C. J. (1989). Reliability of flexible fiberoptic nasopharyngoscopy for evaluation of velopharyngeal function in a clinical population. *Cleft Palate Journal, 26*(3), 217–225; Discussion 225.

D'Antonio, L. L., Muntz, H. R., Marsh, J. L., Marty-Grames, L., & Backensto-Marsh, R. (1988). Practical application of flexible fiberoptic nasopharyngoscopy for evaluating velopharyngeal function. *Plastic and Reconstructive Surgery, 82*(4), 611–618.

David, D. J., White, J., Sprod, R., & Bagnall, A. (1982). Nasendoscopy: Significant refinements of a direct-viewing technique of the velopharyngeal sphincter. *Plastic and Reconstructive Surgery, 70*(4), 423–428.

Federal Register. (1991). Occupational exposure to bloodborne pathogens: Final rule. Occupational and Safety Health Administration, 29 CFR Part 1910.1030, 64175.

Finkelstein, Y., Berger, G., Nachmani, A., & Ophir, D. (1996). The functional role of the adenoids in speech. *International Journal of Pediatric Otorhinolaryngology, 34*(1/2), 61–74.

Finkelstein, Y., Lerner, M. A., Ophir, D., Nachmani, A., Hauben, D. J., & Zohar, Y. (1993). Nasopharyngeal profile and velopharyngeal valve mechanism. *Plastic and Reconstructive Surgery, 92*(4), 603–614.

Finkelstein, Y., Nachmani, A., & Ophir, D. (1994). The functional role of the tonsils in speech. *Archives of Otolaryngology—Head and Neck Surgery, 120*(8), 846–851.

Finkelstein, Y., Talmi, Y. P., Kravitz, K., Bar-Ziv, J., Nachmani, A., Hauben, D. J., & Zohar, Y. (1991). Study of the normal and insufficient velopharyngeal valve by the "Forced Sucking Test." *Laryngoscope, 101*(11), 1203–1212.

Finkelstein, Y., Zohar, Y., Nachmani, A., Talmi, Y. P., Lerner, M. A., Hauben, D. J., & Frydman, M. (1993). The otolaryngologist and the patient with velocardiofacial syndrome. *Archives of Otolaryngology—Head and Neck Surgery, 119*(5), 563–569.

Frosh, A. C., Jayaraj, S., Porter, G., & Almeyda, J. (1998). Is local anaesthesia actually beneficial in flexible fibreoptic nasendoscopy? *Clinics in Otolaryngology, 23*(3), 259–262.

Gereau, S. A., & Shprintzen, R. J. (1988). The role of adenoids in the development of normal speech following palate repair. *Laryngoscope, 98*(3), 299–303.

Golding-Kushner, K. J., Argamaso, R. V., Cotton, R. T., Grames, L. M., Henningsson, G., Jones, D. L., Karnell, M. P., Klaiman, P. G., Lewin, M. L., Marsh, J. L., & et al. (1990). Standardization for the reporting of nasopharyngoscopy and multiview videofluoroscopy: A report from an International Working Group. *Cleft Palate Journal, 27*(4), 337–347; Discussion 347–348.

Gosain, A. K., Conley, S. F., Marks, S., & Larson, D. L. (1996). Submucous cleft palate: Diagnostic methods and outcomes of surgical treatment. *Plastic and Reconstructive Surgery, 97*(7), 1497–1509.

Henningsson, G., & Isberg, A. (1988). Influence of tonsils on velopharyngeal movements in children with craniofacial anomalies and hypernasality. *American Journal of Orthodontics and Dentofacial Orthopedics, 94*(3), 253–261.

Henningsson, G., & Isberg, A. (1991). Comparison between multiview videofluoroscopy and nasendoscopy of velopharyngeal movements. *Cleft Palate Craniofacial Journal, 28*(4), 413–417; Discussion 417–418.

Hirschberg, J., Dejonckere, P. H., Hirano, M., Mori, K., Schultz-Coulon, H. J., & Vrticka, K. (1995). Voice disorders in children. *International Journal of Pediatric Otorhinolaryngology, 32*(Suppl.), S109–S125.

Igawa, H. H., Nishizawa, N., Sugihara, T., & Inuyama, Y. (1998). A fiberscopic analysis of velopharyngeal movement before and after primary palatoplasty in cleft palate infants. *Plastic and Reconstructive Surgery, 102*(3), 668–674.

Karnell, M. P. (1994). *Videoendoscopy: From velopharynx to larynx.* San Diego, CA: Singular Publishing Group.

Karnell, M. P., Ibuki, K., Morris, H. L., & Van Demark, D. R. (1983). Reliability of the nasopharyngeal fiberscope (NPF) for assessing velopharyngeal function: Analysis by judgment. *Cleft Palate Journal, 20*(3), 199–208.

Karnell, M. P., & Langmore, S. (1998). Videoendoscopy in speech and swallowing for the speech-language pathologist. In A. F. Johnson & B. H. Jacobson (Eds.), *Medical speech-language pathology: A practitioner's guide* (pp. 563–584). New York: Thieme.

Karnell, M. P., Rosenstein, H., & Fine, L. (1987). Nasal videoendoscopy in prosthetic management of palatopharyngeal dysfunction. *Journal of Prosthetic Dentistry, 58*(4), 479–484.

Kidder, T. M., Langmore, S. E., & Martin, B. J. (1994). Indications and techniques of endoscopy in evaluation of cervical dysphagia: Comparison with radiographic techniques. *Dysphagia, 9*(4), 256–261.

Kummer, A. W., Billmire, D. A., & Myer, C. M. (1993). Hypertrophic tonsils: The effect on resonance and velopharyngeal closure. *Plastic and Reconstructive Surgery, 91*(4), 608–611.

Kummer, A. W., Curtis, C., Wiggs, M., Lee, L., & Strife, J. L. (1992). Comparison of velopharyngeal gap size in patients with hypernasality, hypernasality and nasal emission, or nasal turbulence (rustle) as the primary speech characteristic. *Cleft Palate Craniofacial Journal, 29*(2), 152–156.

Kunzel, H. J. (1982). First applications of a biofeedback device for the therapy of velopharyngeal incompetence. *Folia Phoniatrica, 34*(2), 92–100.

Langmore, S. E., Schatz, K., & Olsen, N. (1988). Fiberoptic endoscopic examination of swallowing safety: A new procedure. *Dysphagia, 2*(4), 216–219.

Lewin, M. L., Croft, C. B., & Shprintzen, R. J. (1980). Velopharyngeal insufficiency due to hypoplasia of the musculus uvulae and occult submucous cleft palate. *Plastic and Reconstructive Surgery, 65*(5), 585–591.

Lewis, J. R., Andreassen, M. L., Leeper, H. A., Macrae, D. L., & Thomas, J. (1993). Vocal characteristics of children with cleft lip/palate and associated velopharyngeal incompetence. *Journal of Otolaryngology, 22*(2), 113–117.

Lotz, W. K., D'Antonio, L. L., Chait, D. H., & Netsell, R. W. (1993). Successful nasoendoscopic and aerodynamic examinations of children with speech/voice disorders. *International Journal of Pediatric Otorhinolaryngology, 26*(2), 165–172.

MacKenzie-Stepner, K., Witzel, M. A., Stringer, D. A., & Laskin, R. (1987). Velopharyngeal insufficiency due to hypertrophic tonsils: A report of two cases. *International Journal of Pediatric Otorhinolaryngology, 14*(1), 57–63.

MacKenzie-Stepner, K., Witzel, M. A., Stringer, D. A., Lindsay, W. K., Munro, I. R., & Hughes, H. (1987). Abnormal carotid arteries in the velocardiofacial syndrome: A report of three cases. *Plastic and Reconstructive Surgery, 80*(3), 347–351.

Mason, R. M. (1973). Preventing speech disorders following adenoidectomy by preoperative examination. *Clinics in Pediatrics (Phila), 12*(7), 405–414.

McWilliams, B. J., Glaser, E. R., Philips, B. J., Lawrence, C., Lavorato, A. S., Beery, Q. C., & Skolnick, M. L. (1981). A comparative study of four methods of evaluating velopharyngeal adequacy. *Plastic and Reconstructive Surgery, 68*(1), 1–10.

Miyazaki, T., Matsuya, T., & Yamaoka, M. (1975). Fiberscopic methods for assessment of velopharyngeal closure during various activities. *Cleft Palate Journal, 12*, 107–114.

Morris, H. L. (1975). The speech pathologist looks at the tonsils and the adenoids. *Annals of Otology, Rhinology, and Laryngology, 84*(2, Pt. 2, Suppl. 19), 63–66.

Osberg, P. E., & Witzel, M. A. (1981). The physiologic basis for hypernasality during connected speech in cleft palate patients: A nasendoscopic study. *Plastic and Reconstructive Surgery, 67*(1), 1–5.

Pannbacker, M. D., Lass, N. J., Hansen, G. G., Mussa, A. M., & Robison, K. L. (1993). Survey of speech-language pathologists' training, experience, and opinions on nasopharyngoscopy. *Cleft Palate Craniofacial Journal, 30*(1), 40–45.

Peterson-Falzone, S. J. (1985). Velopharyngeal inadequacy in the absence of overt cleft palate. *Journal of Craniofacial Genetics and Developmental Biology* (Suppl. 1), 97–124.

Peterson-Falzone, S. J., & Graham, M. S. (1990). Phoneme-specific nasal emission in children with and without physical anomalies of the velopharyngeal mechanism. *Journal of Speech and Hearing Disorders, 55*(1), 132–139.

Pigott, R. W., Bensen, J. F., & White, F. D. (1969). Nasendoscopy in the diagnosis of velopharyngeal incompetence. *Plastic and Reconstructive Surgery, 43*(2), 141–147.

Pigott, R. W., & Makepeace, A. P. (1982). Some characteristics of endoscopic and radiological systems used in elaboration of the diagnosis of velopharyngeal incompetence. *British Journal of Plastic Surgery, 35*(1), 19–32.

Rich, B. M., Farber, K., & Shprintzen, R. J. (1988). Nasopharyngoscopy in the treatment of palatopharyngeal insufficiency. *International Journal of Prosthodontics, 1*(3), 248–251.

Ross, D. A., Witzel, M. A., Armstrong, D. C., & Thomson, H. G. (1996). Is pharyngoplasty a risk in velocardiofacial syndrome? An assessment of medially displaced carotid arteries. *Plastic and Reconstructive Surgery, 98*(7), 1182–1190.

Rutala, W. A. (1996). APIC guideline for selection and use of disinfectants. *American Journal of Infectious Disease Control, 24*, 313–342.

Shelton, R. L., Beaumont, K., Trier, W. C., & Furr, M. L. (1978). Videoendoscopic feedback in training velopharyngeal closure. *Cleft Palate Journal, 15*(1), 6–12.

Shprintzen, R. J. (1979). The use of multiview videofluoroscopy and flexible fiberoptic nasopharyngoscopy as a predictor of success with pharyngeal flap surgery. In R. Ellis & F. C. Flack (Eds.), *Diagnosis and treatment of palato-glossal malfunction* (pp. 6–14). London: College of Speech Therapists.

Shprintzen, R. J. (1995). Instrumental assessment of velopharyngeal valving. In R. J. Shprintzen & J. Bardach (Eds.), *Cleft palate speech management: A multidisciplinary approach* (Vol. 4, pp. 221–256). St. Louis: Mosby.

Shprintzen, R. J. (1996). Nasopharyngoscopy. In K. R. Bzoch (Ed.), *Communicative disorders related to cleft lip and palate* (Vol. 4, pp. 387-409). Austin, TX: Pro-Ed.

Shprintzen, R. J., & Golding-Kushner, K. J. (1989). Evaluation of velopharyngeal insufficiency. *Otolaryngology Clinics of North America, 22*(3), 519–536.

Shprintzen, R. J., Lewin, M. L., Croft, C. B., Daniller, A. I., Argamaso, R. V., Ship, A. G., & Strauch, B. (1979). A comprehensive study of pharyngeal flap surgery: Tailor made flaps. *Cleft Palate Journal, 16*(1), 46–55.

Shprintzen, R. J., Rakof, S. J., Skolnick, M. L., & Lavorato, A. S. (1977). Incongruous movements of the velum and lateral pharyngeal walls. *Cleft Palate Journal, 14*(2), 148–157.

Siegel-Sadewitz, V. L., & Shprintzen, R. J. (1982). Nasopharyngoscopy of the normal velopharyngeal sphincter: An experiment of biofeedback. *Cleft Palate Journal, 19*(3), 194–200.

Siegel-Sadewitz, V. L., & Shprintzen, R. J. (1986). Changes in velopharyngeal valving with age. *International Journal of Pediatric Otorhinolaryngology, 11*(2), 171–182.

Sinclair, S. W., Davies, D. M., & Bracka, A. (1982). Comparative reliability of nasal pharyngoscopy and videofluorography in the assessment of velopharyngeal incompetence. *British Journal of Plastic Surgery, 35*(2), 113–117.

Skolnick, M. L., Shprintzen, R. J., McCall, G. N., & Rakoff, S. (1975). Patterns of velopharyngeal closure in subjects with repaired cleft palate and normal speech: A multi-view videofluoroscopic analysis. *Cleft Palate Journal, 12*, 369–376.

Taub, S. (1966). The Taub oral panendoscope: A new technique. *Cleft Palate Journal, 3*, 328–346.

Williams, R. G., Preece, M., Rhys, R., & Eccles, R. (1992). The effect of adenoid and tonsil surgery on nasalance. *Clinics in Otolaryngology, 17*(2), 136–140.

Witt, P. D., Miller, D. C., Marsh, J. L., Muntz, H. R., & Grames, L. M. (1998). Limited value of preoperative cervical vascular imaging in patients with velocardiofacial syndrome. *Plastic and Reconstructive Surgery, 101*(5), 1184–1195; Discussion 1196–1199.

Witzel, M. A., & Posnick, J. C. (1989). Patterns and location of velopharyngeal valving problems: Atypical findings on video nasopharyngoscopy. *Cleft Palate Journal, 26*(1), 63–67.

Witzel, M. A., Tobe, J., & Salyer, K. (1988). The use of nasopharyngoscopy biofeedback therapy in the correction of inconsistent velopharyngeal closure. *International Journal of Pediatric Otorhinolaryngology, 15*(2), 137–142.

Witzel, M. A., Tobe, J., & Salyer, K. E. (1989). The use of videonasopharyngoscopy for biofeedback therapy in adults after pharyngeal flap surgery. *Cleft Palate Journal, 26*(2), 129–134; Discussion 135.

Yamaoka, M., Matsuya, T., Miyazaki, T., Nishio, J., & Ibuki, K. (1983). Visual training for velopharyngeal closure in cleft palate patients: A fibrescopic procedure (preliminary report). *Journal of Maxillofacial Surgery, 11*(4), 191–193.

Ysunza, A., Pamplona, M., Femat, T., Mayer, I., & Garcia-Velasco, M. (1997). Videonasopharyngoscopy as an instrument for visual biofeedback during speech in cleft palate patients. *International Journal of Pediatric Otorhinolaryngology, 41*(3), 291–298.

Zajac, D. J., & Linville, R. N. (1989). Voice perturbations of children with perceived nasality and hoarseness. *Cleft Palate Journal, 26*(3), 226–231; Discussion 231–232.

Zwitman, D. H., Sonderman, J. C., & Ward, P. H. (1974). Variations in velopharyngeal closure assessed by endoscopy. *Journal of Speech and Hearing Disorders, 39*(3), 366–372.

PART V

Treatment Procedures: Speech, Resonance, and Velopharyngeal Dysfunction

CHAPTER

Surgical Management of Clefts and Velopharyngeal Dysfunction

David A. Billmire, M.D.

CONTENTS

Cleft lip and palate occur in a spectrum from the abortive form, such as a form fruste of the lip or an asymptomatic submucous cleft of the palate, to a complete bilateral cleft of the lip and palate. Regardless of the degree of involvement, the surgical principles remain the same. The correction must take into account the anatomical and physiological derangement of a complete disruption in embryological development. For example, in a form fruste of the lip, the overlying skin is intact but the underlying muscle, nasal cartilage, and oral sphincter function usually are significantly affected. Therefore, correction requires a complete lip repair. For the same reason, correction of a submucous cleft of the palate requires the same type of repair as a complete cleft.

Although surgical concepts and approaches have become more standardized in the last few years, one will still find a wide range of interpretation of these "standards" across the country and even within a single treatment team. The treatment options, timing, techniques, and philosophies presented here are presented solely as broad general guidelines. Significant variations are present throughout the country and world.

It is important to remember that clefts of lip and palate involve much more that the obvious defect to the lip and roof of the mouth. Their sphere of influence extends to other aesthetic areas, such as the nose and midface; to other anatomical areas, such as the jaws, teeth, the oral sphincter, and velopharyngeal sphincter; to the functional aspects of the airway, hearing, speech, and feeding; and psychologically to one's identity. Surgical repair should seek to achieve a normal anatomical and physiological state as much as possible, which usually results in an improved psychological state as well. The successful treatment of the patient with cleft lip and palate hinges on the treatment team's adherence to and completion of a comprehensive program with well-defined goals and objectives.

Cleft Lip Repair

Timing of the Cleft Lip Repair

There has been considerable debate over the years among surgeons over the appropriate timing for the cleft lip repair, also known as a *cheiloplasty*. At one time, the repair of the cleft lip was often done shortly after birth and before the child was sent home. It was felt that neonatal repair was appropriate because it allowed the mother to better bond with the infant. In addition, from an anesthetic standpoint, neonates were felt to be most physiologically sound immediately after birth before their own physiological systems came on line. Modern pediatric anesthesia has negated the later argument, while the former remains debatable. Although a few cleft palate centers are reintroducing the concept of repair within the first week of life, most centers currently advocate delaying repair and following some variation of the *rule of 10s*. This "rule" is a guideline which says that the infant should be at least 10 weeks of age, weigh at least 10 pounds, and have a hemoglobin of 10 gm prior to the lip repair.

There are several reasons for delaying this initial surgery. These include the fact that cleft lip and palate are often associated with other abnormalities, a number of which are not readily apparent at birth. Delaying surgery allows a longer time for investigation of other potentially serious problems. In addition, an acceptable feeding technique must be established and weight gain assured prior to taking on extensive surgery. Finally, many teams use some form of active or passive presurgical orthopedics to align the cleft. In incomplete clefts and those with a Simonart's band (a band of skin without underlying muscle bridging the cleft just below the nose), this option is usually unnecessary. Delaying surgery allows time for these devices to narrow or better position the cleft segments prior to repair so that a better result can be achieved. Despite the presence of the cleft lip, bonding will occur with the parents, which is crucial to the child's development. Given these considerations, in most cleft palate centers at this time, the initial repair of cleft lip is usually accomplished between 4 weeks and 12 weeks of age.

Presurgical Management

In wide clefts of the lip, whether they are unilateral or bilateral, it is not uncommon to narrow the gap prior to performing the formal repair. Aligning the segments prior to surgical repair can improve the ultimate outcome and result in less tension on the lip repair once it is done.

With a unilateral cleft lip, there are a number of options for aligning the segments. The simplest procedure is to tape the lip with adhesive tape. This may also be used in conjunction with *dental elastics*, which are small rubber bands to add a dynamic component. In some centers, this technique may be used with a palatal molding plate to help guide the segments as they move. This method is usually used over a 4- to 6-week period. It relies heavily on parent cooperation and input.

A second option for aligning the segments is use of an active dental appliance, sometimes referred to as a *Latham appliance* (Georgiade & Latham, 1975; Latham, 1980; Latham, Kusy, & Georgiade, 1976; Millard & Latham, 1990; Millard, Latham, Huifen, Spiro, & Morovic, 1999). (See Chaper 9.) This method uses a two-piece acrylic dental appliance pinned to the greater and lesser segments. On a daily basis, a screw is turned slowly, which draws the two segments together to close the gap. This usually takes about 3 to 4 weeks to accomplish.

The third option for pulling the segments together is a surgical procedure called a *lip adhesion*. This is a simple straight-line lip repair that is performed so that the subsequent lip pressure will draw the segments together. The lip adhesion is usually done at 6 weeks of age followed by the formal lip repair 3 or 4 months later. The decision to use any of the above methods is highly dependent on the experience of the surgeon and the facilities available.

Presurgical treatment options in bilateral cleft lip are similar to those of unilateral clefts. The first is simple taping. A headgear (bonnet) with Velcro elastic bands to draw the premaxilla back into position is a common and long-standing technique. Both the taping and the bonnet methods may be used with a passive molding plate to guide the segments into position. An active Latham appliance may also be used. Like the unilateral device, it is also pinned to the maxilla and dental chain elastics are used to pull the premaxilla back into position. With this appliance, there is also the possibility of expanding the two lateral segments, which are often collapsed together. The chain elastics are usually adjusted by the pediatric dentist. Last, there is the surgical adhesion method, similar to the unilateral procedure, which uses the pressure of the "repaired" lip to draw the premaxilla back into position. One is more apt to see some type of technique used on bilateral lips, as the protrusion of the unrestrained premaxilla and prolabium puts tremendous pressure on the repaired lip.

Techniques for Unilateral Cleft Lip Repair

By examining an unrepaired unilateral cleft lip deformity, one can see that all the structures are present, including the philtral dimple and both of the philtral ridges. The cleft passes just to the lateral side of the philtral ridge. On the cleft side, the lip is short and the cupid's bow is twisted up into the cleft. Early surgical techniques to repair this cleft lip deformity were simple straight-line repairs. This type of repair resulted in a lip that was characteristically short and notched.

Currently, there are two major methods for repairing the unilateral cleft lip: the Millard technique (Trier, 1985b) and the Randall-Tennison technique. Figure 18–1 shows the basic technique for the Millard lip repair and Figure 18–2 is a photograph of this type of repair. With both the Millard and the Tennison-Randall techniques, the philtral ridge is length-

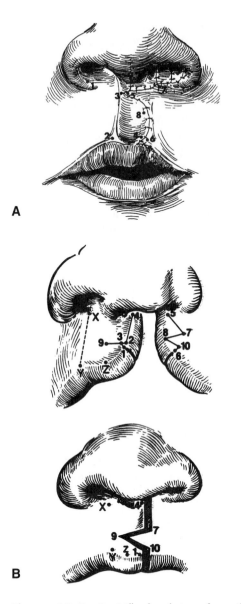

A

B

Figure 18–1. A. Millard technique for unilateral cleft lip repair. From *Cleft lip and Palate: Surgical, Dental and Speech Aspects*, edited by W. C. Grabb, S. W. & Rosenstein & K. R. Bzoch (Eds.), 1971, p. 200. Boston: Little, Brown and Company. Reprinted with permission. **B.** Randall-Tennison technique for unilateral cleft lip repair. From Repair of the Unilateral Cleft Lip: Triangular Flap Repairs, by R. O. Brauer, *Clinics in Plastic Surgery*, 12(4), 1985, p. 597. Philadelphia: W. B. Saunders Company. Reprinted with permission.

ened by inserting a "patch" of tissue into the ridge on the cleft side. This brings the ridge down to match the unaffected side. Because plastic surgeons are not able to do scarless surgery, an attempt is made to place the scars in normally occurring lines and anatomical breaks, such as the philtral ridges.

The Millard technique, or rotation advancement flap, is used in approximately 80% of cases and is perhaps the most anatomical of the repairs (Becker, Svensson, McWilliam, Sarnas, & Jacobsson, 1998). It is known as a "cut as you go" technique because adjustments are constantly made during this procedure to bring the lip into balance. In this technique, the extra tissue or "patch" is inserted at the top of the lip, just beneath the nose. The initial incision is placed along the philtral ridge on the cleft side. As the incision is carried up along the ridge and beneath the nose in a curvilinear manner, the lip opens up and "rotates" down until the cupid's bow is level, hence the rotation part of the name. As the philtrum rotates into the correct position, it leaves a gap at the top of the lip, beneath the nose. Into this gap, tissue is inserted to maintain the length and fill the defect. This is done by advancing tissue from the lateral portion of the lip again beneath the nose (alae in this case) into this gap, hence the advancement portion of the name. By increasing or decreasing the amount of rotation, the lip length may be adjusted. Tissue, which is lateral to the incision on the philtral ridge, is used to lengthen the shortened columella on the cleft side.

The Millard repair, with its "cut as you go" philosophy, is thought by some to be the more difficult of the repairs. Additionally, the tissue is inserted at the point of maximum tension where the underlying structures are relatively fixed to the maxilla. In inexperienced hands, this can often lead to a lip that is too short. In very wide clefts, some will not consider this repair at all or resort to a lip adhesion prior to formal repair. On the plus side, the normal philtral dimple is preserved, the scar follows and mimics the philtral ridge, and by inserting the tissue at the top of the lip, the result is a better nasal

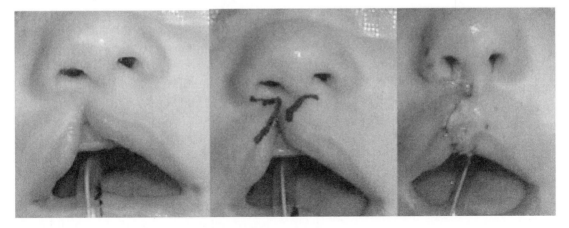

Figure 18–2. Photograph of a unilateral Millard lip repair.

configuration. Revisions when necessary are relatively easy. The most common problem is a lip that is too short. The lip can simply be re-rotated and lengthened. Its advantages far outweigh its disadvantages, and this explains why it is the most widely used repair today.

The Tennison-Randall procedure, or triangular flap technique, is used in about 20% of cases, and follows from an older technique, the LeMesurier repair or quadrilateral flap technique (Figure 18–1). The Tennison-Randall procedure is precise and measured; therefore, it is often referred to a "cookie cutter" technique. Many surgeons like the security of this type of fixed technique. In the Tennison-Randall method, an incision is placed about halfway up through the philtral ridge on the cleft side. This opens a triangular opening (hence the name triangular flap technique) in the inferior portion of the lip and the point of the cupid's bow drops into position. A triangular-shaped flap from the lateral portion of the lip is inserted into this triangular shaped gap. This "patch" of tissue is inserted in the bottom and most mobile portion of the lip. Significant mobilization in the upper portion of the lip, where tension is the greatest, is thereby avoided.

Despite violating both the philtral ridge and philtral dimple, the results from this procedure can be quite good with good lip configu-

ration and a symmetrical cupid's bow. The nasal results are usually not as good, however, because the alar base usually remains somewhat splayed. Subsequent nasal reconstruction is compromised because the tissue in the upper part of the lip will tend to bunch up as the alar base is brought into its proper position and there is little possibility of creating a nostril sill. However, because the extra tissue is inserted in the most mobile portion of the lip, this repair, as previously stated, is often popular in wide clefts.

It is important to remember that the mouth is a sphincter and that clefts can affect both the oral and velopharyngeal sphincters. Just as it is important to reconstruct the velopharyngeal sphincter, it is important to reconstruct the oral sphincter. Although this may seem intuitively obvious, historically it was ignored. When there is a cleft lip, the orbicularis oris muscles of the oral sphincter are divided. Instead of creating a complete ring around the mouth, they are discontinuous and the divided ends are abnormally inserted. In unilateral clefts the orbicularis oris inserts along the *piriform aperture* (the opening at the base of the ala) laterally and the anterior nasal spine (at the base of the columella) medially. In the bilateral cleft, there is no muscle in the prolabial portion and the orbicularis oris abnormally inserts on either side of the piriform aperture at the alar bases. Regardless of the type of repair chosen, these abnormal insertions should be taken down and the muscles realigned into the correct orientation. Failure to do so will result in distortion of the lip on activation, noticeable depressions, and a poor aesthetic result.

In the past, and to a certain extent even today, there has been debate over whether to address the accompanying nasal deformity of the unilateral cleft lip with the initial lip repair. Traditionally, it was felt that the nose should not be operated on in infancy, due to a concern that its growth potential would be adversely affected. In recent years, several surgeons have demonstrated that not only is this concern unfounded, but better long-term results can be achieved by early correction of the nasal deformity at the time of initial lip repair. All the techniques involve some method of repositioning the distorted lower lateral cartilage and malpositioned alar base. Although these early repairs do not obviate the need for secondary surgery, they greatly reduce the initial deformity and lessen the extent of subsequent reconstruction.

Techniques for Bilateral Cleft Lip Repair

Repair of a bilateral cleft lip deformity is a more frustrating and a less successful endeavor when compared to the contemporary unilateral repair. The magnitude of the lip and nasal deformities can present formidable challenges to even the most experienced surgeons. A bilateral complete cleft of the primary palate can result in the unrestrained protrusion of the premaxillary complex. With the premaxilla protruding anteriorly, it is not uncommon for the two lateral segments to collapse behind it. Expansion of the lateral segments is sometimes required to allow the premaxilla to drop back into position. The prolabium (the lip portion of the premaxilla) has no muscle in it and this lack of muscle tension across this portion of the lip results in an appearance of significant "shrinkage."

In the past, the appearance of a diminutive prolabium led to the incorrect assumption that there was a need for extra tissue in this area. This led to a whole host of repairs directed toward adding tissue to the prolabium. This tissue was added beneath the prolabium from the lateral lip elements. The resulting scars were shaped either like a "Y" or a goal post. This was hardly in keeping with the concept of hiding scars in naturally occurring lines. What became evident over time was that when exposed to muscle tension the prolabium would stretch. The resultant lip ended up being tight transversely and very long vertically. The tightness transversely applied significant pressure on an already compromised maxilla resulting in often dramatic retrusion of the upper jaw. In the 1960s, the shortcomings of this type of repair were realized and it was abandoned.

Currently, all contemporary bilateral cleft lip repairs are some variation of a modified straight-line repair. While each repair may boast of having a Z-plasty type component, they all achieve about the same result. The prolabium forms the entire philtral area. Even though the prolabium is small, it is routinely made narrower and the lateral portions or parings are used in some form for eventual columellar lengthening. Immediately after the repair, the lip looks tight and bunched up. Within several weeks, the prolabium begins to stretch out and achieve a more normal size. If care is not taken to initially trim the prolabial segment down, it will be too large once the lip matures.

The two major methods of bilateral cleft lip repair are the Millard technique and some form of the Modified Manchester repair. These repairs are illustrated in Figure 18–3. Both types are essentially straight-line repairs. The major difference between the two procedures are the method in which the white roll of the philtrum is created. In the Millard repair, the white roll comes from the white roll of the lateral elements. In the modified Broadbent-Manchester repair, the white roll from the prolabium is preserved.

Although most surgeons now feel that nasal repair in the unilateral lip can be accomplished with the initial lip repair; this is not the case with the bilateral lip. Several surgeons have attempted to lengthen the columella with the initial repair, but their results are still too early to judge. Most surgeons stage the nasal repair with a bilateral cleft lip. The main problem in bilateral cleft nasal deformity is the lack of sufficient columellar length, and alar splaying, resulting in a nasal tip that is tethered, broad, and lacks normal projection.

Two major methods of columellar lengthening are widely used. The initial lip repair and the handling of the lateral parings usually dictate how the columella will be lengthened. When the prolabium is narrowed, the lateral parings are "banked" or stored in the floor of the nose. They appear as bumps in the floor of the nose. At the second stage of the bilateral repair, an incision is made transversely, curving from alar base to alar base just below the banked parings. As the nose is elevated, two things happen. The floor of the nose (the banked parings) is drawn up into the columel-

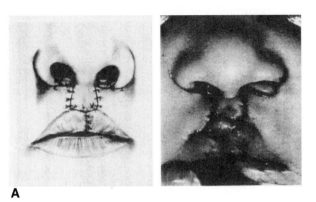

A

Figure 18-3. A. Millard technique for bilateral cleft lip repair. From Repair of Bilateral Cleft Lip: Millard's Technique by W. C. Trier, 1985, p. 617. *Clinics in Plastic Surgery, 12*(4). Philadelphia: W. B. Saunders Company. Reprinted with permission. **B.** Modified Manchester repair for bilateral cleft lip repair. From *Surgical Techniques in Cleft Lip and Palate*, by J. Bardach & K. E. Salyer, 1986, p. 104. Chicago: Year Book Medical Publishers. Reprinted with permission.

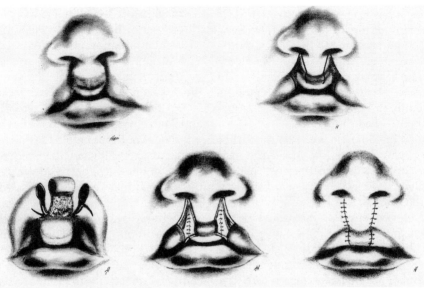

B

la, thereby lengthening it. As the nose moves up, the alae move closer together, narrowing the base of the nose. This type of secondary lip repair is referred to as a Cronin columellar-lengthening procedure.

If no parings were created in the original repair and the full width of the prolabium was used to make the philtral dimple, the resulting dimple will be quite wide once the scars mature. In a sense, the parings were banked in the lip, not the floor of the nose. When this is the case, a forked flap lengthening is used. At the time of the second surgery, the lateral parings are created and raised from the lip. This tissue is then used to lengthen the columella. This is usually the case in a Millard-type approach. Either approach can be used, depending on the configuration of the lip and the site of the excess tissue. Timing of this secondary procedure varies with each surgeon, but usually is done between 9 months and 5 years of age.

Cleft Palate Repair: Palatoplasty

Timing of the Cleft Palate Repair

The timing of the cleft palate repair, also called *pharyngoplasty,* has been even more controversial than timing of the lip repair. A few teams advocate palate repair in the first week of life, but this is extremely controversial. Most centers fall into two major philosophies—early and late. Early is defined as between 6 months and 15 months of age. Late is defined as between 15 months and 24 months.

In general it is acknowledged that the earlier the palate repair is done, the lower the incidence of velopharyngeal insufficiency will be (Witzel, Salyer, & Ross, 1984). However, early repair of the hard palate has raised concerns about the potential effect on the growth of the maxilla, which affects the appearance of the midface. Patients with a history of cleft palate and surgical repair often demonstrate midface retrusion and Class III malocclusion due to a lack of adequate midfacial and maxillary growth. Over the last 50 years, there has been a debate in the literature as to whether this is caused by the inherent nature of the cleft or if it is the result of the surgical repair of the palate. One school of thought has been that midface deficiency is the direct result of the surgical repair of the palate. To avoid the potential adverse effect on facial growth, Schweckendiek (1955) advocated closing the velum only at an early age, usually around 6 months. The hard palate was closed at a later time, usually between 4 to 5 years of age, to avoid scarring of the growing hard palate. Until it was finally surgically closed, the hard palate was usually obturated for speech. The basic philosophy with this technique was that it promoted velopharyngeal closure while avoiding restriction in maxillary growth (Blocksma, Leuz, & Mellerstig, 1975; Dingman & Grabb, 1971; Perko, 1979; Schweckendiek, 1966, 1968, 1983; Schweckendiek & Doz, 1978).

In subsequent studies, the results of this two-stage approach have been found to be less than impressive. Several studies have shown that a high percentage of the patients treated with this method fail to develop acceptable speech and a large number required pharyngeal flaps (Bardach, Morris, & Olin, 1984; Cosman & Falk, 1980; Fara & Brousilova, 1969, 1988; Jackson, McLennan, & Scheker, 1983; Witzel et al., 1984). In addition, the hard palate has been found to be difficult to close when repaired at a later time (Cosman & Falk, 1980; Jackson et al., 1983). Finally, Fara, Brousilova, Hrivnakova, and Tvrdek (1992) reported that, when the second stage was done before the patient is 7 years of age, the results were almost identical to the results of one-stage palate repair performed at the age of 3 to 4 years. They also found that a greater orthodontic effort is needed to achieve an aligned dentoalveolar arch with the two-stage palatoplasty. Ross (1987) reported the results of cephalometric radiographs of 538 males with unilateral cleft lip and palate and compared the results to the age of palate repair.

The results of this study showed that the best facial outcome was found in patients repaired in the teenage years or later. However, the next best outcome was for patients repaired by 11 months or earlier. The worst outcome was with patients who had palate repairs after 20 months. Given these findings, the possible advantages of the two-stage approach in relationship to maxillofacial growth remain difficult to prove and several studies have shown that this delay in hard palate closure has a negative effect on speech. Despite these findings, some centers still promote some variation of this practice.

In addition to the concern about midface growth, there is an additional factor that may delay the palate repair. When there is an extremely wide cleft, some inexperienced surgeons may not be comfortable closing the palate in a single stage. Some feel that closing the velum only will narrow the remaining cleft of the hard palate. As with the classic Schweckendiek technique, the speech results with this delay are less than desirable.

Techniques for Palatoplasty

While the cleft lip repair dates back to antiquity, successful palatal repair dates only from the early 19th century. With the advent of anesthesia and specialized instrumentation, success rates improved dramatically. Achieving a good result in palatal surgery is much more difficult than achieving a good result in lip surgery. Although a palate repair may appear simple in comparison to a lip repair, palate surgery can be quite challenging for several reasons. First, it is technically more demanding than a lip repair. There is a greater chance of mishap (hemorrhage and airway obstruction), and if problems (dehiscence, fistula formation, and excessive scarring) occur, they are more difficult to correct. The potential for airway compromise or excessive bleeding are concerns that may put the patient's life in jeopardy. Second, merely closing the palate is not enough. The palate not only serves as a physical barrier between the mouth and nose, but also must function dynamically for normal speech.

The Von Langenbeck repair is one of the oldest and most successful means of palatal closure and is still popular today (Murison & Pigott, 1992; Trier & Dreyer, 1984). Approximately 60% of palatoplasties performed today are of this type. This repair is illustrated in Figure 18–4. In this repair, an incision is made just inside the gum line, starting just behind the teeth and extending up to the area of the canine tooth. The mucoperiosteum over the bone is carefully raised off the bone and separated in one large layer in conjunction with the velum. The cleft margin is incised and the raw edges are brought together and sewn down the middle. The incisions along the gum line are usually left open. This operation was the procedure of choice until the 1930s. The incidence of velopharyngeal dysfunction with this procedure was reported as high or higher than 40%. It was felt that inadequate physical length was the primary cause of velopharyngeal insufficiency in repaired clefts with this procedure. This set off a search for a procedure that not only closed the opening, but also actively lengthened the palate.

A number of approaches were put forth and promoted. Some were quite horrific, causing problems with growth, wound healing, and airway obstruction. One technique that has somewhat stood the test of time and is still used in a significant percentage of cases is the Wardill-Kilner "V" to "Y" or pushback procedure, which is illustrated in Figure 18–5. In this procedure, the initial incisions are similar to those of the Von Langenbeck procedure except, instead of leaving the mucoperiosteum attached in the front of the mouth, it is cut across as a "V." This frees up the mucoperiosteum of the whole palate and allows it to be pushed back in an attempt to lengthen it. The resultant open area is Y-shaped. Initial reports showed dramatic reduction in the incidence of velopha-

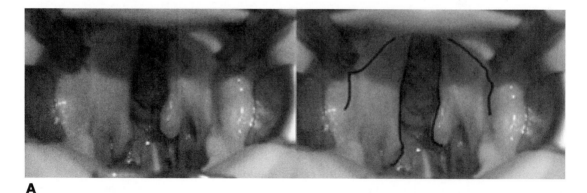

Figure 18–4. A. Photograph of palate marked for Von Langenbeck repair. Anterior palate remains attached forming a bipedicle flap. **B.** Technique of the Von Langenbeck repair. Note lateral relaxing incisions which are left open. (From *Plastic Surgery*, by Joseph McCarthy, 1990, Vol. 4, Fig. 54–12. Orlando, FL: W.B. Saunders Company. Reprinted with permission.)

ryngeal insufficiency. Unfortunately, this has not been borne out over time (Brothers, Dalston, Peterson, & Lawrence, 1995).

Just as a cleft lip disrupts the oral sphincter in the lip and alters the insertion of the sphincteric muscles, a cleft palate also changes the velopharyngeal sphincter. In the patient with cleft palate, the levator veli palatini inserts onto

back of the hard palate instead of fusing together in the midline to form the levator sling. Initial palatal repairs ignored this muscle and did nothing to correct its orientation. More recently, *intravelar veloplasty* (IVVP) or reconstruction of this sling has been advocated (Brown, Cohen, & Randall, 1983; Dreyer & Trier, 1984). Two contemporary repairs pro-

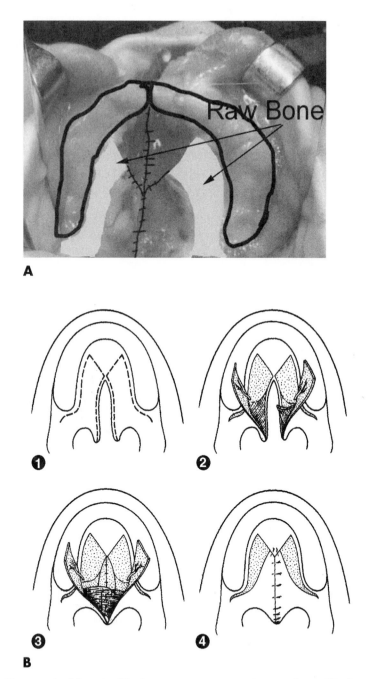

Figure 18–5. A. Photograph of the Wardill-Kilner type repair. **B.** Technique of Wardill-Kilner repair. Palate is lengthened by "pushing" back the mucoperiosteum. The raw area is allowed to fill in by secondary healing (scarring). (From *Plastic Surgery*, by Joseph McCarthy, 1990, Vol. 4, Fig. 54–11. Orlando, FL: W.B. Saunders Company. Reprinted with permission.)

mote the reconstruction of this sling: the two-flap palatoplasty and the Furlow palatoplasty.

The Furlow palatoplasty (Furlow, 1986, 1990), which is shown in Figure 18–6, involves reconstruction of the levator sling, but also lengthens the velum by closing it with a double opposing Z-plasty fashion. The two-flap palatoplasty allows retropositioning of the levator sling, but does not incorporate a Z-plasty in the velum. Initial reports were very encouraging regarding the speech results with these repairs, but it is still too soon to know the long-term results. However, despite the more thorough approach advocated by these two repairs, there is still a 10% to 20% rate of velopharyn-

geal dysfunction in patients with a history of palate repair. Intravelar veloplasty, whether done as an isolated procedure in the treatment of submucous cleft or in conjunction with any type of palatoplasty, has not been as successful as was hoped (Coston, Hagerty, Jannarone, McDonald, & Hagerty, 1986; Jarvis & Trier, 1988). Gunther, Wisser, Cohen, and Brown (1998) reported a better speech outcome with the Furlow palatoplasty than with the intravelar veloplasty. Marsh, Grames, and Holtman (1989) did a prospective study comparing the results of palatoplasty with and without intravelar veloplasty. In that study, they found no difference in the perception of velopharyngeal

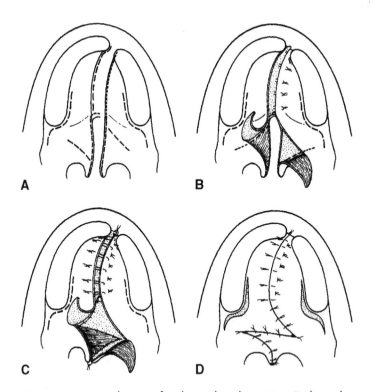

Figure 18–6. Technique of Furlow palatoplasty. Note Z-plasty closure of both nasal side and mirror image on the oral side. (From *Plastic Surgery*, by Joseph McCarthy, 1990, Vol. 4, Fig. 54–9. Orlando, FL: W.B. Saunders Company. Reprinted with permission.)

competence in the two groups. These results suggest that either there is no beneficial effect of intravelar veloplasty or the effect is minimal.

Interpreting the data regarding the effect of each palatoplasty technique on speech is very difficult. There are many variables to consider, including the timing of surgery, the experience and skill of the surgeon, the experience and skill of the speech pathologist, and the very definition of "acceptable" speech. However, there is general agreement that early repair is clearly better than late repair when considering speech results. In addition, experienced surgeons have a lower incidence of growth disturbance. Most experienced cleft palate centers report an incidence of between 17% and 20% of velopharyngeal dysfunction requiring pharyngeal flap surgery.

Fistula Repair Techniques

Fistulas are persistent openings between the nasal and oral cavity. They occur when the palate fails to heal after a palatoplasty. In some cases, a fistula may be deliberately left in the alveolus at the time of the primary palatoplasty and is closed with a bone graft at a later time. Fistulas occur in between about 5% and 30% of reported series. Although fistulas can be asymptomatic, they can also cause significant hypernasality and nasal air emission during speech, and can also cause regurgitation of food and fluids into the nasal cavity during eating. Closure of a fistula can be a daunting task and traditionally carries only a 50% success rate. Fistulas are often blamed on expansion of the dental arch or growth of the patient. Growth and expansion do not cause fistulas, but they commonly reveal ones that already exist.

Closure of fistulas is usually attempted with the use of local autogenous tissue first. If there is not adequate local tissue or if this fails, more complex and difficult procedures may be necessary. Techniques include using turbinates, flaps of tissue from the buccal surface based on

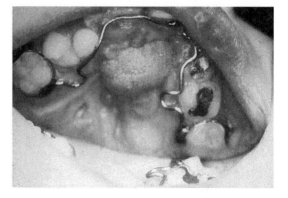

Figure 18–7. Fistula repair with a tongue flap. Note the tongue tissue in the anterior portion of the palate.

the facial artery, and frequently a tongue flap (Figure 18–7) (Argamaso, 1990; Assuncao, 1993; Barone & Argamaso, 1993; Busic, Bagatin, & Boric, 1989; Coghlan, O'Regan, & Carter, 1989; Pigott, Rieger, & Moodie, 1984; Posnick & Getz, 1987; Thind, Singh, & Thind, 1992). With the tongue flap procedure, the dorsum of the tongue is sutured into the fistula and left for about 6 weeks to develop its blood supply. At that point, the tongue flap is severed from the rest of the tongue. Although this leaves scarring on the top of the tongue, it does not adversely affect the movement of the tongue for speech or feeding because the flap does not come from the tongue tip.

Surgery for Velopharyngeal Dysfunction

Velopharyngeal dysfunction following a palatal repair can be due to a number of factors. Scarring as a result of the initial palatoplasty can shorten the velum, making it impossible for it to reach the posterior pharyngeal wall during speech, or the nasopharynx can be deep relative to the position of the velum. In addition, the velum can appear to be of adequate length, but have poor movement due to inadequate muscle insertion or neuromuscular dysfunction. Whether the problem is anatomical or neurological or both, the correction involves introducing something into the velopharyngeal opening to reduce the size of the gap and to take advantage of the velopharyngeal movement that is present.

Successful surgical management of velopharyngeal dysfunction has been a relatively recent accomplishment. In fact, at one time, velopharyngeal dysfunction was primarily treated with prosthetic obturation. In the 1970s, the use of both videofluoroscopy and nasal endoscopy led to a better understanding of the velopharyngeal valve and, therefore, better methods of surgical correction have evolved. At this point, surgical correction of velopharyngeal dysfunction is the norm and prosthetic devices are rarely used for this purpose with children.

Timing of Secondary Surgery

The diagnosis of velopharyngeal dysfunction cannot be made until the child begins to produce connected speech and can adequately cooperate with the speech pathologist. This is typically around the age of 3. Evaluation of velopharyngeal function may include nasendoscopy and/or videofluoroscopy, in addition to the speech pathologist's examination. The speech pathologist's evaluation is the most critical because surgical decisions are based on the auditory perception of the speech rather than instrumental measures. Once an assessment is completed, surgery can be performed if indicated. The earliest this is done is usually around 3½ to 4 years of age. If the patient has a history of Pierre Robin sequence with micrognathia and upper airway obstruction, the surgery may be delayed for a time until the mandible grows or the size of the airway increases. Pharyngoplasty procedures can be performed earlier than age 3, and at one time, one

group advocated simultaneous palatal repair and pharyngeal flap. This is no longer an acceptable practice because it subjected between 40% to 60% of the patients to significant morbidity and a procedure that was not warranted.

Intervention should occur as soon as possible after the diagnosis of velopharyngeal insufficiency or incompetence is made, because a successful outcome is less likely in the older individual who has had velopharyngeal dysfunction for a long period of time. If the patient presents in mid to late adolescence, the success rate will be less than 50% as compared to greater than 90% in the 4- to 5-year-old. In addition to assessing speech and velopharyngeal function in the preschool years, longitudinal follow-up of patients with a history of cleft is critical, because some individuals will present with velopharyngeal insufficiency as the adenoid pad shrinks.

Velopharyngeal dysfunction is a surgical disorder, whether due to an anatomical, or neurological causes. Therefore, therapeutic endeavors through speech therapy are ineffective because they cannot improve an anatomical problem. However, it is important to institute speech therapy as soon as possible to avoid the development of compensatory productions, which can be difficult to eliminate, even after surgical correction. Speech therapy for improvement of articulation placement can be done before the surgery and again after the surgery until these errors are corrected.

Surgical Preparation

Prior to proceeding with a surgical procedure to correct velopharyngeal dysfunction, the patient should undergo a thorough head and neck examination. Particular attention should be paid to the size of the tonsils and the adenoid pad and the presence of micrognathia (small jaw), as is common in Pierre Robin sequence. Enlarged tonsils, adenoid hypertrophy, or micrognathia may portend toward airway obstruction in the immediate postoperative period, as well as long-term problems with sleep apnea. Some centers advocate routine tonsillectomy prior to pharyngeal flap to prevent the tonsils from obstructing the lateral pharyngeal port postoperatively, although this is usually not necessary unless the tonsils are enlarged. If tonsillectomy is indicated, it should precede the flap by at least 6 weeks. Although adenoidectomy is usually not recommended for patients with repaired cleft palate, an adenoidectomy prior to pharyngeal flap placement may allow the surgeon to position the flap higher in the nasopharynx and avoid port obstruction postoperatively. Therefore, because enlargement of the tonsils is often accompanied by enlargement of the adenoids, a conservative adenoidectomy at the time of tonsillectomy is often appropriate. The characteristics of velopharyngeal dysfunction will worsen until the pharyngeal flap is done to correct the velopharyngeal dysfunction.

If the patient has a diagnosis of Velocardiofacial syndrome, a careful examination of the back of the posterior pharyngeal wall may be indicated. One of the phenotypic features of this syndrome is tortuosity of the carotid arteries (D'Antonio & Marsh, 1987; Finkelstein et al., 1993; MacKenzie-Stepner et al., 1987; Ross, Witzel, Armstrong, & Thomson, 1996). As a result, they often course medially beneath the posterior wall of the pharynx, rather than lateral to each side of the pharyngeal wall, putting them in harm's way with a pharyngeal flap. This abnormality can usually be seen at the time of surgery and the vessels avoided, but some advocate preoperative imaging studies or nasopharyngoscopy.

Surgical Techniques: Pharyngeal Wall Augmentation

The velopharyngeal opening that occurs as a result of velopharyngeal dysfunction has led to the search for some type of internal obturation.

When the velopharyngeal opening is small, no more than 10 mm in diameter, posterior *pharyngeal wall augmentation* has been used by some surgeons. With this procedure, an implant is surgically placed or injected in the posterior pharyngeal wall in the area of the velopharyngeal opening. The implant is placed deep in the superior pharyngeal constrictors, but superficial to the prevertebral fascia. Figure 18–8 illustrates velopharyngeal insufficiency prior to the implant and then the closure that occurs with the augmented posterior pharyngeal wall as a result of the implant. Various materials have been reported for posterior pharyngeal wall augmentation including paraffin, cartilage, fascia, fat, silicone, proplast, and polytetrafluoroethylene (Teflon) (Denny, Marks, & Oliff-Carneol, 1993; Furlow, Williams, Eisenbach, & Bzoch, 1982; Gray, Pinborough-Zimmerman, & Catten, 1999; Remacle, Bertrand, Eloy, & Marbaix, 1990; Terris & Goode, 1993; Trigos, Ysunza, Gonzalez, & Vazquez, 1988; Witt et al., 1997; Wolford, Oelschlaeger, & Deal, 1989). Overcorrection is required for all injectable augmentation material because the vehicle solution is absorbed. Complications from implantation of foreign materials in the posterior pharyngeal wall include infections, extrusion, resorption, and even migration of the material after insertion. Granuloma formation has also been associated with Teflon implantation. These implants are not always effective due to the fact that they are often too small or in the wrong location to completely fill the opening. On the other hand, overcorrection can occur, which may result in hyponasality and upper airway obstruction.

Another procedure for pharyngeal wall augmentation is the use of a *rolled flap*. In this case, a flap of tissue is raised from the posterior pharyngeal wall and is rolled up onto itself. This roll forms a bulge on the posterior pharyngeal wall to fill in the velopharyngeal gap (Gray et al., 1999). Some of these techniques have worked, but their overall success rate has been disappointing.

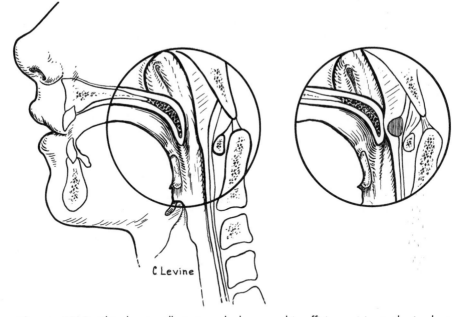

C Levine

Figure 18–8. This drawing illustrates velopharyngeal insufficiency prior to the implant and then the closure that occurs with the augmented posterior pharyngeal wall as a result of the implant.

Surgical Techniques: Pharyngoplasty

A *pharyngoplasty* is a surgical procedure of the pharynx that is designed to correct velopharyngeal dysfunction. Currently, two pharyngoplasty techniques are most commonly used to correct velopharyngeal dysfunction: the pharyngeal flap and the sphincter pharyngoplasty. Both of these techniques are designed to reduce the size of the pharyngeal port so that, during speech, the movement that is present is sufficient to close the entire port.

A *pharyngeal flap* is designed to be a passive, soft tissue obturator that is placed in the middle of the velopharyngeal port (Tharanon, Stella, & Epker, 1990; Trier, 1985a; Vedung, 1995; Wu & Epker, 1990; Yoshida, Stella, Ghali, & Epker, 1992). Figure 18–9 shows a lateral view of a pharyngeal flap. The flap is raised from the posterior pharyngeal wall, and then sutured into the velum. Lateral ports are left on both sides of the flap for normal nasal breathing.

Figure 18–10 shows a superior view (as would be seen through nasopharyngoscopy) of a normal pharynx during nasal breathing, and the same view of a pharynx with a pharyngeal flap during nasal breathing. Note the pharyngeal flap in midline and the open lateral ports on either side for normal nasal breathing. Figure 18–11A and B shows a pharyngeal flap as it would be viewed through nasopharyngoscopy. The pharyngeal flap can be seen in midline and the lateral ports are viewed on either side of the flap.

During speech, the lateral pharyngeal walls move medially to close against the flap, thus closing the lateral pharyngeal ports and the entire pharyngeal opening. Because lateral wall motion is the key to the function of the velopharyngeal mechanism following the placement of the flap, patients with good later-

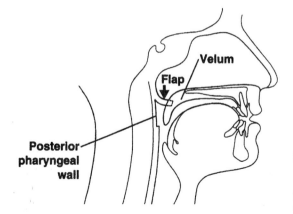

Figure 18–9. A lateral view of a pharyngeal flap. The flap is raised from the posterior pharyngeal wall, and then sutured into the velum. Ports are left on both sides of the flap for normal nasal breathing.

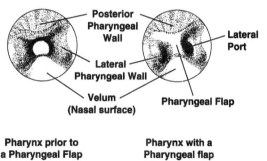

Figure 18–10. A superior view (as would be seen through nasopharyngoscopy) of a normal pharynx during nasal breathing, and the same view of a pharynx with a pharyngeal flap during nasal breathing. Note the pharyngeal flap in midline and the open lateral ports on either side.

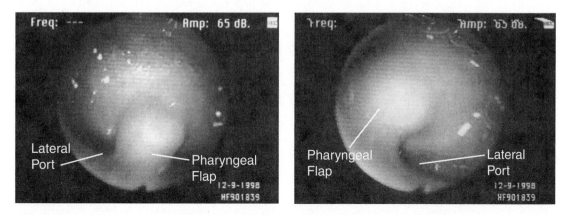

Figure 18–11. A pharyngeal flap as viewed through nasopharyngoscopy. **A.** This photo shows the pharyngeal flap in midline and the lateral ports on either side. **B.** This photo shows a better view of the patient's left lateral port.

al pharyngeal wall movement preoperatively, and particularly those with a sagittal pattern of closure, are particularly good candidates for a pharyngeal flap.

With this procedure, a flap of tissue is dissected from the pharyngeal wall by an incision that begins at the top of the nasopharynx and then goes down to the area near the base of the tongue. The incision then goes across the width of the pharynx between the tonsillar pillars, and then up again so that the base of the flap is connected at the very top of the nasopharynx. The pharyngeal flap includes the mucosal surface and the underlying musculature all the way down to the prevertebral fascia of the spinal column. The blood supply comes in through the attached portion of the flap at the base of the skull. Once the flap is raised, the velum is split up to the hard palate and the flap from the pharynx is elevated and sutured into the velum. A port or opening is left on each side of the flap to allow normal nasal breathing, drainage of nasal secretions, and normal nasal resonance. Stents may be placed in the ports over night to keep them patent, but are removed the next day.

Several factors determine the success of the flap in correcting characteristics of velopharyngeal dysfunction. One factor is the vertical position in the nasopharynx (Skolnick & McCall, 1972). As a general rule, it is important that the flap is set as high as possible, because this is usually the area of maximum lateral pharyngeal wall movement. Although the inferiorly based pharyngeal flap was used at one time, it was found to result in a position that was often too low in the nasopharynx to take advantage of the full extent of lateral pharyngeal wall movement. In contrast, the superiorly based pharyngeal flap has been found to remain higher and in better position in the nasopharynx over time.

The width of the flap is also an important consideration and needs to be based on the extent of lateral pharyngeal wall movement, since this is a primary factor in the success of the flap. The role of lateral pharyngeal wall movement in determining the success of a pharyngeal flap was studied by Argamaso et al. (1980). They evaluated 202 patients with pharyngeal flaps through nasopharyngoscopy and multiview videofluoroscopy. Through these studies they found that, where there was no evidence of velopharyngeal dysfunction following placement of the flap, the sole determiner of velopharyngeal closure was the medial movement of the lateral pharyngeal walls to meet the flap. In cases where the flap failed to correct the velopharyngeal dysfunction, there was an inappropriate degree, level, or symmetry of the lateral pharyngeal wall motion in relation to the position and width of the flap. Lewis and Pashayan (1980) looked for an increase in the degree of lateral pharyngeal wall

motion following placement of a pharyngeal flap in 20 patients. They found that there was no significant difference in the lateral wall motion of their patients postoperatively. On the other hand, Karling, Henningsson, Larson, and Isberg (1999) found a potential for adaptation of pharyngeal wall adduction to different flap widths. They reported that, in patients with limited preoperative lateral pharyngeal wall adduction, pharyngeal wall activity increased in the presence of a narrow flap. When preoperative adduction was pronounced, however, the postoperative activity decreased because of mechanical hindrance by the flap, and the degree of impediment was correlated to the width of the flap. Although this study suggests that there is some adaptation of lateral pharyngeal wall movement to the width of the flap, if the flap is too narrow so that the lateral pharyngeal walls do not close against it, there will be persistent hypernasality or nasal air emission postoperatively.

Patients with a sagittal pattern of closure or good lateral pharyngeal wall movement preoperatively have the best prognosis for total correction of velopharyngeal dysfunction with a pharyngeal flap and can manage with a more narrow flap. In contrast, patients with poor lateral wall motion require a wider flap for total correction. The challenge in these cases is to make the flap wide enough so that the lateral walls can close against it on both sides during speech, yet not so wide that it causes upper airway obstruction with hyponasality and sleep apnea. When there is hypotonia, as in velocardiofacial syndrome, or a compromised airway due to retrognathia, the surgeon may need to compromise perfect speech results for a functional airway.

The *Orticochea sphincter pharyngoplasty* (Orticochea, 1970, 1983, 1997, 1999), also referred to as just a *sphincteroplasty*, is designed to create a dynamic sphincter that encircles a single velopharyngeal port. Because the velopharyngeal valve is a dynamic mechanism that closes off the nasal cavity from the oral cavity during speech, it was felt that superior speech results would be obtained by creating a functional sphincter as opposed to a passive obturator. This procedure has undergone a series of modifications, and in its most current and widely used form, it now exists as the Jackson modification of the Orticochea sphincteroplasty (Jackson, 1985; Jackson, McGlynn, Huskie, & Dip, 1980; Jackson & Silverton, 1977).

The sphincter pharyngoplasty procedure is illustrated in Figure 18–12. In this procedure, bilateral superiorly based myocutaneous flaps are raised from the posterior faucial pillars, which include the palatopharyngeus muscles. These flaps are rotated posteriorly and inset into a transverse incision in the nasopharynx, just at the level of velopharyngeal closure. This effectively narrows the pharynx. A small, superiorly based pharyngeal flap is then raised and attached to the lateral flaps. This leaves a single round opening of about 1 cm in diameter in the center of the pharynx. During speech, the palatopharyngeus muscles work in conjunction with the levator veli palatini muscles to close the opening as a sphincter. Because this procedure results in a narrowing of the lateral border of the velopharyngeal sphincter, it has been advocated for use with poor lateral pharyngeal wall motion or deep lateral pharyngeal recesses, with better closure in the center of the port with the velar movement.

Surgical Complications and Follow-Up Following Pharyngoplasty

Immediately after placement of the pharyngeal flap or sphincteroplasty, there is significant *edema* or swelling in the pharynx. As a result, most patients will exhibit hyponasality and loud snoring during the immediate postoperative period. Snoring is the most common consequence of pharyngoplasty, especially after the pharyngeal flap, and approximately 80% of patients will snore to some extent for the rest of their lives.

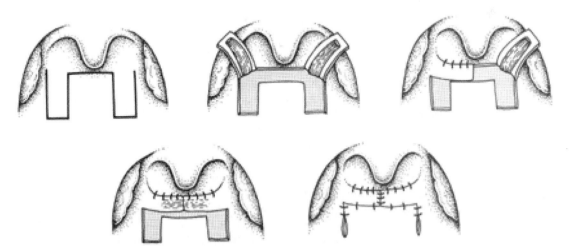

Figure 18–12. Sphincter pharyngoplasty. In this procedure, bilateral myocutaneous flaps are raised from the posterior faucial pillars, which include the palatopharyngeus muscles. These flaps are rotated posteriorly and inset into a transverse incision in the nasopharynx just at the level of velopharyngeal closure. A small superiorly based flap may also be raised and attached to the lateral flaps. This effectively narrows the velopharyngeal port for speech. (From *Plastic Surgery*, by Joseph McCarthy, 1990, Vol. 4, Fig. 58–6. Orlando, FL: W. B. Saunders Company. Reprinted with permission.)

Temporary sleep apnea is another common sequela of the surgery, but this usually resolves within 2 to 6 weeks postoperatively or after the swelling has gone down. Chronic sleep apnea can occur in a small number of patients, however (Tharanon et al., 1990; Trier, 1985a; Vedung, 1995; Wells, Vu, & Luce, 1999; Ysunza, Garcia-Velasco, Garcia-Garcia, Haro, & Valencia, 1993). Chronic sleep apnea is a serious problem and cannot be ignored because it can cause serious health problems if left to continue. Some authors have reported a prevalence of sleep apnea of as high as 10% following pharyngeal flap surgery, but a prevalence of 5% or less is probably more common (personal data). Sleep apnea is the greatest risk for patients who have micrognathia, such as those with Pierre Robin sequence (Abramson, Marrinan, & Mulliken, 1997) or for patients with neurological impairment.

If sleep apnea persists beyond the initial postoperative period, it is usually evaluated with polysomnography during a sleep study. If treatment is indicated, it usually involves continuous positive air pressure (CPAP), which is delivered by mask at night. This positive air pressure keeps the pharynx patent during sleep. Patients with sleep apnea are restudied about every 6 months, and in most cases, the problem will resolve within 1 to 2 years. In refractory cases, however, the flap is taken down. At one time, it was thought that the Orticochea sphincteroplasty did not cause sleep apnea, so this procedure was recommended for patients at high risk. Recent formal studies have shown that, although the risk of sleep apnea following the sphincteroplasty may be less, it still can occur after this procedure (de Serres et al., 1999; Witt, Marsh, Muntz, Marty-Grames, & Watchmaker, 1996).

Following surgery, it is not uncommon for either procedure to require revision or modification. Patients may present within the first year following surgery or may present after many years of normal function with a sudden change in resonance and speech characteristics due to a growth spurt. With the pharyngeal flap procedure, one or both lateral port can become stenosed due to scarring. This can result in hyponasality, upper airway obstruction, and, in severe cases, sleep apnea. For correction, one or both ports need to be opened. More commonly, a port needs to be augmented or closed down for correction of persistent or recurrent hypernasality or nasal air emission. If one port is not closing after the flap is in place, an auxiliary flap can be raised to augment the primary flap on the side of diminished lateral pharyngeal wall motion. With pharyngeal flaps, secondary revisions are relatively uncommon. An appropriately placed pharyngeal flap has a greater than 90% chance for normal speech with speech therapy (our series). The Orticochea sphincteroplasty has a fairly high incidence of secondary revision and the overall success rate has been reported to be less than that of the pharyngeal flap. The success rate with sphincteroplasty for the elimination of hypernasality and nasal air emission has been reported as between 60% to 80% (James, Twist, Turner, & Milward, 1996; Kasten, Buchman, Stevenson, & Berger, 1997; Riski, Ruff, Georgiade, & Barwick, 1992; Riski, Ruff, Georgiade, Barwick, & Edwards, 1992; Roberts & Brown, 1983; Sie et al., 1998; Witt, 1994). One problem may be patient selection. The sphincteroplasty procedure results in a narrowing of the lateral borders of the velopharyngeal port, but there is often a remaining gap in the anterior-posterior dimension (Ren & Wang, 1993). Therefore, it is more appropriate for patients with poor lateral wall movement yet good velar movement. It is unlikely to be successful in cases where there is a short velum or a gap that is primarily in the midline. Other common causes of pharyngoplasty failure include dehiscence, low-lying flaps, and hypotonicity of the velopharyngeal mechanism (Kasten et al., 1997; Witt, Marsh, Marty-Grames, & Muntz, 1995).

Regardless of the pharyngoplasty procedure chosen, the surgery must be followed by a reassessment of the speech so that an appropriate plan of speech therapy can be instituted. Since it takes about 3 months for most of the swelling to resolve and the flap or sphincteroplasty to begin to function, this is the best time for the re-evaluation. Patients and parents must realize that treating velopharyngeal dysfunction is a two-stage process. The surgery is done first to correct the anatomical defect. Following the surgery, speech therapy is required to help the child to eliminate compensatory productions and learn how to use the flap effectively.

Summary

The goals of surgical correction of cleft lip and palate are to normalize feeding, speech, dentition, facial profile, and aesthetics. There are several surgical approaches that can be used to correct each type of deformity. The success of the surgery is dependent on many factors, including the location, size, and severity of the cleft; the type of procedure used; and the experience of the surgeon. With the improvement in surgical techniques in recent years, the functional and aesthetic outcomes of surgery have improved.

Velopharyngeal dysfunction continues to be a risk in the patient with cleft palate, even after successful palate repair. The successful treatment of velopharyngeal dysfunction requires close cooperation and teamwork between the surgeon and the speech pathologist. Failure to work cooperatively may result in unnecessary surgery, unnecessary speech therapy, or both.

References

Abramson, D. L., Marrinan, E. M., & Mulliken, J. B. (1997). Robin sequence: Obstructive sleep apnea following pharyngeal flap. *Cleft Palate Craniofacial Journal, 34*(3), 256–260.

Argamaso, R. V. (1990). The tongue flap: Placement and fixation for closure of postpalatoplasty fistulae. *Cleft Palate Journal, 27*(4), 402–410.

Argamaso, R. V., Shprintzen, R. J., Strauch, B., Lewin, M. L., Daniller, A. I., Ship, A. G., & Croft, C. B. (1980). The role of lateral pharyngeal wall movement in pharyngeal flap surgery. *Plastic and Reconstructive Surgery, 66*(2), 214–219.

Assuncao, A. G. (1993). The design of tongue flaps for the closure of palatal fistulas. *Plastic and Reconstructive Surgery, 91*(5), 806–810.

Bardach, J., Morris, H. L., & Olin, W. H. (1984). Late results of primary veloplasty: The Marburg Project. *Plastic and Reconstructive Surgery, 73*(2), 207–218.

Barone, C. M., & Argamaso, R. V. (1993). Refinements of the tongue flap for closure of difficult palatal fistulas. *Journal of Craniofacial Surgery, 4*(2), 109–111.

Becker, M., Svensson, H., McWilliam, J., Sarnas, K. V., & Jacobsson, S. (1998). Millard repair of unilateral isolated cleft lip: A 25-year follow-up. *Scandinavian Journal of Plastic and Reconstructive Surgery and Hand Surgery, 32*(4), 387–394.

Blocksma, R., Leuz, C. A., & Mellerstig, K. E. (1975). A conservative program for managing cleft palates without the use of mucoperiosteal flaps. *Plastic and Reconstructive Surgery, 55*(2), 160–169.

Brauer, R. O., & Cronin, T. D. (1983). The Tennison lip repair revisited. *Plastic and Reconstructive Surgery, 71*(5), 633–642.

Brothers, D. B., Dalston, R. W., Peterson, H. D., & Lawrence, W. T. (1995). Comparison of the Furlow double-opposing Z-palatoplasty with the Wardill-Kilner procedure for isolated clefts of the soft palate. *Plastic and Reconstructive Surgery, 95*(6), 969–977.

Brown, A. S., Cohen, M. A., & Randall, P. (1983). Levator muscle reconstruction: Does it make a difference? *Plastic and Reconstructive Surgery, 72*(1), 1–8.

Busic, N., Bagatin, M., & Boric, V. (1989). Tongue flaps in repair of large palatal defects. *International Journal of Oral Maxillofacial Surgery, 18*(5), 291–293.

Coghlan, K., O'Regan, B., & Carter, J. (1989). Tongue flap repair of oro-nasal fistulae in cleft palate patients. A review of 20 patients. *Journal of Craniomaxillofacial Surgery, 17*(6), 255–259.

Cosman, B., & Falk, A. S. (1980). Delayed hard palate repair and speech deficiencies: A cautionary report. *Cleft Palate Journal, 17*(1), 27–33.

Coston, G. N., Hagerty, R. F., Jannarone, R. J., McDonald, V., & Hagerty, R. C. (1986). Levator muscle reconstruction: Resulting velopharyngeal competence—A preliminary report. *Plastic and Reconstructive Surgery, 77*(6), 911–918.

D'Antonio, L. D., & Marsh, J. L. (1987). Abnormal carotid arteries in the velocardiofacial syndrome [Letter]. *Plastic and Reconstructive Surgery, 80*(3), 471–472.

Denny, A. D., Marks, S. M., & Oliff-Carneol, S. (1993). Correction of velopharyngeal insufficiency by pharyngeal augmentation using autologous cartilage: A preliminary report. *Cleft Palate Craniofacial Journal, 30*(1), 46–54.

de Serres, L. M., Deleyiannis, F. W., Eblen, L. E., Gruss, J. S., Richardson, M. A., & Sie, K. C. (1999). Results with sphincter pharyngoplasty and pharyngeal flap. *International Journal of Pediatric Otorhinolaryngology, 48*(1), 17–25.

Dingman, R. O., & Grabb, W. C. (1971). A rational program for surgical management of bilateral cleft lip and cleft palate. *Plastic and Reconstructive Surgery, 47*(3), 239–242.

Dreyer, T. M., & Trier, W. C. (1984). A comparison of palatoplasty techniques. *Cleft Palate Journal, 21*(4), 251–253.

Fara, M., & Brousilova, M. (1969). Experiences with early closure of velum and later closure of hard palate. *Plastic and Reconstructive Surgery, 44*(2), 134–141.

Fara, M., & Brousilova, M. (1988). [Long-term experience with 2-stage surgery of cleft palate in total unilateral and bilateral clefts from the aspect of maxillary development]. *Rozhledy v Chirugii, 67*(11), 729–741.

Fara, M., Brousilova, M., Hrivnakova, J., & Tvrdek, M. (1992). Long-term experiences with the two-stage palatoplasty with regard to the development of maxillary arch. *Acta Chirurgiae Plasticae, 34*(3), 138–142.

Finkelstein, Y., Zohar, Y., Nachmani, A., Talmi, Y. P., Lerner, M. A., Hauben, D. J., & Frydman, M. (1993). The otolaryngologist and the patient with velocardiofacial syndrome. *Archives of Otolaryngology—Head and Neck Surgery, 119*(5), 563–569.

Furlow, L. T., Jr. (1986). Cleft palate repair by double opposing Z-plasty. *Plastic and Reconstructive Surgery, 78*(6), 724–738.

Furlow, L. T., Jr. (1990). Flaps for cleft lip and palate surgery. *Clinics in Plastic Surgery, 17*(4), 633–644.

Furlow, L. T., Jr., Williams, W. N., Eisenbach, C. R. D., & Bzoch, K. R. (1982). A long-term study on treating velopharyngeal insufficiency by Teflon injection. *Cleft Palate Journal, 19*(1), 47–56.

Georgiade, N. G., & Latham, R. A. (1975). Maxillary arch alignment in the bilateral cleft lip and palate infant, using pinned coaxial screw appliance. *Plastic and Reconstructive Surgery, 56*(1), 52–60.

Gray, S. D., Pinborough-Zimmerman, J., & Catten, M. (1999). Posterior wall augmentation for treatment of velopharyngeal insufficiency. *Otolaryngology—Head and Neck Surgery, 121*(1), 107–112.

Gunther, E., Wisser, J. R., Cohen, M. A., & Brown, A. S. (1998). Palatoplasty: Furlow's double reversing Z-plasty versus intravelar veloplasty. *Cleft Palate Craniofacial Journal, 35*(6), 546–549.

Jackson, I. T. (1985). Sphincter pharyngoplasty. *Clinics in Plastic Surgery, 12*(4), 711–717.

Jackson, I. T., McGlynn, M. J., Huskie, C. F., & Dip, I. P. (1980). Velopharyngeal incompetence in the absence of cleft palate: Results of treatment in 20 cases. *Plastic and Reconstructive Surgery, 66*(2), 211–213.

Jackson, I. T., McLennan, G., & Scheker, L. R. (1983). Primary veloplasty or primary palatoplasty: Some preliminary findings. *Plastic and Reconstructive Surgery, 72*(2), 153–157.

Jackson, I. T., & Silverton, J. S. (1977). The sphincter pharyngoplasty as a secondary procedure in cleft palates. *Plastic and Reconstructive Surgery, 59*(4), 518–524.

James, N. K., Twist, M., Turner, M. M., & Milward, T. M. (1996). An audit of velopharyngeal incompetence treated by the Orticochea pharyngoplasty [see Comments]. *British Journal of Plastic Surgery, 49*(4), 197–201.

Jarvis, B. L., & Trier, W. C. (1988). The effect of intravelar veloplasty on velopharyngeal competence following pharyngeal flap surgery. *Cleft Palate Journal, 25*(4), 389–394.

Karling, J., Henningsson, G., Larson, O., & Isberg, A. (1999). Adaptation of pharyngeal wall adduction after pharyngeal flap surgery. *Cleft Palate Craniofacial Journal, 36*(2), 166–172.

Kasten, S. J., Buchman, S. R., Stevenson, C., & Berger, M. (1997). A retrospective analysis of revision sphincter pharyngoplasty. *Annals of Plastic Surgery, 39*(6), 583–589.

Latham, R. A. (1980). Orthopedic advancement of the cleft maxillary segment: A preliminary report. *Cleft Palate Journal, 17*(3), 227–233.

Latham, R. A., Kusy, R. P., & Georgiade, N. G. (1976). An extraorally activated expansion appliance for cleft palate infants. *Cleft Palate Journal, 13,* 253–261.

Lewis, M. B., & Pashayan, H. M. (1980). The effects of pharyngeal flap surgery on lateral pharyngeal wall motion: A videoradiographic evaluation. *Cleft Palate Journal, 17*(4), 301–308.

MacKenzie-Stepner, K., Witzel, M. A., Stringer, D. A., Lindsay, W. K., Munro, I. R., & Hughes, H. (1987). Abnormal carotid arteries in the velocardiofacial syndrome: A report of three cases. *Plastic and Reconstructive Surgery, 80*(3), 347–351.

Marsh, J. L., Grames, L. M., & Holtman, B. (1989). Intravelar veloplasty: A prospective study. *Cleft Palate Journal, 26*(1), 46–50.

Millard, D. R., Jr., & Latham, R. A. (1990). Improved primary surgical and dental treatment of clefts. *Plastic and Reconstructive Surgery, 86*(5), 856–871.

Millard, D. R., Latham, R., Huifen, X., Spiro, S., & Morovic, C. (1999). Cleft lip and palate treated by presurgical orthopedics, gingivoperiosteoplasty, and lip adhesion (POPLA) compared with previous lip adhesion method: A preliminary study of serial dental casts. *Plastic and Reconstructive Surgery, 103*(6), 1630–1644.

Murison, M. S., & Pigott, R. W. (1992). Medial Langenbeck: Experience of a modified Von Langenbeck repair of the cleft palate. A preliminary report. *British Journal of Plastic Surgery, 45*(6), 454–459.

Orticochea, M. (1970). Results of the dynamic muscle sphincter operation in cleft palates. *Brtish Journal of Plastic Surgery, 23*(2), 108–114.

Orticochea, M. (1983). A review of 236 cleft palate patients treated with dynamic muscle sphincter. *Plastic and Reconstructive Surgery, 71*(2), 180–188.

Orticochea, M. (1997). Physiopathology of the dynamic muscular sphincter of the pharynx. *Plastic and Reconstructive Surgery, 100*(7), 1918–1923.

Orticochea, M. (1999). The timing and management of dynamic muscular pharyngeal sphincter construction in velopharyngeal incompetence. *British Journal of Plastic Surgery, 52*(2), 85–87.

Perko, M. A. (1979). Two-stage closure of cleft palate (Progress report). *Journal of Maxillofacial Surgery, 7*(1), 46–80.

Pigott, R. W., Rieger, F. W., & Moodie, A. F. (1984). Tongue flap repair of cleft palate fistulae. *British Journal of Plastic Surgery, 37*(3), 285–293.

Posnick, J. C., & Getz, S. B., Jr. (1987). Surgical closure of end-stage palatal fistulas using anteriorly-based dorsal tongue flaps. *Journal of Oral Maxillofacial Surgery, 45*(11), 907–912.

Remacle, M., Bertrand, B., Eloy, P., & Marbaix, E. (1990). The use of injectable collagen to correct velopharyngeal insufficiency. *Laryngoscope, 100*(3), 269–274.

Ren, Y. F., & Wang, G. H. (1993). A modified palatopharyngeous flap operation and its application in the correction of velopharyngeal incompetence. *Plastic and Reconstructive Surgery, 91*(4), 612–617.

Riski, J. E., Ruff, G. L., Georgiade, G. S., & Barwick, W. J. (1992). Evaluation of failed sphincter pharyngoplasties. *Annals of Plastic Surgery, 28*(6), 545–553.

Riski, J. E., Ruff, G. L., Georgiade, G. S., Barwick, W. J., & Edwards, P. D. (1992). Evaluation of the sphincter pharyngoplasty. *Cleft Palate Craniofacial Journal, 29*(3), 254–261.

Roberts, T. M., & Brown, B. S. (1983). Evaluation of a modified sphincter pharyngoplasty in the treatment of speech problems due to palatal insufficiency. *Annals of Plastic Surgery, 10*(3), 209–213.

Ross, D. A., Witzel, M. A., Armstrong, D. C., & Thomson, H. G. (1996). Is pharyngoplasty a risk in velocardiofacial syndrome? An assessment of medially displaced carotid arteries. *Plastic and Reconstructive Surgery, 98*(7), 1182–1190.

Ross, R. B. (1987). Treatment variables affecting facial growth in complete unilateral cleft lip and palate. *Cleft Palate Journal, 24*(1), 5–23.

Schweckendiek, W. (1955). Zur zweiphasigen Gauimenspalten-operation bei primarem Velumerschluss. *Fortschritte Kiefer-und Gesichtschtschirurgie, 1,* 73–76.

Schweckendiek, W. (1966). [The technique of early veloplasty and its results]. *Acta Chirurgiae Plasticae, 8*(3), 188–194.

Schweckendiek, W. (1968). [Early veloplasty and its results]. *Acta Oto-Rhino-Laryngologica Belgica, 22*(6), 697–703.

Schweckendiek, W. (1983). [Primary closure of cleft lip and cleft palate]. *Zahnarztl Prax, 34*(8), 317–320.

Schweckendiek, W., & Doz, P. (1978). Primary veloplasty: Long-term results without maxillary deformity: A twenty-five year report. *Cleft Palate Journal, 15*(3), 268–274.

Sie, K. C., Tampakopoulou, D. A., de Serres, L. M., Gruss, J. S., Eblen, L. E., & Yonick, T. (1998). Sphincter pharyngoplasty: Speech outcome and complications. *Laryngoscope, 108*(8 Pt. 1), 1211–1217.

Skolnick, M. L., & McCall, G. N. (1972). Velopharyngeal competence and incompetence following pharyngeal flap surgery: Videofluoroscopic study in multiple projections. *Cleft Palate Journal, 9*(1), 1–12.

Terris, D. J., & Goode, R. L. (1993). Costochondral pharyngeal implants for velopharyngeal insufficiency. *Laryngoscope, 103*(5), 565–569.

Tharanon, W., Stella, J. P., & Epker, B. N. (1990). The modified superior-based pharyngeal flap: Part III. A retrospective study. *Oral Surgery, Oral Medicine, Oral Pathology, and Endodontics, 70*(3), 256–267.

Thind, M. S., Singh, A., & Thind, R. S. (1992). Repair of anterior secondary palate fistula using tongue flaps. *Acta Chirurgiae Plasticae, 34*(2), 79–91.

Trier, W. C. (1985a). The pharyngeal flap operation. *Clinics in Plastic Surgery, 12*(4), 697–710.

Trier, W. C. (1985b). Repair of bilateral cleft lip: Millard's technique. *Clinics in Plastic Surgery, 12*(4), 605–625.

Trier, W. C., & Dreyer, T. M. (1984). Primary von Langenbeck palatoplasty with levator reconstruction: Rationale and technique. *Cleft Palate Journal, 21*(4), 254–262.

Trigos, I., Ysunza, A., Gonzalez, A., & Vazquez, M. C. (1988). Surgical treatment of borderline velopharyngeal insufficiency using homologous cartilage implantation with videonasopharyngoscopic monitoring. *Cleft Palate Journal, 25*(2), 167–170.

Vedung, S. (1995). Pharyngeal flaps after one- and two-stage repair of the cleft palate: A 25-year review of 520 patients. *Cleft Palate Craniofacial Journal, 32*(3), 206–215; Discussion 215–216.

Wells, M. D., Vu, T. A., & Luce, E. A. (1999). Incidence and sequelae of nocturnal respiratory obstruction following posterior pharyngeal flap operation. *Annals of Plastic Surgery, 43*(3), 252–257.

Witt, P. D., D'Antonio, L. L., Zimmerman, G. J., & Marsh, J. L. (1994). Sphincter pharyngoplasty: A preoperative and postoperative analysis of perceptual speech characteristics and endoscopic studies of velopharyngeal dysfunction. *Plastic and Reconstructive Surgery, 93*(6), 1154–1168.

Witt, P. D., Marsh, J. L., Marty-Grames, L., & Muntz, H. R. (1995). Revision of the failed sphincter pharyngoplasty: An outcome assessment. *Plastic and Reconstructive Surgery, 96*(1), 129–138.

Witt, P. D., Marsh, J. L., Muntz, H. R., Marty-Grames, L., & Watchmaker, G. P. (1996). Acute obstructive sleep apnea as a complication of sphincter pharyngoplasty. *Cleft Palate Craniofacial Journal, 33*(3), 183–189.

Witt, P. D., O'Daniel, T. G., Marsh, J. L., Grames, L. M., Muntz, H. R., & Pilgram, T. K. (1997). Surgical management of velopharyngeal dysfunction: Outcome analysis of autogenous posterior pharyngeal wall augmentation. *Plastic and Reconstructive Surgery, 99*(5), 1287–1296; Discussion 1297–1300.

Witzel, M. A., Salyer, K. E., & Ross, R. B. (1984). Delayed hard palate closure: The philosophy revisited. *Cleft Palate Journal, 21*(4), 263–269.

Wolford, L. M., Oelschlaeger, M., & Deal, R. (1989). Proplast as a pharyngeal wall implant to correct velopharyngeal insufficiency. *Cleft Palate Journal, 26*(2), 119–126; Discussion 126–128.

Wu, J., & Epker, B. N. (1990). The modified superior based pharyngeal flap technique: Part II. An anatomic study. *Oral Surgery Oral Medicine Oral Pathology, 70*(3), 251–255.

Yoshida, H., Stella, J. P., Ghali, G. E., & Epker, B. N. (1992). The modified superiorly based pharyngeal flap: Part IV. Position of the base of the flap. *Oral Surgery Oral Medicine Oral Patholology, 73*(1), 13–18.

Ysunza, A., Garcia-Velasco, M., Garcia-Garcia, M., Haro, R., & Valencia, M. (1993). Obstructive sleep apnea secondary to surgery for velopharyngeal insufficiency. *Cleft Palate Craniofacial Journal, 30*(4), 387–390.

CHAPTER

19

Prosthetic Management

CONTENTS

Individuals with a history of cleft lip, cleft palate, or other craniofacial anomalies often have anatomical problems that affect facial aesthetics, dental arch stability, speech, mastication, and swallowing. Indirectly, these physical and functional problems can also affect the social, emotional, and psychological well-being of the patient in a very negative way.

Historically, patients with cleft lip and palate underwent multiple surgical and habilitative procedures in order to achieve an acceptable aesthetic and functional outcome. Surgical repairs were done later than they are today and the success of the surgical procedures was not as good as it is currently. Despite the best efforts of the surgeon, the patient often had remaining dental and maxillary arch deficiencies and also speech problems due to occlusal anomalies and velopharyngeal insufficiency. Because of these residual problems, prosthetic management was often the most effective form of treatment and, therefore, was commonly used. In recent years however, there has been an increase in the understanding of the nature of craniofacial growth and development. In addition, advancements and improvements in surgical techniques have resulted in greatly improved outcomes. Therefore, prosthetic devices are no longer needed to achieve optimum results in most patients, particularly those who received early and appropriate surgical intervention (Delgado, Schaaf, & Emrich, 1992).

Although surgery is usually the option of choice for correction or improvement of many of these structural and functional problems, there still is a need for prosthetic treatment in certain cases. The overall goal of management, whether it is through surgical or prosthetic treatment, is to obtain the optimum results. However, in choosing a treatment option for the patient, the patient, family, and health care providers must consider not only the expected outcome with each option, but also the total amount of time necessary to achieve results, the risks to the patient, the cost of treatment, and the desires of the patient. A successful treatment option is one that meets the particu-

lar needs and expectations of the patient and the family.

The purpose of this chapter is to discuss the various types of prosthetic devices available for individuals with a history of cleft lip/palate or other craniofacial conditions. Speech pathologists should be well informed about the options for prosthetic management and when it is appropriate for the patient.

Prosthetic Devices

When prosthetic management is chosen for treatment, a prosthesis is made for the patient to help to improve the anatomy through artificial measures. A *prosthesis*, also called a prosthetic device or appliance, is a fabricated substitute for a body part that is missing or malformed. This substitute may be fixed, so that it is essentially permanent, or it can be removable so that the patient can take it out for eating, sleeping, and cleaning. Prosthetic management can also be done on either a temporary basis prior to surgical correction or on a permanent basis.

Construction of a prosthetic device may be done by an orthodontist or pediatric dentist. However, this work is most often done by a prosthodontist who specializes in the construction of these devices. A *prosthodontist* is a dental professional who not only deals with the restoration of teeth, but also deals with the development of appliances to improve the appearance of oral and facial structures and to assist with feeding and velopharyngeal closure. The prosthodontist can be a very important member of a craniofacial team, because regardless of the surgical results, prosthodontists often can improve the speech and appearance of individuals with significant anomalies.

Dental Appliances

Patients with a history of cleft lip that includes the entire primary palate often have missing teeth, particularly in the line of the cleft. Individuals with other craniofacial anomalies are also at risk for missing and malformed teeth, in addition to malocclusion. In these cases, prosthetic management is appropriate. Facial aesthetics and the function of mastication can be improved significantly by the replacement of missing teeth or the correction of malocclusion and other forms of deviant dental anatomy.

There are significant challenges when attempting to replace teeth for individuals with a history of cleft of the primary palate. These challenges may include a shortened upper lip, decreased upper lip mobility due to scarring, protrusion of the premaxilla, spaces created by missing teeth, and supernumerary teeth. Additional problems include jaw discrepancies, an occlusal cant, distortion of the midline of the dentition and face, or scar tissue in the alveolar and palatal areas (Ramstad, 1998). Added to these challenges may be poor dental hygiene, which is common in this population due to psychological and actual neglect.

Replacement of teeth can be done in several ways. A *fixed bridge* is typically used to replace dental segments and complete *dentures* are used when all the teeth need to be replaced. If some of the teeth are to be retained but are not functional, *overlay dentures* are often used. Overlay dentures fit over the existing teeth and usually provide more vertical dimension. The long-term use of this type of denture can place the remaining teeth at risk for decay and periodontal disease due to the forms of retention and the accumulation of plaque. However, some individuals can benefit from overlay dentures. These are individuals who have overclosure of the vertical dimension, resulting in a deep bite. Overlay dentures can increase the vertical dimension to improve function and appearance. These dental appliances also can be combined with any type of speech appliance, if this is also needed.

Although malaligned teeth can make the fabrication of dentures a challenge, tooth extractions are typically avoided unless required for orthodontic purposes. The tooth may serve a purpose in the future, such as providing an anchor for a prosthetic device. Tooth extractions in the cleft area must be especially avoided because it usually results in resorption of the alveolar bone, which will widen and deepen the cleft. This tissue and bone loss may exceed that which can be replaced by a fixed partial prosthesis. Therefore, correction would result in a more complex reconstruction than if the tooth is preserved (McKinstry, 1998a).

Facial Prostheses

Individuals with craniofacial anomalies often demonstrate significant facial defects that affect the person's overall appearance to such a degree that their quality of life is greatly affected. Although surgical intervention often leads to correction, or at least improvement, this is not always the case. Acquired facial defects, due to an injury or ablative surgery for cancer, can be even more challenging to improve with surgery. In these cases, facial prosthetics are used and can result in a dramatic improvement in appearance (Grisius, 1991; Lundgren, Moy, Beumer III, & Lewis, 1993; Schaaf, 1984). Figure 19–1 shows the type of person who can benefit from a facial prosthesis and the result of prosthetic management. This type of rehabilitation can make a major difference in the person's life, allowing the person to function normally in society.

Facial prosthetics can be used to replace any missing or disfigured parts of the facial anatomy. For example, individuals with an aural atresia can benefit from the fabrication of a prosthetic ear. Although the ear will not be functional, it will appear very much like a real ear and thus, the anomaly is not noted by others. The same can be done for the eyes or nose, and even for the cheek (Singh, Bharadwaj, & Nair, 1997). The skilled prosthodontist is able to match skin color, skin tone, skin texture, and overall appearance so that the prosthesis blends in with the natural tissue. Even glossectomy patients can benefit from a specially de-

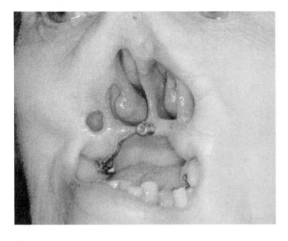

A

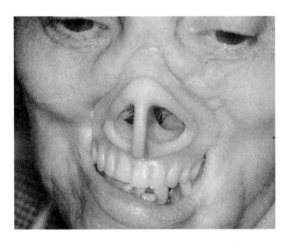

B

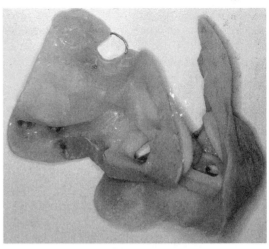

C

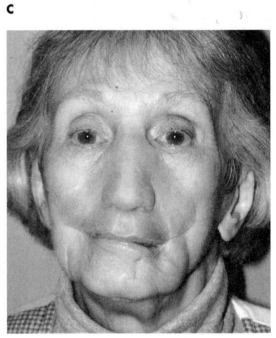

D

Figure 19-1. A. Patient with a history of squamous cell carcinoma. This patient underwent a midface resection that included the anterior maxilla, the upper lip and the nose. A gold bar spans across the defect and is secured and stabilized by dental implants. When in place, the prosthesis attaches to this bar through the use of two retentive pins. **B.** Prosthesis that includes a maxillary obturator and a nasal extension. On the nasal portion, there is a retentive ridge where the silicon prosthesis (nose, cheek and lip) snaps on for retention. **C.** Maxillary and nasal prosthesis in place. The soft tissue prosthesis attaches to this base. **D.** Both the maxillary and soft tissue prostheses in position. When the patient wears her glasses, this helps to further disguise the facial prosthesis.

428

signed prosthesis for the tongue (Aramany, Downs, Beery, & Aslan, 1982; Davis, Lazarus, Logemann, & Hurst, 1987).

Retention of the prosthesis is often accomplished through the use of *osseointegrated implants* (implants that are drilled in the bone) (Beumer, Roumanas, & Nishimura, 1995; Parel, Holt, Branemark, & Tjellstrom, 1986). With the implants in place, the prosthesis can be secured through the use of mechanical clips or magnetic bars. Because of what is involved to secure the device, facial prosthetics work best for adults who are responsible and motivated. They do not work as well for young children who may be less motivated and are certainly less responsible. In addition, periodic modifications and replacement are necessary for children as they grow.

Feeding Obturators

A feeding obturator is a prosthetic appliance that can be used in the first few months of life to assist the infant with cleft palate in feeding normally (Figure 19–2A). The obturator serves to cover the infant's unrepaired cleft palate during feeding. With the obturator in place, the nasal cavity is separated from the oral cavity, which helps to eliminate the regurgitation of liquids into the nose (Figure 19–2B). The feeding appliance keeps the tongue from resting inside the cleft, and it provides a solid surface so that the tongue can achieve compression of the nipple in order to express the milk. The appliance does not obturate the soft palate, however, so it does not help the infant to achieve suction, which would require complete closure (McKinstry, 1998b).

The feeding obturator is fabricated using plaster molds and is made of light-cured resins or acrylic. It is made so that it fits tightly against the roof of the mouth during feeding. Because the infant does not have teeth to anchor the appliance in place, suction against the palate and a tight fit are particularly important.

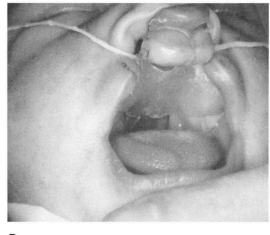

A

B

Figure 19–2. A. An infant feeding obturator. **B.** An infant feeding obturator in place. This type of obturator provides a separation of the nasal cavity from the oral cavity, which helps to eliminate the regurgitation of liquids into the nose. The feeding appliance also keeps the tongue from resting inside the cleft, and it provides a solid surface so that the tongue can achieve compression of the nipple to express the milk.

One or two holes are drilled in the appliance and dental floss is then tied to the appliance through the holes. These "strings" are attached to the appliance to make it easy for the caregiver to remove it following the feeding.

Although obturators are recommended and used in some centers across the country, many other centers feel that they are usually unnecessary. With other simple modifications, infants with cleft palate can feed adequately and gain weight appropriately. Usually, only infants with multiple structural anomalies of the airway or severe brain abnormalities require special feeding devices (Sidoti & Shprintzen, 1995). In fact, there are some obvious disadvantages of using feeding obturators. These include the expense of construction and the increased effort needed to train the parents and the infant in its use. For more information regarding feeding, please see Chapter 5.

Speech Appliances

When surgical correction of velopharyngeal dysfunction or a symptomatic fistula is not an option, prosthetic management is a very good alternative. Prosthetic devices can be developed to close the palate or the velopharyngeal port for speech. Therefore, they can be used effectively with patients who have a history of cleft palate (Gallagher, 1982; Gardner & Parr, 1996). The prosthetic device can improve overall oral resonance by allowing the sound energy to be directed appropriately for speech. This also results in a reduction in nasal air emission and an improvement in intraoral air pressure for consonant production.

Three types of speech appliances can be used to assist with speech production: a palatal obturator, a palatal lift, and a speech bulb obturator. The palatal obturator is used to close defects of the hard palate or velum. In contrast, the palatal lift and speech bulb obturator are used in the treatment of velopharyngeal dysfunction.

Each of these speech appliances is described separately in the following sections.

Palatal Lift

A *palatal lift* prosthesis is a removable device that elevates the velum and holds it in place against the posterior pharyngeal wall for speech (Figure 19–3). This device is positioned so that it elevates the velum at the point of its natural bend. A palatal lift is indicated in cases of velopharyngeal incompetence, where the velum is of sufficient length to achieve closure but does not move well enough to accomplish closure. A palatal lift is not useful if the cause of velopharyngeal dysfunction is a short velum because it does not add to the length or fill in the gap.

Neurological disorders account for the largest number of acquired conditions causing velopharyngeal dysfunction (Posnick, 1977). A palatal lift is very effective in the treatment of individuals with neurological impairment that prevents proper movement, timing and coordi-

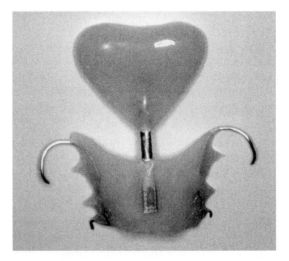

Figure 19–3. A palatal lift. This device is positioned so that it elevates the velum at the point of its natural bend.

nation of velopharyngeal structures. It can be particularly effective for dysarthric patients when hypernasality is the primary contributor to the unintelligibility of speech and articulation, phonation, and respiration are not severely compromised (Bedwinek & O'Brien, 1985; Dworkin & Johns, 1980; La Velle & Hardy, 1979; Marshall & Jones, 1971; Riski & Gordon, 1979; Schweiger, Netsell, & Sommerfeld, 1970; Yorkston, Beukelman, & Traynor, 1988). A palatal lift has even been used successfully with apraxia (Hall, Hardy, & LaVelle, 1990).

The palatal lift device consists of an anterior body that clasps to the teeth, and a fingerlike tail piece that extends to the velum. When treatment is first initiated, the tail piece may reach to the anterior portion of the velum only. As the patient learns to tolerate the device, this extension is gradually lengthened until it reaches the area of the velar dimple at the very least. The extension exerts an upward force against the velum to displace it in a superior and posterior direction. It is important that this tail piece is positioned correctly so that it can push the velum against the posterior pharyngeal wall in the area of maximum lateral pharyngeal wall movement. With the palatal lift in place, the velum is held against the posterior pharyngeal wall at all times. Because this is the appropriate position for speech, additional velar movement during speech is essentially unnecessary. However, the lateral pharyngeal walls must move against the velum to complete closure for speech.

Individuals who have a hyperactive gag reflex or those who are hypersensitive to touch in the area of the soft palate may require desensitization of the area before a palatal lift can be effective. Gentle massage of the soft palate with the index finger can help to increase the person's tolerance for touch in this area. The finger should massage the velum from side to side and then gradually move posteriorly (Daniel, 1982).

One disadvantage of a palatal lift is that, since the velum is held against the posterior

pharyngeal wall at all times, it can potentially interfere with the production of nasal sounds and nasal breathing. Nasal breathing often can be accomplished through openings on either side of the velum, because usually only the middle portion of the velopharyngeal port remains closed. However, hyponasality is often a necessary side effect of forced velopharyngeal closure for adequate oral speech. Fortunately, the palatal lift can be removed during sleep, so sleep apnea is not a concern.

Palatal Obturator

As noted above, a *palatal obturator* is a prosthetic device that can be used to cover an open palatal defect. Figure 19–4A shows a large palatal defect as a result of a maxillectomy for the treatment of cancer. Figure 19–4B shows the palatal obturator in place. The use of a palatal obturator is appropriate if the palatal opening is symptomatic during speech or causes nasal regurgitation during feeding, and surgical correction is not planned in the near future. This prosthetic appliance functions by closing off the nasal cavity from the oral cavity. For speech, this can normalize resonance and improve the ability to impound intraoral pressure for the production of speech.

The most common use of palatal obturators is to cover a palatal fistula. Although palatal fistulas do not occur as frequently as they did in the past, they still are a problem to be dealt with in caring for individuals with a history of cleft palate. When a fistula is present, the surgical closure is often delayed so that it can be done as part of another surgery. With either a delay in surgical correction or a decision not to surgically correct the fistula, obturation can be considered for temporary or permanent correction (Pinborough-Zimmerman, Canady, Yamashiro, & Morales, 1998).

At one time, some treatment centers subscribed to the theory that early cleft palate closure contributed to a reduction in midfacial growth, causing the high incidence of maxillary

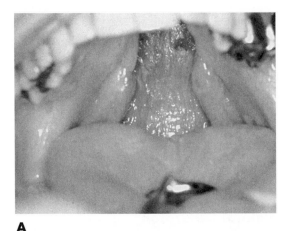

A

B

Figure 19–4. A. This is a patient with a large palatal defect following a maxillectomy for a malignancy. **B.** A palatal obturator. This is a prosthetic device that can be used to cover even a very large open palatal defect. It is appropriate if surgical correction is not indicated or will be delayed and the palatal opening is large enough to be symptomatic during speech or feeding. (This obturator is combined with a speech bulb.)

deficiency in this population (Schweckendiek, 1966, 1968). To counter this effect, these centers opted to close only the velum at an early age and leave the hard palate open until facial growth was complete (around age 14 for girls and age 18 for boys). Therefore, obturators were commonly used to close the clefts of the palate until the palate was ultimately repaired. More recent research has suggested that it is not the

early repair that affects maxillary growth, but rather the inherent deficiency in the maxilla. Therefore, surgical correction of hard palate and velum are now done at the same time, usually around 10 months of age.

Certainly early surgery is the preferred method of treatment to permit normal articulation development. However, when early surgery is not planned for medical reasons, prosthetic management can provide an alternative treatment to promote more normal articulation development, especially if the child receives some speech stimulation (Berkowitz, 1985; Lohmander-Agerskov, Soderpalm, Friede, & Lilja, 1990). The prosthesis should be placed prior to development of meaningful speech to avoid the development of compensatory articulation productions (Dorf, Reisberg, & Gold, 1985).

Although obturators are used less frequently with children, they remain a very important method of treatment for adult patients. They can be effective in covering defects for patients who have undergone ablative surgery due cancer or other maxillary tumors (Myers & Aramany, 1977). They also can be used for those who have had traumatic injuries to the palate. In these cases, surgical correction is usually not an option. Therefore, correction with a prosthetic obturator is a good and effective alternative.

A palatal obturator consists of an acrylic body that looks similar to a dental retainer. However, it has additional acrylic on the top of the appliance, which should fit perfectly into the area of deficiency. The obturator is made to tightly fill in the area of the defect to prevent a leak of air pressure or fluid into the nasal cavity. If the obturator has to be large in order to fill in the defect, it can be hollowed out so that its weight does not cause a problem for retention (Blair & Hunter, 1998).

Speech Bulb Obturator

A *speech bulb obturator,* also known as a *speech aid appliance,* is also a removable device that is used for the treatment of velopharyngeal insufficiency. When the velum is short relative to the depth of the posterior pharyngeal wall, resulting in a velopharyngeal opening during speech, the bulb serves to fill in the pharyngeal space. Figure 19–5A shows a speech bulb obturator. Figure 19–5B shows the same speech bulb in place. The bulb sits in the nasopharynx to occlude the velopharyngeal port during speech. This improves speech and can also improve swallowing, because it eliminates nasal regurgitation. A speech bulb obturator, as with any other type of appliance, can be combined with partial or complete dentures. Figure 19–6A shows a patient with a very short velum and dental implants. A speech bulb that combines a denture is seen in Figure 19–6B. This same prosthesis, with the over dentures, is seen in place in Figure 19–6C.

The speech bulb obturator usually has an oral base section that clasps to the teeth and then a posterior palatal strap with the bulb on the end. The bulb courses upward to fit behind the velum in the nasopharynx. When it is in place, the speech bulb is not visible from an intraoral perspective.

Speech bulb appliances must be removable for several reasons. First, breathing and sleeping could potentially be difficult with the bulb in place. Removal of the appliance at night allows breathing to be normalized and eliminates the risk of sleep apnea. Although the appliance can help to improve swallowing and eliminate nasal regurgitation, some individuals prefer to remove the appliance during meals. Finally, removal of the bulb is necessary so that it can be cleaned for good oral hygiene.

Fabrication of a Speech Appliance

Speech appliances are individually designed to meet the specific needs of the patient. Therefore, they do not all look the same. In fact, there is considerable variation. In addition, dental professionals may differ in some of the techniques and materials that are used. However, there are many commonalties among speech devices in the way that they are designed.

Most speech appliances have an anterior *palatal section*, which is the body portion of the appliance. In some cases, this part of the prosthesis may appear similar to a common ortho-

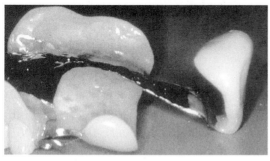

A

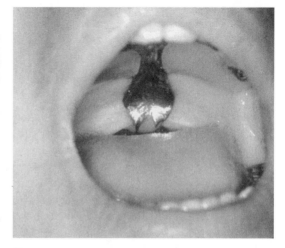

B

Figure 19–5. A. A speech bulb obturator. **B.** The speech bulb obturator in place. The bulb sits in the nasopharynx to occlude the velopharyngeal port during speech. This improves speech and can also improve swallowing, becasue it eliminates nasal regurgitation.

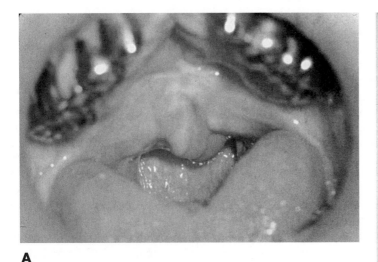

A

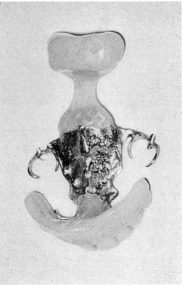

B

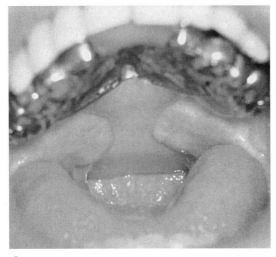

C

Figure 19–6. A. A patient with a very short velum and dental implants. **B.** A speech bulb obturator with dentures. **C.** The speech bulb obturator in place with the over dentures.

dontic retainer. The palatal section is designed to fit snugly against the contours of the individual's teeth and hard palate so that it can resist movement during oral activity. The purpose of this section is to hold the appliance in place against the roof of the mouth. It can also serve as an obturator to close off a defect in the palate.

The palatal section is usually made of either acrylic resins or metal, and is formed from a plaster model of the roof of the mouth. Artificial palatal rugae can also be added to assist with tongue tip orientation and articulation (Gitto, Esposito, & Draper, 1999; Weiss, 1974). This part of the appliance must be made thick enough to avoid easy breakage, but not so thick as to interfere with speech production. The palatal section is held in place by metal wires, which are attached around the teeth for anchorage. The teeth may need to be prepared with buccal lugs on soldered bands, special caps, crowns, or undercuts to adequately retain the wires and the appliance.

The palatal lift and speech bulb appliances are designed to close the middle portion of the velopharyngeal port so that the lateral pharyngeal walls can be more effective in achieving closure against this area during speech. These devices have an extension, or *tail piece*, that projects posteriorly. The palatal appliance is fabricated first, as it forms the basis of the rest of the prosthesis. In designing a palatal lift or speech bulb, the speech pathologist should work closely with the prosthodontist by providing information on speech changes that occur as a result of modifications to the device.

In fabricating a speech bulb obturator, the prosthodontist starts with a small bulb and then slowly adds a thin layer of thermoplastic wax compound until the appropriate size and shape are achieved. This is usually done by putting it in the individual's mouth and having the patient move the head up and down, and back and forth to mold the bulb appropriately. Wax is gradually added to the bulb until it fits comfortably and works effectively in the pharynx. The challenge is to make the bulb fill the space, while keeping it from causing undue pressure against the soft tissue of the pharynx. The individual must be able to move the head without discomfort or irritation of pharyngeal mucosa (Weiss, 1974). Once the form is finalized, the permanent bulb is made of acrylic. If the bulb needs to be large, it may become too heavy for the teeth to bear. When this is the case, the bulb can be hollowed out to make it lighter and more stable.

One of the biggest challenges for the prosthodontist is when a patient with an edentulous maxilla requires a speech aid appliance. Retention and stability of the appliance can be a significant problem without the use of teeth for anchors. Fortunately, recent advances in implant prosthodontics have greatly increased the ability to rehabilitate individuals with intraoral anomalies and an edentulous dental arch (Grisius, 1991; Hudson & Russell, 1994; Lundqvist & Haraldson, 1992; Lundqvist, Haraldson, & Lindblad, 1992; Parel, Branemark, & Jansson, 1986; Parel, Branemark, Tjellstrom, & Gion, 1986). Problems with retention due to a lack of teeth can now be minimized or even resolved with the use of osseointegrated implants. *Osseointegrated implants* are small cylinders (4 mm or less in diameter) that are usually made of titanium. They are fitted into a carefully prepared channel that is drilled into the alveolar bone. At least four implants of a minimum of 10 mm in length are usually recommended in the maxilla of patients with clefts (Ramstad, 1998). Once in place, the bone grows directly to the implant, resulting in osseointegration and a pseudo root. With these implants embedded in the bone, a speech appliance can be attached and retained. Implants can also be used to support dental restorations. A single implant can support a crown to replace an individual tooth. Multiple implants can be used to support restorations of a row of missing teeth or to secure dentures for an entire dental arch.

Depending on the needs of the patient, various combinations of appliances can be constructed. For example, the speech appliance may have an alveolar section with partial or complete dentures. A palatal obturator can be combined with a palatal lift or speech bulb (see Figure 19–4B). (Alpine, Stone, & Badr, 1990) or it can be used with an expansion appliance (Hobson & Clasper, 1995). A maxillary prostheses and mandibular prostheses can also be combined if this results in increased function (Davis et al., 1987). Although these combinations are very beneficial to the patient, the mechanical design of prosthetic appliances should be kept as simple as possible. Wear and tear on the device should be expected and breakage will occasionally occur. Therefore, devices that are simple and easy to repair are best in the long term (Mazahari, 1996). It is also most important that the device is designed so that oral hygiene can be maintained.

Some children and adults learn to accept and tolerate the prosthetic appliance quickly and easily, especially those who are motivated to work for aesthetic or speech improvement. On the other hand, some patients, particularly young children, are less compliant and even resistant to wearing a prosthetic device. In these cases, working through the family is the best avenue for achieving compliance and the inherent benefits of the device. In fact, the success of this form of intervention may depend on the understanding and motivation of the family, and their willingness to work with the patient on habituation of the device and habilitation of the speech. Close cooperation among the surgeon, speech pathologist, and prosthodontist is also necessary to ensure maximal benefits through prosthetic treatment.

Procedures for Assessment and Modification of a Speech Appliance

In comparison to a palatal lift or a speech bulb, a palatal obturator is very easy to fit because the fistula can and should be totally closed. However, for the other appliances, fine adjustments must be made to the appliance so that the velopharyngeal port is closed enough for speech, but not overly closed so that it causes upper airway problems. Achieving an appropriate balance of good speech and normal nasal breathing is the ultimate goal. Therefore, the speech pathologist should provide appropriate feedback to the prosthodontist so that the device can be adjusted for optimal function.

When perceptual measures are used to assess the effectiveness of the speech appliance, the examiner should test the production of pressure-sensitive phonemes, such as plosives, fricatives, and affricates. The examiner could use a listening tube or a See Scape (Pro Ed, Austin, TX) for further information regarding the closure of the velopharyngeal port. If pres-

sure-sensitive sounds can be produced in words and sentences without nasal air emission and there is no evidence of hypernasality, then the velopharyngeal port is closed adequately for speech. The speech pathologist should then assess the ease of nasal breathing with the appliance in place and also test the production of nasal sounds (m, n, ng) in words and sentences. Based on this assessment, the appliance can be modified until an appropriate balance is achieved between closure for oral speech and patency for nasal breathing and the production of nasal phonemes (Rosen & Bzoch, 1997).

In addition to a perceptual assessment of the effect of the appliance, indirect instrumental measures can be used to evaluate the effectiveness of a prosthetic appliance. Aerodynamic measures (Reisberg & Smith, 1985; Riski, Hoke, & Dolan, 1989) and nasometry (Pinborough-Zimmerman et al., 1998; Scarsellone, Rochet, & Wolfaardt, 1999) are indirect instrumental procedures that can give objective information regarding the extent of improvement with the appliance, and the relative normalcy of the speech as a result. They also provide information regarding the patency of the airway while the appliance is in place.

Although a perceptual assessment and indirect instrumental assessment techniques are helpful in evaluating the effect of an appliance, these procedures do not give adequate information if the appliance needs to be adjusted. When adjustments are necessary, the prosthodontist needs to know where the appliance should be augmented and where it should be shaved down. For this information, a direct instrumental approach is needed so that the extent of closure can be visualized. Although a lateral cephalometric X ray or videofluoroscopy could be used (Mazaheri & Hoffman, 1962; Turner & Williams, 1991), radiation risk and limitations in visualization make radiographic techniques less than ideal. Therefore, the best procedure for assessment of velopharyngeal function with the appliance in place is nasopharyngoscopy.

Using nasopharyngoscopy, the extent of velopharyngeal closure with the device in place can be easily determined. The nasal perspective provides valuable information not visible from the oral view. With nasopharyngoscopy, the construction of the prosthesis is more accurate because the examiner can verify the soft tissue-obturator contact during speech (D'Antonio, Muntz, Marsh, Marty-Grames, & Backensto-Marsh, 1988; Karnell, Rosenstein, & Fine, 1987; Rich, Farber, & Shprintzen, 1988; Riski et al., 1989; Turner & Williams, 1991). An optimal fit often requires trial and error and several adjustments to the appliance. If one side of the velopharyngeal port is not closing adequately, then the appliance can be augmented on that side. The patency of the airway can also be evaluated with this technique. At times, the airway must be compromised slightly for the best speech benefit. At other times, perfect speech must be compromised for the sake of the airway. With the benefit of a nasopharyngoscopy view, the device can be modified until closure appears to be optimal for speech and there is an adequate nasal airway.

Clinical Indications and Contraindications for Prosthetic Management

Although surgical correction is usually considered the best option for the treatment of structural defects, there are cases where prosthetic management is more appropriate or necessary. These include patients with a history of cleft for whom surgery must be delayed due to a medical condition or the need to do other procedures first. Prosthetic devices can be used effectively in the management of large soft palate perforations or palatal fistulas. They can also be appropriate for patients with velopharyngeal insufficiency or incompetence secondary to unsuccessful surgical repairs (Hoffman, 1985). For example, if a pharyngeal flap was done, but the lateral ports do not close sufficiently, a device can be made that has a bulb on each side of the flap to fill in the area of the ports (McKinstry, 1998a). If the prosthodontist is routinely consulted in the initial treatment planning, alternatives to surgical management might be considered for patients with high potential for postsurgical failure (McKinstry & Aramany, 1985). Occasionally, individuals will have problems with velopharyngeal function following a uvulopalatopharyngoplasty (UPPP), which is done to alleviate snoring and sleep apnea. When this occurs, prosthetic management is often appropriate, because there is no risk of causing further sleep problems with this form of correction (Finkelstein, Shifman, Nachmani, & Ophir, 1995).

Prosthetic management is particularly useful following cancer treatment, especially if the treatment involved ablative surgery of the maxilla or velum (Myers & Aramany, 1977; Ramsey & Quarantillo, 1977). Patients with oral carcinomas often require resection of other parts of the mouth, including the tongue, the floor of the mouth, or the bone of the mandible. Postoperatively, these patients often encounter problems with chewing, swallowing, and speech. In these cases, prosthetic treatment may include a tongue prosthesis or other prostheses, in addition to the palatal device. Prosthetic management of this type can help to improve articulation, resonance, and swallowing. Socialization is also enhanced through the improved appearance that these prosthetic devices can provide (Aramany et al., 1982).

Patients who exhibit normal velopharyngeal anatomy, but demonstrate velopharyngeal incompetence secondary to neuromotor disorders may not be appropriate surgical candidates (La Velle & Hardy, 1979). However, prosthetic management may be used very effectively. As mentioned before, individuals with dysarthria (Bedwinek & O'Brien, 1985; Dworkin & Johns, 1980; Riski & Gordon, 1979) or apraxia (Hall et al., 1990) may derive significant benefit from a prosthetic device, particularly a palatal lift. This allows the individual to concentrate on anterior articulation and not be concerned about velopharyngeal articulation.

One advantage of using a prosthetic device instead of surgery for the treatment of velopharyngeal dysfunction is that it is not a permanent correction; therefore, in cases where the outcome of correction is unclear, a prosthetic device can be used on a trial basis. The biggest advantage, however, is that this form of management can be used successfully when options for surgical correction have been exhausted or when surgical correction is contraindicated for medical reasons. In addition, prosthetic management is often used very successfully in facilitating the improvement of faulty speech characteristics of individuals with velopharyngeal dysfunction due to neurogenic causes.

Prosthetic management is usually most successful with individuals who have adequate dentition for retention of the device. Good oral hygiene is also very important because the device makes attention to hygiene even more important. Another consideration when trying to fit a palatal lift of speech bulb is the gag reflex. Although the prosthodontist can work to gradually desensitize the patient to the device, a strong gag reflex or oral sensitivity makes successful prosthetic management very difficult, if not impossible, to achieve. Finally, successful prosthetic management is somewhat dependent on good articulation because corrected velopharyngeal function for speech will not improve intelligibility significantly if the articulation is poor.

Although prosthetic devices have been used successfully by many patients for correction of velopharyngeal dysfunction, they have some distinct disadvantages. Unlike surgery, these devices do not result in a permanent correction. In fact, they usually need to be removed at night

and during eating, and with removal, the speech symptoms recur. When they are removed, they can be easily lost or damaged. Of course, manual dexterity or the assistance of others is important for proper insertion and removal of the device. Because of these limitations, removable prosthetic devices are not well suited for patients who are very young, are mentally retarded, or have significant physical handicaps.

Additional disadvantages of prosthetic management are that they may be uncomfortable to wear and can cause ulceration of the surrounding mucosa. As a result, they may be poorly tolerated, especially by children. For a variety of reasons, compliance is often poor with prosthetic devices. In young children, appliances require frequent adjustments as the child grows, and this increases the cost. Finally, retention of appliances can be a challenge for patients with a history of cleft palate or craniofacial anomalies due to irregularities in the dentition and missing teeth. This is a particular problem in treating children who are at the age where there are frequent changes due to dental exfoliation and eruption. Because of these limitations, prosthetic devices are used most frequently with adults and patients who are able to undergo surgical correction usually do opt for surgery after a period of prosthetic management (Marsh & Wray, 1980). However, despite their limitations, prosthetic devices should always be considered for correction of a palatal defect or velopharyngeal dysfunction when surgery is not an option for medical reasons (McKinstry, 1998a).

Prosthetic Management and Speech Therapy

Speech therapy cannot correct velopharyngeal dysfunction or hypernasality. However, once there is sufficient improvement in velopharyngeal function with prosthetic treatment, speech therapy is often required to further improve the speech (Fletcher & Sooudi, 1973; Gallagher, 1982; La Velle & Hardy, 1979.) The presence of a speech appliance does not correct articulation, but it does improve the ability to impound intraoral air pressure, and thus produce oral sounds. Speech therapy is necessary to help the individual to learn to use this air pressure to produce sounds normally. Therapy is also needed to eliminate any compensatory articulation productions that developed prior to the prosthetic management. Finally, speech therapy can be effective in eliminating the nasal rustle (turbulence) that often occurs due to a very small or inconsistent opening with the prosthesis in place.

Prosthetic devices have also been used as a form of therapy to attempt to improve velopharyngeal function. This type of therapy, called *reduction therapy*, is done in hopes of stimulating increased movement of the velopharyngeal structures in order to avoid surgery or reduce the extent of the surgery that is needed. When a palatal lift is used in reduction therapy, the length of the lift is gradually reduced, or the wearing time of the lift is gradually decreased, in hopes of stimulating velar movement. If a speech bulb is used, the size of the bulb is gradually reduced, allowing for the lateral pharyngeal walls to increase mobility and excursion gradually. When reduction therapy is used, the ultimate goal is to improve velopharyngeal function so that surgical management is either not needed, or the extent of management, such as the size of the pharyngeal flap, is reduced. An outcome study of speech bulb reduction therapy at Montifiore Hospital in New York initially revealed some positive results (Golding-Kushner, Cisneros, & LeBlanc, 1995). Of the 31 patients in the study, all of the patients were able to undergo a reduction in the size of the speech bulb, and still maintain normal speech. One question that comes to mind, however, is whether the speech bulb was larger than absolutely needed at the beginning of treatment. Only two of the patients in this study did not need further surgical management, despite the prosthetic treatment. Golding-Kushner has also reported that the results achieved with reduction therapy are not always maintained. Therefore, the true efficacy of this type of treatment remains in question, especially because most individuals who undergo reduction programs still require surgical intervention for correction (Witt et al., 1995; Wolfaardt, Wilson, Rochet, & McPhee, 1993). Considering this fact, and the time and expense of the prosthesis and speech therapy, surgical correction may still be the most appropriate and effective option for correction of velopharyngeal dysfunction.

Summary

Prosthetic management is not required in the habilitation of individuals who have repaired clefts as frequently as in years past. With the advances in surgical procedures and improvement in the timing of surgery, the outcomes of surgical intervention are usually superior to those that can be obtained with prosthetic management. However, in certain cases, there is a definite need for prosthetic management, particularly when surgical intervention is not an option. Prosthetic management can be very effective in improving the individual's appearance, swallowing, and speech. The ultimate goal of prosthetic management is to meet the needs of the patient and to achieve the best possible result.

References

Alpine, K. D., Stone, C. R., & Badr, S. E. (1990). Combined obturator and palatal-lift prosthesis: A case report. *Quintessence International, 21*(11), 893–896.

Aramany, M. A., Downs, J. A., Beery, Q. C., & Aslan, Y. (1982). Prosthodontic rehabilitation for glossectomy patients. *Journal of Prosthetic Dentistry, 48*(1), 78–81.

Bedwinek, A. P., & O'Brien, R. L. (1985). A patient selection profile for the use of speech prostheses in adult dysarthria. *Journal of Communciation Disorders, 18*(3), 169–182.

Berkowitz, S. (1985). Timing cleft palate closure— Age should not be the sole determinant. *Journal of Craniofacial Genetics and Developmental Biology Supplement, 1,* 69–83.

Beumer, J., III, Roumanas, E., & Nishimura, R. (1995). Advances in osseointegrated implants for dental and facial rehabilitation following major head and neck surgery. *Seminars in Surgical Oncology, 11*(3), 200–207.

Blair, F. M., & Hunter, N. R. (1998). The hollow box maxillary obturator. *British Dental Journal, 184*(10), 484–487.

Daniel, B. (1982). A soft palate desensitization procedure for patients requiring palatal lift prostheses. *Journal of Prosthetic Dentistry, 48*(5), 565–566.

D'Antonio, L. L., Muntz, H. R., Marsh, J. L., Marty-Grames, L., & Backensto-Marsh, R. (1988). Practical application of flexible fiberoptic nasopharyngoscopy for evaluating velopharyngeal function. *Plastic and Reconstructive Surgery, 82*(4), 611–618.

Davis, J. W., Lazarus, C., Logemann, J., & Hurst, P. S. (1987). Effect of a maxillary glossectomy prosthesis on articulation and swallowing. *Journal of Prosthetic Dentistry, 57*(6), 715–719.

Delgado, A. A., Schaaf, N. G., & Emrich, L. (1992). Trends in prosthodontic treatment of cleft palate patients at one institution: A twenty-one year review. *Cleft Palate Craniofacial Journal, 29*(5), 425–428.

Dorf, D. S., Reisberg, D. J., & Gold, H. O. (1985). Early prosthetic management of cleft palate. Articulation development prosthesis: A preliminary report. *Journal of Prosthetic Dentistry, 53*(2), 222–226.

Dworkin, J. P., & Johns, D. F. (1980). Management of velopharyngeal incompetence in dysarthria: A historical review. *Clinics in Otolaryngology, 5,* 61–74.

Finkelstein, Y., Shifman, A., Nachmani, A., & Ophir, D. (1995). Prosthetic management of velopharyngeal insufficiency induced by uvulopalatopharyngoplasty. *Otolaryngology—Head and Neck Surgery, 113*(5), 611–616.

Fletcher, S. G., & Sooudi, I. (1973). Joint prosthetics and speech treatment of hypernasality: Report of case. *Journal of the American Dental Association, 87*(7), 1418–1425.

Gallagher, B. (1982). Prosthesis in velopharyngeal insufficiency: Effect on nasal resonance. *Journal of Communication Disorders, 15*(6), 469–473.

Gardner, L. K., & Parr, G. R. (1996). Prosthetic rehabilitation of the cleft palate patient. *Seminars in Orthodontics, 2*(3), 215–219.

Gitto, C. A., Esposito, S. J., & Draper, J. M. (1999). A simple method of adding palatal rugae to a complete denture. *Journal of Prosthetic Dentistry, 81*(2), 237–239.

Golding-Kushner, K. J., Cisneros, G., & LeBlanc, E. (1995). Speech bulbs. In R. J. Shprintzen & J. Bardach (Eds.), *Cleft palate speech management* (pp. 352–363). St. Louis, MO: Mosby.

Grisius, R. J. (1991). Maxillofacial prosthetics. *Current Opinions in Dentistry, 1*(2), 155–159.

Hall, P. K., Hardy, J. C., & LaVelle, W. E. (1990). A child with signs of developmental apraxia of speech with whom a palatal lift prosthesis was used to manage palatal dysfunction. *Journal of Speech and Hearing Disorders, 55*(3), 454–460.

Hobson, R. S., & Clasper, R. (1995). A combined obturator and expansion appliance for use in patients with patent oral-nasal fistula. *British Journal of Orthodontics, 22*(4), 357–359.

Hoffman, S. (1985). Correction of lateral port stenosis following a pharyngeal flap operation. *Cleft Palate Journal, 22*(1), 51–55.

Hudson, J. W., & Russell, R., Jr. (1994). Contributions within dental science to cleft lip/palate management: A literature review. *Compendium, 15*(1), 116, 118–120, 122 passim; Quiz 126.

Karnell, M. P., Rosenstein, H., & Fine, L. (1987). Nasal videoendoscopy in prosthetic management of palatopharyngeal dysfunction. *Journal of Prosthetic Dentistry, 58*(4), 479–484.

La Velle, W. E., & Hardy, J. C. (1979). Palatal lift prostheses for treatment of palatopharyngeal incompetence. *Journal of Prosthetic Dentistry, 42*(3), 308–315.

Lohmander-Agerskov, A., Soderpalm, E., Friede, H., & Lilja, J. (1990). Cleft lip and palate patients prior to delayed closure of the hard palate: Evaluation of maxillary morphology and the effect of early stimulation on pre-school speech. *Scandinavian*

Journal of Plastic and Reconstructive Surgery and Hand Surgery, 24(2), 141–148.

Lundgren, S., Moy, P. K., Beumer, J., III, & Lewis, S. (1993). Surgical considerations for endosseous implants in the craniofacial region: A 3-year report. *International Journal of Oral and Maxillofacial Surgery, 22,* 272–277.

Lundqvist, S., & Haraldson, T. (1992). Oral function in patients wearing fixed prosthesis on osseointegrated implants in the maxilla: 3-year follow-up study. *Scandinavian Journal of Dental Research, 100*(5), 279–283.

Lundqvist, S., Haraldson, T., & Lindblad, P. (1992). Speech in connection with maxillary fixed prostheses on osseointegrated implants: A three-year follow-up study. *Clinics in Oral Implants Research, 3*(4), 176–180.

Marsh, J. L., & Wray, R. C. (1980). Speech prosthesis versus pharyngeal flap: A randomized evaluation of the management of velopharyngeal incompetency. *Plastic and Reconstructive Surgery, 65*(5), 592–594.

Marshall, R. C., & Jones, R. N. (1971, March). Effects of a palatal lift prosthesis upon the speech intelligibility of a dysarthric patient. *Journal of Prosthetic Dentistry,* 327–333.

Mazahari, M. (1996). Prosthetic speech appliances for patients with cleft palate. In S. Berkowitz (Ed.), *Cleft lip and palate with introduction to other craniofacial abnormalities: Perspectives in management* (Vol. 2, pp. 177–194). San Diego, CA: Singular Publishing Group.

Mazaheri, M., & Hoffman, F. A. (1962). Cineradiography speech appliance construction. *Journal of Prosthetic Dentistry, 12,* 571–575.

McKinstry, R. E. (1998a). Cleft palate prosthetics. In R. E. McKinstry (Ed.), *Cleft palate dentistry* (pp. 206–235). Arlington, VA: ABI Professional Publications.

McKinstry, R. E. (1998b). Presurgical management of cleft lip and palate patients. In R. E. McKinstry (Ed.), *Cleft palate dentistry* (pp. 33–66). Arlington, VA: ABI Professional Publications.

McKinstry, R. E., & Aramany, M. A. (1985). Prosthodontic considerations in the management of surgically compromised cleft palate patients. *Journal of Prosthetic Dentistry, 53*(6), 827–831.

Myers, E. N., & Aramany, M. A. (1977). Rehabilitation of the oral cavity following resection of the hard and soft palate. *Transactions of the American Academy of Ophthalmology and Otolaryngology, 84*(5), ORL941–951.

Parel, S. M., Branemark, P. I., & Jansson, T. (1986). Osseointegration in maxillofacial prosthetics: Part I. Intraoral applications. *Journal of Prosthetic Dentistry, 55*(4), 490–494.

Parel, S. M., Branemark, P. I., Tjellstrom, A., & Gion, G. (1986). Osseointegration in maxillofacial prosthetics: Part II. Extraoral applications. *Journal of Prosthetic Dentistry, 55*(5), 600–606.

Parel, S. M., Holt, G. R., Branemark, P. I., & Tjellstrom, A. (1986). Osseointegration and facial prosthetics. *International Journal of Oral and Maxillofacial Implants, 1*(1), 27–29.

Pinborough-Zimmerman, J., Canady, C., Yamashiro, D. K., & Morales, L., Jr. (1998). Articulation and nasality changes resulting from sustained palatal fistula obturation. *Cleft Palate Craniofacial Journal, 35*(1), 81–87.

Posnick, W. R. (1977). Prosthetic management of palatopharyngeal incompetency for the pediatric patient. *Journal of Dentistry for Children, 44*(2), 117–121.

Ramsey, W. O., & Quarantillo, E. P. (1977). Prosthetic obturation subsequent to total resection of the soft palate. A comparison of two case histories. *Journal of the Baltimore College of Dental Surgery, 32*(1), 50–68.

Ramstad, T. (1998). Fixed prosthodontics. In R. E. McKinstry (Ed.), *Cleft palate dentistry* (pp. 236–262). Arlington, VA: ABI Professional Publications.

Reisberg, D. J., & Smith, B. E. (1985). Aerodynamic assessment of prosthetic speech aids. *Journal of Prosthetic Dentistry, 54*(5), 686–690.

Rich, B. M., Farber, K., & Shprintzen, R. J. (1988). Nasopharyngoscopy in the treatment of palatopharyngeal insufficiency. *International Journal of Prosthodontics, 1*(3), 248–251.

Riski, J. E., & Gordon, D. (1979). Prosthetic management of neurogenic velopharyngeal incompetency. *North Carolina Dental Journal, 62*(1), 24–26.

Riski, J. E., Hoke, J. A., & Dolan, E. A. (1989). The role of pressure flow and endoscopic assessment in successful palatal obturator revision. *Cleft Palate Journal, 26*(1), 56–62.

Rosen, M. S., & Bzoch, K. R. (1997). Prosthodontic management of the individual with cleft lip and palate for speech habilitation needs. In K. R. Bzoch (Ed.), *Communicative disorders related to cleft lip and palate* (Vol. 4, pp. 153–168). Austin, TX: Pro-Ed.

Scarsellone, J. M., Rochet, A. P., & Wolfaardt, J. F. (1999). The influence of dentures on nasalance values in speech. *Cleft Palate Craniofacial Journal, 36*(1), 51–56.

Schaaf, N. G. (1984). Maxillofacial prosthetics and the head and neck cancer patient. *Cancer, 54*(11, Suppl.), 2682–2690.

Schweckendiek, W. (1966). [The technic of early veloplasty and its results]. *Acta Chiruriae Plasticae, 8*(3), 188–194.

Schweckendiek, W. (1968). [Early veloplasty and its results]. *Acta Oto-Rhino-Laryngologica Belgica, 22*(6), 697–703.

Schweiger, J. W., Netsell, R., & Sommerfeld, R. M. (1970). Prosthetic management and speech improvement in individuals with dysarthria of the palate. *Journal of the American Dental Association, 80*(6), 1348–1353.

Sidoti, E. J., & Shprintzen, R. J. (1995). Pediatric care and feeding of the newborn with a cleft. In R. J. Shprintzen & J. Bardach (Eds.), *Cleft palate speech management* (pp. 63–74). St. Louis, MO: Mosby.

Singh, V. P., Bharadwaj, G., & Nair, K. C. (1997). Direct observation of tongue positions in speech—A patient study. *International Journal of Prosthodontics, 10*(3), 231–234.

Turner, G. E., & Williams, W. N. (1991). Fluoroscopy and nasoendoscopy in designing palatal lift prostheses. *Journal of Prosthetic Dentistry, 66*(1), 63–71.

Weiss, C. E. (1974). The speech pathologist's role in dealing with obturator-wearing school children. *Journal of Speech and Hearing Disorders, 39,* 153–162.

Witt, P. D., Rozelle, A. A., Marsh, J. L., Marty-Grames, L., Muntz, H. R., Gay, W. D., & Pilgram, T. K. (1995). Do palatal lift prostheses stimulate velopharyngeal neuromuscular activity? *Cleft Palate Craniofacial Journal, 32*(6), 469–475.

Wolfaardt, J. F., Wilson, F. B., Rochet, A., & McPhee, L. (1993). An appliance based approach to the management of palatopharyngeal incompetency: A clinical pilot project. *Journal of Prosthetic Dentistry, 69*(2), 186–195.

Yorkston, K. M., Beukelman, D. R., & Traynor, C. D. (1988). Articulatory adequacy in dysarthric speakers: A comparison of judging formats. *Journal of Communication Disorders, 21*(4), 351–361.

CHAPTER

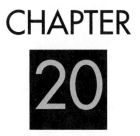

20

Orthognathic Surgery for Craniofacial Differences

Julia Corcoran, M.D.

CONTENTS

Craniofacial differences, including clefting and craniosynostosis syndromes, affect not only soft tissues but also underlying bony tissues. The craniofacial skeleton can be viewed as scaffolding for the soft tissue envelope of the face. If alveolar, palatal, maxillary, or mandibular segments are missing, unstable, or in poor anatomic relationship to one another, the functions of breathing, swallowing, speaking, and chewing can be impaired. Furthermore, the overlying face appears abnormal, drawing unfavorable attention to the patient.

Orthognathic surgery, which involves the bones of the upper jaw (the maxilla) and the lower jaw (the mandible), can address several different problems that occur in these patients. Congenital absence of bone in cleft patients can be corrected by bone grafting to improve the alveolar arch and occlusion. Lack of midfacial growth in cleft patients and the craniosynostosis patients can be compensated for by repositioning the maxilla in a more normal occlusal relationship to the mandible with Le Fort osteotomies (surgical cuts made within bone). An inadequate mandible associated with airway collapse in Pierre Robin sequence or facial asymmetry in facial-auricular-vertebral syndrome (hemifacial microsomia) can be addressed by mandibular advancement through multiple techniques including distraction osteogenesis, osteotomy, or reconstruction with bone grafting. All of these techniques aim to improve both the function of the scaffolding as well as the appearance of the facial soft tissue. This chapter briefly explains these procedures and their potential effects on articulation, resonance, and airway function.

Alveolar Bone Grafting

One of the greatest improvements in care of the patient with cleft lip and palate has been the routine implementation of alveolar bone grafting. While cheiloplasty (lip repair) restores the continuity of the lip muscular sphincter and palatoplasty restores the continuity of the velopharyngeal sphincter, the alveolus is not addressed routinely by either of these procedures. This situation leaves the lesser and greater palatine segments floating free, which usually leads to lateral crossbite on the side of the cleft (the lesser segment). Furthermore, the anterior gap in the arch can lead to loss of the permanent lateral incisor and canine teeth because of lack of supporting bone for the periodontal ligament that secures the tooth within the alveolus. This gap is usually associated with an oronasal fistula in the alveolus with its concomitant problems of discomfort and liquid loss into the nasal cavity (Waite & Waite, 1996).

The crossbite, anterior alveolar gap, and the loss of teeth potentially set the patient up for articulation errors in the production of fricatives and affricates, especially the sibilants. These problems can be addressed by positioning the two alveolar segments in a normal arch alignment and then securing them with a bone graft, which, when healed, provides a stable scaffold for the permanent dentition and the upper lip. Figure 20–1 is a preoperative photo of a patient just prior to the bone graft. Figure 20–2 is a postoperative photo of the same patient following the bone graft.

Timing and Technique of Bone Grafting

The timing of bone grafting is controversial. Repair of the alveolus can be done prior to the eruption of teeth either at the time of palatoplasty or in a separate operation, so-called primary bone grafting. It also can be delayed until the age of mixed dentition when the permanent teeth that will erupt into the grafted area are ready to descend, so-called delayed or intermediate bone grafting. The timing of bone grafting is debated, sometimes quite vigorously, between adherents of each philosophy.

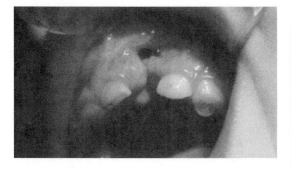

Figure 20–1. The bony cleft in the alveolus can be seen as the dark gap between the teeth. (Photograph courtesy of Delmar Halak, D.D.S.)

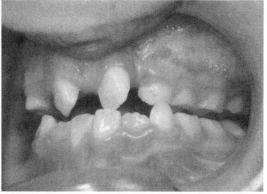

Figure 20–2. The gap has been closed and the gingiva has healed after a successful bone graft. (Photograph courtesy of Delmar Halak, D.D.S.)

Primary bone grafting can be done in one of two ways. A procedure called a *gingivoperiosteoplasty* opens alveolar soft tissues, that is, the gingiva and the underlying periosteum on each edge of the cleft. These raw surfaces are advanced and sewn together. This technique allows the bone progenitor cells found in the gingivoperiosteum to lay down bone as the patient grows. Bone need not be harvested from elsewhere in the body. Sometimes this procedure will provide adequate bonestock to support the permanent dentition. Another technique for primary bone grafting is to use a piece of rib graft as a strut across the alveolar cleft and cover the repair with the gingivoperiosteum.

Surgeons who favor this early, or primary, approach point out that the maxillary arch is aligned appropriately from almost the beginning. The disadvantage to primary bone grafting is that, while bone often will form across the alveolar cleft, it may not be of sufficient quantity or quality to support the permanent dentition, necessitating a delayed or secondary bone graft (Dado, 1993; Santiago et al., 1998). This situation becomes tricky, as the success of bone grafting is directly dependent on the surrounding soft tissues having good blood flow. Scar tissue from the previous primary procedure has a poorer blood supply, hindering the bone engraftment.

Other surgeons favor delaying bone grafting of the alveolus until the permanent dentition begins erupting during the stage of mixed dentition. Delayed or intermediate bone grafting of this type occurs between 6 to 10 years of age when the permanent lateral incisor or the canine tooth roots are about one third developed. These teeth are the ones usually located at the edges of the cleft. If unsupported by adequate bone, the teeth will be lost. Timing of the delayed bone graft depends on which tooth is more at risk, the lateral incisor or the cuspid. The lateral incisor erupts earlier than the canine. The actual age of bone grafting is patient-specific, depending on the anatomy and the child's dental development (Cohen, Polley, & Figueroa, 1993).

The pediatric dentist/orthodontist follows the child through serial radiographs to determine when the tooth roots are mature. While waiting for maturation, the dentist/orthodontist uses an expanding device to put the arch segments into correct alignment. Once aligned, a holding device, such as a retainer or a lingual holding arch of wire, is placed. Bone is harvested from the marrow cavity of the skull or the hip to use as a graft. The edges of the cleft are opened as in a gingivoperiosteoplasty. The floor of the nose is sewn closed and the bone graft is packed into the space. The gingiva is then repaired over the bone graft. This approach also helps build up the bone deficiency in the nasal base and para-alar areas.

Postoperative Complications and Management of Bone Grafting

Certain complications can occur with bone grafting. Bleeding and infection are possible, and are probably the most common adverse occurrences. Inadequate bone engraftment and breakdown of the repair can also happen. During the healing phase, the first 6 weeks after the surgery, the patient's palatal segments are held steady by an orthodontic device. Mastication is limited by placing the patient on a diet of soft and pureed foods. Brushing the teeth is replaced by using antimicrobial mouth rinses and a Water-Pik appliance. About 3 months later when the bone is solidly healed, the orthodontist can then direct the teeth into the appropriate positions along a complete maxillary alveolar arch.

Maxillary Advancement

Patients with cleft lip and palate, facial-auricular-vertebral syndrome, and craniosynostosis syndromes have maxillary growth problems that lead to a concave profile and malocclusion. In cleft patients and synostosis patients, the maxillary arch sits behind the mandibular arch, an Angle's Class III occlusion. A review of the growth patterns of the maxilla and mandible explain why the malocclusion develops.

Children with repaired clefts initially can be placed into a fairly normal occlusal relationship but revert to a Class III relationship. Mandibular growth continues later into life than maxillary growth, which is the normal growth pattern. However, maxillary growth in patients with a repaired cleft frequently is inhibited, presumably because of scar tissue and disturbances to the growth centers from previous surgeries. Eventually the lack of growth in the maxilla and the normal growth in the mandible place the jaws in Class III malocclusion. Children with craniosynostosis syndromes fail to grow normally because the sutures between the facial bones and the skull bones have closed prematurely and stunt the growth.

In addition to these problems, the patient with facial-auricular-vertebral syndrome also has a *cant* (slant in occlusion) to the maxilla, presumably caused by the relationship of the maxilla to the affected hemi-mandible. Normally, the maxilla continues its downward growth until the maxillary teeth meet the mandibular teeth. In the case of facial-auricular-vertebral syndrome, the shortened mandible on the affected side leaves inadequate room for the maxilla on that side to grow.

Common problems with a retrodisplaced or small maxilla include articulation errors, sleep apnea, and hyponasality. The crowding of the maxillary teeth and the relatively narrow arch of the palate in these situations create a constricted oral cavity space. The anatomy of this situation can lead to articulation errors, such as the palatal-dorsal production of consonants and frontal or lateral lisping. The relatively posterior displacement of the maxilla leads to a small pharyngeal space, which allows the tongue to obstruct the entire cavity in the recumbent position, explaining the sleep apnea and hyponasality. A less common problem is a shallow orbit because the cheeks are underdeveloped. The bones affected include not only the maxilla but also the zygoma, as found in the case of Treacher Collins syndrome. Because the orbit is essentially too small, *proptosis* (protrusion) of the globe, with exposure of the cornea, can result in the potential loss of sight. Orthognathic surgery to advance the maxilla can improve these situations. In addition to bringing the midface forward, the maxilla can be rotated to match midlines and tilted to correct cant with the various Le Fort osteotomies.

Maxillary Osteotomies

Le Fort (1901) originally described the naturally occurring fracture planes in the face. These lines of natural weakness in the facial skeleton collapse or break during trauma and are used to describe midfacial fracture patterns. His three labeled levels have been translated so that the surgeon can use these areas to create *osteotomies* (surgical cuts) in the maxilla and then position the bone in a more functional and pleasing position. Figure 20–3 illustrates the levels of the three Le Fort osteotomies.

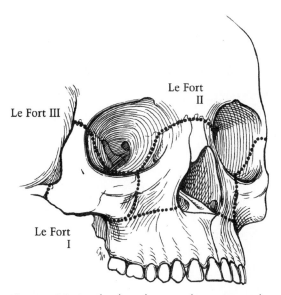

Figure 20–3. This line drawing demonstrates the level of the various Le Fort osteotomies. The Le Fort II osteotomy includes the territory of the Lefort I osteotomy as well. The Le Fort III osteotomy includes the territory of the Le Fort I and Le Fort II osteotomies as well. (From *Grabb and Smith's Plastic Surgery*, edited by James W. Smith and J. Sherrell, 1991, 4th ed., Fig. 12–24, p. 374. Boston: Aston, Little, Brown. Reprinted with permission.)

The most common of these osteotomies is the Le Fort I, which transversely cuts the maxilla just above the tooth roots and the base of the nose, in essence allowing the surgeon to move the lower maxilla and palate as a single unit. One can imagine this movement as an edentulous individual being able to move his denture plate forward and out of his mouth. Figure 20–4A–D, demonstrates the dramatic results of moving this segment of maxilla forward. If the surgeon needs to reposition the bridge of the nose as well as the teeth, as might be the case of patients with Treacher Collins syndrome, a Le Fort II osteotomy includes both the nasal pyramid and the alveolar arch. When the cheeks need to be brought forward to correct proptosis, as might be the case in patients with Apert's syndrome, a Le Fort III osteotomy, which includes cheek bones, orbital rims, nasal pyramid, and alveolar arch, can be used. Figure 20–5A–D shows preoperative proptosis and open bite and the postoperative improvement in a patient with Crouzon's disease after a Le Fort III osteotomy.

The goals of maxillary repositioning include normal occlusion, normal sized oral and pharyngeal resonance cavities, and improved facial proportions. Orthognathic surgery of this magnitude requires careful planning between the orthodontist, surgeon, and speech pathologist.

The orthodontist and surgeon compare the patient's maxillary placement against known normative values by evaluating the *cephalogram*, a standardized lateral radiograph of the craniofacial skeleton. Using these values, they determine how far and at what angle the maxilla must be moved to achieve the desired occlusion and profile. The orthodontist then places the teeth into position using braces. The final planning comes with performing the surgery on plaster cast models to assure surgeon, orthodontist, and patient of the outcome. Splints to be used in the operating room are made from the cast. Once the osteotomies are made, the surgeon can choose to fix the maxilla into the advanced position with metal plates

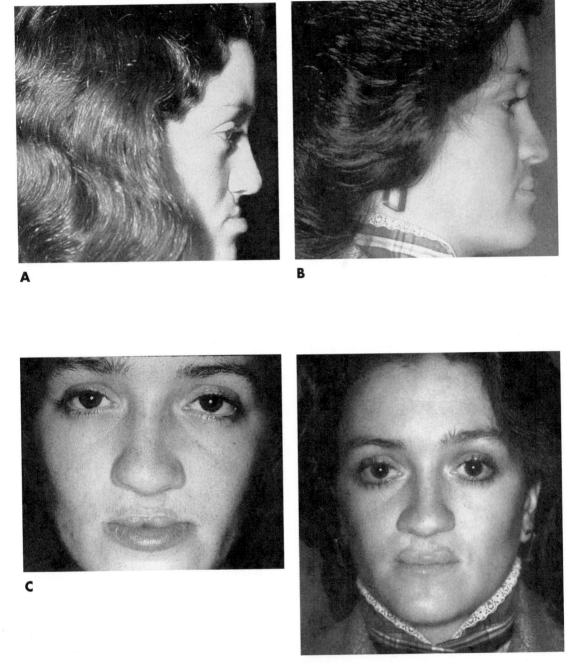

Figure 20–4. The change between the preoperative and postoperative profile after Le Fort I advancement is most remarkable; however, one can appreciate the improved facial harmony on the frontal view, as well. **A** and **C** are preoperative and **B** and **D** are postoperative. (Photographs courtesy of David Billmire, M.D.)

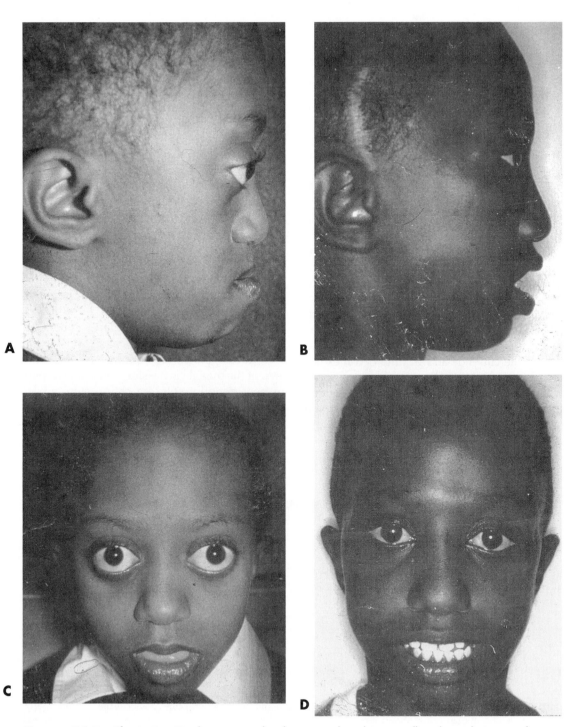

Figures 20-5. After Le Fort III advancement, the changes in the orbits as well as the occlusion are dramatic. **A** and **C** are preoperative and **B** and **D** are postoperative. (Photographs courtesy of David Billmire, M.D.)

and screws. However, if the advancement is unstable or greater than 10 mm, bone grafts are necessary to support the maxilla and to prevent relapse back into its original position.

Postoperatively, these patients may be held in occlusion with wire bands temporarily and then in rubber band ligatures for 6 to 8 weeks while the maxilla heals in its new position. During this period, the patient is kept on pureed and soft diets. Afterwards, final orthodontia can be applied to move the teeth into the most ideal position.

Another method for maxillary advancement is distraction osteogenesis. *Distraction osteogenesis* is a recent development in orthognathic surgery and is used to lengthen bone. This technique involves making a *corticotomy* (a partial cut) or an osteotomy (complete cut through the bone) in a bone, and then slowly pulling apart the cut ends with a mechanical distraction device. New bone is able to regenerate between the cut ends and in time becomes normal bone, obviating the need for bone grafts. When distraction osteogenesis is used, the presurgical planning and surgery to this point are identical. Rather than using plates and screws, however, the surgeon can place a distraction device after making the osteotomies.

This framework provides stability while the maxilla is moved forward gradually. This slow, deliberate advancement (1 mm to 1.5 mm per day) allows the body to lay down new bone growth, which solidly bolsters the maxilla in its new position. Figure 20-6 shows a patient preoperatively, in her distraction device, and her postoperative result. Theoretically, the gradual advancement of the maxilla may allow for progressive adaptation in the velopharyngeal mechanism, although this has not been closely examined to date.

Timing of Orthognathic Surgery

Orthognathic surgery of the maxilla most commonly in synostosis syndrome patients to improve the airway, close the anterior open bite, increase the oral cavity size, and, most importantly, protect the proptotic globes cannot be performed readily until the maxillary sinus is well developed. In the young child, the sinus area of the maxilla is the storehouse for the permanent dentition. Once a child enters mixed dentition, suitable space exists to introduce the surgical saw and allow Le Fort III advancement. Any surgery done at this age probably will not hold up to future growth. The patient

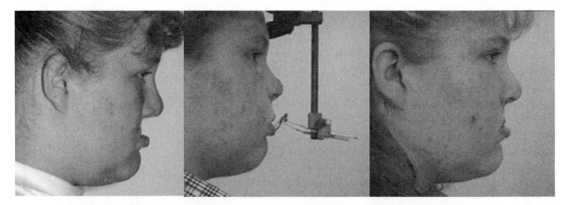

Figure 20–6. Distraction osteogenesis as applied to the midface. The left panel demonstrates the preoperative profile. The middle panel shows the patient at the end of distraction in her halo device. The right panel shows the postoperative results.

will likely need a Le Fort I advancement, or possibly a repeat Le Fort III, in the teenage years to balance the occlusion, improve facial harmony and create a convex profile.

Secondary orthognathic surgery in craniosynostosis patients and orthognathic surgery for the cleft lip and palate patient is usually delayed until facial skeletal maturity and complete eruption of the permanent dentition. The last bone to mature in the facial skeleton is the mandible. Waiting until mandibular growth is complete assures that new maxillary placement will be adequate for facial maturity. Consequently, this type of surgery is delayed in girls until age 15–16 years and in boys until 17–18 years. Prior to Le Fort I maxillary advancement, impacted third molars usually are addressed, although in some cases they can be removed from above at the time of maxillary advancement. Presurgical orthodontia must be complete prior to surgery.

Maxillary Advancement and the Velopharyngeal Mechanism

Advancement of the maxilla, and thus the velum, changes the dimensions of the pharyngeal cavity. With the anterior movement of the velum, there is an increase in the anterior-posterior gap that the velopharyngeal sphincter must close to allow for normal resonance and airflow during speech. Therefore, maxillary advancement can have a negative effect on velopharyngeal function, especially in patients with a repaired cleft palate or submucous cleft. This can result in the development of hypernasality or nasal emission or the worsening of these symptoms if they were present preoperatively (Haapanen, Kalland, Heliovaara, Hukki, & Ranta, 1997; Kummer, Strife, Grau, Creaghead, & Lee, 1989; Maegawa, Sells, & David, 1998; Mason, Turvey, & Warren, 1980; Okazaki et al., 1993; Watzke, Turvey, Warren, & Dalston, 1990). On the other hand, patients

with craniosynostosis syndromes are likely to be hyponasal due to the stenotic suture lines between the facial bones and the cranial base. For these patients, the increased diameter of the sphincter and the reduction of nasal airway resistance often improves or eliminates the hyponasality and upper airway obstruction (Dalston & Vig, 1984).

Planning for speech considerations prior to surgery includes evaluation of articulation, resonance, and velopharyngeal closure. In elective orthognathic cases done for improvement of facial harmony, a simple interview with sampling of speech suffices. Patients with craniofacial differences, however, require more sophisticated evaluations. Clues to tenuous velopharyngeal closure in speech samples include nasal escape during connected speech. In some cases, nasopharyngoscopy should be done to evaluate the anatomy of the velopharyngeal sphincter in this group of patients. Postoperative hypernasality and nasal escape are likely to occur in patients with tenuous velopharyngeal closure preoperatively or with maxillary advancements greater than 10 mm. Patients must be warned preoperatively that hypernasality and nasal escape can occur on a temporary or permanent basis. Many patients have a temporary period of hypernasality that corrects itself as the velopharyngeal structures accommodate to their new anatomic relationships. Other patients will require either a pharyngeal flap or pharyngoplasty to ameliorate the situation.

The second velopharyngeal situation affecting maxillary advancement is the presence of a pharyngeal flap. Patients with a pharyngeal flap already have a history of velopharyngeal dysfunction. They are at increased risk for a recurrence of velopharyngeal dysfunction postoperatively. From a technical point of view, the flap causes more difficulty in bringing the maxilla forward because of soft tissue tethering. To achieve maxillary advancement, some flaps may require division. Over time, patients with a pharyngeal flap prior to maxillary advancement seem to have increased incidence of relapse, that is, retropositioning of the maxilla toward its original location, presumably due to the pull of the scar in the area of the flap.

Maxillary Advancement and Articulation

A primary purpose of maxillary advancement is to normalize the occlusal relationship between the maxillary and mandibular arches. Because malocclusion is a common cause of articulation errors, it stands to reason that the correction of the malocclusion could improve the articulation errors. In fact, several studies have reported improved articulation following maxillary advancement, without intervening speech therapy (Kummer et al., 1989; Maegawa et al., 1998; Mason et al., 1980; McCarthy, Coccaro, & Schwartz, 1979; Vallino, 1990). This improvement is only noted in cases of obligatory errors, where tongue position was normal during production, but the structure was abnormal, causing the distortions. When there are compensatory errors resulting in abnormal tongue position, the maxillary advancement does not improve speech. Instead, speech therapy is required postoperatively for correction of these articulation errors.

Complications of Maxillary Advancement

Complications associated with maxillary advancement include major blood loss requiring massive transfusion, infection of the facial soft tissues, relapse of the maxilla, decreased sensation in the upper lip and midface, loss of teeth, loss of gingiva, persistent malocclusion not correctable with orthodontia, and, most significant to this topic, velopharyngeal insufficiency.

To correct relapse of the maxilla and persistent malocclusion not correctable with orthodontia, maxillary advancement must be performed again, including the presurgical orthodontia.

Loss of gingiva can be improved by periodontal correction. Loss of teeth can be masked with bridgework or other prosthetic replacement. Changes in sensation may correct over time or, more likely, the patient becomes used to the new situation and compensates. Velopharyngeal insufficiency may correct over time or may require a pharyngeal flap or pharyngoplasty.

Mandibular Reconstruction

Management of the mandible can be a significant challenge for surgeons caring for patients with craniofacial differences. Micrognathia is associated with many of the craniofacial differences including the Pierre Robin sequence, Treacher Collins syndrome, and bilateral facial-auricular-vertebral syndrome. A normal mandible appearing prognathic is problematic for patients with craniosynostosis syndromes and with cleft lip and palate. An asymmetric mandible with hypoplastic or absent portions occurs in hemifacial microsomia. An asymmetric mandible and relative prognathism can cause problems with tooth erosion and with articulation but rarely influences the airway or alimentation.

The small, retrognathic mandible frequently causes airway obstruction; problems can range from desaturation during feeding and sleep apnea when supine to complete airway obstruction regardless of position. The initial management of these infants is to provide an adequate airway for vegetative respiration and a method for alimentation. Simple temporizing measures include prone positioning of the baby while sleeping and feeding. More complex methods include placement of a nasal-pharyngeal airway (a so-called trumpet) and gavage feedings through an intermittently placed nasogastric tube. Severe cases may require tracheotomy for airway management and gastrostomy for feeding. Once the airway and feeding issues are solved, the mandibular management is undertaken.

Many of the infants with Pierre Robin sequence will need special positioning and nasal trumpets for a normal airway while feeding and sleeping. Some of the infants will outgrow these needs. Children with severe micrognathia requiring tracheotomy usually require some sort of mandibular advancement to allow decanulation. The earlier decanulation can be done in life, the better the prognosis for speech and language development. Clearly, the presence of the tracheostomy prevents the airflow necessary for speech production. The inability to produce speech normally also affects the development of expressive language skills.

Mandibular reconstruction options are as varied as the surgeons who attempt to solve these problems. The more common methods include distraction osteogenesis, rib graft reconstruction, free tissue microsurgical reconstruction (free-flap), and mandibular osteotomies, the most versatile being the sagittal split osteotomy.

Advancement by Distraction Osteogenesis

Prior to the technique of mandibular distraction, the surgical advancement of the mandible in young patients was rare and fraught with difficulties. Such reconstruction was delayed until later in life, usually at 5 to 6 years of age when the ribs were sufficiently developed to use as struts and grafts. Mandibular distraction osteogenesis has allowed decannulation of patients as young as toddlers (Williams, Maull, Grayson, Longaker, & McCarthy, 1999). McCarthy, Schreiber, Karp, Thorne, and Grayson (1992) presented the first reports of mandibular distraction in children in 1992. Since that time, many different approaches to mandibular distraction have been tried (Cohen, Burstein, & Williams, 1999).

All of the distraction techniques take advantage of the fact that the body will heal a fractured bone by laying down new bone. If the ends of a fracture are gradually separated, the body will lay down new bone in this gap. All distraction procedures produce a fracture, either complete (osteotomy) or partial (corticotomy). To advance the mandible, these cuts are made bilaterally in the non-tooth-bearing area of the mandibular body, the mandibular angle, or in the *ramus*, which is the upturned, perpendicular extremity of the mandible on both sides. After several days of rest, the so-called latent period, the distraction device is activated and the cut ends of the bone are separated gradually, usually 1 to 2 millimeters daily (the active period). Once the desired advancement is achieved, the device is left in place as a scaffold until the new bone has solidified, the so-called resting period. This period is usually equal to or longer than the period of active distraction. The device is then removed. Variations on this procedure include whether the surgeon approaches the patient externally or intra-orally, whether the device is external or internal, whether one or more osteotomies are used, and whether the device can move the mandible in one, two, or three dimensions.

To determine whether advancement has been sufficient to allow decannulation of the patient, the patient is examined prior to end of the active period of distraction. Lateral cephalograms can demonstrate the increased dimensions of the nasopharyngeal cavity. A more certain evaluation is laryngoscopy and bronchoscopy performed in the operating room by a pediatric otolaryngologist who can attend to the other issues that surround chronic airway canulation, including subglottic stenosis, laryngomalacia, and granulation tissue. A more physiologic test of airway adequacy is blocking the cannula temporarily with a valve to see if the child can maintain his airway. Figure 20–7 shows a tracheostomy-dependent child with micrognathia prior to, during, and after distraction.

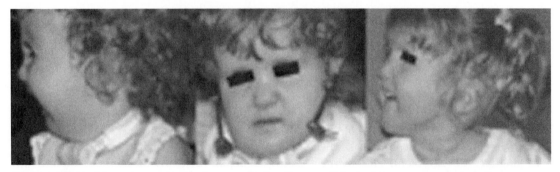

Figure 20–7. Distraction osteogenesis as applied to the mandible. In this case, an external distractor was applied through an intraoral approach. The left panel demonstrates the degree of preoperative micrognathia. The middle panel shows the patient in her distractor. The right panel shows the amount of advancement obtained. Note that the patient has her tracheostomy successfully decannulated. (Photographs courtesy of David Billmire, M.D.)

One of the beauties of distraction osteogenesis is the versatility of the technique. Distraction can be repeated on the same patient should mandibular advancement be needed again as the midface grows. The technique can also be applied unilaterally to rotate the canted, hypoplastic side of the mandible in the facial-auricular-vertebral syndrome patient. Rib graft used to reconstruct a mandible can also be distracted as if it were native mandible (Corcoran, Hubli, & Salyer, 1997).

Complications with distraction are many, but usually minor in nature (Corcoran et al., 1997). The skin surrounding the device can become infected, and on occasion, the device can fail. Unusual complications include facial nerve palsies and fibrous malunion. Distraction, however, has stood the test of time. In the decade since its inception, problems with relapse have not been reported despite frequent application of this novel technique (McCarthy, Stelnicki, & Grayson, 1999).

The changes in velopharyngeal function and articulation, as the mandibular height and relationships change, have been reported by Guyette, Polley, Figueroa, and Cohen (1996). Initially, articulation and resonance may be-

come worse; however, with time resonance can normalize and articulation improve.

Rib Graft Reconstruction

Reconstructive surgeons have taken advantage of the natural structure of the rib with its bony shaft and cartilaginous tip to recreate hypoplastic and absent mandibles, especially in facial-auricular-vertebral syndrome. The child must have adequate-sized ribs, which precludes doing this type of reconstruction prior to 5 to 6 years of age. The cartilage tip is used to mimic the condyle of the mandible and the shaft of the rib to recreate the ramus and body. The graft is fixed to the mandible with plates and/or screws.

This technique has been the mainstay of mandibular reconstruction for several surgical generations. A unique problem with rib grafting is the inability to predict postoperative growth patterns. The graft can partially or completely resorb, leaving the patient without any advancement. Alternatively, it can remain the same size, so that as the child's other facial bones grow, the asymmetry reproduces itself. Rarely, the rib graft can overgrow and create a secondary asymmetry requiring resection of a portion of the graft. Another drawback to rib graft reconstruction of the hypoplastic mandible is its lack of soft tissue replacement. While a rib graft can replace the missing facial height and mandibular length, the soft tissue fullness and contour is not provided by this technique, leaving the patient with an asymmetric appearance.

Free Tissue Transfer (Free Flap) Reconstruction

One of the more elegant solutions to the lack of soft tissue and lack of growth in a rib graft has been the use of a free tissue transfer (free flap) to reconstruct the mandible and overlying soft tissues. The surgeon can harvest bone or bone and soft tissue with their blood vessels and transfer this flap to the mandible, hooking the donor blood vessels into the recipient blood vessels of the face. These small vessels are sewn together with the aid of the operating microscope. The scapula and overlying soft tissue can be used to transfer bone and soft tissue and provide a reliable growth center. If only soft tissue is necessary, many donor sites have been used including the greater omentum from the abdomen.

Mandibular Osteotomies

Many mandibular osteotomies have been designed. The most versatile is the sagittal split osteotomy which allows advancement, set back, and rotation. The surgeon splits the ramus of the mandible between its inner and outer tables, separating the condyle and outer table of the ramus from the body and the inner table (Figure 20–8). The unique advantage to the sagittal split is the large contact area it leaves for the two ends of the mandible to heal, allowing the surgeon to advance, set back, or rotate the segment. The pieces of the mandible are put into their new positions with the aid of splints, as described for maxillary advancement. The surgeon can then secure the segments with wires, screws, or plates.

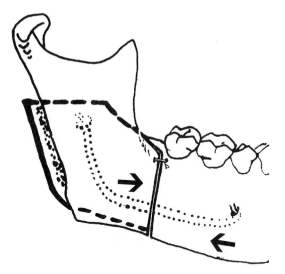

Figure 20–8. This line drawing demonstrates the anatomy of a sagittal split osteotomy and the versatility of either advancement, rotation, or set back that can be obtained. (From *Grabb and Smith's Plastic Surgery*, 4th ed., by J. W. Smith and J. Sherrell, 1991, p. 233 Boston: Aston, Little Brown Company. Reprinted with permission)

Postoperatively the patient must comply with a physical therapy regiment to prevent stiffness of the temporomandibular joint. Proper interoperative positioning of the mandibular segments is essential to prevent temporomandibular joint problems. Depending on the stability of the mandibular movement, the patient may require *intermaxillary fixation*, which involves wiring the mandible against the maxilla to keep it closed, or elastic band therapy. Frequently the patient will be uncomfortable with how the maxillary and mandibular teeth meet. This malocclusion, whether subjective or objective, can usually be improved with postoperative orthodontia.

The technique of sagittal split osteotomy with a rib graft or free flap reconstruction can be applied unilaterally (as in facial-auricular-vertebral syndrome) or applied bilaterally. It can be done in conjunction with a maxillary advancement to improve facial harmony when advancement is limited by soft tissue constraints. It is the workhorse osteotomy of craniofacial reconstruction.

The horizontal mandibular osteotomy for chin advancement, also called a *genioplasty*, is another frequent osteotomy of the mandible. Chin advancement can be done in conjunction with other mandibular or maxillary osteotomies or alone. Although it does not change airway or speech considerations, it does greatly improve facial esthetics.

Summary

The success of reconstruction of children with craniofacial differences is the sum of its parts. With manipulation of the facial bones, significant improvements can be made in the soft tissue contours and the appearance of the child. These bone improvements can also have profound influences on the speech of the child, affecting both articulation and resonance.

References

Cohen, M., Polley, J. W., & Figueroa, A. A. (1993). Secondary (intermediate) alveolar bone grafting. *Clinics in Plastic Surgery, 20*(4), 691–705.

Cohen, S. R., Burstein, F. D., & Williams, J. K. (1999). The role of distraction osteogenesis in the managment of craniofacial disorders. *Annals of the Academy of Medicine, Singapore, 28*(5), 728–738.

Corcoran, J., Hubli, E. H., & Salyer, K. E. (1997). Distraction osteogenesis of costochondral neomandibles: A clinical experience. *Plastic and Reconstructive Surgery, 100*(2), 311–315; Discussion 316–317.

Dado, D. V. (1993). Primary (early) alveolar bone grafting. *Clinics in Plastic Surgery, 20*(4), 683–689.

Dalston, R. M., & Vig, P. S. (1984). Effects of orthognathic surgery on speech: A prospective study. *Amercan Journal of Orthodontics, 86*(4), 291–298.

Guyette, T. W., Polley, J. W., Figueroa, A. A., & Cohen, M. N. (1996). Mandibular distraction osteogenesis: Effects on articulation and velopharyngeal function. *Journal of Craniofacial Surgery, 7*(3), 186–191.

Haapanen, M. L., Kalland, M., Heliovaara, A., Hukki, J., & Ranta, R. (1997). Velopharyngeal function in cleft patients undergoing maxillary advancement. *Folia Phoniatrica et Logopedica, 49*(1), 42–47.

Kummer, A. W., Strife, J. L., Grau, W. H., Creaghead, N. A., & Lee, L. (1989). The effects of Le Fort I osteotomy with maxillary movement on articulation, resonance, and velopharyngeal function. *Cleft Palate Journal, 26*(3), 193–199; Discussion 199–200.

Le Fort, R. (1901). Etude experimental sur les fractures de la machoire superieure. Parts I, II, III. *Revue de Chirurgie de Pari, 23*, 201, 360, 479.

Maegawa, J., Sells, R. K., & David, D. J. (1998). Speech changes after maxillary advancement in 40 cleft lip and palate patients. *Journal of Craniofacial Surgery, 9*(2), 177–182; Discussion 183–184.

Mason, R., Turvey, T. A., & Warren, D. W. (1980). Speech considerations with maxillary advancement procedures. *Journal of Oral Surgery, 38*(10), 752–758.

McCarthy, J. G., Coccaro, P. J., & Schwartz, M. D. (1979). Velopharyngeal function following maxillary advancement. *Plastic and Reconstructive Surgery, 64*(2), 180–189.

McCarthy, J. G., Schreiber, J., Karp, N., Thorne, C. H., & Grayson, B. H. (1992). Lengthening the human mandible by gradual distraction [see Comments]. *Plastic and Reconstructive Surgery, 89*(1), 1–8; Discussion 9–10.

McCarthy, J. G., Stelnicki, E. J., & Grayson, B. H. (1999). Distraction osteogenesis of the mandible: A ten-year experience. *Seminars in Orthodontics, 5*(1), 3–8.

Okazaki, K., Satoh, K., Kato, M., Iwanami, M., Ohokubo, F., & Kobayashi, K. (1993). Speech and velopharyngeal function following maxillary advancement in patients with cleft lip and palate. *Annals of Plastic Surgery, 30*(4), 304–311.

Santiago, P. E., Grayson, B. H., Cutting, C. B., Gianoutsos, M. P., Brecht, L. E., & Kwon, S. M. (1998). Reduced need for alveolar bone grafting by presurgical orthopedics and primary gingivoperiosteoplasty. *Cleft Palate Craniofacial Journal, 35*(1), 77–80.

Vallino, L. D. (1990). Speech, velopharyngeal function, and hearing before and after orthognathic surgery. *Journal of Oral and Maxillofacial Surgery, 48*(12), 1274–1281; Discussion 1281–1282.

Waite, P. D., & Waite, D. E. (1996). Bone grafting for the alveolar cleft defect. *Seminars in Orthodontics, 2*(3), 192–196.

Watzke, I., Turvey, T. A., Warren, D. W., & Dalston, R. (1990). Alterations in velopharyngeal function after maxillary advancement in cleft palate patients. *Journal of Oral and Maxillofacial Surgery, 48*(7), 685–689.

Williams, J. K., Maull, D., Grayson, B. H., Longaker, M. T., & McCarthy, J. G. (1999). Early decannulation with bilateral mandibular distraction for tracheostomy-dependent patients. *Plastic and Reconstructive Surgery, 103*(1), 48–57; Discussion 58–59.

CHAPTER

21

Speech Therapy for the Effects of Velopharyngeal Dysfunction

CONTENTS

Individuals with a history of cleft lip/palate or craniofacial anomalies are at risk for certain speech and resonance disorders secondary to velopharyngeal dysfunction (VPD) and dental malocclusion. Velopharyngeal dysfunction can occur due to a variety of other reasons, in addition to cleft palate.

As has been discussed in other chapters, when the velopharyngeal valve is defective, speech may be characterized by hypernasality and nasal air emission. In addition, inadequate intraoral pressure due to a faulty velopharyngeal valve can result in weak articulation, short utterance length, and the development of compensatory articulation productions. The underlying cause of these speech characteristics is important to determine through perceptual and instrumental methods, because the cause has a direct impact on the selection of the appropriate treatment method.

Appropriate Candidates for Speech Therapy

The most important rule of thumb in determining whether an individual is a candidate for speech therapy is: If the cause of the speech disorder is abnormal structure only, then speech therapy is not appropriate. In fact, for ethical reasons, the speech pathologist must refuse to offer speech therapy for an individual who does not have the structural or physiological ability to succeed with speech therapy. The only exception to the rule is if the structure cannot (or will not) be corrected. In that case, speech therapy is appropriate if the goal is to develop compensatory strategies to improve the overall quality and intelligibility of speech. Given this rule, individuals with a consistent velopharyngeal opening due to velopharyngeal insufficiency are not candidates for speech therapy to improve resonance, intraoral air pressure, or any other obligatory characteristics of velopharyngeal dysfunction. This is due to the fact that

speech therapy will correct abnormal function, but cannot correct abnormal structure.

It may be tempting to try speech therapy with individuals who demonstrate a mild degree of hypernasality or nasal air emission due to a small, yet consistent velopharyngeal gap. As noted previously, Morris (1984) has called this group the "almost-but-not-quite (ABNQ)" group because the gap is small, but the velopharyngeal valve never completely closes. These individuals are generally not stimulable for improvement through articulation therapy. This is because an underlying structural or physiological disorder precludes complete velopharyngeal closure. Therefore, surgical management is more appropriate, even though the opening is small. The decision to consider surgical management should be made based on how much the defect affects the quality and intelligibility of speech. Only the family and patient can determine if its effect on speech warrants surgical intervention. Regardless of the decision about the surgery, speech therapy is not indicated because therapy will not change the structure of the velopharyngeal mechanism.

Now that it is clear which individuals are not candidates for speech therapy, it is important to discuss the criteria for determining which individuals are good candidates. In general, speech therapy is effective in eliminating compensatory articulation productions through articulation therapy. However, hypernasality, nasal air emission, and weak consonants also can be improved or corrected with therapy under very limited conditions. These conditions include:

- *The characteristic is very mild and the child is stimulable.* If there is a very slight degree of hypernasality or nasal air emission, this can indicate a very small velopharyngeal opening, possibly due to poor function. If the child is stimulable for complete closure, a short trial period of speech therapy could be initiated to see if the patient responds to therapy prior to considering surgery.

- *The characteristic is inconsistent or occurs primarily when the child is tired.* If the patient is able to achieve closure most of the time, but occasionally has nasal air emission or assimilated hypernasality, then there is a possibility that improved consistency of closure can be achieved with articulation or biofeedback training. If the patient becomes hypernasal with fatigue, this may be normal (as with whining) or it may suggest tenuous closure and inadequate velar strength to maintain closure. The inconsistency in velopharyngeal closure fits the category that Morris (1984) called "sometimes but not always (SBNA)."
- *The characteristic is due to faulty articulation and the child is stimulable.* If the child is stimulable for a reduction or elimination of the nasal air emission or hypernasality, this is a good prognostic indicator for improvement, if not correction, with therapy. If multiple compensatory articulation errors are noted, yet the child is very stimulable for correct articulatory placement with normal pressure, then the decision regarding surgery should be deferred until after therapy has been initiated (Hoch, Golding-Kushner, Siegel-Sadewitz, & Shprintzen, 1986). Correction of the posterior articulation will eliminate the need for surgery in a small percentage of cases. In fact, the movement of the velopharyngeal structures can be noted to increase with the replacement of those productions with oral phonemes (Hoch et al., 1986; Tomes, Kuehn, & Peterson-Falzone, 1996; Ysunza-Rivera, Pamplona-Ferreira, & Toledo-Cortina, 1991).
- *The characteristic is associated with oral-motor dysfunction,* such as apraxia or dysarthria. If hypernasality or nasal air emission is associated with faulty articulation, then articulation therapy is the obvious method of treatment. When velopharyngeal dysfunction is due to a motor deficit rather than a structural deficit, the prognosis for correction with surgery is guarded. Every effort should be

made to determine if speech therapy can improve speech before considering surgical intervention. Prosthetic management is often indicated in these cases.
- *Surgical correction of velopharyngeal structures has been done, but the individual needs to learn to use the new structure.* Therapy is indicated in most cases of velopharyngeal dysfunction, even if the velopharyngeal dysfunction is treated surgically or with a prosthesis. It is important to remember that changing structure does not change function. The patient may need to be taught appropriate articulatory placement and oral airflow.

If in doubt about whether the individual is a surgical candidate for correction of velopharyngeal dysfunction, a trial period of speech therapy should always be done (Hardin, 1991). The therapy should be short-term, no more than a few months, as it does not take long to determine whether the child will respond. Through therapy, the clinician will be able to determine quickly whether the therapy is going to be effective or whether surgical intervention will be needed. If the individual continues to demonstrate hypernasality or nasal air emission, even with an improvement in articulation, then further evaluation of velopharyngeal function should be done and surgical intervention should be considered. Once the velopharyngeal dysfunction is corrected surgically, speech therapy is usually required to help the individual learn to use the new velopharyngeal mechanism for oral airflow and to correct the remaining compensatory and placement errors.

Muscle Training Techniques

In the last half-century, there have been many experimental attempts to increase velopharyngeal activity, and thus improve velopharyngeal function, through the use of various forms of muscle training. These forms have met with limited success and are generally not accepted today as viable and useful techniques. However, from an historical and clinical perspective, it is important to review what has been found to be unsuccessful, in addition to what has been found to work. Ruscello (1982) provides an excellent review of palatal training procedures that have been tried through 1982.

Nonspeech Exercises

In the 1940s through the early 1960s, it was commonly believed that nonspeech exercises could increase the strength and the voluntary control of the velopharyngeal mechanism for speech. Therefore, clinicians commonly used physical exercises such as blowing, sucking, whistling, cheek puffing, swallowing, and even playing wind instruments in hopes of strengthening the muscles of the velopharyngeal valve for improved function with speech (Berry & Eisenson, 1956; Kanter, 1947; Massengill, Quinn, Pickrell, & Levinson, 1968; Moser, 1942; Van Riper, 1946, 1963; Wells, 1945, 1948). The assumption in using these exercises was that the physiological processes for velopharyngeal closure with these activities are the same as the processes that are used with speech. Unfortunately, these exercises did not seem to be very effective (Powers & Starr, 1974; Ruscello, 1982; Shelton, Hahn, & Morris, 1968). When later research showed significant differences in the closure patterns of speech and nonspeech activities (Flowers & Morris, 1973; McWilliams & Bradley, 1965; Moll, 1965; Peterson, 1973; Shprintzen, Lencione, McCall, & Skolnick, 1974), these nonspeech exercises were abandoned by knowledgeable professionals. Unfortunately, the belief that nonspeech exercises can be useful in training speech has died a slow death. In 1980, Schneider and Shprintzen (1980) surveyed 1000 speech pathologists from the United States and Canada. About 60% responded to the survey, and 65% of those responding

were associated with cleft palate teams. Of those responding, the majority reported that they use some form of blowing, sucking, or swallowing exercises as part of a therapy protocol for velopharyngeal dysfunction. Even today, some clinicians continue to incorporate these exercises in treatment, thinking that they are beneficial.

Temporary Speech Prostheses

Some authors have described the use of a temporary speech prosthesis to stimulate an improvement in velopharyngeal function. Harkins and Koepp-Baker (1948) observed that speech appliances seemed to stimulate velopharyngeal movements in some of their patients. Other authors subsequently suggested the use of "speech bulb reduction therapy" as a means of improving velopharyngeal function (Blakeley, 1964, 1969; Israel, Cook, & Blakeley, 1993; McGrath & Anderson, 1990; Shelton, Lindquist, Arndt, Elbert, & Youngstrom, 1971; Shelton, Lindquist, Chisum, et al., 1968; Weiss, 1971). In this type of therapy, a speech bulb is initially constructed to fill the velopharyngeal gap. Over a period of time, the size of the bulb is gradually reduced, yet the individual is encouraged to continue to achieve velopharyngeal closure. The goal of this therapy is to increase velopharyngeal movement gradually until there is no longer a need for the speech bulb prosthesis. The early studies did not provide strong support for the efficacy of this technique, however.

Golding-Kushner, Cisneros, and LeBlanc (1995) noted that, in the early studies, the effectiveness of the speech bulb reduction technique was judged by the changes in velar elevation, as observed through lateral cephalometric radiographs or lateral cineradiography. They reported that, in their experience, the changes following speech bulb reduction are primarily in the degree of lateral pharyngeal wall motion, which cannot be appreciated on a lateral radiograph. They studied 31 patients between the ages of 3 and 50 who were enrolled in a speech bulb reduction program. By report, these patients had varying degrees of "VPI" so it is uncertain if they had velopharyngeal insufficiency, incompetence, or both. The speech bulb was constructed, evaluated, and modified through the help of nasopharyngoscopy examinations. The mean number of visits for construction of the appliance was 8.3 with a range from 4 to 12 visits. Due to poor compliance with the multiple appointments, only 17 patients completed the program. Of the 17 patients, only 2 had normal speech and resonance following the treatment, but neither of the 2 had a history of cleft or velar abnormality. In addition, both had received speech therapy concurrently with the speech bulb reduction program, so it is impossible to know which treatment resulted in the improvement. Even though their speech remained abnormal, 10 of the 17 patients showed increased lateral pharyngeal wall movement, although for some the increases were noted only when the bulb was in place.

An argument could be made that the speech bulb reduction therapy can increase lateral pharyngeal wall motion so that, if a pharyngeal flap is done, it does not need to be very wide or obstructing. However, the increase in lateral wall motion can (and often does) occur in the same way once the flap is in place. With the time involved, the expense, the trauma of nasopharyngoscopy for children, and the effort expended in speech bulb reduction therapy, this may not be a valid rationale for its use. Certainly, further research on the efficacy of this method is needed before it should be commonly used in the treatment of individuals with velopharyngeal dysfunction.

Wolfaardt and colleagues (Wolfaardt, Wilson, Rochet, & McPhee, 1993) studied the effects of systematic reduction of the use of a palatal lift appliance worn by 32 patients. During this reduction therapy, the patients also received speech therapy and feedback training.

They reported that, at the end of the therapy, 14 were able to discontinue wearing the appliance. There is no information on the type of velopharyngeal dysfunction, however, so the effect of speech therapy on the improvement must be taken into consideration.

Direct Stimulation

Cole (1971, 1979) described treatment methods that stimulated the velum and/or pharyngeal muscles and called these "direct training methods." Cole theorized that these techniques increase muscle activity by teaching the patient to be able to control an essentially involuntary process. Several investigators have attempted to increase velar and pharyngeal wall movement through the use of some form of stimulation.

Lubit and Larsen (1969, 1971) suggested the use of a device described as a "palatal exerciser." The device consisted of a bite block, an inflatable rubber bag, and a hand pumping bulb. The patient was instructed to put the device in the mouth and then pump up the bag until it was inflated, pushing the velum up against the posterior pharyngeal wall. Practice was carried out daily with several sessions per day. Out of 28 cases, only 1 patient showed a positive change in speech, but this was not in the area of nasality. Of course, one concern about this method is that there really was no exercise involved. In fact, the velum was elevated passively, so muscle strengthening could not really take place.

Massengill and colleagues (Massengill, Quinn, & Pickrell, 1971) reported the use of "palatal stimulators," which were essentially palatal lifts. They reported a reduction in the size of the velopharyngeal opening in their five patients after wearing these stimulators for about a year, although an opening still remained in all patients.

Tudor and Selley (1974) described the use of a device that had a palatal body and then a U-shaped extension that made contact with the velum at rest. Elevation of the velum activated an electrical circuit, which then turned on an external monitoring light. These investigators used this device to try to train increased velar movement through visual feedback. They reported that their patients developed closure with this device, but this was not transferred to connected speech. Selley and colleagues (Selley, Zananiri, Ellis, & Flack, 1987) later speculated that the device may have reduced tongue humping, which increased oral airflow.

Several studies investigated the effectiveness of electrical stimulation in increasing velopharyngeal movement. Yules and Chase (1969) reported that direct electrical stimulation of the velum, along with tactile stimulation, resulted in improved velopharyngeal closure and a reduction in nasal air emission in 24 of their 30 patients. In addition, 60% of the 24 patients also eliminated hypernasality. However, this result has never been replicated. In fact, Weber, Jobe, and Chase (1970) used the same form of electrical stimulation with 34 patients over a period of 12 months. They found this technique to be ineffective in reducing nasal air emission or hypernasality during speech. Peterson (1974) reported one subject's response to electrical stimulation during a single session. The results showed some effect of the stimulation on movement, but inconsistent movement patterns were observed.

Tash and others (Tash, Shelton, Knox, & Michel, 1971) described the use of touch stimulation of the lateral pharyngeal walls to increase movement. As a result of this stimulation, their subjects were able to increase control of lateral pharyngeal wall movement, but the effect on closure for speech was not significant and speech was not improved for the abnormal speakers.

Continuous Positive Airway Pressure (CPAP)

A continuous positive airway pressure (CPAP) device is an instrument that consists of a flow generator, a valve mechanism, a hose, and a nasal mask. Airflow and air pressure are delivered to the nasal cavity, and thus the pharynx, through the hose and nasal mask. CPAP has been found to be useful in the treatment of individuals with obstructive sleep apnea (OSA) because the positive pressure prevents the collapse of the pharyngeal airway during sleep.

In 1991, Kuehn (1991) described the use of CPAP as a means for treating hypernasality. He suggested that CPAP could provide resistance training for the velopharyngeal muscles by having them work actively against the positive air pressure. Based on the principles of exercise physiology, CPAP therapy is designed to overload the muscles by subjecting them to a greater level of resistance than usual. The positive air pressure provided by CPAP results in greater resistance than atmospheric pressure, and thus, the muscles of the velum must work harder against this pressure to achieve velopharyngeal closure for speech. Once the muscles adapt to a certain level of pressure, the pressure is increased, which also increases the resistance. Once more, the muscles must work harder to adapt to this increase in pressure. Through this progressive resistance training, the muscles are thought to gain strength and become more resistance to fatigue. This strengthening of the musculature could therefore improve velopharyngeal closure.

CPAP therapy is done by having the individual place the mask over the nose and set the pressure to the desired level. The individual should feel the pressure as fullness in the nose. The muscle exercises used during the therapy are actually a form of speech drillwork. The individual begins with the production of 50 vowel, nasal consonant, oral consonant, vowel strings (i.e., "imbi"). The second syllable with the oral consonant is emphasized during production. These syllables are designed to lower the velum during the nasal consonant and then cause rigorous elevation of the velum to achieve closure for the oral sound. As the oral sound is produced, the velopharyngeal musculature must work hard to overcome the resistance of the positive pressure. This process has been likened to a power lift in weight training because the velopharyngeal muscles have to work against the resistance of the air pressure to elevate (Tomes et al., 1996). These syllable strings are followed by the production of a list of six sentences with pressure-sensitive phonemes. The entire sequence is then repeated until the session time expires.

Kuehn (1991) suggested a CPAP training protocol that starts with a pressure of 3 cmH_2O and a 10-minute treatment session. The individual does the exercises once each day and 6 days per week over an 8-week period. The amount of pressure and the length of exercise time is gradually increased so that the individual is practicing 24 minutes a day at a pressure of 7 cmH_2O by the end of the 8 weeks. At the end of the treatment period, the effectiveness of the therapy is evaluated. If there is no change in velopharyngeal function or speech, the individual is referred for physical management.

Kuehn, Moon, and Folkins (1993) compared electromyographic activity of the levator veli palatini during the use of CPAP and with atmospheric air pressure only. There was a significant increase in the activity of the levator muscle with an increase in the intranasal pressure, suggesting that this muscle actively reacts to the resistance. This was suggested as evidence to support the use of CPAP therapy as a means to increase the strength of the velopharyngeal musculature.

Kuehn listed several advantages of the CPAP technique, including the fact that it is noninvasive, easy to use, and can be done at home (Kuehn, 1991, 1997). Some caveats of this form of treatment might include the fact that patient selection is very important. Even on a theoretical basis, muscle strengthening will not improve velopharyngeal insufficiency, because it cannot change the structure of the mechanism. CPAP therapy will not be effective if the hypernasality or nasal air emission is due to mislearning or faulty articulation. This form of treatment is best suited for cases with velopharyngeal incompetence when there is poor velar movement. However, it is unlikely to be successful if there is more than mild to moderate velopharyngeal incompetence. Further research is needed to clearly define the effects of CPAP on individuals with mild velopharyngeal incompetence, and whether short-term improvements are sustained once the CPAP therapy is terminated.

Biofeedback Techniques

Biofeedback is a technique for making unconscious or autonomic physiological processes perceptible to the senses in order to manipulate them by conscious mental control. Biofeedback techniques are based on the principle that a desired response can be learned when it is determined that a specific thought process can produce that physiological response. Different types of biofeedback techniques have been used in medicine for years and have been found to be effective in many ways, such as reducing tension, decreasing heart rate, and even decreasing pain. In recent years, biofeedback techniques have been applied in speech pathology, particularly in the area of voice (McGillivray, Proctor-Williams, & McLister, 1994; Prosek, Montgomery, Walden, & Schwartz, 1978; Rossiter, Howard, & DeCosta, 1996; Stemple, Weiler, Whitehead, & Komray, 1980), fluency (Davis & Drichta, 1980; Weiss, Carson, & Brady, 1979), and dysarthria (Gentil, Aucouturier, Delong, & Sambuis, 1994; Murdoch, Pitt, Theodoros, & Ward, 1999; Nemec & Cohen, 1984; Rubow, Rosenbek, Collins, & Celesia, 1984; Rubow & Swift, 1985). Biofeedback techniques have also been used in an attempt to train the velopharyngeal mechanism to increase movement in order to achieve closure.

There are several ways to provide biofeedback to help the individual to determine what needs to be done to achieve a desired result with the velopharyngeal mechanism. The feedback can be auditory, visual, or tactile-kinesthetic. Many of the techniques used in traditional speech therapy use a form of biofeedback. For example, the air paddle and the See Scape (Pro-Ed, Austin, TX) provide visual biofeedback, while a tape recorder provides auditory feedback. Feeling the placement of a /t/ prior to attempting a /tsss/ is a form of tactile-kinesthetic feedback.

Perhaps the most effective form of biofeedback, particularly with children, is visual biofeedback. Visual biofeedback is usually easier to discriminate and judge; and some forms, such as a graph, do not disappear after the production is completed. Several of the instruments that are used in the diagnosis of resonance and velopharyngeal dysfunction are also useful in providing concrete, visual feedback regarding the individual's efforts to achieve velopharyngeal closure.

Aerodynamics

Pressure-flow instrumentation has numerous speech therapy applications. It can be used to provide feedback for phoneme-specific nasal air emission and can be very helpful in eliminating glottal stops and pharyngeal stops. With posterior compensatory productions, there is usually no oral pressure (see Figure 15–20). Pressure-flow instrumentation can provide visual feedback to help facilitate a change in placement of articulation for such compensations. The modification of a mid-dorsum palatal stop, for example, may be facilitated by placement of a pressure catheter behind the alveolar ridge. A lingual-alveolar placement for stop production will dramatically result in the appearance of oral air pressure pulses. Negative practice may also be implemented by instructing the speaker to revert to the mid-dorsum place of articulation once lingual advancement has been accomplished. Inappropriate nasal air emission may also be targeted in this fashion. Although the use of devices such as the See Scape will also provide feedback, pressure-

flow instrumentation has the advantage of providing for objective documentation of therapy progress.

Aerodynamic instrumentation can also be useful in providing feedback regarding breath support. With the use of a mouthpiece and pneumotachograph, real-time feedback of respiratory parameters, such as inspiratory volume and maximum phonation volume, can be monitored by the patient. To isolate the effect of inadequate respiratory support from velopharyngeal dysfunction, the nostrils can be plugged for one measurement and then open for another. The prolongation of voiceless continuants, such as /s/, may be especially helpful to discriminate between respiratory and velopharyngeal factors.

Nasometry

Nasometry is an excellent biofeedback instrument. Because it is updated every 8 milliseconds, it provides the individual with visual feedback that is essentially real-time regarding the amount of nasal acoustic energy that is generated during speech. This can be displayed in the form of either a bar graph (histogram) or a contour display. On both types of displays, the height of the graph increases with an increase in nasal acoustic energy. The speech pathologist can set tangible goals for the child during the treatment process and the child can receive immediate feedback on his or her success in attaining those goals.

The type of display that is used in therapy depends on the type of speech sample. The bar graph is best when working on individual phonemes, as it displays only one production at a time. The clinician can begin by having the child produce a prolonged /m/ and then a sustained "ah" in order to see the difference in the graphic display. The clinician can then determine an appropriate threshold line, which will serve as the child's visual target. If the child typically achieves around 30% nasalance on a particular phoneme, the examiner might place the bar at 25% and have the child repeat the phoneme without going over the bar. The target can be adjusted downward as the child becomes more proficient in reaching the goal. The contour display is most appropriate for use with connected speech because it consists of a 4-second time axis. The filled contour display is most visually appealing and, therefore, is best for use in therapy. If left in the normal mode, the goal is to keep the contour as low as possible, which reflects a decrease in nasal energy and/or an increase in oral energy. Since most children naturally want to make the contour as high as possible, the clinician can invert the display so that 0% is at the top and 100% is at the bottom. This way, the child must produce the high "mountains" as the goal.

The Nasometer software includes games designed to be used as part of a therapy protocol. These games are visually appealing and fun for children of all ages. The games help to break the monotony of repetitive practice and provide additional motivation and rewards for success. The software also includes lists of sentences that are useful in therapy. These sentences are grouped according to phoneme and degree of difficulty in achieving velopharyngeal closure. Since statistics regarding performance are automatically generated with each speech sample, the clinician can use these objective data to determine the child's ability to achieve each goal. The clinician can also track the child's progress over time with serial records.

The Nasometer is particularly useful in eliminating a nasal rustle (turbulence), since this is usually due to a small, inconsistent velopharyngeal opening. It is also useful in remediating phoneme-specific nasal air emission. It has been suggested that this form of biofeedback can even be used to modify resonance in certain cases of velopharyngeal incompetence (Heppt, Westrich, Strate, & Mohring, 1991). The clinician must keep in mind, however, that

biofeedback will only be successful if the individual is anatomically and physiologically capable of achieving normal velopharyngeal closure. Therefore, if progress is not made within a reasonable amount of time (no more than a few months), the child should be referred for physical management.

Photodetection

Dalston (1982) described a method to provide visual feedback to patients using a "photodetector." This device uses a light source below the velopharyngeal valve and a light detector above the valve. Feedback is provided to the patient by measuring the amount of light that is transmitted through the velopharyngeal valve during speech. Dalston reported that, in a small group of normal and abnormal speakers, the subjects were able to alter velopharyngeal movements to some degree. This therefore raised the possibility of using photodetection as a means for biofeedback. Photodetection has not become widely used since that time, however.

Nasopharyngosopy

Traditional speech therapy procedures rely on the use of auditory feedback and, in some cases, tactile feedback, to help the individual to achieve and then maintain appropriate speech production. Several authors have reported that nasopharyngoscopy can be a useful tool in therapy because it can provide visual feedback regarding the actions of the velopharyngeal mechanism during speech (Hoch et al., 1986; Rich, Farber, & Shprintzen, 1988; Shelton, Beaumont, Trier, & Furr, 1978; Siegel-Sadewitz & Shprintzen, 1982; Witzel, Tobe, & Salyer, 1988, 1989; Ysunza, Pamplona, Femat, Mayer, & Garcia-Velasco, 1997). In fact, nasopharyngoscopy is the only practical technique that allows direct visualization of the velopharyngeal structures and their function during unimpeded connected speech (Witzel et al., 1989). Nasopharyngoscopy has the advantage of being well-tolerated by most patients, and it can be repeated whenever necessary without any risk to the patient. Videofluoroscopy, which is the other technique to visualize the velopharyngeal structures, is not only impractical and too expensive for use in therapy, but the radiation risk prohibits its use for therapy.

The use of visual feedback assumes that the abnormal speaker may not "know how" to move the velum and pharyngeal walls to achieve closure under certain circumstances. Nasopharyngoscopy can be useful by providing visual feedback, which is associated with the neuromuscular signal during velopharyngeal movement. This can result in some active control of the velopharyngeal movements for opening and closing the valve. Of course, this implies that there is a role for learning in velopharyngeal function and that an individual may be able to change or increase movement when there is defective valving due to physiological causes related to mislearning.

The biofeedback procedure begins by helping the patient to identify the velopharyngeal structures on the video monitor. The person is then instructed to swallow, blow, or better yet produce a sound repetitively that results in complete closure. The action of the velopharyngeal mechanism is pointed out and the patient is encouraged to try to identify the sensation of the movement and closure of the port. Therapy then focuses on achieving velopharyngeal closure for the phonemes where closure is normally incomplete. This is done by changing the place of production for these sounds. Most commonly, the sibilant phonemes, particularly /s/, are defective. The fastest and easiest method to obtain closure on sibilants (if it is physically possible) is to have the patient produce a /t/ repetitively and watch the closure. The individual is then instructed to produce the /t/ with the teeth closed. Next, the patient is asked to prolong the /t/ with the teeth closed so that it is actually a /tssss/, while watching and feeling the effects of closure.

Before long, the patient is usually able to produce the /s/ in isolation and sometimes in words with this visual feedback. This can usually be done in one short session. It is sometimes helpful to have the patient go back and forth between the "good production" and the "bad production" to be able to feel, see, and hear the difference. This helps to develop voluntary control. Once the placement is achieved and the sound can be reproduced with correct placement easily, then the patient is ready for traditional speech therapy where the production is established first in syllables, then in words and sentences, and finally in connected speech.

As a biofeedback tool, nasopharyngoscopy is appropriate for patients who have the physical ability to achieve velopharyngeal closure, but are unable to do so on a consistent basis. It is therefore used effectively with individuals who demonstrate inconsistent velopharyngeal closure or phoneme-specific nasal air emission (Witzel et al., 1988). Nasopharyngoscopy can also be useful in helping patients to increase lateral pharyngeal wall movement following a pharyngeal flap procedure (Siegel-Sadewitz & Shprintzen, 1982; Witzel et al., 1989; Ysunza et al., 1997).

Speech Therapy Techniques

Although research continues in an effort to find methods to increase velopharyngeal movement through various "exercises," there tends to be general agreement that physical management, through surgical correction or a prosthesis, is still the most effective means to correct velopharyngeal dysfunction. Unless the velopharyngeal dysfunction is due to mislearning, speech therapy is usually not effective. Certainly, training of the velopharyngeal muscles has very limited applicability at this time. Speech therapy does have an important role in the habilitation of the speech of individuals with velopharyngeal dysfunction, however. The correction of misarticulation and other sequelae of velopharyngeal valving disorders must be done through the therapy process. This is usually most effective after the correction of the structure has been done.

The speech therapy techniques used with resonance disorders or compensatory productions are not magical, and they are really not very different from the techniques that are used in basic articulation therapy. As with any form of articulation therapy, the goal of therapy is to establish appropriate placement for each speech sound. In this case, it is also important to establish normal oral air pressure and airflow. Fortunately, this usually occurs naturally with a change in placement, unless there is a structural problem that requires surgical intervention. Several authors have reported that, with the use of compensatory productions, the velopharyngeal valve may remain open. Correction of the placement of these productions can result in an increase in velopharyngeal activity. Therefore, if the patient is stimulable for improvement with a change in placement, it is wise to attempt to correct these errors prior to considering surgical intervention (Ysunza, Pamplona, & Toledo, 1992; Ysunza-Rivera et al., 1991).

The following sections describe some specific therapy techniques that can be used with the common characteristics of velopharyngeal dysfunction. These techniques are offered as suggestions only. Further research is needed before the efficacy of techniques to alter resonance and the sequelae to velopharyngeal dysfunction can be determined.

Hypernasality

Hypernasality is very difficult, and most often impossible, to correct with therapy because it is usually due to a significant velopharyngeal opening. Therefore, the speech pathologist will rarely, if ever, provide speech therapy for pa-

tients with hypernasality. There are some techniques that can encourage oral resonance, however, and may be effective with hypernasality secondary to dysarthria.

Therapy Suggestions

- *Auditory Discrimination Training.* Have the child listen to hypernasal speech and then normal oral speech. This can be done by simulating both or by presenting different samples on a tape recorder. The best way to do this however is to use a "listening tube" (Figure 21–1). With this technique, the child puts one end of the tube at the entrance to a nostril and the other end near his or her ear. When hypernasality occurs, it is very audible and loud. The child is then ask to try to make adjustments in articulation to reduce or eliminate the sound in his or her ear.

- *Visual Feedback.* Any instrument that provides visual biofeedback can be used to try to increase oral resonance. This includes the

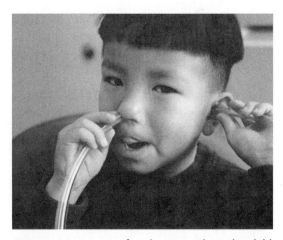

Figure 21–1. Use of a "listening tube." The child places one end of the tube at the entrance to a nostril and the other end by the ear. When hypernasality or nasal air emission occur, they can be heard loudly through the tube. This provides excellent auditory feedback.

Nasometer, pressure-flow instrumentation, and nasopharyngoscopy.

- *Tactile-Kinesthetic Training.* Have the child try to raise and lower the velum during the production of vowel sounds to produce nasal/oral contrasts. This can increase velar sensation and control. If this is hard, the velum can be mechanically raised with a tongue blade as the child is producing vowel sounds. The vowel "ah" is the best to use because the mouth is most open for that sound. Then have the patient attempt to raise the velum on his own to match the sound. (If there is a significant difference in resonance with elevation using the tongue blade, the patient may be a good candidate for a palatal lift.)

- *Tactile Feedback.* Have the child lightly touch the side of his or her nose to feel for vibration during the production of nasal phonemes (Figure 21–2). Then ask the child to feel for vibration during the production of oral sounds. If vibration is still felt, have the child try to eliminate this vibration as he or she works on various vowels and voiced pressure phonemes.

- *Lower the Back of the Tongue.* Have the child produce individual vowel sounds and then words with the back of the tongue down during the production of the vowels. Make sure that the back of the tongue is not abnormally elevated during articulation. To assist with this type of articulation, have the child yawn to forcibly lower the back of the tongue and raise the velum. Then have him produce vowel sounds and anterior consonants, keeping the same movement in mind.

- *Increase Oral Activity and Volume.* Increasing vocal effort has been shown to decrease velopharyngeal orifice size (McHenry, 1997). This may be due to the fact that increasing anterior oral activity increases posterior oral (thus velar) movement. Oral activity and the resulting resonance is the difference between "mumbling" and normal speech. Increased mouth opening can reduce oral resistance and increase oral resonance. Increasing volume al-

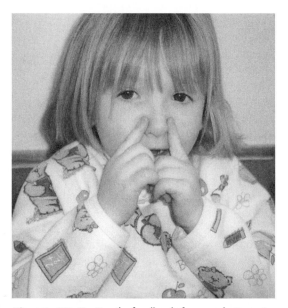

Figure 21–2. Tactile feedback for nasal air emission or hypernasality. By having the child lightly touch the side of his or her nose, the child will be able to feel the vibration that occurs with hypernasality or nasal air emission.

so tends to increase overall oral activity. However, the ultimate goal is a normal degree of oral activity and a normal volume level.

Nasal Air Emission

Nasal air emission occurs when there is audible emission of the airstream through the nasal cavity during the production of pressure-sensitive phonemes (plosives, fricatives, affricates). Nasal emission, nasal turbulence or rustle, a nasal snort, and the accompanying nasal grimace should all be targets of the speech therapy.

Therapy Suggestions

- *Auditory Feedback.* Make the child aware of the nasal air emission. This can be done by simulating this characteristic, or by having the child listen to and identify his own nasal air emission on a tape recorder. Again, the "listening tube" is the best method for auditory feedback because when nasal air emission occurs, it is heard clearly and even loudly through the tube (see Figure 21–1).

- *Tactile Feedback.* Have the child feel the sides of his or her nose for vibration during the repetitive production of pressure-sensitive phonemes or during the production of sentences with these sounds (no nasals). Ask the child to carefully produce these sounds or sentences without the vibration that occurs with nasal air emission (see Figure 21–2).
- *Visual Feedback.* Place an air paddle under the nares during the production of pressure-sensitive phonemes to help the child to see the nasal air emission (Figure 21–3). Ask the patient to produce the same sounds without moving the air paddle. Another method is to use a See Scape (Pro-Ed, Austin, TX; Figure 21–4). With the nasal olive in place in the

nares, the foam stopper will rise during the production of nasal phonemes, with nasal breathing at the end of the utterance, and during the production of oral sounds if there is accompanying nasal emission. Other forms of visual biofeedback can also be used, such as the Nasometer, pressure-flow instrumentation, or nasopharyngoscopy.

- *Cul-de-Sac Technique.* The child is asked to pinch his or her nostrils during the production of pressure sounds to eliminate the nasal air emission (Figure 21–5). The child is told to feel the increase in oral airflow and pressure. The child is then instructed to produce the sounds in the same way with the nostrils unoccluded.

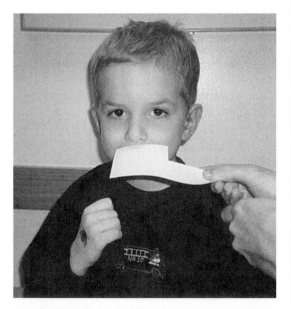

Figure 21–3. Air Paddle. Place a paper "air paddle" under the nares during the production of pressure-sensitive phonemes to help the child to see the nasal air emission if it occurs during the production of oral sounds.

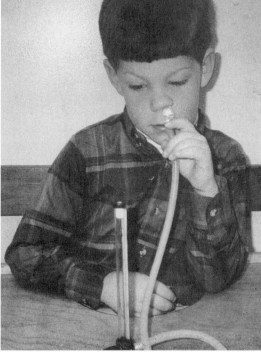

Figure 21–4. Use of the See Scape. The child is instructed to put the nasal olive in one nostril. The child is then asked to try to produce pressure consonants repetitively without allowing the foam stopper to rise in the tube.

- *Light, Quick Contacts.* Ask the child to produce light, quick contacts during the production of pressure-sensitive phonemes. This helps to eliminate the backup of air pressure in the nasopharynx and reduces the occurrence of nasal air emission.

Weak Consonants

When there is inadequate intraoral breath pressure, consonants become very weak in intensity and are occasionally omitted. Therefore, correction involves decreasing nasal air emission (as noted above) and increasing oral air pressure.

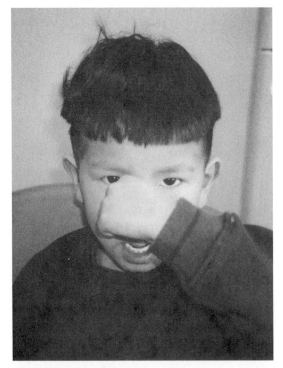

Figure 21–5. Cul-de-Sac Technique. The child is asked to pinch his or her nostrils during the production of pressure sounds to eliminate the nasal air emission. The child is told to feel the increase in oral airflow and pressure. The child is then instructed to produce the sounds in the same way with the nostrils unoccluded.

Therapy Suggestions

- *Increase Volume and Oral Activity.* Have the child increase volume and oral activity to increase the force of articulation, the oral air pressure and airflow, and velar movement.
- *Visual Feedback.* Place an air paddle in front of the child's mouth during the production of pressure-sensitive phonemes. Have the child try to produce the sounds with enough pressure to force the air paddle to move. Visual biofeedback instrumentation can also be used.
- *Tactile Feedback.* Have the child place his or her hand in front of your mouth as you produce plosives in a forceful manner. Have the child feel the air pressure as you produce each sound. Then have the child place his hand in front of his own mouth to do the same.

Compensatory Articulation Productions

Compensatory articulation productions are usually developed by an individual because the normal productions are too difficult to produce due to inadequate air pressure and they do not result in an adequate acoustic product. The compensatory productions are easier to produce and usually result in better use of the airflow and, thus, an improvement in intelligibility. Therefore, changing placement to eliminate compensatory productions is not easy in the presence of persistent velopharyngeal dysfunction. If surgical correction of the velopharyngeal valve is planned, it is often better to wait until after the surgery before beginning therapy. On the other hand, if the examiner finds that the patient is stimulable for a change in placement, and this results in an elimination of the nasal air emission, then therapy should be done prior to considering surgical intervention. The abnormal articulation may be a learned variation, rather than a true compensatory error due to velopharyngeal dysfunction.

Therapy Suggestions

Glottal stops as a substitution for plosives:

- Have the child whisper the syllable, which will prevent vocal fold adduction for a glottal stop.
- Have the child produce voiced and voiceless plosives slowly, followed by an aspirate /h/ before the vowel to eliminate the glottal stop (i.e., p-ha for pa).
- Modify voice onset time by delaying the voicing on the voiced plosive, or by delaying voicing on the vowel that follows a voiceless plosive (which is similar to the technique above).
- Have the child place a hand on his or her neck during the production of a glottal stop and then a prolonged vowel or nasal consonant. Have the child try to produce the plosive with the smoothness of the vowel or nasal consonant and without the "jerk" of the glottal stop.

Pharyngeal plosives as a substitution for plosives:

- Work on the placement of bilabial and lingual-alveolar plosives first. Ask the child to produce a yawn to get the base of the tongue down and the velum up. Have the child use anterior articulation with a posterior yawn movement to produce the sounds. Once these are mastered, work on velar plosives.
- Establish placement for velar plosives by starting with an /ng/. Then have the child push with the back of the tongue to produce the plosive.
- Work on an upward movement of the back of the tongue, rather than a posterior movement during production.

Pharyngeal fricatives as a substitution for sibilant sounds:

- Have the child produce fricative sounds first with the nostrils occluded and then open to get the feel for oral rather than pharyngeal airflow.
- Work on /s/ by having the child produce a hard /t/ with the teeth closed. Increase the duration of the production until it becomes /ts/ and then /tssss/. Finally, eliminate the /t/ component.
- Work on the /sh/ sound by having the child produce a big sigh with the teeth closed and lips rounded. Try to increase the force of oral air pressure. Work on the /ch/ sound by going from a /t/ with the teeth closed or trying a loud sneeze sound with the teeth closed. Once this sound is mastered, work on the /j/ by adding voicing.
- Place a straw at the point of the central incisors. Encourage the child to produce the sound with airflow through the straw.

For a nasal /l/ or /ng/ substitution:

- Ask the child to produce a yawn to get the base of the tongue down and the velum up. With the yawn, have the tongue tip go up to produce the /l/. Gradually eliminate the use of the yawn.

For mid-dorsum palatal stops:

- Have the patient bite on a tongue blade so that it is between the canine or molar teeth. Make sure it is back far enough to depress the middle part of the tongue to prevent a dorsal production. Have the child produce lingual-alveolar sounds in front of the tongue blade and velar sounds behind the tongue blade.

Hyponasality or Cul-de-Sac Resonance

When there is blockage somewhere in the vocal tract, due to such conditions as enlarged tonsils, enlarged adenoids, deviated septum, or stenotic naris, there may be either a mixture of

Case Report: Speech Therapy for Hypernasality Due to a Conversion Disorder

Jessica. had a history of normal speech and language development. She had an adenoidectomy at the age of 6, but this had no effect on speech or resonance. At the age of 12, she underwent a tonsillectomy due to tonsillar hypertrophy and chronic tonsillitis. The mother reported that Jessica didn't talk for about 2 weeks after the tonsillectomy in response to the pain. Once she did start to talk, marked hypernasality was noted. In addition, she was having difficulty drinking and was experiencing significant nasal regurgitation.

One month following the tonsillectomy, Jessica was seen for an evaluation. She was found to demonstrate a severe degree of hypernasality with significant nasal air emission. Consonants were very weak in intensity and pressure. In addition, utterance length was short due to the significant degree of nasal air emission and the loss of air pressure. A nasometric assessment showed a severely high degree of nasalance (Zoo = 92.40, mean 15.53, *SD* 4.86). All of this suggested a severe degree of velopharyngeal dysfunction.

An oral examination revealed no evidence of a submucous cleft through visual inspection or palpation. However, an assessment of oral-motor function showed very poor velar movement during phonation. During swallowing of thin liquids, there was a delay in the initiation of the swallow, and the tongue base was obviously forward, causing a gulp. Significant nasal regurgitation was noted to occur with each swallow. The patient attempted to compensate for this by closing her nose during the swallow, or holding something under her nose to catch the liquid.

A nasopharyngoscopy assessment showed very poor velar movement. As a result, a very large, midline velopharyngeal gap remained during speech production. In addition, the tongue was held forward during articulation and swallowing, thus exacerbating the hypernasality and nasal regurgitation. An inspection of the velum on the nasal surface showed normal morphology and no evidence of velar abnormality.

Based on the examination results, it was concluded that this was a case of an hysterical conversion disorder. It was surmised that this occurred secondary to the attempt to avoid or alleviate pain just following the tonsillectomy. After a few weeks, this speech pattern had become habituated. Therefore, a short period of intensive speech and swallowing therapy was recommended.

Jessica was seen for seven half-hour sessions over a period of 4 weeks. The following techniques were used in therapy:

- Puffing the cheeks with air.
- Biofeedback using the Nasometer
- Biofeedback using the See Scape
- Palpation of the velum to increase tolerance and decrease sensitivity.
- Drinking with the tongue back against the velum.
- Yawning to bring the back of the tongue down and the velum up.
- Blowing with the cheeks puffed.
- Producing a /t/ sound and then prolonging it with teeth closed to produce an /s/.

Gradual progress was noted during the first few sessions, but significant improvement occurred between the fifth and sixth sessions. A sampling of nasometric scores shows the improvement.

- Evaluation: Zoo = 92.40
- Session 1: Zoo = 57.96
- Session 2: Zoo = 64.00
- Session 5: Zoo = 46.91
- Session 6: Zoo = 14.51, Nasals = 68.17).

During the sixth session, the mother reported that Jessica's speech seemed to have improved overnight and was back to normal. During the session, she was noted to have normal resonance and no nasal emission. She was able to blow normally and whistle and she was able to swallow without gulping or nasal regurgitation. This improvement was maintained; therefore, Jessica was discharged from therapy after the seventh session.

hypernasality and hyponasality or cul-de-sac resonance. Whenever there is blockage, it requires medical or surgical intervention. Speech therapy will not correct resonance that is due to this type of structural cause. If there is intermittent hyponasality due to the timing deficits of apraxia, however, then nasal-oral contrasts could be used to improve the timing and coordination of velopharyngeal function for connected speech.

Timetable for Intervention and Goals

Infants and Toddlers

During the first few weeks of life, feeding is necessarily the first priority. Most infants with cleft lip, and even those with cleft palate, soon develop adequate feeding skills, even though some minor modifications of the nipple or bottle may be needed. If there are additional structural or neurological problems, however, the infant may have more complex problems that affect feeding. In those cases, the speech pathologist should assist in the development of a feeding program to assure adequate nutrition, while trying to enhance oral-motor development as much as possible. Once effective feeding has been established, the next priority is language development.

In the first few years of life, the child is learning about the world and developing language for the first time. The parent or caregiver should concentrate on stimulating language so that first receptive language and then expressive language skills develop appropriately. The speech pathologist for the cleft palate/craniofacial team is responsible for counseling families on language stimulation during this critical period of time. The families should always be given written information, including a home language-stimulation program to use as a guide (Hardin, 1991). Because the parents are the primary instructors of language for the child, they should be advised on how to be most effective in that job (Hahn, 1989; O'Gara & Logemann, 1990; Phillips, 1990). If language does not develop normally, or if there are problems with the physical prerequisites for speech, therapy should be initiated immediately.

The parents should be told that during the first 3 years, they should concentrate on the quantity of speech, not the quality. However, there are some things that they can do to stimulate early phonemic development. Parents should be shown how to encourage vocalizations by imitating the child's cooing and babbling. If there was a cleft palate, they should be instructed on how to encourage the production of plosives once the cleft is repaired.

Preschool Children

By the age of 3, most children are communicating with complete sentences, although errors in syntax and morphology are common. The child should also have developed the use of nasal and plosive sounds, and should also be using fricatives and even affricate phonemes. Therefore, this is an appropriate time to evaluate speech, resonance, and velopharyngeal function and, if indicated, begin treatment. If it is determined that secondary surgical intervention is needed, this is usually done between the ages of 3 and 5. Speech therapy can be initiated prior to correction of the structure and work can begin of the correction of articulation placement errors. However, if the structure is corrected first, the therapy will be easier and less frustrating for the child. In addition, progress will be much faster, and as a result, the therapy will be more cost-effective because there will be more "bang for the buck."

Whenever possible, the parents or caregivers should be encouraged to observe therapy and, if possible, videotape the session for the other spouse to view at home. The speech pathologist should work closely with the parents and even the siblings to involve them in the therapy process as much as possible. Progress will be much faster if the parent is involved and there is practice in between the therapy sessions (Pamplona, Ysunza, & Uriostegui, 1996).

With the physical management and speech therapy in the preschool years, the goal should be to attain age-appropriate speech, or close to

it, by the time the child enters kindergarten. This is important for several reasons. First, preschool children are more receptive to correcting abnormal speech patterns than older children due to the "critical period" and "habit strength" factors. In addition, funding for private speech therapy through medical insurance is very limited for school-aged children because they are eligible for services in the schools. Unfortunately, children with a history of cleft or craniofacial anomalies do not always get the services that they need through the schools. This is related to the size of the school caseloads, the break in the summer, and the fact that the school speech pathologists must be generalists, and therefore, they usually do not have the specialty expertise in this area. Fortunately, with early intervention services, most children with a history of cleft lip or palate are able to attain age-appropriate or acceptable speech by the time they reach school-age.

School-Aged Children

As noted previously, school-aged children who continue to have speech problems typically receive speech and language services through their school. At this point, velopharyngeal dysfunction, if it was present, should have been corrected. If there is evidence of velopharyngeal dysfunction in this age group, the child should be referred immediately to a specialist, preferably someone with a craniofacial center, for further evaluation of velopharyngeal function. In most cases, significant gains in speech therapy cannot be achieved without the correction of the velopharyngeal dysfunction first.

When therapy is required in this age group, it is usually for the correction of any remaining articulation errors, which are commonly related to dental abnormalities or malocclusion or language problems. Typical errors due to the malocclusion include a lateral lisp, a frontal lisp, or the use of a mid-dorsum palatal stop for lingual-alveolar sounds. These errors may be either compensatory or obligatory. Either way, correction is difficult, if not impossible, as long as the structural anomaly is still present. The dilemma is that the malocclusion may not be correctable until the child undergoes a maxillary advancement after facial growth is complete, which is usually after age 14 for girls and age18 for boys. In the meantime, the speech distortion persists. The speech pathologist should consider very carefully if the child is appropriate for therapy in these cases. Although it is hard to wait, the speech may self-correct with a correction in malocclusion especially if the errors are obligatory. If they do not, therapy is appropriate after the surgery.

Some cleft palate or craniofacial centers offer summer camps for their school-aged patients who continue to demonstrate speech problems that are correctable with therapy (Schendel & Bzoch, 1979). The purpose of the camp is to provide intensive speech therapy, while giving the children opportunities to interact with others who have similar problems and experiences. These speech camps are usually overnight camps of 6 to 12 weeks duration so that the children remain with their peers during most of the summer. During the day, speech pathologists provide intensive individual and group therapy and this can be done with real-life communication experiences. The children are also able to work on some of their psychosocial issues through individual and group sessions with a psychologist or counselor. The positive atmosphere of the camp and the development of friendships can help to motivate and modify the attitudes of many of these children. This model is especially beneficial for children who live in rural or thinly populated areas where services are not readily available. It is also helpful for children who are receiving inconsistent or inadequate therapy services through their school.

Because there are many apparent advantages of a summer speech therapy camp, it may seem unusual that more centers do not provide this type of program. Unfortunately, as many advantages as this type of setting can offer, there are an equal number of disadvantages and obstacles. Having a summer camp requires an enormous amount of planning, coordination, time, and effort from the trained professional staff of the cleft palate/craniofacial team. Finding an appropriate and safe facility can be particularly challenging. The camp requires the expenditure of a significant amount of money for adequate materials and resources. Finding qualified and experienced speech pathologists for the short summer session is very difficult. The camp must purchase liability insurance and malpractice insurance. Overall, the expenses of providing the camp program are enormous and are not totally reimbursable by insurance or fees. Therefore, outside funding must be obtained. Many of the patients have problems with transportation, with funding, and once they are there, with homesickness. Even getting the patients to commit to that length of time is hard when most kids are involved in sports and other activities during the summer. The final concern is that the efficacy of a short-term intensive therapy program is unclear. There is no research to show the long-term gains from this type of program. Because of these various problems and concerns, the camp that was sponsored by the Craniofacial Center at Cincinnati Children's Hospital Medical Center has been discontinued.

Adolescents and Adults

Occasionally, an older child or an adult will decide to seek improvement in his or her speech. In many cases, the primary problem is uncorrected velopharyngeal dysfunction. Therefore, surgical or prosthetic intervention should be done prior to initiating speech therapy, unless there are learned errors that affect velopharyngeal function. The physical management should improve or eliminate the hypernasality or nasal air emission. However, the prognosis for normal speech at these ages is somewhat guarded for several reasons. First, the force of habit strength cannot be underestimated. In addition, the older patient has developed a self-monitoring system so that modifying speech and resonance to change what is perceived as "normal" can be very difficult. Speech therapy after the surgery is also challenging for the same reasons. Therefore, to be successful, the patient needs to be highly motivated to make his or her speech better.

The Ultimate Goal

In past generations, the goal of treatment for most individuals with a history of cleft palate was acceptable or intelligible speech, because normal speech was not always obtainable. With increased knowledge of the nature of the velopharyngeal mechanism, and with the advances in surgical techniques and even therapy techniques over the past few decades, most individuals born with cleft palate can expect to ultimately attain normal speech with no evidence of hypernasality. Normal speech production and resonance with no evidence of "cleft palate speech" should therefore be the goal when the structural anomaly is the only cause of the abnormal speech. If there is concomitant neurological dysfunction, including pharyngeal hypotonia, dysarthria, or apraxia, then the prognosis for perfect speech is more guarded because surgical correction cannot affect movement. Regardless, all efforts should be made to achieve normal speech, not just "acceptable speech considering the velopharyngeal mechanism."

Summary

Speech therapy is an appropriate treatment option for correction of the articulation disorder that results from velopharyngeal dysfunction. Speech therapy will not correct velopharyngeal insufficiency, since this is due to a structural defect, and its efficacy with even mild velopharyngeal incompetence is also questionable. Instead, physical management, usually sur-

gery, is necessary to correct the velopharyngeal dysfunction first. When in doubt regarding the appropriate recommendation, however, a trial period of speech therapy can be done to determine the individual's stimulability and response to therapy. It is always recommended that the speech pathologist who is inexperienced in this area consider consultation with a more experienced speech pathologist. Therapy should continue as long as the child is making progress. If the child is not responding to the therapy and continues to have characteristics of velopharyngeal dysfunction, it is very important to refer the child to a craniofacial anomaly team or specialist for further evaluation of velopharyngeal function. Surgical intervention or revision may be necessary.

References

Berry, M. F., & Eisenson, J. (1956). *Speech disorders: Principles and practices of therapy*. New York: Appleton-Century-Crofts.

Blakeley, R. W. (1964). The complementary use of speech prostheses and pharyngeal flaps in palatal insufficiency. *Cleft Palate Journal, 1*, 194.

Blakeley, R. W. (1969). The rationale for a temporary speech prosthesis in palatal insufficiency. *British Journal of Disorders in Communication, 4*(2), 134–139.

Cole, R. M. (1971). Direct muscle training for the improvement of velopharyngeal function. In K. Bzoch (Ed.), *Communicative disorders related to cleft lip and palate* (pp. 250–256). Boston: Little, Brown.

Cole, R. M. (1979). Direct muscle training for the improvement of velopharyngeal activity. In K. Bzoch (Ed.), *Communicative disorders related to cleft lip and palate* (2nd ed., pp. 328–340). Boston: Little, Brown.

Dalston, R. M. (1982). Photodetector assessment of velopharyngeal activity. *Cleft Palate Journal, 19*(1), 1–8.

Davis, S. M., & Drichta, C. E. (1980). Biofeedback theory and application in allied health: Speech pathology. *Biofeedback and Self Regulation, 5*(2), 159–174.

Flowers, C. R., & Morris, H. L. (1973). Oral-pharyngeal movements during swallowing and speech. *Cleft Palate Journal, 10,* 181–191.

Gentil, M., Aucouturier, J. L., Delong, V., & Sambuis, E. (1994). EMG biofeedback in the treatment of dysarthria. *Folia Phoniatrica et Logopedia, 46*(4), 188–192.

Golding-Kushner, K. J., Cisneros, G., & LeBlanc, E. (1995). Speech bulbs. In R. J. Shprintzen & J. Bardach (Eds.), *Cleft palate speech management* (pp. 352–375). St. Louis, MO: Mosby.

Hahn, E. (1989). Directed home language stimulation program for infants with cleft lip and palate. In K. R. Bzoch (Ed.), *Communicative disorders related to cleft lip and palate* (3rd ed., pp. 313–319). Boston: Little, Brown.

Hardin, M. A. (1991). Cleft palate. Intervention. *Clinics in Communication Disorders, 1*(3), 12–18.

Harkins, C., & Koepp-Baker, H. (1948). Twenty-five years of cleft palate prosthesis. *Journal of Speech and Hearing Disorders, 13,* 23.

Heppt, W., Westrich, M., Strate, B., & Mohring, L. (1991). [Nasalance: A new concept for objective analysis of nasality]. *Laryngorhinootologie, 70*(4), 208–213.

Hoch, L., Golding-Kushner, K., Siegel-Sadewitz, V. L., & Shprintzen, R. L. (1986). Speech therapy. In B. J. McWilliams (Ed.), *Current methods of assessing and treating children with cleft palates* (pp. 313–326). New York: Thieme.

Israel, J. M., Cook, T. A., & Blakeley, R. W. (1993). The use of a temporary oral prosthesis to treat speech in velopharyngeal incompetence. *Facial and Plastic Surgery, 9*(3), 206–212.

Kanter, C. E. (1947). The rationale for blowing exercises for patients with repaired cleft palates. *Journal of Speech Disorders, 12,* 281.

Kuehn, D. P. (1991). New therapy for treating hypernasal speech using continuous positive airway pressure (CPAP). *Plastic and Reconstructive Surgery, 88*(6), 959–966; Discussion 967–969.

Kuehn, D. P. (1997). The development of a new technique for treating hypernasality: CPAP. *American Journal of Speech-Language Pathology, 6*(4), 5–8.

Kuehn, D. P., Moon, J. B., & Folkins, J. W. (1993). Levator veli palatini muscle activity in relation to intranasal air pressure variation. *Cleft Palate Craniofacial Journal, 30*(4), 361–368.

Lubit, E. C., & Larsen, R. E. (1969). The Lubit palatal exerciser: A preliminary report. *Cleft Palate Journal, 6,* 120–133.

Lubit, E. C., & Larsen, R. E. (1971). A speech aid for velopharyngeal incompetency. *Journal of Speech and Hearing Disorders, 36*(1), 61–70.

Massengill, R., Jr., Quinn, G. W., & Pickrell, K. L. (1971). The use of a palatal stimulator to decrease velopharyngeal gap. *Annals of Otology, Rhinology, and Laryngology, 80,* 135–137.

Massengill, R., Jr., Quinn, G. W., Pickrell, K. L., & Levinson, C. (1968). Therapeutic exercise and velopharyngeal gap. *Cleft Palate Journal, 5,* 44–47.

McGillivray, R., Proctor-Williams, K., & McLister, B. (1994). Simple biofeedback device to reduce excessive vocal intensity. *Medical and Biological Engineering Computing, 32*(3), 348–350.

McGrath, C. O., & Anderson, M. W. (1990). Prosthetic treatment of velopharyngeal incompetence. In J. Bardach & H. L. Morris (Eds.), *Multidisciplinary management of cleft lip and palate* (pp. 809–815). Philadelphia: W. B. Saunders.

McHenry, M. A. (1997). The effect of increased vocal effort on estimated velopharyngeal orifice area. *American Journal of Speech-Language Pathology, 6*(4), 55–61.

McWilliams, B. J., & Bradley, D. (1965). Ratings of velopharyngeal closure during blowing and speech. *Cleft Palate Journal, 2,* 46.

Moll, K. L. (1965). A cinefluorographic study of velopharyngeal function in normals during various activities. *Cleft Palate Journal, 2,* 112.

Morris, H. L. (1984). Types of velopharyngeal incompetence. In H. Winitz (Ed.), *Treating articulation disorders: For clinicians by clinicians* (p. 211). Baltimore: University Park Press.

Moser, H. (1942). Diagnostic and clinical procedures in rhinolalia. *Journal of Speech Disorders, 7,* 1.

Murdoch, B. E., Pitt, G., Theodoros, D. G., & Ward, E. C. (1999). Real-time continuous visual biofeedback in the treatment of speech breathing disorders following childhood traumatic brain injury: Report of one case. *Pediatric Rehabilitation, 3*(1), 5–20.

Nemec, R. E., & Cohen, K. (1984). EMG biofeedback in the modification of hypertonia in spastic dysarthria: Case report. *Archives of Physical Medicine and Rehabilitation, 65*(2), 103–104.

O'Gara, M. M., & Logemann, J. A. (1990). Early speech development in cleft palate babies. In J. Bardach & H. L. Morris (Eds.), *Multidisciplinary management of cleft lip and palate* (pp. 717–726). Philadelphia: W. B. Saunders.

Pamplona, M. C., Ysunza, A., & Uriostegui, C. (1996). Linguistic interaction: The active role of parents in speech therapy for cleft palate patients. *International Journal of Pediatric Otorhinolaryngology, 37*(1), 17–27.

Peterson, S. J. (1973). Velopharyngeal closure: Some important differences. *Journal of Speech and Hearing Disorders, 38,* 89.

Peterson, S. J. (1974). Electrical stimulation of the soft palate. *Cleft Palate Journal, 11,* 72–86.

Phillips, B. J. (1990). Early speech management. In J. Bardach & H. L. Morris (Eds.), *Multidisciplinary management of cleft lip and palate* (pp. 732–736). Philadelphia: W. B. Saunders.

Powers, G. L., & Starr, C. D. (1974). The effect of muscle exercises on velopharyngeal gap and nasality. *Cleft Palate Journal, 11,* 28.

Prosek, R. A., Montgomery, A. A., Walden, B. E., & Schwartz, D. M. (1978). EMG biofeedback in the treatment of hyperfunctional voice disorders. *Journal of Speech and Hearing Disorders, 43*(3), 282–294.

Rich, B. M., Farber, K., & Shprintzen, R. J. (1988). Nasopharyngoscopy in the treatment of palatopharyngeal insufficiency. *International Journal of Prosthodontics, 1*(3), 248–251.

Rossiter, D., Howard, D. M., & DeCosta, M. (1996). Voice development under training with and without the influence of real-time visually presented biofeedback [Letter]. *Journal of the Acoustical Society of America, 99*(5), 3253–3256.

Rubow, R. T., Rosenbek, J. C., Collins, M. J., & Celesia, G. G. (1984). Reduction of hemifacial spasm and dysarthria following EMG biofeedback. *Journal of Speech and Hearing Disorders, 49*(1), 26–33.

Rubow, R., & Swift, E. (1985). A microcomputer-based wearable biofeedback device to improve transfer of treatment in parkinsonian dysarthria. *Journal of Speech and Hearing Disorders, 50*(2), 178–185.

Ruscello, D. M. (1982). A selected review of palatal training procedures. *Cleft Palate Journal, 19*(3), 181–193.

Schendel, L. L., & Bzoch, K. R. (1979). Advantages of intensive summer training programs. In K. R. Bzoch (Ed.), *Communicative disorders related to cleft lip and palate* (2nd ed., pp. 318–327). Boston: Litttle, Brown.

Schneider, E., & Shprintzen, R. J. (1980). A survey of speech pathologists: Current trends in the diagnosis and management of velopharyngeal insufficiency. *Cleft Palate Journal, 17*(3), 249–253.

Selley, W. G., Zananiri, M. C., Ellis, R. E., & Flack, F. C. (1987). The effect of tongue position on division of airflow in the presence of velopharyngeal defects. *British Journal of Plastic Surgery, 40*(4), 377–383.

Shelton, R. L., Beaumont, K., Trier, W. C., & Furr, M. L. (1978). Videoendoscopic feedback in training velopharyngeal closure. *Cleft Palate Journal, 15*(1), 6–12.

Shelton, R. L., Hahn, E., & Morris, H. L. (1968). Diagnosis and therapy. In D. R. Spriestersbach & D. Sherman (Eds.), *Cleft palate and communication* (pp. 225–268). New York: Academic Press.

Shelton, R. L., Lindquist, A. F., Arndt, W. B., Elbert, M., & Youngstrom, K. A. (1971). Effect of speech bulb reduction on movement of the posterior wall of the pharynx and posture of the tongue. *Cleft Palate Journal, 8,* 10–17.

Shelton, R. L., Lindquist, A. F., Chisum, L., Arndt, W. B., Youngstrom, K. A., & Stick, S. L. (1968). Effect of prosthetic speech bulb reduction on articulation. *Cleft Palate Journal, 5,* 195–204.

Shprintzen, R. J., Lencione, R. M., McCall, G. N., & Skolnick, M. L. (1974). A three dimensional cinefluoroscopic analysis of velopharyngeal closure during speech and nonspeech activities in normals. *Cleft Palate Journal, 11,* 412–428.

Siegel-Sadewitz, V. L., & Shprintzen, R. J. (1982). Nasopharyngoscopy of the normal velopharyngeal sphincter: An experiment of biofeedback. *Cleft Palate Journal, 19*(3), 194–200.

Stemple, J. C., Weiler, E., Whitehead, W., & Komray, R. (1980). Electromyographic biofeedback training with patients exhibiting a hyperfunctional voice disorder. *Laryngoscope, 90*(3), 471–476.

Tash, E. L., Shelton, R. L., Knox, A. W., & Michel, J. F. (1971). Training voluntary pharyngeal wall movements in children with normal and inadequate velopharyngeal closure. *Cleft Palate Journal, 8,* 277–290.

Tomes, L., Kuehn, D., & Peterson-Falzone, S. (1996, April). Behavioral therapy for speakers with velopharyngeal impairment. *NCVS Status and Progress Report, 9,* 159–180.

Tudor, C., & Selley, W. G. (1974). A palatal training appliance and a visual aid for use in the treatment of hypernasal speech. *British Journal of Disorders of Communication, 9,* 117–122.

Van Riper, C. (1946). *Speech correction: Principles and methods.* New York: Prentice-Hall.

Van Riper, C. (1963). *Speech correction: Principles and methods* (4th ed.). New York: Prentice-Hall.

Weber, J., Jobe, R. P., & Chase, R. A. (1970). Evaluation of muscle stimulation in the rehabilitation of patients with hypernasal speech. *Plastic and Reconstructive Surgery, 46,* 173–174.

Weiss, C. E. (1971). Success of an obturator reduction program. *Cleft Palate Journal, 8,* 291–297.

Weiss, T., Carson, L. F., & Brady, J. P. (1979). Effects of training schedule and biofeedback on speech dysfluency. *American Journal of Psychiatry, 136*(3), 342–344.

Wells, C. (1945). Improving the speech of the cleft palate child. *Journal of Speech Disorders, 10,* 162.

Wells, C. (1948). Practical techniques for speech training for cleft palate cases. *Journal of Speech and Hearing Disorders, 13,* 71.

Witzel, M. A., Tobe, J., & Salyer, K. (1988). The use of nasopharyngoscopy biofeedback therapy in the correction of inconsistent velopharyngeal closure. *International Journal of Pediatric Otorhinolaryngology, 15*(2), 137–142.

Witzel, M. A., Tobe, J., & Salyer, K. E. (1989). The use of videonasopharyngoscopy for biofeedback therapy in adults after pharyngeal flap surgery. *Cleft Palate Journal, 26*(2), 129–134; Discussion 135.

Wolfaardt, J. F., Wilson, F. B., Rochet, A., & McPhee, L. (1993). An appliance based approach to the management of palatopharyngeal incompetency: A clinical pilot project. *Journal of Prosthetic Dentistry, 69*(2), 186–195.

Ysunza, A., Pamplona, C., & Toledo, E. (1992). Change in velopharyngeal valving after speech therapy in cleft palate patients. A videonasopharyngoscopic and multi-view videofluoroscopic study. *International Journal of Pediatric Otorhinolaryngology, 24*(1), 45–54.

Ysunza, A., Pamplona, M., Femat, T., Mayer, I., & Garcia-Velasco, M. (1997). Videonasopharyngoscopy as an instrument for visual biofeedback during speech in cleft palate patients. *International Journal of Pediatric Otorhinolaryngology, 41*(3), 291–298.

Ysunza-Rivera, A., Pamplona-Ferreira, M. C., & Toledo-Cortina, E. (1991). [Changes in valvular movements of the velopharyngeal sphincter after speech therapy in children with cleft palate. A videonasopharyngoscopic and videofluoroscopic study of multiple incidence]. *Boletin Medico del Hospital Infantil de Mexico, 48*(7), 490–501.

Yules, R. B., & Chase, R. A. (1969). A training method for reduction of hypernasality in speech. *Plastic and Reconstructive Surgery, 43*(2), 180–185.

Glossary

ablative surgery: surgery that involves removal of a part, such as a portion of the hard palate, due to a malignancy.

acrocentric: when the centromere of a chromosome is very close to one end of the chromosome.

active speech characteristics: see *compensatory errors*.

acute otitis media: bacterial infection of the middle ear.

adenoid: a normal collection of unencapsulated lymphoid tissue that is found on the posterior pharyngeal wall of the nasopharynx on the skull base; also called the *pharyngeal tonsil*.

adenoid facies: facial characteristics due to airway obstruction secondary to adenoid enlargement; characteristics include an open mouth posture, anterior tongue position, the mandible in a forward or downward position, facial elongation, suborbital coloring and puffy eyes, and the appearance of pinched nostrils.

adenoidectomy: surgical procedure to remove the adenoids; done to resolve recurrent infection, improve eustachian tube function, or eliminate upper airway obstruction.

adenotonsillectomy: a surgical procedure where both the tonsil and adenoid tissue are removed; done to resolve recurrent infection, improve eustachian tube function, or eliminate upper airway obstruction.

adipose: fat tissue.

aerodynamics: a branch of physics that deals with the mechanical properties of air and other gases in motion, the properties that set them in motion, and the results of that motion.

affricate sounds: pressure-sensitive consonants that require a build-up of intraoral air pressure and then slow release through a narrow opening; are produced as a combination of a plosive and fricative; includes /ch/ and /j/.

ala nasi: (pl. alae) Latin for "wing;" the outside curved part of the nostril.

alar base: the area where the ala meets the upper lip.

alar rims: the part of the nose that surrounds the opening to the nostril on either side.

alleles: the alternative forms or variations of a given gene that are found at the same locus on an homologous chromosome.

almost-but-not-quite (ABNQ): a term used to refer to a small, yet consistent velopharyngeal gap.

alveolar bone graft procedure: a surgical procedure of grafting bone, often from the iliac crest (hip bone), into the cleft site to stimulate new bone formation; this helps to repair the alveolar ridge, serves as the missing nasal floor and piriform (nasal) rim, and provides bone for eruption of teeth.

alveolar ridge: the portion of the maxilla and mandible that form the base and the bony support for the teeth; also called the *alveolus*, or simply the gum ridge.

alveolus: the socket of the tooth; also used as another word for *alveolar ridge*.

amniotic bands: strands of tissue from the amnion (membrane surrounding the embryo and fetus) that have ruptured and float in the amniotic cavity; these strands can attach to limbs, the head, or other body parts and act as tourniquets, cutting off blood supply to developing structures, resulting in amputations of limbs and digits, cleft lip, and encephalocele if the cranium is involved.

Angle's classification system: differentiates normal occlusion and three types of malocclusion.

ankyloglossia: a condition where the lingual frenulum is short or has an anterior attachment, resulting in restricted movement of the tongue tip; also known as *tongue-tie.*

anotia: absence of the external auditory canal.

anterior crossbite: a condition where a maxillary tooth or teeth are inside the mandibular arch; may involve any or all of the anterior teeth, such as the central incisors, lateral incisors, or canines; commonly seen in patients with dental or skeletal Class III malocclusion.

anterior nasal spine: the anterior point of the maxilla that corresponds to the base of the columella.

anterior-posterior (AP) view: see *frontal view.*

anticipation: in genetics, the tendency for a disorder to have earlier age of onset or more severe manifestations in successive generations.

antimongoloid slant: downward slant of the eyes.

apnea: see *sleep apnea.*

apraxia (of speech): (adj. apraxic) characterized by difficulty executing volitional oral movements and difficulty in sequencing oral movements for connected speech; can result in an inability to adequately coordinate velopharyngeal movement with the other subsystems of speech (respiration, phonation, and articulation); also called *dyspraxia* or *verbal apraxia.*

articulators: the oral structures that move to modify the airstream during speech; these include the lips, jaws (including the teeth), tongue, and velum.

association: in genetics, when two or more abnormalities appear together frequently but have not yet been classified together as a syndrome.

ataxia: an inability to coordinate muscle activity during voluntary movements; usually due to disorders of the cerebellum or posterior columns of the spinal cord.

atlas: the first cervical vertebrae; articulates with the occipital bone and rotates around the dens of the axis.

atresia: (adj. atretic) congenital absence or closure of any bodily orifice (opening, passage, or cavity); see *aural atresia.*

atrial septal defect (ASD): congenital discontinuity of the tissue that separates the upper chambers of the heart.

atrophy: shrinkage or degeneration of a structure.

attention deficit-hyperactivity disorder (ADHD): a cluster of behavioral characteristics involving impaired attention, distractibility, impulsivity, and hyperactivity; there appears to be a genetic basis to this disorder that affects the biochemical function in the brain.

audio: related to the sense of hearing.

audiologist: a professional who is responsible for testing hearing and middle-ear function; the professional who works in conjunction with the otolaryngologist in the monitoring, evaluation, and treatment of hearing loss associated with middle-ear disease, structural anomalies, or neurological anomalies that affect hearing recognition and perception.

auditory: pertaining to the sense of hearing or organs of hearing.

auditory atresia: see *aural atresia.*

auditory cortex: part of the brain that provides an awareness of sound.

auditory tube: see *eustachian tube.*

aural: related to the ear or hearing.

aural atresia: congenital closure of the auditory canal that usually results in a conductive hearing loss; also called *auditory atresia.*

auricle: the external ear; also known as *pinna* or *concha.*

autosomal recessive: traits that are manifest only when the trait is present in both copies of a gene.

autosome: (adj. autosomal) any chromosome that is not a sex chromosome.

backing of phonemes: a compensatory articulation strategy characterized by the production of most phonemes with the back of the tongue, and with the velum or with the posterior pharyngeal wall.

base view: X-ray view that allows the examiner to see the entire velopharyngeal sphincter during connected speech, as if looking up through the port; the relative contributions of the velum, the lateral pharyngeal walls, and posterior pharyngeal wall to closure can be determined; also called an *en face view*.

Bell's palsy: facial paralysis due to an infection.

bicuspids: teeth that typically have two cusps.

bifid uvula: a congenital split or cleft in the uvula; a stigmata that is frequently associated with a submucous cleft palate.

biofeedback: a technique for making unconscious or autonomic physiological processes perceptible to the senses in order to manipulate them by conscious mental control; techniques are based on the learning principle that a desired response can be learned when it is determined that a specific thought process can produced the desired physiological response.

body section (of a prosthetic device): the anterior or palatal portion of a speech appliance that fits snugly against the contours of the individual's mouth and teeth; the purpose of the body section is to hold the appliance in place against the roof of the mouth or to serve as an obturator to close off a defect in the palate.

bone graft procedure: see *alveolar bone graft procedure*.

brachycephaly: a short skull.

brachydactyly: abnormally short digits (fingers or toes).

Brodie crossbite: occurs when the lingual cusps of all the maxillary posterior teeth are buccal to the mandibular teeth.

buccal (adj.): for the buccinator muscle of the cheeks; pertaining to, in the direction of, or adjacent to the cheek; the part of the dental arch that is posterior to the canine teeth and on the side of the teeth.

buccal crossbite: occurs when one or more maxillary teeth are positioned buccally such that the maxillary lingual cusps reside buccal to the mandibular cusps.

buccal sulcus: (pl. sulci) the area between the cheeks and teeth.

canines: teeth that have one point or cusp; also known as *cuspids*.

cant: a slant, as in dental occlusion.

canthus: (pl. canthi) the angle or corner of the eye.

caries: decay in the teeth, resulting in cavities.

cell cycle: the process of preparing for and undergoing cell division.

central fossa: (pl. fossae) the valley between the buccal cusp to lingual cusp of a tooth.

central sleep apnea: suspension of breathing during sleep due to medullary depression, which inhibits respiratory movement.

centromere: the area of constriction of a chromosome that divides the chromosome into two pairs of arms.

cephalogram: a lateral radiograph of the craniofacial skeleton; used in the planning of orthognathic surgery.

cephalometric radiographs: standardized lateral skull films used to measure the jaw relationship and the soft tissue profile of the forehead, nose, lips, and chin.

cheiloplasty: cleft lip repair.

choana: the opening on each side of the posterior part of the vomer that leads from the nasal cavity into the nasopharynx.

choanal atresia: congenital closure of the choana.

choanal stenosis: a narrowing of the choana.

cholesteatoma: a mass of keratinizing squamous epithelium and cholesterol in the middle ear, usually resulting from chronic otitis media.

chromosome: one of the bodies in the cell nucleus that contains genes; consists of a single linear double strand of DNA with associated proteins that function to organize and compact the DNA in a cell-for-cell division; the 46 chromosomes (23 pairs) contain the complete set of instructions for cell replication and differentiation.

cine study: see *cineradiography*.

cineradiography: radiography of an organ in motion; an old method for evaluating velopharyngeal function by recording multiple views on motion picture film in order to observe several dimensions; often referred to as a *cine study*.

circular pattern: pattern of velopharyngeal closure that occurs when all of the velopharyngeal structures contribute equally, and the closure pattern resembles a true sphincter.

circumvallate papilla: a line of prominent taste buds that makes an inverted "V" on the posterior tongue.

Class I occlusion: normal dental arch relationship, although the teeth may be misaligned; the mesiobuccal (front outside) cusp of the first maxillary molar fits in the buccal (outside) groove of the first mandibular molar.

Class II malocclusion: abnormal dental arch relationship where the mesiobuccal (front outside) cusp of the first maxillary molar is *anterior* to the buccal (outside) groove of the first mandibular molar; the maxillary arch is protrusive and too far in front of the mandibular arch.

Class III malocclusion: abnormal dental arch relationship where the mesiobuccal (front outside) cusp of the first maxillary molar is posterior to the buccal (outside) groove of the first mandibular molar; the maxillary arch is retrusive and too far behind the mandibular arch.

cleft: an abnormal opening or a fissure in an anatomical structure that is normally closed.

cleft lip: a congenital malformation that occurs in utero during the first trimester of pregnancy and involves a fissure of the lip and sometimes alveolus.

cleft muscle of Veau: refers to abnormal velar muscle insertion due to a cleft palate; the levator veli palatini muscle does not interdigitate in the midline and both this paired muscle and the palatopharyngeus muscles are inserted abnormally onto the posterior border of the hard palate, rendering them essentially nonfunctional.

cleft palate: a congenital malformation that occurs in utero during the first trimester of pregnancy and involves a fissure in the soft palate and sometimes the hard palate.

cleft palate team (CPT): a team of professionals that consists of a surgeon, an orthodontist, a speech-language pathologist, and one additional specialist according to the requirements of the American Cleft Palate-Craniofacial Association; other team members may include an audiologist, dentist, geneticist (dysmorphologist), nurse, oral surgeon (maxillofacial surgeon), and others.

clinodactyly: deflection or curvature of the digits (fingers or toes).

co-articulation: an abnormal consonant production characterized by one manner of production with simultaneous valving at two places of production.

cochlea: a part of the inner ear that is composed of a bony spiral tube that is shaped as a snail's shell and is responsible for hearing.

coding region: portions of a gene that determine the amino acid sequence for a polypeptide.

cognition: (adj. cognitive) refers to the individual's ability to engage in conscious intellectual activities, such as thinking, reasoning, imagining, or learning.

coloboma: a congenital defect, especially of the eye, which often involves a notch of the eyelid margin; usually affects the lower lid.

columella: the "little column" at the lower portion of the nose that separates the nostrils; cartilage and mucosa that are located under the nasal tip and at the lower end of the nasal septum.

compensatory errors: articulation gestures that are the individual's response to velopharyngeal dysfunction (or dental malocclusion), rather than the direct result of velopharyngeal dysfunction; also known as *active speech characteristics.*

complete cleft lip: involves the entire lip through the nostril sill and the alveolus (or dental arch) all the way to the area of the incisive foramen.

concha: (pl. conchae) a structure that is comparable to a shell in shape, such as the auricle or pinna (or auricle) of the ear or the turbinated bone within the nose; see *turbinates.*

conductive hearing loss: a type of hearing loss due to a blockage or problem with sound conduction to the inner ear.

condyle: the rounded articular surface of the bone, such as in the jaw joint.

congenital: a disease or deformity that is present at birth and may be the result of an inherited (genetic or chromosomal) condition, or may be due to something that occurred during the pregnancy (exogenous factors).

congenital palatal insufficiency (CPI): velopharyngeal dysfunction with no history of cleft palate, no apparent evidence of submucous cleft, or other known etiology.

consanguinity: mating between related individuals.

consulting team: a team of professionals whose members provide opinions regarding the total care of the patient; the opinions and recommendations are forwarded to the treating professionals for follow-up.

contiguous gene syndromes: syndromes caused by deletions large enough to contain several genes, but too small to be seen on routine cytogenetic analysis.

continuous positive airway pressure (CPAP): an instrument that delivers continuous airway pressure to the nasopharynx by means of a hose and nasal mask; used primarily in the treatment of sleep apnea to prevent pharyngeal collapse; has also been used to provide resistance training to strengthen the velopharyngeal musculature when there is velopharyngeal incompetence.

coronal pattern: a pattern of velopharyngeal closure that is accomplished primarily by the posterior movement of the velum against a broad area of the posterior pharyngeal wall and the possible anterior movement of the posterior pharyngeal wall; there is less contribution of the lateral pharyngeal walls during closure with this pattern.

corticotomy: a partial cut in the bone.

craniofacial anomaly: a structural or functional abnormality that affects the cranium or face.

craniofacial team (CFT): a team of professionals that consists of a craniofacial surgeon, an orthodontist, a mental health professional, and speech-language pathologist according to the requirements of the American Cleft Palate-Craniofacial Association; other members may include a neurosurgeon, an ophthalmologist, and others.

craniosynostosis: abnormal development of the cranial skeleton due to premature ossification of one or more cranial sutures, resulting in malformation of the skull with growth; the shape of the skull depends on the sutures that are involved; can cause raised intracranial pressure (ICP) and mental retardation if not treated; can be syndromal, due to genetic factors, or nonsyndromal.

crossbite: a type of dental malocclusion where a maxillary tooth or teeth are inside the mandibular teeth; when the normal overlap of the upper teeth to the lower teeth is reversed, so that the lower teeth overlap the upper teeth buccally; can be anterior or lateral.

cryptorchidism: undescended testes.

cul-de-sac resonance: abnormal resonance during speech, which occurs when the transmission of acoustic energy is trapped in a blind pouch in the vocal tract with only one outlet; the speech is perceived as muffled due to the fact that the sound is contained in a cavity with no direct means of escape.

cupid's bow: the shape of the top of the upper lip, which includes a rounded configuration with an indentation in the middle.

cusp: the point on a tooth.

cuspids: teeth that have one point or cusp; also known as *canines.*

cytogenetics: the branch of genetics that is concerned with the structure and function of the cell, particularly the chromosomes; molecular cytogenetics allows extremely small genetic abnormalities to be detected.

cytokinesis: the separation of the cell cytoplasm to form two distinct cells with separate cell membranes.

deciduous teeth: primary or "baby" teeth.

deep bite: when the upper teeth overlap more than 25% of the lower teeth; the lower incisors may be in contact with the alveolar ridge of the palate.

deformation: (syn. deformity) birth defect that arises as a result of abnormal mechanical or physical forces in the fetal environment on an otherwise normal structure; usually results in the abnormal shape or form of a completely formed organ or structure, such as clubfoot.

deformity: see *deformation.*

dehiscence: breakdown of a surgical repair.

deletion: in genetics, absence of a piece of a chromosome or genetic material; often results in multiple malformations and developmental handicaps.

denasality: abnormal resonance due to a lack of vibration of the sound energy in the nasal cavity; total nasal airway obstruction and the resultant effect on resonance.

dental arch: the curved structure in the maxilla and mandible that consists of the alveolar ridge and teeth.

dental elastics: small rubber bands used to add a dynamic component for pulling teeth or bony segments together.

dental implants: cylindrical shaped pieces of titanium that can take the place of a missing tooth's root and are able to support crowns and prosthetic devices.

dental occlusion: the manner in which the maxillary teeth and mandibular teeth fit together, or the bite; in normal occlusion the upper arch overlaps the lower arch.

dentition: the teeth taken all together.

dentures: removable prosthetic teeth that replace an entire dental arch.

deoxyribonucleic acid (DNA): a nucleic acid made up of building blocks called nucleotides; contained in the nuclei of animal and vegetable cells and is the component of chromosomes; each DNA molecule contains many genes, which contain hereditary information; consists of two strands that wrap around each other in the shape of a twisted ladder or double helix.

dermatoglyphics: creases on the hands or changes in the fingerprints that can give clues to early developmental problems.

diastasis: a separation between two normally joined structures; as in separation of the levator veli palatini muscles when there is a submucous cleft palate.

diastema: a space or opening between the teeth, usually the upper central incisors.

differential pressure: the difference in pressure between the nasal cavity and the oral cavity during speech, as measured simultaneously through aerodynamic instrumentation.

direct measures: instrumental procedures that allow the examiner to visualize the anatomical and physiological defects that cause velopharyngeal dysfunction; includes videofluoroscopy and nasopharyngoscopy procedures.

disruption: a morphologic defect resulting from an extrinsic breakdown or interference with a normal developmental process.

distal (adj.): the direction away from the midline, following the curvature of the dental arch.

distraction osteogenesis: a method for increasing bone length; involves making a corticotomy in the middle of a bone, then slowly pulling the cut ends apart (distracting) with a mechanical device; new bone is able to regenerate between the cut ends, obviating the need for bone grafts; can be used for maxillary or mandibular advancement.

dolichocephaly: long, narrow skull seen with prematurity.

dominant inheritance: when only one gene is needed for expression of a trait (i.e., brown eyes); when one allele from one parent is expressed over a contrasting allele from the other parent.

dorsum: the top surface, as on the tongue.

double helix: coiled ladder of a DNA molecule that consists of two polymers of nucleotides.

duplication: when part of a chromosome is duplicated, often resulting in multiple malformations and developmental handicaps.

dysarthria: a motor speech disorder that affects the oral articulators and is characterized by abnormalities of muscular strength, range of motion, speed, accuracy, and tonicity due to a neurological injury or insult; speech is very slow and characterized by inaccurate movement of the articulators.

dysmorphogenesis: (adj. dysmorphic) the process of abnormal tissue formation, resulting in abnormally formed features.

dysmorphology: the study of abnormal shape or form.

dysphagia: abnormality or difficulty in swallowing.

dysphonia: (adj. dysphonic) refers to voice disorder that results in an alteration in the normal phonatory quality of the voice; characterized by breathiness, hoarseness, low intensity, and glottal fry.

dysplasia: an abnormal organization of cells into tissues and the outcome of the process.

dyspraxia: see *apraxia (of speech)*.

eardrum: see *tympanic membrane*.

ectopic tooth: a normal tooth that erupts in an abnormal position.

edema: an excessive amount of fluid in cells and tissues, causing swelling.

encephalocele: a congenital gap in the skull with herniation of brain tissue into the nose or palate.

endogenous: a factor from within the organism rather than from the environment, such as the genetic makeup of the organism.

endoscope: a specialized, flexible fiberoptic instrument that consists of an eyepiece at the end of a long tube or scope; used for examination of an internal canal or organ; can be used for evaluation of the velopharyngeal mechanism, pharynx, or larynx; a type of endoscope is a *nasopharyngoscope*.

endoscopy: a procedure that allows the visualization of the interior of a canal or hollow organ by means of a special instrument, usually called an *endoscope*.

en face view: see *base view*.

epibulbar dermoid: a cyst on the eyeball.

epicanthal folds: folds of tissue that extend from the upper eyelid to the lower part of the orbit at the inner canthus or corner of the eye.

epiphyseal dysplasia: underdevelopment or abnormality of the long bones of the extremities.

eustachian tube: the tube that connects the middle ear with the nasopharynx; usually closed at the pharyngeal end at rest, but opens with swallowing and yawning due to the action of the tensor veli palatini muscle; allows ventilation of the middle ear, equalization of air pressure on both sides of the tympanic membrane, and drainage of fluids; also known as the *auditory tube*.

exogenous: a factor that is outside an organism and is not indigenous to that organism, such as drugs or smoke.

exons: portions of the DNA in a gene function in the transcribed RNA template to direct the incorporation of amino acids into a protein.

exophthalmos: protrusion of one or both globes of the eye beyond the socket due to either congenital or pathological factors that provide pressure behind the eye; often associated with craniosynostosis involving the coronal suture.

exorbitism: excessive protrusion of the globe of the eye from its socket due to shallow orbits.

expressive language: the ability to generate and then transmit a message.

expressivity: the extent to which a gene is apparent in the phenotype.

external auditory canal: a skin-lined canal of the external ear that leads to the eardrum.

external ear: part of the ear that is comprised of the pinna and the external auditory canal.

fascia: a sheet of fibrous tissue that encloses muscles and muscle groups.

faucial pillars: bilateral curtainlike structures in the posterior portion of the oral cavity; the anterior faucial pillar is formed as the velum curves downward toward the tongue and the posterior faucial pillar is just behind the anterior pillar.

faucial tonsils: lymphoid tissue that is located on either side of the mouth between the anterior and posterior faucial pillars; also referred to as merely *tonsils*.

fiberoptic endoscopic evaluation of swallowing (FEES): a procedure where a flexible endoscope is used in the evaluation of swallowing disorders; involves the transnasal passage of an endoscope for viewing of the pharyngeal and laryngeal structures to study the integrity of airway protection during swallowing.

fistula: (pl. fistulae or fistulas) an abnormal hole or passage from one epithelialized cavity to another epithelialized cavity; exam-ples included an oronasal (palatal) fistula or tracheoesophageal fistula.

fixed bridge: permanently placed prosthetic teeth typically used to replace dental segments.

fluorescent in situ hybridization (FISH): a procedure used in a cytogenetic laboratory that involves the use of a nucleic acid probe labeled with a fluorescent dye to localize a specified submicroscopic segment of DNA; used to determine deletion of parts of chromosomes, as in the diagnosis of velocardiofacial syndrome.

foramen: (pl. foramina) a normal hole or opening in a bony structure or membranous structure; often serves as a passageway to allow blood vessels and nerves to pass through to the area on the other side.

forme fruste: a partial or arrested form of a cleft lip where the overlying skin is intact, but the underlying muscle, nasal cartilage, and oral sphincter function usually are significantly affected.

fovea palati: (pl. foveae palati) one of the bilateral midline depressions at the junction of the hard and soft palate that are the openings to minor salivary glands.

frenulum: (pl. frenula) a small frenum; see *frenum* and *lingual frenulum*.

frenum: (pl. frena or frenums) a narrow fold of mucous membrane that connects a fixed structure to a movable part and serves to check undue movement; see *frenulum* and *lingual frenulum*.

fricative sounds: pressure-sensitive sounds that require a gradual release of air pressure through a small opening; includes /f/, /v/, /s/, /z/, /sh/, /th/.

frontal view: an X-ray view that allows the examiner to visualize the lateral pharyngeal walls at rest and during speech; the orientation of this view is as if one is looking straight through the nose; also called the *anterior-posterior* view or simply the AP view.

gamete: a sex cell, either an ovum or sperm cell.

gastrostomy (G) tube feeding: a method of parenteral feeding through the use of a tube that is place directly into the stomach through an opening that is surgically created.

gene: (adj. genetic) a functional unit of heredity that is submicroscopic, resides at a specific location or locus on a chromosome, and is capable of reproducing itself with each cell division; consists of a sequence of nucleotide bases in a molecule of deoxyribonucleic acid (DNA).

genetics: the science of patterns of heredity.

genioplasty: horizontal mandibular osteotomy for chin advancement.

genome: consists of chromosomes and DNA and contains a complete set of instructions for cell replication and differentiation for an organism; see *Human Genome Project.*

genotype: the genetic constitution of an individual.

gingivoperiosteoplasty: a procedure to close the cleft of the alveolus with raised gingival flaps and the underlying periosteum on each edge of the cleft; raw surfaces are advanced and sewn together to allow the bone progenitor cells to lay down bone as the patient grows.

glossopexy: a surgical procedure that involves suturing the tongue tip to the bottom lip to help to keep the airway open in patients with glossoptosis.

glossoptosis: the posterior displacement of the tongue in the pharynx; can cause airway obstruction.

glossus: related to the tongue.

glottal plosive: see *glottal stop.*

glottal stop: a compensatory articulation production characterized by forceful adduction of the vocal folds and the build-up and release of air pressure under the glottis, resulting in a grunt type sound.

greater segment: palatal segment on the non-cleft side.

hair cells: sensory cells, as in the organ of hearing, that have hairlike properties.

hard palate: a bony structure that serves as the roof of the mouth and floor of the nasal cavity and separates the oral cavity from the nasal cavity.

hemangioma: a congenital anomaly in which a proliferation of blood vessels results in a large mass.

hemifacial microsomia: lack of development of the bones on one side of the face; results in various degrees of both unilateral mandibular hypoplasia and facial weakness.

hemihypertrophy: where one side of the body grows faster than the other side.

heterogeneity: the mutation of different genes leading to the same phenotype.

heterogeneous: a characteristic where more than one gene can cause the same clinical features.

heterozygous: having two different copies or alleles of a gene at the same locus on a pair of homologous chromosomes.

holoprosencephaly: failure of the forebrain to divide into the two hemispheres; often accompanied by a midline deficit in facial development or a midfacial cleft.

homozygotes: persons with two identical copies of a gene.

homozygous: when genes have two similar alleles.

horizontal plates: paired plates of the palatine bones located just behind the transverse palatine suture line; forms the posterior portion of the hard palate, ending with the protrusive posterior nasal spine.

Human Genome Project: an international initiative whereby researchers from all over the world are collaborating to compile a comprehensive map of the human genome.

hypernasality: a resonance disorder that occurs when sound enters the nasal cavity inappropriately during speech; the perceptual quality of speech is often described as just "nasal," muffled, or characterized by mumbling; is particularly perceptible on vowels.

hyperplasia: (adj. hyperplastic) overdevelopment of a structure; an increase in the number of cells in a tissue or organ, not related to tumor formation, whereby that body part is larger than normal.

hypertelorism: excessive distance between two paired organs, such as the eyes.

hypertrophy: (adj. hypertrophic) overgrowth of a structure.

hypoglycemia: low blood sugar.

hyponasality: a type of abnormal resonance that occurs when there is a reduction in nasal resonance during speech due to blockage in the nasopharynx or in the entrance to the nasal cavity; particularly affects the production of the nasal consonants (m, n, and ng).

hypopharynx: part of the pharynx, or throat, which is below the oral cavity and extends from the epiglottis inferiorly to the esophagus.

hypoplasia: (adj. hypoplastic) underdevelopment or defective formation of a tissue or organ, usually due to a decrease in the normal number of cells.

hypospadias: where the orifice of the penis is proximal to its normal location.

hypotelorism: narrow-spaced eyes.

hypotonia: (adj. hypotonic) a lack of adequate muscular tonicity or tension.

ideogram: a schematic drawing of the banding pattern of a chromosome.

idiopathic: a condition that appears without apparent cause or etiology.

imprinting: when some genes function differently, depending on whether they were inherited maternally or paternally.

incidence: in epidemiological terms, refers to the number of new cases of a disease or disorder in a given population, such as the number of persons becoming ill with a certain disease.

incisive foramen: a hole in the bone that is located in the alveolar ridge area of the maxillary arch, just behind the central incisors, and forms the tip of the premaxilla.

incisive papilla: the slight elevation of the mucosa at the anterior end of the raphe of the palate.

incisive suture lines: embryological suture lines in the hard palate that go between the lateral incisors and canines and meet posteriorly at the area of the incisive foramen; the suture lines that separate the premaxilla.

incisors: teeth that are somewhat shovel shaped; their biting surfaces are thin knife-like edges.

incomplete penetrance: the lack of a recognizable phenotype in an individual who carries a gene for an autosomal dominant trait.

incus (anvil): one of the ossicles in the middle ear; articulates with the malleus and the stapes.

indirect measures: instrumental procedures that provide object data regarding the results of velopharyngeal function, such as airflow, air pressure, or acoustic output, but do not allow visualization of the structures; includes nasometry and aerodynamic instrumentation.

infant oral orthopedics: see *palatal orthopedics.*

inner ear: part of the ear that consists of the cochlea and semicircular canals.

intelligence: relates to the ability to learn; a prerequisite for normal language development.

interdisciplinary team: a group of professionals from various disciplines who work together to coordinate the care of a patient through collaboration, interaction, communication, and cooperation.

intermaxillary fixation: wiring the mandible against the maxilla to keep it closed and in place; often done for a period of time after orthognathic surgery.

intermaxillary palatine suture line: see *median palatine suture line.*

interosseous dental implants: implants that are imbedded in the bone so that a speech appliance or denture can be attached and retained.

interphase: the time between cell divisions.

intonation: refers to the frequent changes in pitch throughout an utterance, as controlled by subtle changes in vocal fold length and mass.

intraoral air pressure: a build-up of air pressure in the oral cavity that provides the force for the production of oral consonants, particularly plosives, fricatives and affricates.

intravelar veloplasty (IVVP): a surgical reconstruction of the levator veli palatini sling during palatoplasty for correction of a cleft of the velum.

introns: the portions of a gene's DNA sequence that are removed from the RNA transcript before it is transported to the cytoplasm for translation.

inversions: when a portion of a chromosome is turned 180° from its usual orientation; may not be associated with any abnormalities in the individual because the total amount of genetic material may be unchanged.

karotype: a gross chromosome analysis that is done by drawing blood, growing the cells in a culture, analyzing the white blood cells, photographing the chromosomes and then arranging the chromosomes in pairs for display and assessment.

labial (adj.): relating to the lip; the outer part of the dental arch that touches the lip.

labial tubercle: the prominent projection on the inferior border, or free edge, of the midsection of the upper lip.

labioversion: when the upper incisors are displaced anteriorly, with overjet greater than 2 mm, causing the maxillary incisors to protrude out toward the lips.

labyrinthitis: inflammation of the labyrinth, which is sometimes accompanied by vertigo and deafness.

laminar airflow: airflow through the nasal cavity that is steady and smooth due to the lack of significant resistance.

laminography: use of a radiograph to measure distances and angles between particular landmarks.

language: refers to the meaning or message that's conveyed back and forth during communication.

laryngeal web: a congenital anomaly that consists of a band of tissue between the vocal folds, usually in the anterior portion of the larynx, and causes respiratory stridor.

laryngomalacia: abnormally soft cartilage in the epiglottis and aryepiglottic folds at birth, resulting in loud inspiratory stridor that is particularly pronounced when the infant cries or breathes deeply.

lateral cephalometric X rays: still radiographs of the head taken in the sagittal plane.

lateral pharyngeal walls: the side walls of the throat.

lateral view: an X-ray view that shows the velum and posterior pharyngeal wall in a midsagittal plane; the orientation of the lateral view is as if we were able to look through the side of the head to view these structures from the side.

Latham appliance: a two-piece acrylic dental appliance that is used prior to the lip and alveolus repair to close the gap between the greater and lesser maxillary segments from a wide cleft of the primary palate.

Le Fort I osteotomy: a surgical cut in the bone that transversely separates the maxilla just above the base of the nose so that the maxilla and palate can be moved as a single unit.

Le Fort II osteotomy: a surgical cut in the bone that includes both the nasal pyramid and the alveolar arch.

Le Fort III osteotomy: a surgical cut in the bone that includes cheek bones, orbital rims, nasal pyramid, and alveolar arch.

lesser segment: palatal segment on the cleft side.

levator sling: the levator veli palatini muscles from each side interdigitate and blend together to form a muscle sling.

levator veli palatini: paired muscle that forms the main muscle mass of the velum, primarily responsible for velar elevation.

lingual: related to the tongue; the inner part of the upper and lower dental arch that is in contact with the tongue.

lingual frenulum: (pl. frenula) a narrow fold of mucous membrane that extends from the floor of the mouth to the midline of the under surface of the tongue; see *frenum* and *frenulum*.

lingual tonsils: a mass of lymphoid tissue located at the base of the tongue that extends to the epiglottis.

linguoversion: when the upper teeth are inside the lower teeth; also known as *anterior crossbite* or *underjet*.

lip adhesion: a simple, straight-line surgical procedure to temporarily repair a cleft lip; this procedure is performed so that the subsequent lip pressure will draw the segments together, making the final repair more successful.

lip pits: depressions in the bottom lip that are usually bilateral and are associated with Van der Woude's syndrome with cleft palate.

lobulated tongue: the tongue appears to have multiple lobes, with fissures between each lobe.

lower esophageal sphincter (LES): sphincter at the base of the esophagus that relaxes to allow a bolus to enter the stomach.

macro: large.

macroglossia: large tongue.

macrostomia: a large mouth opening, often due to failure of fusion between the maxillary and mandibular process of embryonic development of the face.

mala: (adj. malar) relating to the cheek or cheekbone (zygomatic bone).

malar hypoplasia: lack of cheekbone development.

malformation: defect in basic embryological plan due to chromosomal or genetic factors.

malleus (hammer): one of the ossicles in the middle ear; is firmly attached to the tympanic membrane and articulates with the incus.

malocclusion: improper dental or skeletal relationship of the maxillary and mandibular arches so that the arches do not close together normally.

mandibular hypoplasia: lack of mandibular development, causing a small, retrusive mandible; see *micrognathia* and *retrognathia*.

mastoid cavities: a section of the temporal bone that is porous and located just behind the ear.

mastoiditis: inflammation or infection in any part of the mastoid process.

maxillary hypoplasia: lack of development of the maxilla, causing midface retrusion or deficiency and concavity of the midface.

maxillary retrusion: characterized by a small upper jaw (maxilla) relative to the lower jaw (mandible); a common anomaly, especially in individuals with repaired cleft lip and palate secondary to the inherent deficiency in the maxilla due to the cleft and the possible restriction in maxillary growth with the surgical repair; also known as *midface deficiency*.

meatus: an opening, channel or passageway; usually the external opening of a canal; see *nasal meatus*.

median palatine raphe: the thin white line that can often be seen running longitudinally down the middle of the velum.

median palatine suture line: embryological suture line that begins at the incisive foramen and ends at the posterior nasal spine; separates the paired palatine processes of the maxilla and the horizontal plates of the palatine bones; also known as *intermaxillary palatine suture line*.

meiosis: a special process of cell division that results in gametes (spermatocytes or oocytes) with 23 chromosomes rather than the 46 that are found in somatic cells.

mesial (adj.): the direction toward the midline, following the curvature of the dental arch.

messenger RNA (mRNA): ribunucleic acid (RNA) that has had the introns removed and is transported from the nucleus to the cytoplasm to function as a template for protein synthesis.

metacentric: chromosomes with a centrally located centromere.

metopic: related to the forehead or anterior portion of the cranium.

micro: small.

microcephaly: small head circumference in comparison to age-matched peers.

microglossia: small tongue.

micrognathia: a small or hypoplastic mandible; see *mandibular hypoplasia*.

micropenis: small penis.

microphthalmia: small eyes.

microstomia: a small mouth opening.

microtia: hypoplasia or absence of the external ear (pinna or auricle); often accompanied by aural atresia (a blind or absent external auditory meatus).

middle ear: a hollow space within the temporal bone.

middle-ear effusion: collection of fluids within the middle ear space due to the eustachian tube dysfunction.

mid-dorsum palatal stop: an abnormal articulation production that is often compensatory for anterior oral cavity crowding; produced as a stop consonant that is articulated with the middle of the dorsum against the middle of the hard palate; is usually substituted for the lingual-alveolar sounds (t and d), for the velar sounds (k and g), and in some cases, for sibilant sounds (s, z, sh, ch, and j); also called a *palatal dorsal production*.

midface deficiency: see *maxillary retrusion*.

midface retrusion: concavity of the midface due to maxillary hypoplasia.

mitosis: the process of separating duplicated chromosomes and reconstitution of two cell nuclei.

mixed resonance: a combination of hypernasality, hyponasality, or cul-de-sac resonance during connected speech.

modified barium swallow (MBS): see *videofluoroscopic swallowing study (VSS)*.

Moebius syndrome: involves specific cranial nerve damage with weakness affecting the oral and facial musculature.

molars: teeth that are designed for grinding; on each side of the maxillary and mandibular arch, there are the first molars (6-year molars), the second molars (12-year molars), and the third molars (wisdom teeth); upper molars have four cusps, two buccal and two palatal (or lingual) cusps and lower molars have five cusps, three buccal and two lingual cusps.

mongoloid slant: upward slant of the eyes.

monosomy: absence of an entire chromosome of a pair of homologous chromosomes.

morphogenesis: the process of embryonic tissue formation.

mosaicism: an anomaly of chromosome division resulting in the presence of cells with two or more different genetic makeups, or a different number of chromosomes, in a single individual.

mucoid effusion: a thick, mucuslike fluid in the middle ear.

mucoperiosteum: tissue that consists of a mucous membrane and periosteum; covers the hard palate.

mucosa: see *mucous membrane*.

mucous membrane: (adj. mucosal) the lining tissue of the nasal cavity, oral cavity, and pharynx; consists of stratified squamous epithelium and lamina propria; also known as *mucosa*.

mucus: a clear, viscid secretion of the mucous membranes.

multidisciplinary team: a group of professionals from various disciplines who work independently in evaluating and treating patients with complex medical needs; members of this type of team have well-defined roles and cooperate with each other, but there is little communication and interaction among the team members.

multifactorial inheritance: a characteristic in the phenotype that is the result of a combination of many genes at different loci and/or factors from the environment; the combination of genes and other factors all have a small added effect to form the characteristic in the phenotype.

musculus uvulae: a paired muscle that creates a bulge on the posterior nasal surface of the velum during phonation; during contraction, this bulge provides additional bulk and stiffness to the nasal side of the velum and helps to fill in the area between the velum and posterior pharyngeal wall, to contributing to a firm velopharyngeal seal.

mutation: a change in the sequence of base pairs in the DNA molecule that is reflected in subsequent divisions of the cell; a change in the chemistry of the gene that is reflected in the subsequent genotype and phenotype.

mutation: a change in the sequence of a molecule of DNA; mutation can be as small as a substitution of a single base pair or as large as the deletion of an entire chromosome.

myopia: nearsightedness.

myringotomy: a surgical puncture of the tympanic membrane so that fluid can be drained or suctioned out of the middle ear.

naris: (pl. nares) nostril.

nasal air emission: an inappropriate flow of the airstream through the nose during speech, causing distortion of the speech; usually caused by velopharyngeal dysfunction; also called *nasal escape*.

nasal airway resistance: attenuation of the nasal airflow due to any condition that obstructs or restricts the patency of the nasopharynx or nasal cavity.

nasal bridge: the bony structure that is located between the eyes and corresponds to the middle of the nasofrontal suture; also known as *nasion*.

nasal grimace: a muscle contraction during speech that is typically noted either above the nasal bridge (in the area between the eyes) or around the nares; occurs as an overflow muscle reaction when there is an attempt to achieve velopharyngeal closure; usually accompanied by nasal air emission.

nasal meatus: any of the three passages in the nasal cavity that lie directly under a nasal concha; see *meatus*.

nasal molding: a method of repositioning the nasal septum and ala in the infant prior to cleft lip repair; usually involves an intraoral/nasal appliance combined with taping.

nasal regurgitation: reflux of fluids into the nasopharynx and nasal cavity during drinking or vomiting.

nasal root: where the nose begins at the level of the eyes.

nasal rustle: a fricative sound that occurs as air pressure is forced through a partially opened velopharyngeal valve causing the airflow to become turbulent and resulting in bubbling of secretions above the opening; also called *nasal turbulence*.

nasal septum: a wall separating the nasal cavity into two halves; consists of the vomer bone, the perpendicular plate of the ethmoid, and the quadrangular cartilage and is covered with mucous membrane; see *septum*.

nasal sill: the base of the nostril opening.

nasal sniff: an uncommon compensatory articulation production that is produced by a forcible inspiration through the nose; usually substituted for sibilant sounds, particularly the /s/, and typically occurs in the final word position.

nasal snort: a burst of nasal air emission that is produced by a forcible emission of air pressure through the nares during consonant production, resulting in a noisy, sneezelike sound.

nasal turbulence: see *nasal rustle*.

nasalance score: represents the relative amount of nasal acoustic energy in the person's speech as determined by the Nasometer; the ratio of nasal acoustic energy over total (oral plus nasal) acoustic energy during speech as determined through the use of the Nasometer; the score represents the mean of the percentage points that are calculated for an entire speech passage.

nasalization of oral phonemes: an obligatory error due to an open velopharyngeal valve.

nasendoscopy: see *nasopharyngoscopy*.

nasion: see *nasal bridge*.

nasogastric (NG) tube: a tube placed through the nose and down to the stomach and used for feeding.

nasogastric (NG) tube feeding: a method of feeding through the use of a tube that is placed in the nose and goes down to the stomach.

nasogram: a contour display on a computer screen that represents the nasalance results of the spoken passage on the Nasometer.

Nasometer: a computer-based instrument (Kay Elemetrics, Inc., Pinehurst, NJ) that measures the relative amount of nasal acoustic energy in a patient's speech.

nasopharyngeal airway: a tube that used to improve the airway of infants, such as those with Pierre Robin sequence; the tube is placed in the nose of the infant in such a way that one end sticks out of the nose and the other end extends to below the region of tongue obstruction.

nasopharyngoscope: a type of endoscope that is used for examination of the pharynx, larynx, and velopharyngeal mechanism.

nasopharyngoscopy: a minimally invasive endoscopic procedure that allows visual observation and analysis of the velopharyngeal mechanism or larynx during speech through the use of a scope (nasopharyngoscope) that is inserted through the nose until it reaches the nasopharynx; can be used to evaluate velopharyngeal function, phonation, or swallowing; also called *nasendoscopy* or *video endoscopy*.

nasopharynx: the part of the pharynx, or throat, that lies above the soft palate and just behind the nasal cavity.

nondisjunction: the failure of one or more chromosomes to separate in cell division.

nonpneumatic activities: as they relate to the velopharyngeal valve: swallowing, gagging, and vomiting.

nosocomial infections: infections that are acquired while in the hospital.

nucleotides: building blocks of DNA that consist of a 5-carbon sugar chemically bonded to a phosphate group and a nitrogenous base.

obligatory errors: speech characteristics that are the product of structural abnormality or dysfunction; includes hypernasality, nasal air emission, weak consonants, and short utterance length; also known as *passive speech characteristics*.

oblique view: X-ray view that allows the examiner to see the lateral pharyngeal walls and velum during connected speech; used primarily if the base view cannot be obtained due to enlarged adenoids or the inability to hyperextend the neck.

obstructive sleep apnea (OSA): a period during sleep when the individual is exerting muscular forces to inspire, but is unsuccessful in moving air into the lungs due to a blockage in the pharynx; often caused by enlarged tonsils, enlarged adenoids, or pharyngeal hypotonia during sleep.

obturator: a generic term to describe a device that can be used to cover a hole; see *palatal obturator*.

occlusal cant: a sloping, transverse occlusal plane caused by impaired vertical maxillary growth on one side, which is compensated by vertical alveolar growth in the mandible on the same side; common in patients with unilateral cleft lip/palate and those with hemifacial microsomia.

occlusion: the relationship between the maxillary and mandibular teeth when the jaws are closed as when biting.

occult submucous cleft: a defect in the velum that is under the mucous membrane and not visible on the oral surface; this defect can usually be viewed on the nasal surface of the velum through nasopharyngoscopy.

ocular: related to the eyes.

oligogenic model: a variation of the multifactorial model of inheritance, where a trait may be determined by the interaction of multiple genes with little environmental influence; a small number of genes may contribute most of the risk.

omphalocele: where part of the intestines may be outside of the abdomen in the region of the umbilical cord.

open bite: occurs when one or more maxillary teeth fail to occlude with the opposing mandibular teeth; primarily affects the anterior dentition (anterior open bite) and less commonly the posterior dentition (lateral open bite).

ophtha: related to the eyes.

optic: related to the eyes.

oral frenulae: oral tissue webs.

oral manometer: an instrument that was used in the past to provide a gross measurement of airflow abilities during blowing or negative pressure during sucking; the patient was required to blow into a catheter or suck the catheter; this is no longer considered valid because information is now available about the physiological differences between blowing or sucking activities and speech.

oral resonance: the result of the sound energy vibrating (resonating) in the oral cavity during speech.

orbicularis oris: the muscle that encircles the mouth and serves to close the lips.

organ of corti: the part of the inner ear where the mechanical energy introduced into the cochlea is converted into electrical stimulation.

orogastric tube feeding: a method of feeding through the use of a tube that is placed in the mouth and goes down to the stomach.

oronasal fistula: see *palatal fistula.*

oropharyngeal isthmus: the opening from the oral cavity to the pharynx; bordered superiorly by the velum, laterally by the faucial pillars, and inferiorly by the base of the tongue.

oropharynx: the part of the pharynx, or throat, that lies below the soft palate at the level of the oral cavity or just posterior to the mouth.

orthodontist: the professional who is responsible for aligning misplaced teeth and correcting discrepancy in jaw size to improve the dental and facial aesthetics and the function of the dentition.

orthognathia: (adj. orthognathic) the study of the causes and the treatment of conditions related to malposition of the bones of the jaw.

orthognathic surgery: surgery that involves the bones of the upper jaw (the maxilla) and the lower jaw (the mandible).

Orticochea sphincteroplasty: see *sphincter pharyngoplasty.*

osseointegrated implants: implants that are inserted in the bone; used for retention of bridges and prosthetic devices.

ossicles: (adj. ossicular) three small bones in the middle ear that conduct sound energy from the tympanic membrane to the cochlea; include the malleus, incus, and stapes.

osteotomies: surgical cuts in a bone so that the bone can be placed in a more functional and appropriate position.

otic: relating to the ear (otitis, otolaryngologist, otorrhea, microtia, etc.).

otitis media: a bacterial infection and inflammation of the middle ear.

otitis media with effusion: an inflammation of the middle ear that is accompanied by a build-up of fluids.

otolaryngologist: the physician who is responsible for monitoring middle-ear function and treating middle-ear disease, assessing and treating anomalies and disease of the oral cavity, pharynx, nasal cavity, and upper airway and lower airway; also known as the ear, nose and throat specialist (ENT).

otorrhea: a type of ear disease with discharge.

otoscope: an instrument used to visualize the tympanic membrane.

overbite: the vertical overlap of the upper and lower incisors; can be measured in millimeters but is often reported as a percentage of coverage of the lower incisors by the upper incisors; normal overbite is approximately 2 mm or about 25%; greater amounts are called either deep overbite, or *deep bite.*

overjet: the horizontal relationship between the upper and lower incisors; typically measured in millimeters from the labial surface of the lower incisor to the labial surface of the upper incisor with the teeth in occlusion; a normal amount of overjet is about 2 mm with upper incisors and lower incisors in light contact; excessive overjet is where the maxillary incisors are labioverted or stick out toward the lips.

overlay dentures: dentures that fit over the existing teeth and usually provide more vertical dimension.

palatal (adj.): the inner part of the upper and lower arch that is in proximity to the surface of the hard palate.

palatal fistula: a hole or opening in the palate that goes all the way through to the nasal cavity; may be the result of a breakdown of the area of a previously repaired cleft, the result of maxillary expansion, or even growth; also called *oronasal fistula.*

palatal lift: a prosthetic appliance that can be used to raise the velum for speech in cases where the velum is long enough to achieve velopharyngeal closure, but does not move well, often due to neurological impairment.

palatal obturator: a prosthetic appliance that can be used to cover an open palatal defect, such as an unrepaired cleft palate or a palatal fistula; this device can be used to improve an infant's ability to achieve compression of the nipple for suction or can be used to close a palatal defect for speech.

palatal orthopedics: a method used to align the alveolar segments in both unilateral and bi-lateral clefts of the palate prior to surgical correction; also known as *infant oral orthopedics.*

palatal section (of a prosthesis): the body portion of a prosthetic appliance that fits over the palate.

palatal vault: the rounded dome on the upper part of the oral cavity.

palatal-dorsal production: see *mid-dorsum palatal stop.*

palate: the bony and muscular partition between the oral and nasal cavities.

palatine aponeurosis: a sheet of fibrous tissue located just below the nasal surface of the velum and extending about 1 cm posteriorly from its attachment on the posterior border of the hard palate; consists of periosteum, fibrous connective tissue, and fibers from the tensor veli palatini tendon; provides an anchoring point for the velopharyngeal muscles and adds stiffness to that portion of the velum; also called *velar aponeurosis.*

palatine processes: paired bones of the maxilla that are just behind the incisive suture lines and form the anterior three quarters of the maxilla.

palatine tonsils: masses of lymphoid tissue between the anterior and posterior faucial pillars on both sides of the oral cavity; also called simply the *tonsils.*

palatine torus: see *torus palatinus.*

palatoglossus: paired muscles that act antagonistically to the levator veli palatini to depress the velum or elevate the tongue; these muscles contribute to lowering the velum for the production of nasal speech sounds.

palatomaxillary suture line: see *transverse palatine suture line.*

palatopharyngeus: paired muscle of the pharynx; the horizontal fibers are thought to be associated with the sphincteric action of the velopharyngeal valve, assisting with velopharyngeal closure by pulling the lateral pharyngeal walls medially to narrow the pharynx.

palatoplasty: palate repair.

palpebra: (pl. palpebrae, adj. palpebral) eyelid.

palpebral fissures: opening between the eyelids.

panendoscope: an older illuminated instrument that included an optical tube that is placed in the mouth and turned upward for visualization of the velopharyngeal sphincter; no longer used.

paresis: (adj. paretic) weakness of muscle movement; partial or incomplete paralysis.

partial trisomy: duplication of a piece of a chromosome rather than the entire chromosome so that there is a part of a chromosome with the pair.

Passavant's ridge: a shelflike ridge that projects from the posterior pharyngeal wall into the pharynx during speech; occurs as a result of contraction of specific fibers of the superior pharyngeal constrictor muscles; found in normal speakers and speakers with velopharyngeal dysfunction.

passive speech characteristics: see *obligatory errors.*

pedigree: pictorial representation of family members and their line of descent; used by geneticist to analyze inheritance, particularly for certain traits or anomalies.

penetrance: the frequency of the expression of a genotype in a phenotype; if the trait does not appear 100% of the time when the gene is present, then it is said to have reduced penetrance.

periosteum: a thick, fibrous membrane that covers the surface of bone.

peripheral sleep apnea: see *obstructive sleep apnea.*

perpendicular plate of the ethmoid: the bone that projects down to join the vomer and lies between the vomer and the quadrangular cartilage; forms part of the nasal septum.

pharyngeal affricate: a compensatory articulation production that is produced when the tongue is retracted so that the base of the tongue articulates against the pharyngeal wall; is the combination of either a pharyngeal plosive or a glottal stop and a pharyngeal fricative.

pharyngeal flap: a type of pharyngoplasty designed to be a passive soft tissue obturator of the middle of the velopharyngeal sphincter to improve or correct velopharyngeal function.

pharyngeal fricative: a compensatory articulation production that is produced when the tongue is retracted so that the base of the tongue approximates, but does not touch, the pharyngeal wall; a friction sound occurs as the air pressure is forced through the narrow opening that is created between the base of the tongue and pharyngeal wall.

pharyngeal plexus: a network of nerves that lies along the posterior wall of the pharynx and consists of the pharyngeal branches of the glossopharyngeal and vagus nerves, which provide motor innervation for the velar muscles that contribute to velopharyngeal closure.

pharyngeal plosive: a compensatory articulation production that is produced with the back of the tongue articulating against the pharyngeal wall; also called *pharyngeal stop.*

pharyngeal stop: see *pharyngeal plosive.*

pharyngeal tonsil: see *adenoid.*

pharyngeal wall augmentation: an implant that is surgically placed or injected in the posterior pharyngeal wall, or a rolled flap on the pharyngeal wall; placed in the area of the velopharyngeal opening to correct velopharyngeal dysfunction.

pharyngoplasty: a surgical procedure of the pharynx that is designed to correct velopharyngeal dysfunction.

pharynx: (adj. pharyngeal) the walls of the throat between the esophagus and nasal cavity.

phenotype: the manifestations of a genotype; range of characteristics associated with a genetic syndrome.

philtral columns: the raised lines on either side of the philtrum, which are embryological suture lines that are formed as the segments of the upper lip fuse.

philtrum: (adj. philtral) a long dimple or indentation that courses from the columella down to the upper lip and is bordered by the philtral columns on each side.

phonation: the sound generated by the vocal folds as they vibrate.

phoneme-specific nasal air emission (PSNAE): nasal air emission that is due to velopharyngeal mislearning rather than a structural or physiological cause; occurs due to the use of a posterior nasal fricative as a substitution for oral sounds; usually substituted for sibilant sounds, particularly s/z.

Pierre Robin sequence: a congenital condition that consists of micrognathia, glossoptosis, and cleft palate; there is often upper airway obstruction for several months after birth.

pinna: the delicate cartilaginous framework of the external ear; functions to direct sound energy into the external auditory canal; also known as the *auricle* or *concha*.

piriform aperture: literally means pear-shaped opening; the opening to the nostril or nasal cavity.

pyriform aperture stenosis: narrowing of the anterior nasal openings.

plagiocephaly: asymmetric or abnormal skull shape.

pleiotropy: the phenomenon where a single gene can affect multiple unrelated systems.

plosive sounds: pressure-sensitive consonants that require a build-up of intraoral pressure prior to a sudden release; include /p/,/b/, /t/, /d/, /k/, /g/.

pneumotachograph: an airflow device that consists of a flowmeter and a differential pressure transducer; one of the components of aerodynamic instrumentation to measure velopharyngeal orifice area or nasal resistance.

pneumatic activities: as they relate to the velopharyngeal valve: blowing, whistling, sucking, and speech.

polycythemia: an increase in the normal number of red blood cells.

polydactyly: extra fingers and/or toes.

polymorphism: variability in genes that contributes to the uniqueness of individuals.

polysomnography: a type of sleep study.

posterior crossbite: involves any combination of teeth distal (posterior) to the canines where the maxillary teeth are inside the mandibular teeth; usually occurs because the maxilla is too narrow.

posterior nasal fricative: an abnormal articulation production that is produced with the velum somewhat down so that air pressure goes through a velopharyngeal opening, creating a friction sound with audible nasal air emission; typically used as a substitution for sibilant sounds, particularly s/z; associated with *phoneme-specific nasal air emission* (PSNAE).

posterior nasal spine: a protrusive projection in the middle of the posterior border of the hard palate.

posterior pharyngeal wall: back wall of the throat.

preauricular tags: projection of scalp and skin tags from the area of the ear to the cheek.

premaxilla: a triangular-shaped bone that is bordered on either side by the incisive suture lines; this bony segment normally contains the central and lateral maxillary incisors.

premolars: teeth that typically have two cusps, although they may sometimes have three.

pressure equalizing (PE) tubes: see *ventilation tubes*.

pressure-flow technique: procedure using aerodynamic instrumentation to evaluate the dynamics of the velopharyngeal mechanism during speech; also used to evaluate nasal respiration and to quantify upper airway obstruction through measurements of nasal airway resistance.

prevalence: in epidemiological terms, refers to a measure of existing cases of a disorder in a given population.

primary dentition: stage of dental development where there are 10 teeth in the upper arch, 10 teeth in the lower arch and usually spacing between all of the primary teeth.

primary palate: the lip and palate anterior to the incisive foramen; includes the lip and alveolus.

prognathia: (adj. prognathic) protrusive mandible caused by mandibular hyperplasia.

prognathism: having a large mandible.

prolabium: the tissue that normally makes up the central portion of the upper lip between the philtral columns but is isolated when there is a bilateral cleft lip.

proptosis: (adj. proptotic) protrusion of the eyeball.

prosthesis: (adj. prosthetic) a fabricated substitute for a body part that is missing or malformed; also called a prosthetic device.

prosthodontist: a dental professional who deals with the restoration of teeth and the development of appliances to replace or improve the appearance of oral and facial structures or to assist with feeding and velopharyngeal closure.

provisionally unique syndromes: patterns of multiple anomalies in what appears to be an underlying syndrome, although a diagnosis cannot be made because the pattern is not one that has been previously described or reported.

psychologist: the professional who assesses a patient's psychosocial needs, and assists the patient and family in dealing with the medical, social and emotional challenges that occur due to the patient's anomalies.

pterygoid process: a part of the sphenoid bone that contains the medial pterygoid plate, the lateral pterygoid plate, and the pterygoid

hamulus, all of which provide attachments for muscles in the velopharyngeal complex.

purines: nitrogenous bases of nucleotides in a DNA molecule that consists of adenine and guanine.

ptosis: drooping of the eyelids.

purulent effusion: the fluid in the middle ear that is like pus.

pyrimidines: nitrogenous bases of nucleotides in a DNA molecule that consist of thymine and cytosine.

quad helix: a palatal expansion device that consists of bands on the most posterior molars, and frequently the primary canines, which are connected by a palatal spring that has two posterior and two anterior loops.

quadrangular cartilage: the cartilage that forms the anterior nasal septum and projects anteriorly to the columella.

radiography: the use of the roentgen rays (X rays) to image internal body parts.

ramus: the upturned, perpendicular extremity of the mandible on both sides.

raphe: (pronounce rayfay) a line of union between two bilaterally symmetric structures; the palatine raphe is the midline of the mucosa of the hard palate that runs from the incisive papilla posteriorly over the entire length of the hard palate.

rapid palatal expander: a palatal expansion device that consists of two or four molar bands and a jackscrew connecting them in the middle of the palate; turning the screw creates the necessary force to widen the dental arches.

receptive language: the understanding of a message that is sent.

recessive inheritance: a trait that is expressed only in individuals who are homozygous for the gene involved in that they have inherited the same gene for the trait from both parents (e.g., blue eyes); when the same allele is needed from both parents for expression of a trait.

reduction therapy: a form of speech therapy where a prosthetic device is used to stimulate the movement of the velopharyngeal structures to avoid the need for surgery, or reduce the extent of the surgery needed.

replication: the process of making two identical DNA molecules from one, resulting in two double strands, each containing one original and one complementary newly synthesized strand of DNA.

resonance: the quality of the voice that results from the vibration of sound in the pharynx, oral cavity, and nasal cavity.

retrognathia: (adj. retrognathic) when one or both jaws is located posterior to its normal position; usually used in reference to a retrusive mandible; associated with micrognathia (mandibular hypoplasia).

reverse pull headgear: a device used to advance the maxilla and improve an anterior crossbite.

ribonucleic acid (RNA): a nucleic acid which is found in the nucleus and cytoplasm of all cells.

ribosomes: organelles within the cell that function in protein synthesis.

right sided aortic arch: abnormality where the aortic arch is on the right side rather than the left.

rhinomanometry: procedure for measuring nasal airway resistance; involves measurement of the pressure encountered by air passing through the nasal cavity.

rolled flap: a flap of tissue is surgically raised from the posterior pharyngeal wall and is rolled up on to itself to form a bulge on the posterior pharyngeal wall; used to fill in a velopharyngeal gap.

rotameter: used for the calibration of the pneumotachograph; uses a compressed air supply to provide a known rate of airflow.

rugae: folds, ridges, or creases in a structure; the transverse ridges in the mucosal covering of the hard palate.

rule of 10s: a guideline for the appropriate time for a cleft lip repair, which says that the infant must be at least 10 weeks of age, 10 pounds, and have a hemoglobin of 10 gm prior to the lip repair.

saccule: a sensory organ within the inner ear that provides a sensation of acceleration.

sagittal pattern: the least common pattern of velopharyngeal closure; the lateral pharyngeal walls move medially to meet in midline to effect closure; the velum may move to close against the lateral pharyngeal walls rather than against the posterior pharyngeal wall.

sagittal plane: the median, longitudinal plane of the body; a plane of view for x-ray procedures.

salpingopharyngeal folds: folds that originate from the torus tubarius at the opening to the eustachian tube on both sides of the pharynx and then course downward to the lateral pharyngeal wall; consist of glandular and connective tissue.

salpingopharyngeus: paired muscle that arises from the inferior border of the torus tubarius and courses vertically along the lateral pharyngeal wall and under the salpingopharyngeal fold; is not felt to have a significant role in achieving velopharyngeal closure given its size and location.

scaphocephaly: skull that is oblong from front to back; caused by premature closure of the sagittal suture.

secondary palate: structures that are posterior to the incisive foramen, including the hard palate (excluding the premaxilla) and the velum.

semicircular canals: the loop-shaped tubular parts of the inner ear that provide a sense of spatial orientation; the loops are oriented in three planes at right angles to each other.

sensitivity: the extent to which a test is able to correctly identify positive results; proportion of true positive results as intended to be revealed by a test.

sensorineural hearing loss: a type of hearing loss due to a problem with the creation of nerve impulses within the inner ear or the transmission of the nerve impulses through the brainstem to the auditory cortex.

septum: a thin wall separating two cavities; see *nasal septum.*

sequence: the occurrence of a pattern of multiple anomalies within an individual that arise from a single known or presumed prior anomaly or mechanical factor; where one anomaly leads to the development of the other anomalies as in Pierre Robin sequence.

serous effusion: fluid in the middle ear that consists of a very thin, watery liquid.

sex chromosomes: the 23rd pair of chromosomes (X and Y) that function in determining gender.

sialorrhea: drooling.

sibilant sounds: speech sounds that are produced by the friction of air pressure as it is emitted anteriorly through the incisors; includes /s/, /z/, /sh/, /ch/, /zh/, and /j/.

Simonart's band: a strand of soft tissue in the area of the cleft lip that is due to partial, yet incomplete, embryonic fusion of the upper lip.

single tooth crossbite: a crossbite that involves only one upper and one lower tooth.

sleep apnea: cessation of respiration during sleep due to upper respiratory obstruction or central (neurogenic) causes, or a combination of both.

soft palate: see *velum.*

sometimes-but-not-always (SBNA): a term for an individual who demonstrates inconsistent velopharyngeal closure; the individual may be able to achieve total closure with effort, but has difficulty maintaining closure consistently and over a prolonged period of time.

somia: refers to body.

specificity: the extent to which a test correctly identifies true negative results; the proportion of individuals with negative test results for what the test is intended to reveal.

speech aid appliance: see *speech bulb obturator.*

speech bulb obturator: a prosthetic device that can be considered when the velum is too short to close completely against the posterior pharyngeal wall; this device consists of a retaining appliance and a bulb (usually of acrylic) that fills in the pharyngeal space for speech; also known as a *speech aid appliance.*

sphincter pharyngoplasty: a type of pharyngoplasty to create a dynamic sphincter that encircles the velopharyngeal port; also known as the *Orticochea sphincteroplasty.*

stapes: one of the ossicles in the middle ear; acts as a piston to create pressure waves within the fluid-filled cochlea.

stenosis: an abnormal narrowing or stricture of a canal (e.g., choanal stenosis, pharyngeal stenosis, or subglottic stenosis).

stoma: the surgical opening into the trachea through which the patient can breathe following a tracheostomy.

stomia: refers to the mouth.

stress: related to increased muscular effort and subglottic pressure during the production of a syllable; stressed syllables are produced with greater articulatory precision, are longer in duration, and are higher in pitch and intensity than unstressed syllables.

submetacentric: when the centromere of a chromosome is closer to one end than the other.

submucous cleft palate: a congenital defect that affects the underlying structures of the palate, while the structures on the oral surface are intact; can involve the muscles of the velum and also involve the bony structure of the hard palate.

succedaneous teeth: secondary or permanent teeth.

suckling: an early form of sucking characterized by extension-retraction movements of the tongue.

superior pharyngeal constrictor: paired muscle of the pharynx; the upper fibers are responsible for the medial displacement of the lateral pharyngeal walls to effectively narrow the velopharyngeal port.

supernumerary tooth: an extra tooth; usually erupts in the line of the cleft.

syndactyly: fusion or webbing of the digits (fingers and/or toes).

syndrome: a pattern of multiple anomalies or malformations that regularly occur together and are pathogenically related and, therefore, have a common known or suspected cause; craniofacial syndromes (involving the head and face) cause affected individuals to look alike, even when there is no family relationship (e.g., Down syndrome).

synostosis: abnormal fusion or premature fusion of the two or more normally separated bones; see *craniosynostosis*.

tailpiece (of a prosthetic device): the part of a palatal lift or speech bulb appliance that extends posteriorly to either raise the velum or close the nasopharynx behind the velum.

telecanthus: increased distance between the medial canthi of the eyelids.

temporomandibular joint: the joint of the mandible and temporal bone.

tensor veli palatini: paired muscles that are felt to be responsible for opening the eustachian tubes to enhance middle ear aeration and drainage.

teratogen: an external chemical or physical agent, such as cigarette smoke, drugs, viruses, or radiation, that can interfere with normal embryological development and result in congenital malformations.

tetralogy of Fallot: most common congenital heart defect; includes ventricular septal deviation (VSD), dextroposition (right-sided) aortic arch, right ventricular hypertrophy, and pulmonary stenosis; often associated with a syndrome.

TONAR: developed by Fletcher in 1970, this was the first instrument to measure nasal and oral acoustic energy during speech; predecessor to the Nasometer.

tongue-tie: see *ankyloglossia*.

tonsillectomy: surgical procedure to remove the tonsils; done to resolve recurrent infection or to eliminate oral cavity obstruction.

tonsils: see *faucial tonsils*.

torus palatinus: a normal variation, not an abnormality, that consists of a prominent longitudinal ridge, or exostosis, on the oral surface of the hard palate in the area of the median palatine suture line; found most often in Caucasians, particularly those of northern European descent, and reportedly common in the North American Indian and Eskimo populations.

torus tubarius: a ridge in the nasopharyngeal wall, posterior to the opening of the eustachian tube, caused by the projection of the cartilaginous portion of this tube.

Towne's view: a radiographic view that is sometimes used as an alternative to the base view because it also provides an en face orientation; it allows the examiner to look down into the port.

tracheoesophageal (TE) fistula: congenital opening between the trachea and the esophagus; causes aspiration during feeding.

tracheostomy: a surgical procedure that involves placement of a tube directly in the trachea; done to relieve upper airway obstruction, which can be life-threatening.

transcription: the process of creating a strand of RNA that is complementary to a given strand of DNA.

transdisciplinary team: an interdisciplinary team where members understand the other disciplines and how they relate to the total care of the patient; this understanding of the various disciplines allows them to be able to see the "big picture" in the care of the patient.

transducers: as part of aerodynamic instrumentation, used to convert the detected air pressure or flow into electical signals for further processing.

translocations: the result of a transfer of genetic material between two or more chromosomes; may not be associated with any abnormalities in the individual because the total amount of genetic material may be unchanged.

transverse palatine suture line: an embryological suture line that separates the paired palatine processes of the maxilla, which form the anterior three quarters of the maxilla, and the paired horizontal plates of the palatine bones; also known as the *palatomaxillary suture line.*

treating team: the team members provide a consultation regarding the total care of the patient and also offer treatment.

trigonocephaly: the top of the skull is triangular-shaped with a pointed forehead.

trisomy: a condition where there is an extra chromosome in an homologous pair of chromosomes; for example, trisomy 21 or Down syndrome in humans is a condition where the cell contains 47 rather than 46 chromosomes.

tubercle (of the lip): the somewhat prominent point at the inferior border of the midsection of the upper lip.

turbinates: bony structures in the nose that are covered with mucosa; the superior and middle turbinates are parts of the ethmoid bone and the inferior turbinate, which is the largest, is part of the sphenoid bone; see *concha.*

turbulent flow: airflow through the nasal cavity that is affected by obstacles, irregularities, and convolutions.

tympanic membrane: thin tissue that separates the outer ear from the middle ear; transmits sound energy through the ossicles to the inner ear; also called the *eardrum.*

underjet: a reversal of the normal incisor position, with the maxillary incisors lingua-verted or facing inward toward the tongue; also called *linguoversion* or *anterior crossbite.*

Universal Blood and Body Fluid Precautions (UBBFP): guidelines for infection control that were developed by the Centers for Disease Control and Prevention (CDC) in Atlanta.

upper esophageal sphincter (UES): the upper end of the esophagus that normally is closed, but stretches open as the bolus travels through the hypopharynx and into the esophagus.

utricle: a sensory organ within the inner ear that provide a sensation of acceleration.

U-tube water manometer: a device that consists of a U-shaped glass tube partially filled with water and is used for the calibration of pressure transducers.

uvula: a teardrop-shaped structure that is typically long and slender and hangs freely from the back or free edge of the velum; it has no known function.

uvulopalatopharyngoplasty (UPPP): a surgical procedure for the treatment of the obstructive sleep apnea in adults; involves the excision of the remaining tonsil and resection of the free margin of the soft palate and uvula; the anterior and posterior tonsillar pillars are sewn together to open the oropharyngeal inlet.

Van der Woude's syndrome: includes cleft palate and bilateral lip pits, which are small depressions in the bottom lip; has a 50% recurrence risk for future pregnancies.

variable expressivity: variability in the clinical presentation (phenotype) of patients with a particular genetic disorder; a gene can result in variations in the phenotype from a very pronounced effect in one individual to a barely noticeable effect in another.

velar aponeurosis: see *palatine aponeurosis.*

velar dimple: the area on the oral side of the velum where it bends during phonation or velopharyngeal closure; can be noted through an intraoral examination.

velar eminence: a bulge on the nasal surface of the velum during phonation which comes from the musculus uvulae muscles; can be seen through nasopharyngoscopy.

velar fricative: a compensatory articulation production that is produced with the back of the tongue in the same position as for the production of a /y/ sound so that a small space is created between the back of the tongue and the velum; a fricative sound is produced as air is forced through that small opening.

velar stretch: the process where the velum elongates as it elevates to achieve velopharyngeal closure.

velo-adenoidal closure: the velum commonly closes against the adenoid during speech in children who have a prominent adenoid pad.

velopharyngeal dysfunction (VPD): a generic term that is used to describe abnormal velopharyngeal function, regardless of the cause.

velopharyngeal inadequacy (VPI): a generic term that is used to describe abnormal velopharyngeal function, regardless of the cause.

velopharyngeal incompetence (VPI): a neuromotor or physiological disorder that results in poor movement of the velopharyngeal structures.

velopharyngeal insufficiency (VPI): an anatomical or structural defect that precludes adequate velopharyngeal closure by causing the velum to be short relative to the posterior pharyngeal wall.

velopharyngeal mislearning: inadequate velopharyngeal closure due to faulty learning of appropriate articulation patterns.

velum: the part of the palate that is located in the back of the mouth and consists of muscles that are covered by the same mucous membrane as the hard palate; frequently referred to as the *soft palate*.

ventilation tubes: small tubes that are surgically inserted in the eardrum to provide an alternate route for air to enter the middle ear for ventilation if the eustachian tube is nonfunctional; also called *pressure equalizing (PE) tubes*.

ventral surface: the lower surface, as of the tongue.

ventricular septal defect (VSD): congenital discontinuity of the tissue that separates the lower chambers of the heart.

verbal apraxia: see *apraxia (of speech)*.

verbal language: meaning or message that is conveyed through speech.

vermilion: the red pigmented portion of the upper and lower lips.

video endoscopy: see *nasopharyngoscopy*.

videofluoroscopic speech study: an evaluation of the velopharyngeal mechanism and other oral and pharyngeal structures during speech using videofluoroscopy.

videofluoroscopic swallowing study (VSS): a radiographic procedure that allows an overall view of the oral, pharyngeal, and esophageal phases of swallowing as well as the interactions between the phases; also referred to as a *modified barium swallow (MBS)*.

videofluoroscopy: a radiographic procedure used to examine deep structures of the body during movement; the images are recorded on a videotape.

vocal nodules: bilateral, circumscribed enlargements on the vocal folds that are the result of abuse, overuse, or misuse of the voice; commonly seen in patients with mild velopharyngeal dysfunction due to the strain in the vocal tract with attempts to achieve velopharyngeal closure; can also occur secondary to the use of compensatory articulation productions, particularly glottal stops.

vomer: a flat bone of trapezoidal shape that is positioned so that it is perpendicular to the palate; the inferior border meets the nasal surface of the maxilla in midline and forms the inferior and posterior portion of the nasal septum.

Waldeyer's ring: a complex of lymphoid tissue, including the adenoids, tonsils, and lingual tonsil, which encircles the pharynx and plays a role in the immune system.

W-arch: a variation of the quad helix palatal expansion device.

well-type manometer: similar to a U-tube water manometer but provides for the direct reading of applied pressures; has a calibrated reservoir filled with water or oil and is used for the calibration of pressure transducers.

white roll: the white border tissue that surrounds the red tissue, or vermilion, of the upper and lower lips.

X-linked inheritance: an inherited trait from genes located on the X chromosome; the trait is usually more pronounced or is lethal in males because males have only one X chromosome as opposed to females who have two X chromosomes.

zona pellucida: a bluish area in the middle of the velum that is the result of abnormal insertion of the levator veli palatini muscles, effectively causing the velum to be thin and almost transparent in appearance.

APPENDIX

A

Resources for Information and Support

Resources for information regarding cleft lip and palate and craniofacial anomalies are available from a variety of sources. The following is a list of some of the national organizations that can be helpful in providing information and resources. This list is not inclusive by any means. In fact, there are many local and state organizations that can provide information and support. Information on other organizations and resources can be found on many of the web sites listed.

AboutFace is an organization of individuals and families who have experienced the challenges of facial differences. This organization provides emotional support, information services, and educational programs about living with facial differences. AboutFace focuses on syndromes and conditions, psychosocial issues, public awareness, and integration issues. It provides a variety of resources, including newsletters, videotapes, and publications. There is a national chapter network for local access and networking. For further information:

Phone: (800) 665-FACE (3223)

Fax: (416) 597-8494

e-mail: info@aboutfaceinternational.org

Web site: http://www.aboutfaceinternational.org

Children's Craniofacial Association offers assistance with doctor referrals and nonmedical assistance. There are annual family retreats and educational programs. The organization has publications about various craniofacial syndromes.

Phone: (800) 535-3643

Fax: (972) 240-7607

e-mail: char_smith@prodigy.net

Web site: http://www.childrenscraniofacial.com

Let's Face It is an information and support network for people with facial differences, their families, and professionals. Once a year, this organization publishes an extensive manual of organizations and resources for individuals with facial difference. To be placed on their mailing list, just send an e-mail address. For further information:

Phone: (360) 676-7325

e-mail: letsfaceit@faceit.org

Web site: http:// www.faceit.org/letsfaceit/

Parents Helping Parents (PHP) is a parent-directed family resource center serving children with special needs, their families, and the professionals who serve them. This organization provides parent and professional training on how to begin and maintain a parent support network. Publications are available for training and information.

Phone: (408) 727-5775

e-mail: alexandra@php.com or nancy@php.com

Web site: http://www.php.com

The **American Cleft Palate-Craniofacial Association** (ACPA) is a professional organization, founded in 1943, which includes all disciplines involved in the care and treatment of cleft palate and craniofacial anomalies. Members are from the United States and from over 40 countries all over the world. Membership is open to individuals who are qualified to treat or conduct research in the areas of cleft lip, cleft palate, and other craniofacial anomalies.

The ACPA is dedicated to the study and treatment of all aspects of craniofacial anomalies, including cleft lip and palate. The organization has worked toward establishing standards of care for patients with craniofacial anomalies. Clinical and research information is shared through its quarterly *Cleft Palate-Craniofacial Journal*. Annual professional meetings are held at various locations around the country for the purpose of sharing and exchanging clinical information and the latest research findings. For more information:

Phone: (919) 933-9044

Fax: (919) 933-9604

e-mail: cleftline@aol.com

Web site: http://www.cleft.com

The **Cleft Palate Foundation** (CPF) is a group that is associated with the American Cleft Palate-Craniofacial Association. The CPF has the mission of serving as a resource to families and professionals around the country. Services include a 24-hour toll-free phone number (CLEFTLINE) that is available to both families and professionals who are seeking information about the evaluation or treatment of individuals with cleft lip, cleft palate, or other craniofacial birth defects. In addition, the CPF provides consumers with booklets on all aspects of cleft lip and palate (available in English and Spanish), craniofacial anomalies, and related syndromes. They provide a bibliography for parents of children with cleft lip/palate and a catalog of informational videocassettes. They can refer families to local and national support groups. Finally, the CPF provides consumers with a list of guidelines for choosing a medical team for cleft palate or craniofacial care, and also provides listings of qualified cleft and craniofacial anomaly teams in the patient's area. For more information:

Phone: (919) 933-9044

Cleftline: (800) 24-CLEFT (800-242-5338)

Fax: (919) 933-9604

e-mail: cleftline@aol.com

Web site: http://www.cleft.com

FACES: The National Craniofacial Association is a nonprofit organization that serves children and adults with craniofacial disorders by acting as a clearinghouse of information on specific disorders and available resources, providing networking opportunities with other families, publishing a quarterly newsletter, and providing financial assistance to families who cannot afford to travel away from home to a specialized craniofacial medical center. For further information:

Phone: (423) 266-1632, (800) 332-2373

Fax: (423) 267-3124

e-mail: faces@mindspring.com

Web site: http://www.faces-cranio.org

Wide Smiles is a nonprofit organization that is supported through contributions. Its purpose is to provide resources for individuals and family members with a history of cleft lip and palate. For more information:

Phone: (209) 942-2812

Fax: (209) 464-1497

e-mail: info@widesmiles.org

Web site: http://www.widesmiles.org

APPENDIX

B

Selected Bibliography for Parents

This list was compiled by the Parent/Patient Liaison Committee of the Cleft Palate Foundation (CPF). The committee stresses that no single pamphlet is appropriate in its entirety for any given child. They advise parents to consult with their health care providers for a better understanding of the written material as it applies to their child's specific needs.

Publications from the Cleft Palate Foundation

Contact: 104 S. Estes Drive, Suite 204, Chapel Hill, NC 27514; Phone: (800) 24-CLEFT

Booklets

Cleft Lip and Palate: The First Four Years, 1998. 24 pp. $2.00.
Labio Hendido y Paladar Hendido: Los Cuatro Primeros Anos, 1999. 20 pp. $2.00.
Cleft Lip and Palate: The School-Aged Child, 1998. 32 pp. $2.00.
Information for the Teenager Born with a Cleft, 1997. 12 pp. $2.00.
Cleft Lip and Palate: The Adult Patient, 1998. 31 pp. $2.00.
Feeding an Infant with a Cleft, 1999. 15 pp. $2.00.
Como Alimentar a un Bebe con Paladar Hendido, 1998. 20 pp. $2.00.
The Genetics of Cleft Lip and Palate, 1998. 7 pp. $2.00.
Moebius Syndrome, 1998. 18 pp. $2.00.
Hemangiomas and Vascular Malformations, 1999. 25 pp. with color photos. $2.50.
For Parents of Newborn Babies with Cleft Lip/Cleft Palate, 1997. 4 pp. $0.25.
A los Padres de los Bebes Recien Nacidos con Labio Leporino/Paladar Hendido, 1988. 4 pp. $0.25.
Audiovisual and Supplemental Resource Catalog, 1998. 50 pp. $1.00.

Single copies of all publications are free for patients and their families. CPF offers discounts for bulk orders. Call for shipping and handling fees. Prices are subject to change.

Free Factsheets

Information about Choosing a Cleft Palate or Craniofacial Team
Information about Dental Care
Information about Financial Assistance
Information about Crouzon Syndrome (Craniofacial Dysostosis)
Information about Pierre Robin Malformation Sequence
Information about Submucous Cleft Palate
Information about Treacher Collins Syndrome (Mandibulofacial Dysostosis)
Information about Treatment for Adults with Cleft Lip and Palate
Bone Grafting the Cleft Maxilla
Replacing a Missing Tooth
Answers to Common Questions about Scars
Letter to the Parent of a Child with a Cleft
Letter to a Teacher

Publications from the American Cleft Palate-Craniofacial Association (ACPA)

Contact: 104 S. Estes Drive, Suite 204, Chapel Hill, NC 27514; Phone: (919) 933-9044

Cleft Palate-Craniofacial Journal. Published six times per year. Contact your local medical library.
Parameters for Evaluation and Treatment of Patients with Cleft Lip/Palate or other Craniofacial
   Conditions, 1993, 32 pp.
The Cleft and Craniofacial Team, 1993,and 6 pp. $1.50.

Information Published by Other Sources

Order these items directly from their publishers. This list is not all-inclusive; other resources
and organizations are also available to assist you. *Listing in the following bibliography does not
imply endorsement or support of the item or organization by the Cleft Palate Foundation, and CPF is not
liable for the consequences of medical advice provided by them.*

AboutFace, *AboutFace Newsletter.* AboutFace International, 123 Edward St., Suite 1003, Toronto, Ontario,
   M5G 1E2, Canada. Phone: (800) 665-FACE. Membership: $20/year. Other publications available.
Berkowitz, S., *The Cleft Palate Story,* 1994. Quintessence Publishing, 551 N. Kimberly Dr., Carol Stream, IL
   60188-1881. Phone: (800) 621-0387. Fax: (630) 682-3288. 219 pp. ISBN 0867152591. $24 + S&H.
Charkins, H., *Children With Facial Difference: A Parent's Guide,* 1996. Woodbine House, 6510 Bells Mill Rd.,
   Bethesda, MD 20817. Phone: (800) 843-7323 or (301) 897-3570. 361 pp. $16.95.
Craniofacial Center, University of Illinois at Chicago, *Feeding Your Special Baby,* 1982. (English and Spanish
   versions.) University of Illinois Craniofacial Center, 811 S. Paulina, Chicago, IL 60612-4353. Phone: (312)
   996-7546. $1.75, or 6 copies for $10. Videos also available on this topic and others.
Let's Face It, *Resources for People With Facial Difference.* Annual Directory. Send self-addressed 9×12 enve-
   lope with $3.20 stamp to: Let's Face It, P.O. Box 29972, Bellingham, WA 98228-1972.
Lipman, K., *Don't Despair Cleft Repair,* 1999 edition. Parent memoir. Karen Lipman, 2179 Morning Sun Ln.,
   Naples, FL 34119. Phone: (941) 517-1752. Email: lipbook@aol.com. 76 pp. w/ pictures. $25 + $3 S&H.
MacDonald, S., *Caring for Your Newborn.* Prescription Parents, 22 Ingersoll Rd., Wellesley, MA 02181.
   Phone: (781) 431-1398. $1.95.

MacDonald, S., *Hearing and Behavior in Children With Cleft Lip and Palate.* Prescription Parents, 22 Ingersoll Rd., Wellesley, MA 02181. Phone: (781) 431-1398. $1.95 each.

Mead Johnson, *Looking Forward: A Guide for Parents of the Child With Cleft Lip and Palate.* Mead Johnson, 2404 Pennsylvania St., Evansville, IN 47721. 37 pp. Free through doctors' offices.

Miller, N., *Nobody's Perfect: Living and Growing With Children Who Have Special Needs,* 1997. Brookes Publishing, P.O. Box 10624, Baltimore, MD 21285. Phone: (800) 638-3775. 307 pp. $21.

Moller, K., C. Starr, and S. Johnson, *A Parent's Guide to Cleft Lip and Palate,* 1990. University of Minnesota Publication. Contact: University of Chicago Press, 11030 S. Langley Ave., Chicago, IL 60628. Phone: (800) 621-2736 or (773) 568-1550. ISBN 0816614911. 131 pp. $16.95 + $3.50 UPS S&H.

Peckinpah, S.L., *Rosey . . . The Imperfect Angel,* 1991. Scholars Press. Hardcover children's book. Dasan Productions. Phone: (800) 348-4401. Available through major bookstores. 32 pp. $15.95.

St. John's Hospital Cleft Palate Center, *If Your Baby Has a Cleft,* 1990. 30 min. video. Contact: Barbara Wasilewski, St. John's Hospital Child Study Center, Attn: Cleft Palate Center, 1339 20th St., Santa Monica, CA 90404. Phone: (310) 829-8150. $25 to rent, $58 to buy (includes tax).

Wicka, D., and M. Falk, *Advice to Parents of a Cleft Palate Child,* 1982. Charles Thomas Publisher, 2600 S. 1st St., P.O. Box 19265, Springfield, IL 62794-9265. Phone: (217) 789-8980. 80 pp. $23.95 + $5.50 S&H.

Wide Smiles, *Wide Smiles Magazine.* Joann Greene, Wide Smiles, P.O. Box 5153, Stockton, CA 95205-0153. Phone: (209) 942-2812. Web site: www.widesmiles.org. $20/year.

Wynn, S., *Team Approach to Children With Cleft Lip and Palate.* Item 75001. 32 pp. $5. Contact: Maxishare, P.O. Box 2041, Milwaukee, WI 53201. Phone: (800) 444-7747.

Wynn, S., *How to Feed Babies With a Cleft.* 14 min. video. $19 for families, $89 for institutions. Rentals also available. Contact: Maxishare, P.O. Box 2041, Milwaukee, WI 53201. Phone: (800) 444-7747.

Index